THE DEVELOP[INHALATION AN.

Barbara M. Duncum

Royal Society of Medicine Press Ltd
London · New York

First published by Oxford University Press, London, 1947.

This edition published 1994 by Royal Society of
Medicine Press Ltd, 1 Wimpole Street, London
W1M 8AE, on behalf of the History of Anaesthesia Society.

British Library Cataloguing in Publication Data
A catalogue record for this book is
available from the British Library

ISBN 1-85315-225-0

Printed and bound in Great Britain by Marston Book Services Limited, Oxford

DUNCUM REVISITED

SOON after its appearance in 1947, Barbara Duncum's *The development of inhalation anaesthesia* was acknowledged to be a superb scholarly guide to its subject. Over forty years later that judgement is still intact. That the book's reputation remains untarnished in the critical academic world of the history of medicine today is high praise indeed. A fact which makes its production in the relative historical doldrums of the 1940s appear all the more extraordinary. How did this authoritative text come to be written? In 1931 after reading history at London University, Barbara Duncum (then Pycraft) joined the staff of the Wellcome Historical Medical Museum in Wigmore Street, London (it moved to the new Wellcome Building in Euston Road in 1932). The Wellcome Museum had an idiosyncratic flavour deriving from the passions and perspectives of its founder, the ageing Sir Henry Wellcome, pharmaceutical entrepreneur and collector.[1] Although the Museum employed scholars it had little or no relationship with university departments. Indeed academic history of medicine scarcely existed in Britain. Most of that great generation of British physicians and surgeons who were medical historians and bibliophiles, such as Sir Clifford Allbutt and Sir D'Arcy Power, were dead or elderly. Charles Singer, Britain's leading historian of medicine, was increasingly concentrating his interests on the history of science.[2] In fact Duncum did not meet Singer until after her book was published, when he offered his congratulations over afternoon tea in the Singers' private sitting-room at Brown's Hotel, Albemarle Street. At the Wellcome Museum, Duncum collaborated with another employee, A. W. Haggis, on the sort of disparate subjects which characterized the Museum's work in those years: cinchona, bishops' licences, medical illustrations on rood-screens.

---

[1] Skinner, G. M. 'Sir Henry Wellcome's Museum for the science of history', *Med. Hist.*, 1986, 30, 383–418.

[2] Webster, C. 'Medicine as social history: changing ideas on doctors and patients in the age of Shakespeare', in Stevenson, L. (ed.) 1982. *A celebration of medical history*. Baltimore and London. 103–26.

An opportunity for change came in 1938. In 1946 Lord Nuffield had offered to endow four new chairs in medical subjects at the University of Oxford. The proposal to include anaesthetics amongst these scandalized the medical hierarchy. Nonetheless Nuffield got his way and on February 1 1937 Robert Reynolds Macintosh was appointed to the Chair of Anaesthetics.[3] In 1938 Duncum was recruited by Macintosh to the multidisciplinary team he was assembling in the department. Duncum was employed, primarily, to write the opening historical chapter for the textbook Macintosh was projecting. Her duties in the department, however, were, as might be imagined in the chaotic years before and during the second world war, various. She completed the historical chapter for Macintosh's *Essentials of general anaesthesia* which was published by Blackwell Scientific Publications in 1940. Macintosh had been impressed by Duncum's approach and encouraged her to extend and deepen her work and present it for a D.Phil. This she did, the work being done mainly in the evenings at the Radcliffe Science Library. In 1945 she was awarded the degree. Turning the thesis into a book seemed an obvious way to proceed. In 1947 the Wellcome Historical Medical Museum became interested and Oxford University Press produced the book for the Wellcome Foundation Ltd. Not long afterwards Duncum moved to the Nuffield Foundation in London, where she worked on a project investigating the functions and design of hospitals. From 1960 onwards she was engaged in various researches connected with the Foundation and medicine. She retired in 1975.

Duncum's book was soon acknowledged to be authoritative. Reviewing it in *Isis* Chauncey Leake said that it "offers the most important information on the development of anaesthetic apparatus and technique of any history of anaesthesia which has yet appeared".[4] From Yale John Fulton, distinguished physiologist and keen student of early anaesthesia, sent her a congratulatory telegram. In retrospect the achievement is all the more impressive, for scholarly literature in the history of anaesthesia was rare at this time. From the very early days of anaesthesia, recounting its history had been a source of intense activity. Much of this history, however, was far from dispassionate. Indeed most of it was produced in support of individual or national priority claims. Many of the productions therefore, interesting as historical documents

[3] Beinart, J. 1987. *A history of the Nuffield Department of Anaesthetics, Oxford 1937–87.* Oxford.
[4] *Isis*, 1947–48, **38**, 132.

themselves, were of little use as histories. This concentration on the early years of anaesthesia was perpetuated in the twentieth century. What happened after the introduction of ether in 1846 and chloroform in 1847 seemed of little interest.[5] The scarcity of good secondary sources available is evident from Duncum's footnotes. A book-length history of anaesthesia had appeared in 1938. But it was a sensationalizing account, whose style and lack of scholarship Duncum vigorously eschewed.[6] Around 1946, the centenary of Morton's demonstration of ether anaesthesia, a clutch of commemorative general histories and special studies appeared.[7] Although some were relatively scrupulous in their use of sources none approached Duncum in depth and rigour. None had appeared early enough for her to use.

Duncum organized her work in chapters which tackled different topics: agents, individuals, institutions, scientific developments. Using this approach Duncum was able to present the history of anaesthesia in a detailed and many-sided way. Too much history of anaesthesia before this time had been myopic. According to who was writing the history what emerged as central was, for example, the apparatus, the practitioners or the physiology. Duncum took in all these aspects and more, linking together practice, research, technological innovation and associated scientific and, to some extent, social changes.

Some of the material Duncum used was relatively accessible and indeed possibly not unknown to a few readers. Her organization of it, however, made it possible to see a main theme and a number of sub-plots which had not been constructed before. This was the case, for instance, in the complex history of chloroform death. The latter was a source of continuing controversy in the nineteenth century, between anaesthetists who designated its cause as respiratory and those who decreed it to be cardiac in origin. It was a dispute which she traced through various committees, medical journals and the complex history of the Hyderabad Commissions of the 1890s. Here, as elsewhere, Duncum's approach was to quote lengthy sections from original material. This was a technique that proved particularly revealing when she dealt with sources that were

[5] See Osler, W. 'The first printed documents relating to modern surgical anaesthesia', *Proc. Roy. Soc. Med. (Sect. Hist. Med.)*, 1918, 11, 65–9 ; Fulton, J. F. and Stanton, M. E. 1946 *The centennial of surgical anesthesia ; an annotated catalogue of books and pamphlets . . . exhibited at the Yale Medical Library.* New York.

[6] Fülöp-Miller, R. [1938]. *Triumph over pain.* New York.

[7] See the works listed by Leake, *op. cit.*, note 4.

not well known or readily accessible to her readers. For example, in 1930 Henry Wellcome had produced a Centenary Exhibition to display the original papers and other material of the early nineteenth-century general practitioner Henry Hill Hickman. These had been acquired and comprehensively described in 1912 by C. J. S. Thompson, first curator of the Museum.[8] However, the present day interest in Hickman and his experiments undoubtedly stems from Duncum's re-examination and publication of long quotations from the papers themselves. Similarly she explored and reproduced material from Joseph Clover's manuscripts in the possession of Macintosh's department. Many of these Macintosh later presented to the History Library of the University of British Columbia in Vancouver.

Duncum was not only interested in detail however. She was the first historian to expose the broad geographical and temporal patterns in anaesthetic usage in the nineteenth century. There were plenty of first-hand impressions by anaesthetists of changing fashions in the agents and apparatus employed. But there was no overall survey taken from the literature. Duncum demonstrated the uptake of ether, its declining use in the face of chloroform, then the reappraisal of ether, first in America, then in England and finally on the continent. On this pattern she superimposed another: the revival of nitrous oxide in the 1860s and the mixed anaesthesia boom of the 1870s.

The development of inhalation anaesthesia set a standard in anaesthetic history writing to which any subsequent author needed to aspire in order that his or her work might be considered a scholarly contribution to the literature. There is still much to be done in the history of anaesthesia. The high ground of theory and practice needs cultivation. The low ground of everyday anaesthetic life, ordinary practice, economics, instrument making, etc. remains relatively untilled. Whichever path potential researchers choose, however, Duncum's text is a mandatory starting point. Its reissue is not only a delight, but a necessity.

Christopher Lawrence

Senior Lecturer
Wellcome Institute for the History of Medicine
February 1994

[3] Lawrence, C. and Lawrence, G. 1987. *No laughing matter: historical aspects of anaesthesia.* London, Wellcome Institute for the History of Medicine/Science Museum.

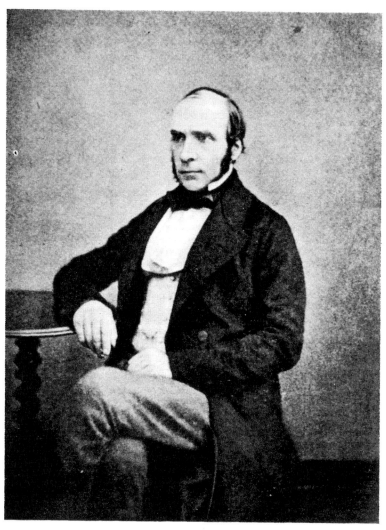

JOHN SNOW (1813–58)

Physician and first Specialist Anaesthetist. He was among the first to carry out researches upon the physiological effects of volatile anaesthetics and the first to base the design of an inhaler upon conclusions reached in the course of such experiments.

THE DEVELOPMENT OF
INHALATION ANAESTHESIA

With Special Reference to the Years
1846–1900

BARBARA M. DUNCUM

D.PHIL.(Oxon)
OF THE NUFFIELD DEPARTMENT OF ANAESTHETICS,
UNIVERSITY OF OXFORD: FORMERLY OF THE
WELLCOME HISTORICAL MEDICAL MUSEUM

Published for
THE WELLCOME HISTORICAL MEDICAL MUSEUM
By GEOFFREY CUMBERLEGE
OXFORD UNIVERSITY PRESS
LONDON   NEW YORK   TORONTO
1947

OXFORD UNIVERSITY PRESS
AMEN HOUSE, WARWICK SQUARE
LONDON, E.C.4

Edinburgh Glasgow New York
Toronto Melbourne Cape Town
Bombay   Calcutta   Madras
GEOFFREY   CUMBERLEGE
PUBLISHER   TO   THE   UNIVERSITY

PRINTED IN GREAT BRITAIN
3445,6438

PREFACE

MY first aim in writing this book has been to trace the beginnings and to follow the development of those concepts and practices which have gone to the making of the science and art of inhalation anaesthesia as it is to-day. The search led back into the seventeenth and eighteenth centuries and forward into the present century ; nevertheless this book is chiefly concerned with the period between the winter of 1846 and the end of the year 1900, which comprises the first phase of modern anaesthetic history. In this phase the introduction of a gas or the vapour of a volatile drug into the body by way of the respiratory tract was generally considered to be by far the most important of all known means of achieving anaesthesia, and was the method almost exclusively used. In the succeeding phase, which still continues, anaesthesia by inhalation has become only one of several accredited methods in common use.

My secondary aim has been to show, during the whole period under review, how current beliefs and current happenings which at first sight appear unconnected or only remotely connected with anaesthesia, affected its evolution.

To illustrate the character of the various trends of thought which prompted those who concerned themselves with the theory and practice of inhalation anaesthesia during its first phase, I have attempted to build up the history in a series of quotations from contemporary literature, British, American, and Continental. The sources from which these quotations and translations have been made include medical journals and periodical publications such as year-books, the proceedings and transactions of scientific societies, theses and reports submitted to various learned institutions, text-books and monographs, and manuscript notes and letters in the possession of the Nuffield Department of Anaesthetics, University of Oxford, and the Wellcome Historical Medical Museum, London. The abbreviated titles given in the references are according to *A world list of scientific periodicals published in the years 1900–33* (Oxford University Press, 1934).

The fact of my working as a member of the Nuffield Department of Anaesthetics gave me the opportunity of research for this study, and I am very grateful to Professor R. R. Macintosh and to my colleagues for help in its preparation ; in particular, Dr. S. L. Cowan read and criticized my manuscript with unfailing patience and insight. I have also to thank especially Dr. K. J. Franklin, Dean of the School of Medicine in the University of Oxford, for advice and encouragement. The actual research work was made pleasant and inestimably easier by the facilities allowed me at the Radcliffe Science Library, and by the kindness of the staff.

This, the centenary year of the general adoption of anaesthesia in surgery, seems an appropriate time to consider the history of inhalation anaesthesia in detail, and I am grateful to the Wellcome Foundation for including this work as a Publication of the Wellcome Historical Medical Museum. In revising the proofs I have adopted many suggestions made by the Oxford University Press Reader, and my husband has given me much help.

I have had also the invaluable advice of my friend A. W. Haggis, of the Wellcome Historical Medical Museum, whose sudden death in April of this year is a source of deep grief to me. This book owes much to his wide knowledge of the history of medicine and to his experience in the preparation of works for publication.

The illustrations are listed with their sources, and I am indebted to the various persons concerned for so readily giving me permission to reproduce them. In particular I should like to thank Mme. A. Klobukowski for the photograph of her father, Paul Bert (Fig. 102) ; Mr. Frank Coleman for the photograph of Alfred Coleman (Fig. 76) ; Dr. C. C. Clay, Assistant Director of the Massachusetts General Hospital, Boston, for the photograph of Morton's inhaler (Fig. 12) ; and the Harvard Medical Library for permission to reproduce the portrait of Jackson (Fig. 13). I must also thank Messrs. Macmillan & Co., the publishers of Hewitt's *Anaesthetics and their administration*, and Messrs. H. K. Lewis, the publishers of Buxton's *Anaesthetics : their uses and administration*, and of Davis's *Guide to the administration of anaesthetics*, from which books many of my illustrations are taken.

BARBARA M. DUNCUM

Oxford
September 1946

CONTENTS

PART FIVE
CONTINENTAL DEVELOPMENTS

PART SIX
THE BEGINNING OF MODERN ANAESTHESIA

LIST OF ILLUSTRATIONS

INTRODUCTION

Economic and Social Background—The Use of Ether established for Surgical Anaesthesia—Introduction of Chloroform—Anaesthesia on the Continent of Europe, 1847 to *c.* 1870—John Snow's Influence upon English Anaesthesia—The Revived Use of Nitrous Oxide—Ether revived in England—Antisepsis, Asepsis, and Surgical Developments—Ether revived in Germany and France—Teaching of Anaesthesia ; Specialization—Open Ether ; Endotracheal Anaesthesia—Non-Inhalation Anaesthesia—English Attitude towards Anaesthetic Questions, *c.* 1900.

Economic and Social Background

THE year 1846, in which anaesthesia at last became established as an essential part of surgical practice, comes at the beginning of a period, roughly a quarter of a century in extent, of violent national and international disturbances affecting not only the European but also the North American Continent. These disturbances appear to have exerted so considerable an influence over the development of anaesthesia as to warrant an outline of their nature.

The twenty-five years preceding 1846 had everywhere been peaceful ; but during that comparatively short space of time the cumulative effects of intensive industrialization had so altered man's way of life that he suddenly found himself confronted with social and political problems, arising out of changed conditions, which demanded immediate solution. The magnitude of these problems he had not clearly foreseen, and since he was without experience of any comparable situation he was ill-equipped to deal satisfactorily with them.

A characteristic feature of this period of rapid development was the concentration of a large proportion of the steadily multiplying population into towns. The towns themselves continually expanded to accommodate new industries and new inhabitants, but they did so hastily and inadequately, without systematic planning or, indeed, any enlightened supervision or control. Overcrowding in mean surroundings was inevitable and this immediately raised grave problems of public health and hygiene. By the eighteen-thirties existing facilities for such essential public services as, for example, the disposal of sewage and of refuse, the maintenance of an ample and reasonably unpolluted water supply and the provision of space for the burial of the dead were all grossly insufficient.

Although the exact interrelation between population living under crowded conditions and the spread of disease was imperfectly understood, a close connexion between the two was made evident by the pandemic appearance of Asiatic cholera in Europe and North America during the eighteen-thirties, and its periodic reappearance.[1] The severity of these and other epidemics was the most potent factor in compelling governments to intervene in matters relating to public health and hygiene and to initiate measures first of control and ultimately of reform.

The industrial revolution began in England during the reign of George III, and it was here that the characteristic symptoms of political and economic unrest were most clearly defined. But, in the eighteen-thirties and forties, a national uprising was averted by the timely introduction of measures of reform and a providential revival in trade, due to a variety of causes, and during the remainder of the nineteenth century the popular demands were gradually satisfied by a series of compromises.

The urgency of problems affecting the health of the nation led to the establishment, during the eighteen-thirties, of various commissions of investigation. Overwork, under-nourishment because of low wages and the high price of bread, and unhygienic environment were obviously lowering the resistance of the people to illness. Industry itself was creating new types of occupational disease and of trauma. The first Factory Act was passed in 1833, yet the full horrors of existing conditions were not realized until the publication of reports [2] from the commissioners during the eighteen-forties. Then a public outcry was raised against the exploitation of labour, particularly female and child labour, in industry and against the living conditions forced upon the working classes. Between 1842 and 1848 Peel's Government, which had come into office in 1841, made serious

---

[1] John Snow (see frontispiece) was the first, in 1848, to put forward the suggestion that cholera is transmitted through drinking-water contaminated with sewage from persons already infected with the disease. (Snow, J. 1849. *The mode of communication of cholera.* London.) In 1854 Snow was able to give a practical demonstration of the truth of his theory. During the cholera outbreak in the Broad Street district of Westminster he persuaded the local authorities to remove the handle of the Broad Street pump, whereupon the virulence of the outbreak abated.

[2] *E.g.* Edwin Chadwick's report *On the sanitary conditions of the labouring population of Great Britain* (1842) ; his report on urban burials (1843), and the report of the Royal Sanitary Commission (1843–5).

attempts to check the worst abuses by legislation,[1] and fiom this time onwards local authorities, also, began gradually to shoulder their responsibilities in controlling and reforming social conditions.

In 1846 the Corn Laws were repealed. The removal of the tariff on foreign grain and the production of a cheap loaf led to an immediate improvement in living conditions for the poor. This coincided with a general revival in trade, and wages began to rise. The crisis was over, and England was indeed about to embark on a period of such unprecedented material prosperity (in some degree affecting all classes) and apparently unassailable national security that the glory of her various institutions tended to eclipse their faults. Her geographical situation and her preponderance in important spheres of world trade (as, for instance, in the export of coal) allowed her for the remainder of the nineteenth century to stand aloof from the political and economic struggles of other nations, save when she chose to intervene to enhance her prestige.

In the course of the nineteenth century matters relating to public health came increasingly under the control of both central and local government. The medical services available for the individual, however, remained fundamentally unchanged from those existing at the close of the eighteenth century although of necessity they became modified by the general trend of development in national life. For the aged poor and the destitute the Poor Law authorities provided infirmaries and sick wards financed by local rates ; but the general hospitals, many of which were old foundations, continued to be supported by voluntary contributions from the public. To the general hospitals was added an increasing number of hospitals devoted to special branches of treatment.

Medical education preserved its national tradition of being clinical rather than academic ; the most important factor in the student's training was the experience which he gained in the wards and operating theatres of the hospitals at one or other of the teaching centres—London, Edinburgh, Glasgow and Dublin.

The general practitioner continued to be the most important figure in English medicine and from his ranks the hospitals appointed their honorary officers. The system was in many ways excellent. It encouraged the personal element in medicine,

[1] Mines Act, 1842 ; Factory Act, 1844 ; Ten Hours Bill, 1847 ; Public Health Act, 1848.

giving scope for individuality in outlook and in method and making the association between the medical man and his patient a close one. During the nineteenth century individuality in outlook showed itself particularly in a tendency to specialize. The principal shortcomings of the system were a certain lack of co-ordination among the various branches of medicine and allied sciences and a reluctance on the part of physicians and surgeons to adopt major changes in traditional procedure such, for example, as Lister's antiseptic method in surgery (see pp. 26–31) and, towards the close of the century, the administration of anaesthetics otherwise than by inhalation (see pp. 38–50).

Partly because English constitutional government was fundamentally sound, partly because England commanded a world market for her goods which brought increased prosperity at a critical juncture, she was able to control the democratic demands of her people and to initiate reform gradually. On the Continent of Europe such political and economic advantages were either less positive or were non-existent; during the course of 1848 the social and political grievances of many Continental peoples reached a pitch of intensity which the machinery of government could not control and the situation deteriorated into widespread revolt.

In France the climax came in February 1848, when the monarchy of Louis Philippe was overthrown and the Second Republic, under the presidency of Louis Napoleon, was set up. By 1852, however, the revolutionary spirit had given place to reaction and Louis Napoleon was made Emperor by popular election. For eight years his rule was autocratic ; his aim was to appease the people through the aggrandisement of France herself. He developed industry and trade and invested the national wealth in impressive undertakings such as the erection of public buildings and the construction of docks. Education came once more under the control of the Church and scientific thought was discouraged, except in so far as it might be of practical value in State undertakings. Instead of the intellectual freedom which France had known since the eighteenth century, her people were now encouraged to seek material prosperity.

The enhanced prestige which France gained among her neighbours through her part in the Crimean War led Louis Napoleon in 1859 to champion the cause of Italy, with which he had real sympathy, against Austrian domination. A free and united Italy finally emerged from the struggle, but the part which

Napoleon played was a vacillating one and in France the war led to a revival of demands for democratic reform. Civil unrest was intensified in 1862 by Napoleon's abortive attempt to establish Maximilian of Austria upon the throne of Mexico. In order to retain his Empire Napoleon was forced to make concessions to the working classes, allowing the formation of co-operative societies and of trades unions. Popular agitation reached a belated climax during 1870 when France, divided against herself by the opposing Liberal and Catholic factions, was precipitated into war with Prussia.

In France, as in most countries, the State had been compelled, during the early eighteen-forties, to assume control in matters broadly relating to public health. Hospitals, also, came directly under State control, being administered as public charities.

During the two decades of Napoleon's rule intellectual life suffered a decline. From the point of view of practical medicine, however, this decline was not serious because the French medical tradition, like the English, had always been clinical rather than academic.

An important feature of French scientific circles, and one which differed from English usage, was the free exchange of ideas between men working in different fields of knowledge. This was made possible by the ease with which professional men could become members of the two great national institutions, the Académie des Sciences and the Académie de Médecine, or could present papers setting out their views to be read before members in the course of a meeting. In England, Fellowship of the Royal Society remained exclusive of all save experts of the first distinction, and although numerous societies existed in connection with particular branches of knowledge these, too, remained each one a closed circle of specialists.

The February Revolution of 1848 in France had been immediately followed by the March Days Revolution in Berlin, and rioting simultaneously broke out in Vienna in sympathy with German popular demands for universal franchise and improved social conditions. Unrest spread through the Austrian Empire; in northern Italy, in particular, Lombardy and Venetia revolted.

But, as in France, revolution gave place to reaction about 1852. Austria's hold upon her Empire became as firm as, and more repressive than, before. Germany was closer knit into a Federal State for the mastery of which Austria and Prussia vied with each other. During the eighteen-fifties, however, Prussia so cultivated her natural bent for militarism that the Prussian army was converted into the most powerful military force in Europe and by the eighteen-sixties Bismarck, now in power, was already manœuvring to drive Austria from the confederation and to make Prussia all-powerful not only in Germany but in Europe.

In 1866 war broke out between Austria and Prussia from which Prussia emerged victorious, and Austria withdrew her influence from German affairs. Bismarck then turned his attention to preparation for war with France. By 1870 Prussia was ready and war was deliberately negotiated by Bismarck. As he had planned, the war resulted in a powerful and united German Empire, temporarily without further territorial claims, and in the collapse of Louis Napoleon's regime in France.

Germany immediately set about consolidating her position. Hitherto the German States had been mainly agricultural. From 1871 onwards, under the leadership of Prussia, Germany became an increasingly important industrial power and a land of large towns. The new home policy of the State set great importance upon the bodily well-being of the working classes. During the eighteen-eighties Germany set an example to the rest of the world by introducing State insurance of workers against accident, sickness and old age. It was at this period, too, that German surgery achieved a stage of development which, for a time, outstripped that of any other nation. This was partly due to the technical brilliance of German surgeons, who had trained in the hard school of war surgery, partly to their foresight in immediately adopting Lister's antiseptic precautions and from them, later evolving asepsis.

A sound factor in German medicine was the importance laid upon the study of chemistry and physics as a starting point in the approach to medical problems. But medical education itself was hampered by didactic methods of teaching which kept the student in the lecture room and as a mere spectator at the bedside and in the operating theatre.

The recovery of France from the disaster of the Franco-Prussian War was necessarily slow. After the surrender of the Emperor in 1870, rioting took place in Paris and the Third Republic was established. The Senatorial elections of 1879 gave the Republicans ascendancy over the Clerical Party and in 1880 the reorganization of education was undertaken by the

State. A revivification of university life immediately followed. But although France gradually regained something of her lost prestige, Paris, which represented France as no other capital city represented its country as a whole, was no longer the intellectual centre of the world. By the close of the nineteenth century world power lay chiefly in the grasp of Britain, Germany and the United States of America.

During the first half of the nineteenth century the United States were subject to the same rapid process of internal development as Europe. Through the preoccupation of Europe in the Napoleonic Wars, new markets had been opened to the cotton trade of the Southern States, to the food-producing Middle States and to the industrial undertakings of the North. The resulting prosperity gave rise, as elsewhere, to a sudden increase in population which was still further inflated by a stream of immigrants seeking escape from the hard and troubled conditions of life in the Old World. In the late eighteen-thirties migration to the West, with gathering momentum, entered its final phase, which came to a close only during the eighteen-nineties when practically the whole territory had been settled.

The frontier, perpetually advancing westward, was the most important factor in American life during the nineteenth century ; it meant a succession of new towns springing up where before there had been no permanent habitation, without any background of tradition either to help or to hinder their development. Everything had to be done the quickest, most expedient way and the pace of life was further quickened by the extension of railway and river-steamboat services and the introduction of agricultural and industrial machinery. Life in the new settlements was at first little more than an arduous round of primitive and essential tasks, but as the land and new industries became productive so the material comforts, by which the age set much store, were introduced. Such widely scattered communities had of necessity to be self-governing and since the members were all engaged in the task of making a livelihood from common opportunities, democratic principles prevailed.

The war against Mexico (1846–8) resulted in the annexation of California to the States. When in the course of 1848 it became known that gold had been found there fresh streams of settlers poured in, not only from other States in the Union but immigrants, also, fresh from Europe. Whereas in February 1848 there were some 2000 Americans in California, by the end of 1850 the number was estimated to have risen to 80,000.

During the eighteen-fifties business speculation artificially intensified the rate of territorial and commercial expansion until it so far exceeded the actual needs of the population that in 1857 people became panic-stricken about the safety of their investments, and commercial depression resulted.

In 1846 the balance of political power had been fairly evenly distributed between the Southern States, where negro slavery was general, and the Northern States of the Union, where it was not countenanced. By 1858 this balance no longer existed, because to the original States of the North had been added the anti-slave States of the North-West, giving a majority in political representation. The tension between North and South arising out of this situation reached breaking point in 1860 when it became known that Lincoln, who was bitterly opposed to slavery, was President-elect. South Carolina and six other States then seceded from the Union. In 1861 a state of war was declared between North and South ; but when peace came, in 1865, the new democratic order triumphed. The next twenty years were devoted to political reconstruction and intensified commercial development and although, once again, expansion tended to be pushed beyond the immediate capacity of the nation to consolidate, nevertheless by 1885 America had set her house in order. She emerged from her long period of self-absorption and began to take an interest in world affairs.

By 1847 the general standard of medical education in America was found to have deteriorated from the standards (based upon those of Edinburgh University) which the medical schools of the Eastern States had set during the second half of the eighteenth and earlier years of the nineteenth centuries. In that year, 1847, the American Medical Association was formed. Its aim was, by organizing medical opinion on a representative basis, to bring pressure to bear upon the average practitioner to improve his skill and upon the medical schools to raise the level of knowledge which the graduating student must reach. Despite this effort no great national contribution to medicine was made by America until after 1885, although valuable individual contributions were made.

During the half century, 1846 to 1896, the characteristic and the most important figure in American medicine was the general practitioner—the man with the small-town surgery and the immense, scattered, country visiting round, whose knowledge was largely empirical and whose experience was entirely clinical.

The Use of Ether established for Surgical Anaesthesia

The final acceptance of the principle of surgical anaesthesia appears to have become inevitable by the eighteen-forties. That the time was at last ripe is shown by the fact that C. W. Long, in 1842, and Horace Wells, in 1844, had independently, but through making similar chance observations, hit upon the idea of inhaling, in the one case a vapour, in the other a gas, to obtund surgical pain. It was largely fortuitous, however, that the principle should have been generally adopted during the winter months of 1846–7. W. T. G. Morton, who had profited by the experience of Wells, happened to be successful in his public demonstration of etherization on October 16, 1846, so that the surgeons of the Massachusetts General Hospital became permanently interested and supported his claim. The patronage of two of the most distinguished among contemporary American medical men, the surgeon, John Collins Warren, and the Professor of Materia Medica, Jacob Bigelow, gained for etherization an immediate and almost unquestioning acceptance both at home and abroad.

As was to be expected, the use of etherization had an immediate effect upon surgical practice. In the latter half of the eighteenth century John Hunter related the study of surgery to that of physiology and pathology and created a science where before there had been only a skilled craft. His pupil, Astley Cooper, during the first quarter of the nineteenth century laid the foundations of experimental surgery, but because of the uncontrollable factor of pain, much of the knowledge which he gained from his constant dissections of the cadaver could not be applied in operating upon the living body.

Etherization immediately removed the necessity for haste on the part of the surgeon in order to make the duration of suffering for the patient as short as possible. The patient ready for the surgeon was now, to all outward appearances, insensible or nearly so. But, owing to various shortcomings in the inhalers at first used—particularly a tendency to freeze up and to offer resistance to breathing—and to the diffidence and hesitancy with which inexperienced administrators applied even the most dilute

1*

ether vapour, the patient was often so lightly anaesthetized that surgical stimuli provoked responses which sometimes culminated in uncontrollable excitement. Even when the patient remained tranquil he was seldom sufficiently deeply anaesthetized for his muscles to be completely relaxed.

When, however, in November 1847, little more than a year after the adoption of etherization, James Young Simpson sub-stituted chloroform for ether vapour, the potency of the drug and the simple but effective method of applying and re-applying it from a folded cloth, provided the surgeon with a patient in whom the degree both of unconsciousness and of muscular relaxation could be controlled. It was then that conservative surgery—the preservation by careful dissection of as much of the living tissues as possible—began rapidly to be developed.

' Besides the great benefit conferred by chloroform in the prevention of pain, it probably confers still greater advantages by the extension which it gives to the practice of surgery ',

wrote John Snow, who very frequently acted as anaesthetist for William Fergusson, a pioneer of the conservative method.

' Many operations take place in children which could not be performed in the waking state ; excision of joints and tedious operations for the removal of necrosed bone are often performed on persons who would be altogether unable to go through them except in a state of anaesthesia ; and the moving of stiff joints by force is an operation now frequently performed although it would probably not have been thought of if narcotism by inhala-tion had not been discovered. The surgeon also obtains the ready assent of his patient to a number of other operations, where it would either not be obtained, or not at the most favourable time, if the patient had to suffer the pain of them.' [1]

The fact that chloroform readily subdued the patient gave the administrator the feeling that he was master of the anaes-thetic. He gained confidence and began to profit by experience. From observations made during an increasing number of satis-factory administrations in which certain manifestations of the action of chloroform on the body appeared to remain consistently reproducible, medical men were able to build up for themselves a routine for successful administration.

During the course of the year 1848 such routine practices collectively began to acquire definite national characteristics and

[1] Snow, J. 1858. *On chloroform and other anaesthetics.* London. 263.

these, to a considerable extent, showed the influence of prevailing conditions in national life.

In the United States the technique of anaesthesia had already, in February 1847, assumed the characteristics which it retained until the close of the century.

A serious disadvantage of the sponge-filled glass flask used by Morton during his early administrations of ether at the Massachusetts General Hospital (see Fig. 12) was that the patient had to breathe entirely by mouth through a small, valved tube held between his lips, his nostrils being pinched shut by an assistant. When it became known that Morton was applying for letters patent to protect this inhaler the surgeons of the Hospital discarded its use and instead poured ether freely on to a small, bell-shaped sponge which was then applied over both the mouth and nose of the patient. Because they believed implicitly in the safety of ether they did not hesitate to force the vapour upon the patient, disregarding his initial resistance to its irritating qualities. These methods proved so successful that even when Morton relaxed the patent in the Hospital's favour no return was made to the use of an inhaler, and the example set in Boston was followed by surgeons elsewhere.

After Simpson's recommendation of the use of chloroform the drug was tried in the United States. But, in the Northern States, the simple method of ' pushing ' the ether during induction had overcome those difficulties which in Europe retarded development during 1847 and, after fatalities had occurred which appeared to be due to chloroform, there seemed no justification for persevering in its use.

Chloroform was preferred, however, in the Southern States of the Union. The climate of the South may possibly have weighed against the use of the more volatile drug ; but the following explanation was given in 1904, by R. Villeneuve, quoting observations made by Dr. Francis Munch, of Paris :

' In the Northern States of the Union ether only is used, while chloroform is preferred in the South. The reasons for this exclusiveness are of an historical nature. It is from local pride that Boston has remained faithful to ether. One knows, indeed, that it was at the Massachusetts General Hospital in that city that ether was first employed. The neighbouring cities, New York, Philadelphia, Baltimore, have followed its example and influence. In fact the influence of Harvard University on the intellectual development of the United States has always been considerable ; its medical school, with that of the University of Pennsylvania, has long been one of the only two important medical centres in the North.

' In the South chloroform is preferred on account of the influence of New Orleans. For until recent years one could scarcely practise surgery in New Orleans unless one had been to Paris. And in Paris the anaesthetic of choice is chloroform.' [1]

A notable exception to the rule that ether was far more frequently used than chloroform in the Northern States of America during the nineteenth century was afforded by anaesthetic practice during the Civil War (1861–5). In the official *Medical and surgical history of the war of the rebellion*,[2] the following statement occurs :

' From the rapidity of its effects, and from the small quantity required—quantities which can only be appreciated at their proper value by the field surgeon when surrounded by hundreds of wounded anxiously awaiting speedy relief—chloroform was preferred by nearly all field surgeons, and their testimony as to its value and efficiency is almost unanimous, although all recommend the greatest care in its administration. . . . The nature of the anaesthetic employed was indicated in 8900 cases, viz. chloroform in 6784, ether in 1305 and chloroform and ether in 811 cases.'

No doubt because patients' skin was often frozen, and thus more easily chafed from direct contact with the ether-saturated sponge, the custom of improvising a cone by some simple method such as folding up a towel or a sheet of paper, and placing the sponge in its apex, soon became general in the United States.

These principles of anaesthetic technique, the rejection of all but the simplest utensils and the resolute administration of strong ether vapour, had not only the sanction of intellectual leaders in the old-established medical centres of the Eastern States but the approval of men practising among the new settlements and advancing frontier outposts of the Middle and Western States. For these men, many of whom had received scanty medical training, the tools of their craft necessarily had to be cheap, simple and reasonably foolproof. Ether anaesthesia appeared admirably to conform to such requirements. That anaesthesia

[1] Villeneuve, R. 1904. *L'Anesthésie et les anesthésiques usuels.* Paris. 157.
[2] *Medical and surgical history of the war of the rebellion.* Washington, 1883, 2 (iii), 887.

could be looked upon as a science needing an expert to apply it clinically was, to the average American, either unthinkable or ridiculous. In American hospitals so foolproof was etherization considered that it was entrusted to a nurse, or more often still it was one of the less interesting routine duties to which junior medical students were relegated. Only during the last quarter of the nineteenth century, when America was finally throwing off the intense self-absorption of the ' frontier period ' and when her surgeons were coming under the powerful influence of rapidly developing German surgery, did more far-sighted men begin to appreciate, as the Germans themselves had already begun to do, the need for introducing new conceptions and new methods into anaesthesia.

The Introduction and Establishment of Chloroform

In the spring of 1847 James Miller, Professor of Surgery at Edinburgh, learned of Warren's use of a sponge for administering ether. News of etherization, together with a Squire's inhaler (see Fig. 17), had first reached Miller from London, from his former chief, Liston himself, the first British surgeon to make use of ether ; nevertheless, after trying Warren's method, Miller adopted it and his example was followed by James Young Simpson, Professor of Midwifery, and other of his colleagues. This established a precedent in Scotland for resolutely administering ether by the simplest means, as in America, and when, towards the close of the same year, 1847, Simpson introduced the use of chloroform the same principles were applied. Chloroform was poured freely upon a folded handkerchief or pad of material which was then held over the patient's face.

Whereas the Americans were able to claim that ether was safe in any hands, even those of a novice, it quickly became apparent that chloroform could be extremely dangerous. Because, while the first casualties ascribed to chloroform were occurring in England, the United States, and France, no such casualties occurred at Edinburgh, Simpson and his colleagues formed the opinion that chloroform was perfectly safe so long as the Edinburgh method [1] was implicitly followed—a belief to

---

[1] The method was modified by Simpson himself about 1860. He had found that in careless hands the pad was often held in such a way that it prevented sufficient dilution of the chloroform vapour with air. He therefore used a single layer of towel held puffed out into a fan-shape and laid lightly over the patient's nose and mouth. On this, liquid chloroform was dropped, not poured (see pp. 192–3).

which Scottish surgeons stoutly adhered for the remainder of the nineteenth century.

Edinburgh had long been one of the great centres of surgical teaching. During his surgical training each student was attached to a senior surgeon for a definite period as one of a team of student-assistants, the junior members of which were known as ' dressers ', the seniors as ' clerks '. After the introduction of the use of anaesthesia it became customary to entrust the task of ' chloroforming ' the patient to each clerk in rotation. Fixed rules for his guidance were drawn up and in these he was expected to be perfect so that it was unnecessary for the surgeon to supervise him during the course of an operation (cf. p. 539). Although this method of teaching did not foster an interest in the further study of anaesthesia, it nevertheless produced medical men each of whom, within the somewhat narrow limits of the prescribed routine, was capable during the remainder of his professional career of chloroforming a patient satisfactorily. Such a grounding as this in a simple method of making a patient insensible to pain was particularly valuable to the country practitioner who, on his rounds, had to take all his instruments with him on horseback or in his gig and single-handed had often first to chloroform his patient and then operate.

During 1847 anaesthetic methods passed through similar phases of development in England and on the European Continent. Attempts were made to copy or improve upon the construction of Morton's patented inhaler. But although considerable ingenuity went to the making, the performance of these early ether inhalers, almost without exception, was poor. This chiefly accounts for the alacrity with which administrators turned from ether to chloroform anaesthesia in November 1847.

At Lyons, however, a return to the use of ether was made during 1848, after chloroform deaths had occurred. Naples followed the example set at Lyons, and in the Austrian sphere of influence, particularly in Vienna, mixtures of chloroform and ether, poured on to a folded cloth, were used. The re-adoption of ether by the Lyonnais surgeons was simplified by the fact that a satisfactory way of administering it—by pouring it into a bag the mouth of which was then held over the patient's nose and mouth (see Fig. 24)—had already been found (see pp. 204–7).

Elsewhere on the Continent the prestige of chloroform remained almost unshaken until the last decade of the nineteenth century.

Anaesthesia on the European Continent, 1847 to c. 1870

In France the approach to anaesthetic problems was twofold. On the one hand was the clinical approach of the surgeons, on the other the academic approach of the physiologists who, early in 1847, became deeply interested in the anaesthetic state because it threw fresh light upon problems already being studied in connection with the function of the central nervous system. Although collaboration between the academic scientist and the clinician was a characteristic and important feature in the development of anaesthesia in France, this collaboration was not close. The typical form which it took was for the scientist to initiate research upon some physiological, physical or chemical problem the solving of which involved the experimental use of anaesthetic agents and the anaesthetic state. If in the course of his investigations the scientist arrived at conclusions which he considered potentially valuable to clinical anaesthesia he embodied them in a paper. This was then read at a meeting of one or other of the learned societies (and, as a rule, published in the proceedings) with the recommendation that the new evidence should be turned to practical account by surgeons. Less commonly the scientist made his suggestion directly to a surgeon known to him. In either case, it was generally left to the surgeon to work out the technique of application.

This lack of close collaboration was due to the surgeons themselves who (with few exceptions) were not interested in studying anaesthesia but wished to have at their command the most effective method of producing what they had learned by experience gave the most favourable operating conditions—an insensible and relaxed patient.

Once the use of chloroform had become established in France, anaesthesia was quickly reduced to a simple routine. Although, during 1848, the surgical instrument makers put various mechanical inhalers on the market, these were not popular and the folded cloth on to which chloroform was poured, as Simpson himself had advocated, was used almost everywhere, except in the Navy, where surgeons preferred a cardboard cone, containing lint to absorb the liquid chloroform, the base of which fitted over the patient's nose and mouth (see Fig. 47).

Ultimate responsibility for the administration of an anaesthetic rested with the surgeon and induction was usually begun
by him. But in order that his attention should not be distracted
from what he considered the far more important task of operating,
it was customary for him to decide upon a satisfactory method of
anaesthetic procedure and then so thoroughly to drill two or
three of the house surgeons in the routine that whichever of them
happened to be available could be left, once the administration
was satisfactorily under way, to carry it through unsupervised.
A second house surgeon, without special training, was entrusted
with the task of watching the pulse and keeping the administrator informed of its behaviour. Some surgeons, for example
Sédillot and others at Strasbourg, employed a permanent
assistant, often without medical training, to accompany them
to all operations to administer the chloroform. This system,
however, was regarded with disapproval in Paris.[1]

On the whole, the French system was less satisfactory than the
Scottish. In both countries anaesthesia was under the control
of the surgeon and so far as practice in the larger hospitals was
concerned, was not dissimilar ; but while in Scotland each
medical student was trained to give a reasonably efficient anaesthetic by the routine method, in France the student, when he
qualified, was unpractised in the art of anaesthesia. He would
probably receive a single lecture on the administration of anaesthetics and the reactions most commonly to be observed in
the patient, but during his clinical training in the operating
theatre his attention was expected to be concentrated upon
the surgeon's hands, not upon the subordinate carrying out the
necessary but otherwise insignificant task of keeping the patient
anaesthetized.

The complete failure of some French surgeons, even as late
as 1868, to recognize the importance of anaesthesia was commented upon with astonishment in England, by the editor of the
Medical Times :

‘ M. Giraldès informs us that we have not mistaken the
purport of his observations, and that it is a fact that in
many of the secondary provincial towns in France patients
still undergo operations without being submitted to any anaesthetic agent. This is even the case in so important a town as
Amiens, in which there is a School of Medicine, and where

[1] Cf. Guyon, F. 1873. *Éléments de chirurgie clinique*. Paris. 171–4.

the Surgeons, or, at all events, the senior Surgeon, never employ anaesthetics.'[1]

During the first two decades of the general use of anaesthesia in surgery the scientific prestige of France was still the greatest in Europe, and it was French anaesthetic practice which, broadly speaking, was originally taken as a model by the other nations of the European Continent. With them, also, research into anaesthetic problems was left to the academic investigator, the surgeons regarding anaesthesia merely as a useful adjunct to their craft. Administration was reduced to a simple routine by the surgeons and was then entrusted to an assistant, and the medical student was left all but uninstructed in anaesthesia.

It seems probable that this, the typical Continental attitude towards anaesthesia during the greater part of the half century 1846-96, was largely brought about by the prevailing political and social conditions. When Simpson first proposed the use of chloroform, Europe was in a ferment of unrest ; soon afterwards revolution broke out and nowhere was there either the desire or the opportunity seriously to question Simpson's method. The early good opinion of chloroform anaesthesia was confirmed by the experience of surgeons during the Crimean War when, under the most trying conditions, the drug was satisfactorily administered to a far greater number of seriously injured patients than normal peace-time practice could have provided in the same space of time. For the next thirty or so years the spirit of the times was utilitarian and surgeons found no imperative reason to alter the routine of chloroform anaesthesia which was familiar to them and to their assistants and reasonably adequate for their needs.

John Snow's Influence upon English Anaesthesia

Nineteenth century anaesthetic practice in England had a more strongly marked individuality than that of any other country. Two features particularly distinguish it—the existence, from the beginning, of the specialist anaesthetist and the persistent development and routine use of mechanical inhalers.

The first professional anaesthetist was the Yorkshireman, John Snow, and how this calling came into being was described by Benjamin Ward Richardson in his biographical introduction to Snow's book, *On chloroform and other anaesthetics* (London,

[1] *Med. Times, Lond.*, 1868, ii, 9.

1858). Referring to the medical events of the year 1846, Richardson wrote :

' In this year, the news came over from America that operations could be performed without pain under the influence of sulphuric ether.

' The fact was just such an one as would at once attract the earnest attention of Dr. Snow. It was a physiological, as well as a practical fact. It was rational in its meaning, and marvellously humane in its application. The question once before him, was in a scientific sense his own. His previous experimental studies on respiration and asphyxia [1] had prepared him for this new inquiry. He lost no time, therefore, in investigating the new fact ; he took it up for its own sake, however, not from any thought, at the time, of a harvest of gold.

' The first inhalations of ether in this country were not so successful as to astonish all the surgeons, or to recommend etherization as a common practice. The distrust arose from the manner in which the agent was administered. Dr. Snow at once detected this circumstance ; and . . . remedied the mistake by making an improved inhaler. He next carried out many experiments on animals and on himself, and brought the administration to great perfection. One day, on coming out of one of the hospitals (I am giving the narrative as he gave it to me), he met Mr. —— (a druggist whom he knew) bustling along with a large ether apparatus under his arm. " Good morning!" said Dr. Snow. " Good morning to you, doctor!" said the friend ; " but don't detain me, I am giving ether here and there and everywhere, and am getting quite into an ether practice. Good morning, doctor!" " Good morning to you!" Rather peculiar! said the doctor to himself; rather peculiar, certainly! for the man has not the remotest chemical or physiological idea on the subject. An " ether practice! If he can get an ether practice, perchance some scraps of the same thing might fall to a scientific unfortunate." Consequently, with his improved inhaler, Dr. Snow lost no time in asking to be allowed to give ether at St. George's Hospital. He got permission to give it there to the out-patients, in cases of tooth-drawing. Dr. Fuller, of Manchester Square, standing by, was surprised to see with what happy effects ether was administered when administered properly. A day or

---

[1] On October 16, 1841, Snow read his first paper, at a meeting of the Westminster Medical Society. It was entitled ' Asphyxia and on the resuscitation of new-born children.' ' The object of the paper ', wrote Richardson, ' was to introduce to the Society a double air-pump, for supporting artificial respiration, invented by a Mr. Read, of Regent Circus. . . . There was also a sentence or two on the cause of the first inspiration which is well worthy of note.' (B. W. Richardson in his introduction to Snow, J. 1858. *On chloroform and other anaesthetics.* London. xi.)

two afterwards, an operation having to be performed, and the surgeon (I believe, Mr. Cutler) not approving of the ether in the way in which it had previously acted, Dr. Fuller remarked on the superiority of Dr. Snow's mode of administering it ; and the result was, that he was asked to give it on operating days. He did so with great success. He administered it at University College with the same success. Liston, then the leading operator, struck with the new man who came before him in such an able and unaffected way, took him by the hand ; and from that time the ether practice in London came almost exclusively to him. Science for once put assumption in its right place.' [1]

That the English professional tradition in anaesthesia, thus founded by Snow, was able to become firmly established was largely due to the tenor of life—peaceful, prosperous and un-hurried—during the Victorian era.

Snow was the first to carry out experiments on the physiology of the anaesthetic state and then to construct an inhaler for clinical use, the design of which was based upon conclusions reached in the course of his researches. He insisted that in administering an inhalation anaesthetic the administrator must have control over the concentration of anaesthetic vapour in the anaesthetic-air mixture reaching the patient's lungs, and he claimed that the only sure means of achieving this was to use an inhaler, such as his own (see Figs. 29 and 30), which could be easily and accurately regulated to deliver the required mixture. But to use such an inhaler safely and successfully the adminis-trator must be a man of skill and judgment with at least some scientific understanding of the more important physiological processes involved.

In November 1847, ' having satisfied himself personally as to the effects and greater practicability of chloroform, he [Snow] at once commenced its use, and forgot sooner almost than others all predilections for ether '.[2]

Deaths due to chloroform which soon occurred in the hands of others, merely strengthened Snow in his belief that, unless some completely innocuous anaesthetic agent could be found, administration should be entrusted only to the expert, who should employ the additional safeguard of an accurately regulating inhaler. Snow himself, in the latter part of 1847, designed a chloroform inhaler, based on the same principles as his ether

[1] Richardson, in Snow, J. 1858. *On chloroform and other anaesthetics.* London. xiii *et seq.* [2] *Ibid.* xvi.

inhaler, and regulated to deliver a maximum of 5 per cent. chloroform vapour in the inhaled air (see Fig. 41).

Richardson wrote of Snow :

' The fact that in almost every fatal case from chloroform the result had occurred from the action of the narcotic on the central organ of the circulation, was never absent from his thoughts. An agent having this effect, however intrinsically valuable, was not to be put in the hands of every person for administration. " There would be a great uproar," he remarked on one occasion, " if a student were to undertake on the operating table to tie the femoral artery, and were to open the femoral vein. Yet at some of our hospitals, the administration of chloroform has been entrusted to the porter, who would only grin in ignorance, if informed that each time his services were required, he performed the grand act of suspending for a time the oxidation of the whole body, and of inducing a temporary death ; and who would tell you, if you asked him the composition of chloroform, that it was smelling stuff." He spoke this from no selfish feeling, but with that kind of regret which an educated engineer would feel, on referring to the fact of a railway porter who, knowing nothing of steam, how to put it on, when to take it off, or why it propelled, had mounted an engine and driven a host of confiding passengers to their destruction. This is the way in which he expressed himself, and it would be difficult to show that he was not correct.' [1]

To discover the perfect substitute for chloroform anaesthesia remained Snow's dearest wish.

' He continued steadily to investigate the effects of various volatile agents for the production of insensibility, and arrived by frequent experiment to such a degree of positive knowledge regarding agents of this class, that the composition and boiling point of any new chemical body having been supplied, he could predict whether or not its vapour would produce narcotism by inhalation. . . . His grand search was for a narcotic vapour which, having the physical properties and practicability of chloroform, should, in its physiological effects, resemble ether in not producing, by any accident of administration, paralysis of the heart.

' He paid considerable attention to the subject of local anaesthesia, and tried numerous methods for attaining to a knowledge of a perfect local anaesthetic. He performed experiments with freezing mixtures, with chloroform ; and for the production of

[1] Richardson, in Snow, J. 1858. *On chloroform and other anaesthetics.* London. xxviii.

rapid and efficient benumbing by cold, he tried, in 1854, the effects of applying solid carbonic acid to the skin ; . . . but he was never satisfied with them, and soon relinquished the inquiry, in order to concentrate his energies on the discovery of what he felt sure must be discovered ultimately,—an anaesthetic which might be inhaled without destroying consciousness.' [1]

Although Snow's teaching was very far from being put into practice generally in England his professional prestige was great, both with medical men and, after he had twice anaesthetized Queen Victoria herself,[2] with the public, so that his views were widely accepted as embodying an ideal of anaesthetic conduct.

In provincial towns and in country practice particularly, Simpson's original method of chloroforming the patient was by far the most commonly used. But at the time of Snow's death, in 1858, in many London hospitals and some of the larger provincial hospitals, his inhaler, or some similar piece of apparatus, was regularly used and the custom of appointing a general practitioner interested in anaesthetics to attend the hospital regularly, in the intervals of his private practice, in the capacity of honorary 'chloroformist' was steadily growing. Thus the administration of anaesthetics came increasingly into the hands of qualified and experienced men, some of whom were anxious and able to develop the theoretical as well as the practical side of their specialty.

By the early eighteen-sixties it had become evident that the search, undertaken by Snow and others, for the perfect substitute for chloroform was not soon to be successful. It was equally evident that something ought to be done to put a stop to or at least check the shocking frequency with which deaths occurred under chloroform anaesthesia. The Royal Medical and Chirurgical Society of London, therefore, appointed a committee to investigate the physiological action of chloroform.

In the course of the investigation two parallel series of experiments were done on animals, one series with chloroform, the other with ether. From these it was concluded that, as an anaesthetic, ether was far safer than chloroform because, when an overdose of ether was given, the respiration always stopped

[1] Richardson, in Snow, J. 1858. *On chloroform and other anaesthetics.* London. xxvii, xxviii, xxx.
[2] The occasions were the birth of Prince Leopold, in 1853, and the birth of Princess Beatrice, in 1857.

before the action of the heart and it was usually possible to revive the animal by applying artificial respiration ; but when an overdose of chloroform was given the action of the heart stopped before the respiration and the animal could not be revived. The committee in its report, made in 1864, nevertheless stated that ether anaesthesia was impracticable from a clinical point of view on account of its immoderate slowness in producing the anaesthetic state and the frequent turbulence, during the induction period, of the subject being etherized. (These were the very reasons which had led to the rejection of ether for chloroform in the autumn of 1847. Since then ether had rarely been used in England and, although the American preference for the drug was known, the English still had no practical experience of a satisfactory technique for administration.)

On the horns of a dilemma—the danger of chloroform anaesthesia and the impracticability of ether anaesthesia—the committee compromised and suggested that chloroform should be diluted by mixing it in various proportions with ether, or with ether and alcohol. Such mixtures did not immediately become popular, but a certain number of men began to make use of anaesthetic sequences. The majority induced anaesthesia with chloroform and then changed over to ether, claiming that they thus used the safer agent for maintenance yet avoided a troublesome induction. A few reversed the sequence, having noticed that chloroform appeared most frequently to be fatal in the early stages of anaesthesia but nevertheless gave extremely satisfactory deep anaesthesia (see pp. 258–64).

The chief importance of these anaesthetic mixtures and sequences lay in the fact that their adoption made a break with the tradition which had grown up in Snow's time, that the ideal anaesthetic to replace all others would one day be discovered. Although the search was by no means abandoned, after 1864 anaesthetists began to wonder if, in fact, the exclusive use of any single anaesthetic agent or method of procedure, however excellent, could solve every anaesthetic problem.

The Revived Use of Nitrous Oxide

In 1862 Gardner Quincy Colton (at whose demonstration of the exhilarating effects of nitrous oxide Wells, in 1844, had hit upon the idea of inhaling the gas to obviate the pain of a dental extraction) was still making his living by touring the United States giving pseudo-scientific lectures on popular subjects. At a certain town in his circuit he was persuaded by the chance request of an old lady to administer gas to her while her dentist extracted some teeth. Although since 1844 Colton had always included in his lectures the story of Wells's first use of the gas, he had never again, until then, administered it for an extraction. So successful was he, however, that other patients presented themselves. On his return to the same town a year later, Colton found the dentist, whom he had instructed in making and administering nitrous oxide, in so prosperous a way of business as anaesthetist-dentist, that he himself decided to give up the less lucrative profession of lecturer. He went to New York and there founded the Colton Dental Association. He and a staff of assistants then devoted themselves exclusively to administering nitrous oxide and extracting teeth. The success of this venture was immediate. Soon branches were established in other American cities and the use of gas in dentistry became widespread in the United States.

In the course of 1867 an International Exhibition and the first International Congress of Medicine were held in Paris. Colton, while attending these, deeply interested a fellow-countryman, T. W. Evans, whose dental practice was among the most fashionable in Paris, in nitrous oxide anaesthesia. In the following year, 1868, Evans came to London for the sole purpose of teaching English dentists to make and use the gas. He installed his generating apparatus in his suite at the Langham Hotel and drew off supplies of the gas into rubber bags. These he took round with him to various demonstrations arranged by the leading London dentists. When he finally returned to Paris, Evans presented £100 to the Odontological Society of Great Britain to be devoted to research on nitrous oxide and the development of apparatus for administering it clinically.

Dentists and anaesthetists were not slow to take advantage of this generosity. Everyone had been impressed by Evans's demonstrations, but even while these were in progress J. T. Clover (since Snow's death the leader of the anaesthetic profession) and others, perceived how the American apparatus could be bettered. Moreover, by the autumn of 1868, the London firms of Coxeter and Barth had both succeeded in compressing the gas into metal cylinders and an efficient commercial service for supplying and refilling the cylinders was gradually established, so that by 1870 nitrous oxide in an easily portable form and at small cost was available to almost all dentists and anaesthetists who wished to use it.

Ether revived in England

In 1872 another American, an ophthalmologist from Boston, named B. Joy Jeffries, came to England on the occasion of an international ophthalmological congress held in London. He declared that ever since he had visited Europe as a medical student, during the eighteen-fifties, he had thought it regrettable that chloroform should be in daily use while ether was completely neglected. At a meeting of the congress he read a paper on ether anaesthesia and subsequently arranged to give a number of demonstrations of the American ' towel cone ' method of administration.

In order to prove the perfect safety of ether Jeffries poured the drug lavishly into the cone and impressed upon his audience that so long as the patient was warned to expect a feeling of suffocation and to inhale deeply in spite of it, and so long as the administrator applied the cone with determination, ignoring the patient's struggles, then anaesthesia could be rapidly and effectively established. No doubt this procedure appeared somewhat lacking in refinement to the chloroformists ; but the majority were already sufficiently convinced (by the findings of the Chloroform Committee of 1864) of the safety of ether to be prepared to try a method which certainly overcame the very difficulties which had prevented them from using the drug.

Within a year of Jeffries's visit the use of ether was becoming general among professional anaesthetists in hospital practice, and even some of those who were by no means convinced that ether was in any way superior to chloroform were forced to use the former in deference to popular opinion.

During the course of 1873, as experience in the use of ether increased, more and more anaesthetists discarded the American method and reverted to the use of inhalers, increasing numbers of which, designed on entirely new principles, were appearing on the market.

Three distinct factors may account for this deep-rooted Victorian preference for inhalers. First, there was the Englishman's natural bent for mechanical invention and the trust which, whether as administrator or patient, he placed in the use of apparatus as a sure means of reducing human error. There was also the importance which he attached to personal comfort, so that even as a preliminary to a surgical operation he no doubt found reassurance in breathing the anaesthetic from an inhaler made by some reputable firm from good glass and plated metal and having a facepiece, plush-lined or with a padded rubber rim, to fit his cheeks snugly. Whether or not the apparatus had been thoroughly cleansed even of the grosser soiling of previous use does not appear to have troubled him greatly.

But undoubtedly the principal cause of the English preference for inhalers was the existence of the professional anaesthetist. Because, in England, able, qualified men chose to act as administrators it was never necessary to reduce anaesthesia to the simplest possible routine so that it could be applied by the inexpert. The professional anaesthetist liked to work out his own technique, overcoming particular anaesthetic difficulties as they arose, either by designing a special piece of apparatus for himself or by modifying apparatus invented by his colleagues. Since these men constantly devoted some part of their time to anaesthesia most of them were sufficiently familiar with anaesthetic machines to be able to master the intricacies of even the most elaborate.

From about 1873 onwards ether became the anaesthetic of choice for general surgery, but chloroform continued to be used in obstetrics, except where surgical intervention was necessary, and nitrous oxide was used in dentistry. About 1876 the value of Clover's new apparatus for the gas-ether sequence which he had devised and begun to use even before Jeffries's visit (see p. 312), began to be appreciated by other anaesthetists, because induction with gas was more pleasant and rapid than with ether alone, even when given from the improved types of inhaler available.

At the time of Clover's death, in 1882, further tendencies towards selection in the choice of anaesthetic were becoming noticeable. Because of the frequency with which chest complications were found following ether anaesthesia,[1] chloroform

---

[1] Two principal reasons to-day held to be responsible for the occurrence of post-operative chest complications are :

(a) the lack of a preliminary dose of atropine to control the excessive secretion of mucus due to ether ; and

(b) the fact that patients recovering from abdominal operations (a type of operation undertaken with increasing frequency during the last quarter of the nineteenth century) are liable to become ' chesty ' no matter what anaesthetic has been used, because the pain of the wound deters them from breathing properly and from coughing productively.

These reasons, however, began to be appreciated only during the first decade of the present century.

had been reinstated as a more suitable anaesthetic for any patient whose condition predisposed him to develop a ' post-operative chest '. Old people, as a class, came within this category. Chloroform was customarily administered, also, to young children, who were popularly supposed (like parturient women) to be immune from cardiac syncope due to its use. Some surgeons claimed that chloroform provided better operating conditions than ether for reducing dislocations and in eye surgery. This general rejection of ether in special types of case gave those anaesthetists who had never willingly accepted it an opportunity to return to the use of chloroform in all cases. Still other anaesthetists revived the use of anaesthetic mixtures such as the Chloroform Committee of 1864 had recommended, and complicated (but often quite pointless) sequences were attempted (see pp. 461–2).

Clover's death left English anaesthetic practice temporarily without leadership and during the eighteen-eighties little real progress was evident.

Antisepsis, Asepsis and Surgical Developments

After October 1846, although directly etherization had become an established practice patients more readily submitted to surgical operations, and although, when chloroform anaesthesia had been substituted for etherization, surgeons were able to attempt delicate and protracted procedures, nevertheless the prognosis for the patient's final recovery grew worse rather than better. For as the number of operations performed increased, so hospital gangrene, pyaemia, erysipelas, tetanus and similar conditions, popularly known under the collective name *hospitalism*, increased also.

Writing upon hospitalism, in the eighteen-sixties, James Young Simpson stated :

' In the Edinburgh Infirmary, out of the first 99 cases in which limbs were amputated [during the eighteenth century], 8 of the patients died, or 1 in 12. Out of the first 30 amputations for disease in the Glasgow Infirmary, 1 patient only died. At the present day, in these now greatly-enlarged and palatial hospitals, the mortality from the same operations has latterly become higher than 1 in every 3 operated upon. . . . This increase is traceable, I believe, chiefly or entirely to our system of huge and colossal hospital edifices, and to the hygienic evils which that system has hitherto been made to involve.' [1]

In an address read at Belfast in 1867, upon the same subject, Simpson said :

' The man laid on an operating-table in one of our surgical hospitals is exposed to more chances of death than the English soldier on the field of Waterloo.
' Dr. Bristowe and Mr. Holmes of London, in visiting the Parisian hospitals in order to draw up a report upon them for the medical officer of the Privy Council (Mr. Simon [2]), obtained from the government official archives the results of the major amputations of the limbs . . . during the year 1861 in all the Parisian hospitals taken as a whole. The mortality among those operated upon was as high as 1 in 1½ ; or 3 out of every 5 died . . . nearly double the death-rate which attends upon the same operations in our large and metropolitan British hospitals, in which the mortality is fully 1 in 3 ; while, as Mr. Simon points out . . . '' in the London hospitals [the special death-rate from amputations] is half as high again as in the country hospitals.'' ' [3]

Simpson claimed to have stated, as long ago as 1848 :

' There are few or no circumstances which would contribute more to save surgical and obstetric patients from phlebitic and other analogous disorders, than a total change in the present system of hospital practice. I have often stated and taught, that if our present medical, surgical and obstetric hospitals were changed from being crowded palaces . . . into villages or cottages, with one, or at most two, patients in each room, a great saving of human life would be effected ; and if the village were constructed of iron (as is now sometimes done for other purposes), instead of brick or stone, it could be taken down and rebuilt every few years—a matter apparently of much moment in hospital hygiene.' [4]

Simpson seemed in doubt as to the rationale of this argument. But during 1846 Ignaz Philipp Semmelweis, assistant in the obstetrical clinic of the Vienna Medical School where the medical

[1] Simpson, J. Y. 1871. *Anaesthesia, hospitalism and other papers.* Ed. by W. G. Simpson. Edinburgh. 289.
[2] Simon, J. 1887. *Public Health Reports,* **2,** 128 ; Sixth Report, 1863 (iv) ' Hospital hygiene, especially in relation to the so-called traumatic infections, and to the spread of contagious fevers.'
[3] Simpson, J. Y. 1871. *Anaesthesia, hospitalism and other papers.* Edinburgh. 291.
[4] *Ibid.* 290.

students received their training, had been struck by the fact that the mortality was there nearly three times as great as in the clinic where the midwives trained. After careful observation Semmelweis concluded that in his clinic the women were being contaminated by infected matter carried on the hands of students coming straight from the dissecting room to examine them. He further concluded that any form of decayed organic material might cause blood poisoning, and when, in 1847, he insisted that everyone before undertaking any manual procedure on a patient must wash hands and instruments in a solution of 1 ounce of chlorinated lime in $1\frac{1}{2}$ pints of water and that infected and healthy women must be segregated, the incidence of infection rapidly decreased.[1]

By about 1863 the possibility of the spread of infection in hospitals, not only directly from patient to patient, but through contamination by soiled objects such as bedding and even wall surfaces in the wards, was beginning to be widely recognized. Florence Nightingale's reforms in hospital management and her newly-trained nurses from the school at St. Thomas's Hospital, opened in 1862 (for England, certainly the most important outcome of the Crimean War), had already effected enormous improvements in the attention given to the patient's toilet and the regular cleansing and ventilation of the wards.[2] But the operating theatre itself was still untouched by such innovations.

In March 1867 Joseph Lister, then Professor of Surgery in the University of Glasgow, published an article in the *Lancet*,[3] ' on a new method of treating compound fracture, abscess, etc., with observations on the conditions of suppuration '. In this article Lister referred to Pasteur's researches upon putrescence and suggested that since the mischief is caused by airborne microbes—

' it appears that all that is requisite is to dress the wound with some material capable of killing these septic germs, provided that any substance can be found reliable for this purpose, yet not too potent as a caustic.

' In the course of the year 1864,' he continued, ' I was much struck with an account of the remarkable effects produced by

---

[1] Cf. Neuburger, M. 1943. *British medicine and the Vienna school.* London. 74–5.
[2] Cf. Simon, J. 1887. *Public Health Reports*, **2**, 149, 154, 165.
[3] *Lancet*, 1867, i, 326.

carbolic acid upon the sewage of the town of Carlisle, the admixture of a very small proportion not only preventing all odour
from the lands irrigated with the refuse material, but, as it was
stated, destroyed the entozoa which usually infest cattle fed upon
such pastures.

' My attention having for several years been much directed to
the subject of suppuration, more especially in its relation to
decomposition, I saw that such a powerful antiseptic was peculiarly
adapted for experiments with a view to elucidating that subject,
and while I was engaged in the investigation the applicability of
carbolic acid for the treatment of compound fracture naturally
occurred to me.

' My first attempt of this kind was made in the Glasgow
Royal Infirmary in March, 1865, in a case of compound fracture
of the leg. It proved unsuccessful . . . but subsequent trials
have more than realised my most sanguine anticipations.'

In opening abscesses, in the early cases, the incision was
made beneath a rag dipped in a solution of carbolic acid in
boiled linseed oil. Lister explained that ' the instant the knife
is withdrawn the rag is dropped back upon the skin as an antiseptic curtain '. Crystallized carbolic acid, liquefied by the
addition of a few drops of water, was then introduced ' into all
accessible recesses of the wound by means of a piece of rag '.
The wound was then dressed with ' glazier's putty ', made by
mixing a solution of carbolic acid in linseed oil with carbonate
of lime. ' This is spread upon a piece of sheet block tin about
six inches square. . . . The tin thus spread with putty is placed
upon the skin so that the middle of it corresponds to the position
of the incision. . . . The tin is then fixed securely with adhesive
plaster, the lowest edge being left free for the escape of discharge
into a folded towel placed over it and secured by a bandage.' [1]

Between 1868 and 1870 Lister slightly modified this somewhat
drastic treatment ; instead of using the acid at full strength, he
irrigated the wound with a 1 in 20 solution of carbolic acid in
water, then covered it with two or three layers of oiled silk
smeared on both sides with carbolic acid in linseed oil. Upon
these he placed an overlapping pad of lint, soaked in the oily
solution and over this a layer of gutta-percha. Next a carbolized
towel was wrapped round, then an outer layer of gutta-percha
or oiled silk.[2]

In 1870 Lister began to use the carbolic spray—adapting for

[1] *Lancet*, 1867, ii, 95, 353.   [2] *Brit. med. J.*, 1870, ii, 243.

the purpose an apparatus used by Richardson for local anaesthesia
—which ' threw over the part [being operated upon] a cloud of
spray of 1 to 40 carbolic lotion '.[1] By 1875 the spray had been
made to work automatically by steam pressure. For wound
dressing Lister now used simply a pad of 8 layers of carbolized
gauze with a sheet of thin mackintosh beneath the uppermost ;
chloride of zinc or boracic acid (an especial favourite of Lister's)
were often applied to the wound in place of carbolic.[2]

    Although these elaborate precautions against infection were
taken, during the early years of antisepsis Lister paid little or no
attention to the general state of cleanliness in the operating
theatre. J. R. Leeson, who went as a student from the newly
rebuilt St. Thomas's Hospital in London, to study under Lister
at Edinburgh (where the latter had become Professor of Surgery
in 1869, in succession to Syme), in later years recalled that :

' The operating theatre was grimed with the filth of decades ;
I suppose it was occasionally cleaned but such process was never
in evidence. There was but one window, the large one to the
north, which lighted it, but it was never opened. . . . Many of
the students came straight from the dissecting room. The operating-table looked as though it was never washed and around its
base sawdust was sprinkled.
    ' No one dreamt of washing his hands before commencing
work. . . . No one ever took off his coat ; occasionally the
professor would turn up his cuffs ; but the assistants never ;
probably they would have considered it a breach of etiquette as
assuming an unwarranted importance. . . . One marvels that
early antiseptic surgery survived at all, but it was saved by
carbolic ; everything was soaked in 1 in 20, hands, instruments,
and patient's skin. . . .
    ' Moreover, the whole scene of an operation, or dressing was
enveloped in its spray, which dispersed its globules into every
nook and cranny of the wound, and our faces and coat-sleeves
often dripped with it.
    ' Towels soaked in 1 in 20 . . . were placed around the
wound. I never remember them so used in London, but Lister
never worked without them ; he would pin them carefully with
(carbolized) safety-pins around the part, leaving a window in
which he worked ; he was very fond of safety-pins.' [3]

    Lister's antiseptic methods were not readily accepted in
Great Britain. Even J. Y. Simpson, whose interest in wound

[1] *Brit. med. J.*, 1871, i, 30.   [2] *Lancet*, 1875, i, 365, 401, 603.
[3] Leeson, J. R. 1927. *Lister as I knew him*. London. 107, 108.

infection was of long standing, instead of encouraging Lister, in 1867 wrote a long letter to the *Lancet* [1] merely to point out that the use of carbolic acid in surgery was not new.

Leeson, referring to his student days at St. Thomas's, which he entered in October 1871, about a year before joining Lister in Edinburgh, wrote :

' It was at St. Thomas's that I first smelt carbolic acid and became familiar with the old sticky yellow gauze, and yet the demonstration of its failure seemed complete. Had not carbolic acid been sprinkled upon the wound and carbolic gauze applied as a dressing ? and yet a few days later the patient's temperature was high and he had had a rigor ! He was evidently no better than if he had been treated by the old methods ! ' [2]

In the late eighteen-sixties the antagonism between Prussia and France, which Bismarck was so carefully fostering, led German surgeons in search of new ideas from abroad to look to Edinburgh rather than to Paris, as they had formerly done, and to interest themselves in the work of such men as Syme, Simpson and Lister himself. When war broke out in 1870 the Germans were prepared to apply Lister's antiseptic pastes and dressings in the field dressing stations and base hospitals. The experience of antisepsis thus gained under the exacting conditions of war convinced German surgeons that the method was valuable and worth developing when peace came.[3]

Lister described, in 1870, ' A method of treatment applicable to wounded soldiers in the present war ', and in 1875 he visited Germany and discussed antiseptic methods with her leading surgeons. Among his most important supporters were Karl Thiersch, of Leipzig ; Richard von Volkmann, Professor of Surgery at Halle ; Adolf von Bardeleben of the Charité in Berlin ; and Langenbeck, under whose tutelage most of the leading surgeons of Germany had grown up.[4]

The *British and Foreign Medico-Chirurgical Review* [5] commented upon Lister's German tour :

' . . . Professor Bardeleben uses Lister's treatment carefully. . . . He opens abscesses under spray and attends to all the

---

[1] *Lancet*, 1867, ii, 546.
[2] Leeson, J. R. 1927. *Lister as I knew him.* London. 11.
[3] Cf. *Sanitäts-Bericht über die deutschen Heere im Kriege gegen Frankreich, 1870–1.* Berlin, 1890, **3** (iii) *Die Verwundungen durch Kriegswaffen.* 37, 38.
[4] *Brit. med. J.*, 1875, ii, 769.   [5] *Brit. foreign med. Rev.*, 1875, **56**, 278.

minutiae, making free use of drainage tubes and carbolized sponges.

'Langenbeck lately performed an operation in Professor Lister's presence with antiseptic precautions for the first time. It is not often that a man so distinguished and at an advanced age is ready to try new ways. Nussbaum at Munich has found, after the use of antiseptic methods, a great decrease in the amount of pyaemia in hospital gangrene.

'On the other hand, we have conflicting opinions as to the power of antiseptic dressing in preventing erysipelas. . . .'

In France antiseptic methods were introduced into practice in 1869 by Just Lucas-Championnière, who had studied them under Lister in Glasgow during 1868. He returned to Scotland in 1875 and made a further, intensive study, particularly of Lister's methods of wound dressing.[1]

From 1868 onwards many reports of the success of antisepsis reached Britain from distinguished surgeons in various parts of Europe [2] and an increasing stream of foreign visitors came to Edinburgh to see Lister at work.

Although the practice of disinfecting hands, instruments, dressings and the patient's skin by rinsing them with some kind of antiseptic solution was widely accepted abroad, Lister's spray was less popular. Not only was its use inconvenient but by chilling and irritating the tissues it frequently caused serious forms of dermatitis. As a result of experience with the simpler procedure of observing strict antiseptic cleanliness, more and more surgeons became converted to the view, held by Theodor Billroth, for example, that the danger of wound infection from the surrounding atmosphere could be safely ignored.[3] By the eighteen-eighties the spray was almost entirely discarded except by Lister himself and a few other surgeons, in particular J. N. Nussbaum in Munich and Edmund Rose in Berlin [4] and many antiseptic substances in addition to those suggested by Lister were in use. By the close of the eighteen-eighties antisepsis had given place to asepsis.

The initiative in bringing about this change was taken by

[1] Lucas-Championnière, J. 1880. *Chirurgie antiseptique. Principes, modes d'application et résultats du pansement de Lister.* Paris. 2.

[2] Cf. *Lancet*, 1868, ii, 299 ; *New Sydenham Soc. Biennial Retrosp. Med. Surg.*, 1868–70, 199, 204 ; *Brit. med J.*, 1870, i, 557.

[3] Billroth, T. 1883. *General surgical pathology and therapeutics.* (Trs. by C. E. Hackley.) London. 115.

[4] Nussbaum, J. N. 1887. *Leitfaden zur antiseptischen Wundbehandlung.* Stuttgart. 46 ; *Dtsch. Z. Chir.*, 1884, **19**, 36.

the brilliant body of German surgeons who, taking advantage of the high ratio of immunity from accidental wound infection which became apparent immediately antiseptic methods were adopted, had been gradually developing visceral surgery, hitherto undertaken only in desperate cases and with small chance of the patient's ultimate survival. In dealing with the delicate tissues of the abdominal cavity it was obvious that even the blandest antiseptic substances must be avoided. It was well known, however, that bacteria could be readily destroyed by heat, and during the eighteen-eighties an elaborate routine for the sterilization of every object brought into contact with the wound was evolved. Gustav Neuber organized his private hospital in Kiel wholly upon aseptic lines and a similarly comprehensive aseptic routine was later elaborated and standardized by Ernst von Bergmann, who had served as a military surgeon, first in the Prussian army during the war of 1870, then in the Russian army during the Russo-Turkish War of 1877-8. In 1878 he accepted the Chair of Surgery at Würzburg and when in 1882 he succeeded Langenbeck in Berlin, his ideas upon aseptic procedure had already taken definite shape. He introduced steam sterilization in 1886.

The Franco-Prussian War, which played so important a part in establishing the use of antiseptic methods, came at a most inopportune time from the point of view of anaesthetic development on the Continent.

In France the war interrupted the general adoption of nitrous oxide, which in any case was progressing but slowly, partly, no doubt, because the American type of apparatus, introduced by Colton and Evans in 1867, was both costly and cumbersome, but also because the theory that nitrous oxide was not a true anaesthetic but merely an asphyxial agent was widely believed (see p. 310). In Germany, dentists, a few among whom had tentatively adopted the use of nitrous oxide, were conscripted into the army as general surgeons and during the war emergency used chloroform exclusively.[1]

During the two decades immediately following the Franco-Prussian War, when Germany was consolidating her new Empire both internally and in relation to other countries, the intensive development of surgery and the accompanying transition from

[1] Cf. *Sanitäts-Bericht über die deutschen Heer im Kriege gegen Frankreich 1870-1.* Berlin, 1890. **3** (iii), 31.

2

antiseptic to aseptic procedure engrossed the attention of her medical profession. Neither in Germany nor in France was anaesthesia considered more than a subsidiary part, although an important one, of surgery. In France, however, there was a revival of interest in anaesthesia during the twenty years immediately following the Franco-Prussian War, which was directly due to the influence of the physiologists Claude Bernard and Paul Bert.

Bernard, as an outcome of work upon the physiological action of morphine, about 1869 suggested the clinical use of 'mixed anaesthesia'—an injection of morphine[1] as a preliminary to chloroform inhalation in order to reduce the amount of chloroform required to produce and maintain anaesthesia. Mixed anaesthesia was eagerly adopted by those French surgeons who keenly feared the possibility of producing chloroform syncope in their patients through overdosage, yet continued to administer the drug because they knew of no entirely satisfactory substitute for it.

Bert, in 1878, completed a series of researches in connection with the physiological effects of variations in barometric pressure on the gases of the blood. He proceeded to apply certain conclusions drawn from these researches to the problem of nitrous oxide anaesthesia.

In reintroducing the use of nitrous oxide for dental purposes, Colton had believed it necessary to administer 100 per cent. gas in order to obtain adequate anaesthesia ; this belief was for many years unquestioningly accepted by the great majority of medical men. Bert pointed out that such an exclusion of air from the patient's lungs made asphyxia inevitable ; he suggested, however, that if the gas, instead of being administered at normal atmospheric pressure, were administered under a positive pressure of two atmospheres, then 50 per cent. air could be combined with 50 per cent. nitrous oxide. Asphyxia would not then occur and anaesthesia, he claimed, could be indefinitely prolonged.

A mobile pressure chamber was constructed to accommodate patient, surgeon and assistants and this 'anaesthetic car' plied between the various hospitals of Paris for some time before it was finally abandoned as inexpedient (see Fig. 103).

---

[1] It is noteworthy that the injection of morphine with a Pravaz syringe (see p. 376 n.) was extensively used on the battlefield during 1870–1. (Cf. *Sanitäts-Bericht über die deutschen Heere im Kriege gegen Frankreich, 1870–1.* Berlin, 1890. **3** (iii), 30.)

In 1883 Bert suggested that equally effective anaesthesia might be produced more simply if a proportion of oxygen were mixed with the nitrous oxide at atmospheric pressure. Almost immediately he then turned his attention to the question of safe percentages of chloroform in anaesthetic mixtures. In fact the technique of administering nitrous oxide-oxygen mixtures was developed not by the French but independently by the obstetrician S. Klikowitsch of St. Petersburg,[1] and by Viennese and German dentists and then by Hewitt, in England, during the late eighteen-eighties and early nineties (see pp. 481–9).

Bert's work on chloroform-air mixtures, although it was applied in practice by a few French surgeons with whom he had personal contact, exercised a more important influence upon English anaesthetists during the revival of the use of chloroform in the late eighteen-nineties and the first decade of the present century (see pp. 372–4).

Ether revived in Germany and France

In 1890 the Tenth International Congress of Medicine was held in Berlin. The English visitors were as astonished to see von Bergmann's paraphernalia for aseptic surgery—the steam sterilizing plant, the instruments made blade and haft in one piece, the glass-topped operating table, the surgeons' galoshes —as they were to observe that chloroform anaesthesia was still exclusively used in Berlin and apparently everywhere in Germany. During the Congress Professor Horatio C. Wood, of Philadelphia, who, like the English, thought the Germans' reliance upon chloro-form a pity, read a paper on anaesthesia. In the course of it he quoted statistical evidence showing the very much smaller in-cidence of death under ether than under chloroform anaesthesia.

As an indirect outcome of Wood's paper statistics were inde-pendently compiled over a period of several years by the surgeon Ernst Julius Gurlt, working on behalf of the German Surgical Society. The figures which he was able to adduce weighed heavily in favour of ether and this evidence was supported by the actual experience of ether anaesthesia gained by a few German surgeons. These men, in the late eighteen-eighties, had followed either the Swiss surgeon Julliard's example (set in 1877) of giving ether from a large wire mask with an impermeable outer cover (see Figs. 107–112), or that of the Danish surgeon

[1] *Arch. Gynaek.*, 1881, **18**, 81.

Wanscher who, about 1884, had introduced the use of ether at Copenhagen, using an inhaler based upon Ormsby's (see Fig. 113).

By 1894 a large number of German surgeons were giving ether anaesthesia a thorough trial and by about 1896 surgeons in France began to wonder whether they, too, might not be well advised to follow suit.

The Teaching of Anaesthesia ; Specialization

The jubilee of inhalation anaesthesia was celebrated in the autumn of 1896. Only in Great Britain had that half century been uninterrupted in its course. On the Continent of Europe and in the United States of America it was sharply divided into two nearly equal parts—first the period of alternating revolt and reaction culminating in war, then the period of peaceful reconstruction and consolidation.

The English anaesthetist could trace the development of his specialty from 1846 to 1896 as an ordered sequence of events still in progress, and the Scottish surgeon might congratulate himself upon fifty years of almost unchanged anaesthetic tradition. But on the Continent, particularly in Germany, and in the United States, where the example of German surgical development was exercising a profound influence, changes in surgical practice which had taken place within the preceding ten years served to accentuate the fact that little or no advance had been made in anaesthesia since the inception of its use. The need for development was suddenly both obvious and urgent.

While many Continental and American surgeons now envied the English system of employing only specialist anaesthetists in major surgery, the English themselves were regretting the shortcomings of their own medical training which, no less than the Continental and the American, made little provision for educating the medical student in anaesthesia. In England this need for grounding each student in anaesthesia was dictated by the intricacies of the specialty itself. In the course of the preceding ten years the new leadership of such men as Hewitt and Dudley Buxton had been increasingly felt. They insisted that it was not sufficient to master the technique of administering one or possibly two anaesthetic agents. Even the general practitioner must be prepared to assess his cases individually, to choose from among the principal agents—ether, chloroform and nitrous oxide, alone or in some combination—the one he considered best suited to the type of operation and the condition of the patient, and be able to administer it with assurance from the apparatus commonly used for the purpose.

Abroad, on the other hand, anaesthetic procedure had recently appeared too crude for the delicate, often protracted, operations undertaken. Surgeons acutely felt the need for highly skilled men to whom the exacting task of keeping a patient satisfactorily anaesthetized throughout, say, an upper abdominal operation, could be entrusted.

In England after 1896 the initiative in anaesthetic development continued to lie with anaesthetists ; on the Continent it remained in the hands of the surgeons. But in America, although the influence of the surgeons still predominated, at the close of the nineteenth century the specialist anaesthetist had already appeared and had come to stay.

Open Ether ; Endotracheal Anaesthesia

One of the first refinements in the technique of inhalation anaesthesia to become apparent in America under the new surgical regime was the use of an open mask for ether. This, the ' open-drop ' method, which had long been familiar in Europe in connection with chloroform, was independently adopted for ether by the Germans at the close of the century.

Marin Théodore Tuffier's researches on chest surgery, begun in 1896, and his use of laryngeal intubation and controlled insufflation, to prevent the ill-effects of pneumothorax while the chest wall was open, led other surgeons—Doyen in France, and, more particularly, Kuhn in Germany, and Rudolph Matas in America—to work upon similar lines. In order to control pneumothorax and at the same time to maintain anaesthesia, these men adopted and modified the Fell-O'Dwyer apparatus for endotracheal anaesthesia already in use in America and on the Continent, during the eighteen-nineties, to enable the throat to be packed off to prevent the aspiration of debris in operations involving the oro-nasal cavity.

A further development in thoracic surgery and anaesthesia adapted to it was the use of Sauerbruch's negative pressure cabinet (1904) within which the surgeon and his assistants operated. This was superseded by Brauer's positive pressure cabinet which enclosed the patient's head and the anaesthetist's hands only. Then, in 1909, Meltzer and Auer of the Rockefeller

Institute devised their method of insufflation anaesthesia. The method was applied clinically by Elsberg in 1910 and this may be taken as the starting point of modern endotracheal anaesthesia.

Non-Inhalation Anaesthesia.

Throughout the half century 1846 to 1896 general anaesthesia produced by making the patient inhale into his lungs a vapour, a gas or a combination of the two, was the method of paramount importance and the only one universally accepted. Because of grave disadvantages found to be associated with it, however, many men both hoped and worked for the discovery of some satisfactory method of anaesthesia which would not directly involve the respiratory tract. Several such methods were tried, but until 1884 none proved entirely feasible.

As early as 1847, Nikolai Ivanovich Pirogoff, the Russian military surgeon, had considerable success with the insufflation of ether vapour into the rectum. The idea was revived by Mollière of Lyons in 1884.

About 1858 a dentist in Philadelphia named Francis, and several dentists in France and England attempted to produce anaesthesia for dental extractions by means of a galvanic current. The method was also tried by Velpeau and others, in minor surgery. It was generally concluded, however, that the electricity did no more than provide a counter-irritant shock to the surgical pain and the matter was dropped.[1]

In 1859 Paul Broca claimed (as Elliotson and Esdaile had done during the eighteen-forties) to have induced a state of hypnosis in his patient sufficiently profound to allow a surgical operation (the opening of an abscess) to be painlessly performed. Broca used Braid's [2] method of hypnosis.[3]

In 1874 Oré, Professor of Physiology at Bordeaux, injected a solution of chloral hydrate into the radial vein of a man suffering from traumatic tetanus and induced sufficiently deep general anaesthesia for the removal of a finger nail. (See footnote, p. 385.)

[1] Cf. Arch. gén. Méd., 1858, ii, 623, 631.
[2] James Braid, who practised medicine in Manchester, hypnotized his patients by causing them to stare fixedly at some bright object (' I generally use my lancet case ', he wrote), held about 8 to 15 inches from the eyes and a little above eye level. In the majority of Braid's cases the aim of his hypnotic treatment was psychothera- peutic, but he claimed to have extracted teeth painlessly from hypnotized patients. (Braid, J. 1843. Neurypnology. London. 27–9, 250–60.)
[3] Bull. Soc. Chirurgie Paris, 1859, 10, 247.

For a time it appeared that the injection of chloral by the intravenous route might become established as a valuable anaesthetic procedure, but when deaths occurred from it the method was hastily dropped and remained in disrepute until 1909 when Burkhardt began to experiment with intravenous chloroform, ether and paraldehyde.

James Arnott of Brighton, in 1848, having noticed that ' there are many operations in which the only source of pain is the incision of the skin and more in which this is the principal source ', overcame this particular type of pain in minor surgery by gradually refrigerating the superficial tissues.[1] This he did by laying on the skin ' a small pig's bladder . . . containing tepid water '. He then dropped into it pounded ice and finally a little salt, ' so as to bring the temperature considerably below freezing point. The water or dissolved ice is occasionally drawn off from the bladder '. After about 15 or 20 minutes, ' when all sensation had ceased ', the operation was performed.[2]

In 1866 Benjamin Ward Richardson devised a spray, worked by a hand bellows, which blew a finely atomized cloud of sulphuric ether on to the patient's skin where it immediately vaporized, and in so doing refrigerated the superficial tissues sufficiently for minor surgery to be done painlessly. This spray achieved considerable popularity in France.[3]

During the course of the next twenty-five years various agents, including Richardson's rhigolene (a petroleum distillate), ethyl bromide and, latterly, ethyl chloride, were used with a spray, chiefly by dentists on the Continent.

In 1884 Carl Koller introduced the use of cocaine as a local anaesthetic, and the reading of his first paper on the subject at an ophthalmological congress in Heidelberg marks the inception of the modern period in anaesthetic practice.

Writing in 1928 Koller himself stated :

' Up to 1884 the only method of local anesthesia known and not very frequently practiced was the Richardson ether spray . . .

[1] The anodyne use of cold was well known during the mediaeval period and afterwards. It is mentioned, for example, by Avicenna (980–1037) (Gruner, O. C. 1930. *A treatise on the canon of . . . Avicenna.* Lond. 320) and by Thomas Bartholin (1616–80). Bartholin stated that Severinus, of Naples, taught him that snow rubbed on or held against the flesh caused sufficient numbness to allow the cauterizing or cutting of the part by the surgeon without the patient feeling pain. (Bartholinus, Th. 1661. *De nivis usu medico.* Copenhagen. 132–3.)
[2] *Lancet*, 1848, ii, 98.
[3] *Retrosp. practical Med.*, 1866, **53**, 369 ; *Un. méd., Paris*, 1866, **30**, 226, 276, 322, 525.

used for operations on subcutaneous abscesses and for similar operations of short duration. At that time I was an intern and house surgeon on the staff of the Allgemeine Krankenhaus in Vienna. . . . The immediate cause for my approaching the question of local anesthesia was the unsuitability of general narcosis for eye operations ; for not only is the cooperation of the patient greatly desirable . . . but the sequelae of general narcosis—vomiting, retching and general restlessness—. . . frequently . . . constitute grave danger to the operated eye. . . .

'Sometime in the summer of 1884 [Sigmund] Freud, who had become interested in the physiologic systemic effects of cocaine, asked me to undertake with him a series of experiments . . . on our muscular strength . . . and the like. . . .

'The fact that cocaine locally applied paralyzed the terminations and probably the fibres of the sensory nerves had been known for twenty-five years before it came to the attention of some one interested and desirous of producing local anesthesia for the performance of operations.

'It is not correct, as was said at the time, that I discovered this important fact by accident, a drop of the solution coming by chance into my eye. . . . When in the course of preparing for the physiologic experiments, I realized that I had in my possession the local anesthetic which I had been previously searching for, I went at once to Sticker's laboratory, made a solution of cocaine and instilled a drop in the eye of a frog, and afterwards of a guinea-pig. I found the cornea and conjunctiva anesthetic. . . . Afterwards I repeated these experiments on myself, some colleagues and many patients.

'I made the first preliminary communication . . . [on] Sept. 15, 1884, at the meeting of the German Ophthalmologic Society of Heidelberg. . . . Later, on October 17, I read a more elaborate paper before the Gesellschaft der Aerzte of Vienna.'[1]

After the reading of Koller's papers cocaine was rapidly adopted as a local anaesthetic. Solutions were instilled into the conjunctiva, painted upon mucous surfaces, sprayed on to the skin or injected subcutaneously, to allow minor surgical procedures to be painlessly performed.

In October of the following year (1885), after preliminary experiments on dogs, J. Leonard Corning, a New York neurologist who had for some time been interested in the local medication of the spinal cord, reported the case of a patient of his, suffering from spinal weakness and seminal incontinence.

[1] *J. Amer. med. Ass.*, 1928, **90**, 1742.

·I was bent upon abolishing reflex action and annulling sensory conduction in the cord,' Corning wrote.

'To this end I injected thirty minims of a three-per-cent. solution of the hydrochlorate of cocaine into the space situated between the spinous processes of the eleventh and twelfth dorsal vertebrae. As there was no numbness, tingling, or other evidence of modified sensibility after the lapse of six or eight minutes, I again injected thirty minims of the solution at the same spot and in the same manner. About ten minutes later the patient complained that his legs " felt sleepy " ; and, on making a careful examination with the wire brush [attached to a faradic battery], I found that sensibility was greatly impaired. Currents which caused lively sensations of pain and reflex contractions in the upper extremities were disregarded and barely perceived in the lower limbs. . . . Fifteen or twenty minutes later the anesthesia had increased in intensity, and, although there were some evidences of diffusion on the part of the anesthetic, the impairment of sensibility was principally limited to the lower extremities. . . . The passage of a sound, though usually accompanied by considerable pain remained almost unperceived. . . .

'Whether the method will ever find an application as a substitute for etherization in genito-urinary or other branches of surgery, further experience alone can show. Be the destiny of this observation what it may, it has seemed to me, on the whole, worth recording.' [1]

Although between 1885 and 1899 a considerable amount of experimental work was carried out, tending to prove the clinical practicability of spinal anaesthesia, it was not until 1899 that August Bier of Kiel, after experimenting upon himself and his assistant, was able to report six operations which he had performed on patients under low spinal anaesthesia. In the same year Tuffier in Paris, and Rudolph Matas of New Orleans, followed Bier's example. By 1900 many surgeons were busy testing the new method, often with a lack of circumspection in their methods against which Bier protested in vain.

The earliest experiments on ' nerve blocking ', also called ' regional anaesthesia ', and in German *Leitungsanästhesie* (' conduction anaesthesia '), by injecting cocaine in solution into the path (or into the fibres) of a sensory nerve trunk in order to produce anaesthesia of the field of its peripheral distribution, were made by William Stewart Halsted, in New York, in the winter of 1884–5. Halsted, according to Rudolph Matas, then performed ' a major operation . . . under regional anaesthesia,

[1] *N.T. med. J.*, 1885, **42**, 483.

2*

. . . in which he had freed the cords and nerves of the brachial plexus by blocking its roots in the neck with cocaine solution '.

So little publicity did he give to this achievement, however, that regional anaesthesia did not come into general use until 1900, when Harvey Cushing ' rediscovered the principle of nerve blocking and applied it successfully in operations on hernia ; he was utterly unaware ', Matas stated on Cushing's own authority, ' that his chief had ever made studies on cocaine of any sort—so reticent was Dr. Halsted about this matter and so little did questions of priority interest him '.[1]

In 1885 Leonard Corning made the discovery that if, when cocaine was injected, the circulation of blood through the injected area was interrupted by a tourniquet, the effect of the cocaine was intensified ; this meant that a reduced and therefore less toxic dose could be given.   Oberst and his pupil Pernice, and others, applied this technique, during the late eighteen-eighties and the eighteen-nineties, to surgery of the fingers and toes.

The only method of local anaesthesia to become firmly established for major surgery before the close of the nineteenth century was ' infiltration anaesthesia ', to which the names of the Frenchman, Paul Reclus, and the German, C. L. Schleich, are attached.   The method consisted in completely infiltrating the tissues with an anaesthetic solution to a suitable depth in the immediate field of operation, by making a series of successive overlapping injections.

When Reclus began his researches, in 1886, he used a 20 per cent. solution of cocaine.   In the course of the next few years he gradually reduced the strength of his solution to 2 per cent. cocaine, then to 1 per cent., and finally, by 1903, to 0·5 per cent.[2]

Schleich, who began his researches about 1891, regularly made use of three solutions, strong, medium and weak, which, besides cocaine, contained sodium chloride and morphine.[3]

At the close of the nineteenth century the majority of German surgeons was still far from adopting Schleich's infiltration anaesthesia ; nevertheless, the method was in regular use in many important hospitals in Germany.   The revived use of ether had not proved an unqualified success, for although it reduced the

[1] *Johns Hopk. Hosp. Bull.*, 1925, **36**, 4.
[2] Reclus, P. 1903. *L'Anesthésie localisée par la cocaine.* Paris. 5.
[3] Schleich, C. L. 1899. *Schmerzlose Operationen.* Berlin. 186.

number of anaesthetic deaths on the table, some surgeons maintained that it caused as many or more post-operatively from chest complications and they also feared that it damaged the kidneys.

With reference to infiltration anaesthesia, Schleich wrote in 1899 :

' My friend Briegleb, at Worms, has rightly pointed out that " if each German surgeon carried out only 10 operations a year using [my] method then (reckoning 20,000 surgeons in Germany), 200,000 general anaesthesias would be avoided ; thus in each year alone—according to the conservative statistics of the Surgical Congresses (1 death in 2000 general anaesthesias)—100 human lives would be saved." ' [1]

The surgeon, Johann von Mikulicz (see footnote, p. 421), after keeping comparative case records over a four-year period (1896–1900), showed that the incidence of post-operative pneumonia following, for example, thyroidectomy and upper and lower abdominal operations, averaged about the same after local as after general anaesthesia. Nevertheless, the opinion held by Schleich and his supporters that local anaesthesia was greatly to be preferred to inhalation anaesthesia, exercised a considerable influence upon contemporary thought. Moreover, pharmacological researches were in progress to discover local anaesthetic drugs less toxic than cocaine and therefore more suitable for general adoption. Of the early substitutes for cocaine the most successful was beta-eucaine, particularly recommended, in 1898, by Heinrich Braun of Leipzig.[2]

Apart from any consideration of the relative advantages and disadvantages of the two types of anaesthesia—inhalation and non-inhalation—the development of local techniques was intrinsically interesting to Continental and also to American surgeons who, hitherto, had been in the unsatisfactory position of bearing the responsibility for the results of inhalation anaesthesia, a method which it was inexpedient for them to apply personally.

The English Attitude towards Anaesthetic Questions

While on the Continent of Europe and in the United States of America attention was thus turned to entirely new methods of

[1] Schleich, C. L. 1899. *Schmerzlose Operationen*. Berlin. 145.
[2] Cf. Dumont, F. L. 1903. *Handbuch der allgemeinen und lokalen Anaesthesie*. Berlin and Vienna. 182, 183, 221–34.

anaesthesia, the English were once more reviewing the pros and cons of chloroform anaesthesia. Interest in the subject had been mildly rekindled during the eighteen-eighties, by the suggestion (independently made by several physiologists, in Great Britain and in France) that chloroform syncope was due to cardiac inhibition caused by the drug stimulating the vagal nerves and could be avoided simply by paralyzing them with a preliminary dose of atropine.

Hard upon the physiological researches arising out of this suggestion came the dogmatic criticism of English methods of chloroform anaesthesia made, in 1888, by Edward Lawrie, Residency Surgeon at Hyderabad. Lawrie's assertion that the Scottish disregard for the behaviour of the heart and concentration upon the behaviour of the respiration during chloroform anaesthesia was an infallibly safe procedure, caused a storm which raged with considerable fury for several years. The experiments carried out by the members of the Second Chloroform Commission called together in Hyderabad in 1889, at the Nizam's request, appeared to confirm Lawrie's original contention. Despite the fact that Thomas Lauder Brunton, who had been sent to Hyderabad by the *Lancet* to represent the English point of view, concurred in the Commission's findings, English anaesthetists were not satisfied and independent researches were undertaken in this country.

These, particularly the cross-circulation experiments devised by Gaskell and Shore, showed the Hyderabad Commission to have erred in concluding that chloroform always affected respiration before affecting the heart's action. Nevertheless further researches, upon the trend of which Paul Bert's recommendation of a 2 per cent. chloroform-air mixture (see pp. 446–50) had a considerable influence, convinced the English that very low percentages of chloroform—lower than those advocated by Snow (see p. 188) and by Clover (see p. 242)—could be administered with safety.[1]

In addition to researches on chloroform initiated in the laboratory, the Hyderabad controversy indirectly occasioned a general survey of clinical practice, carried out by means of a questionnaire addressed to 'anaesthetists throughout the king-

---

[1] In 1911, however, A. Goodman Levy put forward the suggestion that most deaths from chloroform, far from being due to overdosage, were caused by ventricular fibrillations occurring in lightly anaesthetized patients (see pp. 452–6).

dom '. This survey was undertaken by a special committee appointed by the British Medical Association in 1891.

By 1893 all the returns had been received, but although interim reports were issued the committee's analysis of the data was not published until 1901. Anaesthetists by this time had accepted and begun to put into practice the recent suggestion made by the physiologists that very low percentages of chloroform might safely be employed. The committee's report, therefore, which to be commensurate with the time and energy expended upon it should have been an important one, in fact dealt with methods already superseded.

By comparison with the newly found vitality of anaesthetic practice abroad, English practice, which for half a century had been the most highly developed and progressive in the world, at the opening of the new century appeared in grave danger of stagnating, and among certain members of the medical profession a feeling of frustration in regard to anaesthetic matters was becoming evident. This feeling is reflected in an editorial commentary upon the report of the British Medical Association's Anaesthetics Committee, which appeared in the *Journal* in March 1901 :

'It must be admitted that the practical administration of anaesthetics still remains before the profession as a problem inadequately met. Its data remain still insufficiently determined. Mr. George Eastes, in his address to the Society of Anaesthetists, published in our columns on February 23rd, gave an excellent summary of the painstaking latest report from the Anaesthetics Committee. It is to be feared that, despite the labour and judicial caution largely evident in the report, most practical men will rise from the perusal of Mr. Eastes's address with a feeling of disappointment. . . . The inquiry as its fruit yields little, if indeed any, advance in knowledge on a subject about which the profession is keenly anxious to know more. The finding that chloroform is on the whole more dangerous than the other anaesthetic drugs in ordinary use is no doubt important, but merely endorses what is well-known to the profession. As its final and single " general conclusion ", the Committee finds " that by far the most important factor in the safe administration of anaesthetics is the experience which has been acquired by the administrator ". What the elements are on which experience founds the judgment which has skill to guide it the report does not seem to be able definitely to state. . . . For years past the profession in general has been acutely aware that, for surgical anaesthesia, it is advantageous to have an administrator of such large experience as to make him more or less a specialist. But it had hoped that cumulative experience of that kind could be of a scientific nature, and impart definite rules of guidance helpful to and applicable by all. . . . The annual death-roll from surgical anaesthesia is an increasing one. The number of deaths registered as due to anaesthetics in England and Wales is now more than double what it amounted to ten years ago. . . .

'The art of anaesthesia is, it must be confessed, still in the stage of almost pure empiricism. In that stage the secret of skill is always, from want of radical knowledge, hard to impart or transmit, for its true basis is generally not rightly guessed even by its own possessor. But in a matter so important as surgical anaesthesia the profession cannot rest until it obtains definite knowledge, quantitative and scientific, chemical " measures " rather than personal " impressions ", intelligible to and accessible to every member of the profession. For the conduct of deep anaesthesia may at any time fall to the lot of—thrust itself as an imperative duty upon—any member of the profession wherever the surgeon has to work. . . .' [1]

Although in the opening year of the twentieth century, the impartial observer could perceive a decline of inspiration in the development of inhalation anaesthesia in England, the specialist anaesthetist appeared unaware of any such deterioration. Nor did he seem able fully to appreciate the significance of the development of non-inhalation anaesthesia taking place abroad. Tuffier's use of spinal anaesthesia, for example, was described in a special article, ' from a correspondent', in the *Lancet*, January 12, 1901 ; in the course of the article the writer commented :

' To judge by the most recent *résumé* of the subject in [*La Presse médicale*, November 7, 1900] one would almost think that the final cry of " Eureka " had been raised and that a general anaesthetic had been found to largely replace chloroform and ether, free from both their dangers and their inconveniences. Here and there, however, a few warning voices have been raised, and it is interesting to note that England, with her characteristic conservative caution, is lagging behind the general movement.' [2]

In the previous year the *Lancet*, in a leader on Schleich's infiltration anaesthesia, had expressed the opinion :

' It must be conceded that, valuable as the method is, it should be used as an adjuvant to, rather than as a supplanter of, general anaesthetics.' [3]

[1] *Brit. med. J.*, 1901, i, 655.   [2] *Lancet*, 1901, i, 137.   [3] *Ibid.* 1900, ii, 271 .

A further example of the continued preoccupation with inhalation anaesthesia shown by the English specialist anaesthetist despite fundamental changes in practice taking place even in England, is furnished by the *Transactions* of the Society of Anaesthetists.[1] From these it appears that up to 1901, and indeed long after, the subject of non-inhalation methods had never been broached at a meeting of the Society, although Schleich's ' mixtures ' for inhalation anaesthesia had been freely discussed (see p. 523).

In 1899, however, Arthur E. Barker, Professor of the Principles and Practice of Surgery at University College, London, and Surgeon to University College Hospital, had given a clinical lecture, in which he said :

' For the last eight or nine months I have occasionally been operating on patients for various surgical conditions without using either chloroform or ether, trusting rather to one or other form of " local infiltration analgesia ". . . . During all this period I have been endeavouring to make myself familiar with the whole subject of infiltration analgesia by every means in my power. Having seen the method employed abroad where it is largely used and having been much impressed by it, it was only rational to get hold of the best and most recent of the now very numerous monographs on the subject and to study them carefully both as regards the physiological and physical theories advanced and the details of the practical application of the latter advocated in them.'

During 1899 Barker performed 53 operations under infiltration anaesthesia, including 15 for the radical cure of hernia, a gastroenterostomy, an exploration for carcinoma of the gall-bladder and 4 cases of ' goitre '.

' Of course ', wrote Barker, ' the 53 cases . . . form but a small group in proportion to the number of operations done in the course of the year in which I have used general anaesthesia, but as far as they go they are fairly representative.' [2]

So far as the average surgeon and the occasional anaesthetist were concerned, at the opening of the twentieth century local anaesthesia for minor surgery, produced by spraying a volatile agent on to the skin or mucous membrane, and by spraying, painting or subcutaneously injecting cocaine, was a long-

[1] Cf. *e.g.* p. 49 and footnote.
[2] *Lancet*, 1899, i, 282 ; *ibid.* 1900, i, 156.

established procedure. That considerable interest had been aroused among such medical men by reports of Schleich's infiltration anaesthesia and the synthesis of drugs less toxic than cocaine (particularly beta-eucaine) is shown by the very frequent appearance in the journals of requests for guidance in applying the latest methods.[1]

During the first half of the year 1901 a correspondence indicative of the difference in attitude between the surgeon and the specialist anaesthetist was conducted in the *Lancet*, on ' local *versus* general anaesthesia in abdominal surgery '. The correspondence was started by Thomas H. Morse, consulting surgeon to the Cromer Hospital.

Morse reported five cases in which badly shocked patients had had the abdomen successfully opened and closed under superficial local anaesthesia (produced by the ether spray, the ethyl chloride spray and by the injection of eucaine). In a sixth case the patient, suffering from intestinal obstruction, died under general anaesthesia (ether) from inhaling faecal vomitus.

Sydney H. Long, of Norwich, and Joseph Blumfeld wrote to the *Lancet*, pointing out that all six operations could have been performed with perfect safety under general anaesthesia and that shock should not be considered a contraindication to the use of general anaesthesia. Both men refused to be drawn into any discussion of the fact that Morse had used local anaesthesia successfully in his five cases.

' In the abdominal operations which I have seen performed under local anaesthetics ', wrote Blumfeld, ' though no pain was felt the reflex effects of manipulation of abdominal contents were enough to impede the surgeon and distress the patient, and shock was certainly no less than it would have been under general anaesthetics properly administered.'

This provoked a letter from S. Johnson Taylor, of Norwich, who wrote :

' In spite of the strictures of Dr. S. H. Long and Dr. J. Blumfeld, I think Mr. T. J. Morse has done well to draw attention to a subject which as yet has not received sufficient attention at the hands of the profession and is, in fact, practically in its infancy.

' Possibly, if every medical man called upon to assist a surgeon

[1] See *e.g. Brit. med. J.*, 1899, ii, 1524 ; *ibid.* 1901, i, 999, 1455.

in the performance of a critical and urgent operation were as able an anaesthetist as Dr. Long or Dr. Blumfeld, the subject of local anaesthesia might not be worth further consideration. These gentlemen naturally consider the subject mainly from their own special point of view. . . . I am quite aware that Mr. Morse is only one pioneer in this direction, but his efforts deserve encouragement rather than the strictures they have met with at the hands of his critics, who mainly discuss his opening statements on the causation of shock after operations . . . but, shock or no shock, local anaesthesia appears to me to have come to stay. Mr. A. E. Barker was, I believe, one of the very first to use this method. We may look forward, I trust, to hearing the results of his extended experience of the subject ere long.' [1]

Not only was the specialist anaesthetist taking no part in the development of non-inhalation anaesthesia at the beginning of the present century, but so steeped in tradition was he that he was still debating the question, ' Is chloroform more dangerous than ether ? ' [2] apparently with as little hope as ever of reaching any final conclusion.

From the specialist anaesthetist's point of view, however, it no doubt seemed unnecessary to try to acquire proficiency in methods of local anaesthesia which already called for a far more expert knowledge of anatomy than he was likely to be able to command without considerable study. He may well have believed, with more than fifty years' cumulative experience of inhalation anaesthesia to draw upon, that he had so thoroughly mastered this particular art that he could confidently expect in every case to produce results not merely equally satisfactory but often more satisfactory than could ever be achieved by any non-inhalation method.

In the chapters which follow an attempt has been made to analyse in detail the various phases through which the evolution of inhalation anaesthesia passed from its origin to the close of the nineteenth century.

It so happened that the opening of the twentieth century coincided with the beginning of a new phase in the history of anaesthesia. In this phase, beyond which anaesthesia has not yet passed, Continental surgeons and the surgeons and anaesthetists of the United States of America readily accepted and rapidly developed spinal anaesthesia and new methods of local

[1] *Lancet*, 1901, i, 1322, 1493, 1569, 1627, 1712, 1791.
[2] See *Trans. Soc. Anaesth.*, 1903, **5,** 36.

anaesthesia. Some of these methods, since 1901, have been cautiously adopted by British surgeons ; but the British anaesthetist has shown, and indeed still shows, a certain reluctance to admit any permanent rival to the supremacy of inhalation anaesthesia—the method in which he has always excelled.

Note on Sources

In the preparation of this chapter I am indebted generally to the following works for the social and economic background : Sir G. M. Trevelyan, *History of England* ; H. A. L. Fisher, *A history of Europe* ; *The Cambridge modern history*, vol. vi, ' The eighteenth century ', vol. vii, ' The United States ', vol. xi, ' The growth of nations ', vol. xii, ' The latest age '. For the general medical background I have used Charles Singer, *A short history of medicine*, and Fielding H. Garrison, *An introduction to the history of medicine* (4th edition).

PART ONE

THE PREPARATORY PERIOD

CHAPTER I

RESPIRATION AND PNEUMATICS

Development of the Study of Physiology and Pneumatic Chemistry during the Seventeenth and Eighteenth Centuries—Pneumatic Medicine—Davy's Researches on Nitrous Oxide—The Inhalation of Nitrous Oxide and of Ether Vapour as a form of Entertainment.

Development of the Study of Physiology and Pneumatic Chemistry during the Seventeenth and Eighteenth Centuries

SURGICAL anaesthesia produced by inhaling a gas or the vapour of a volatile drug was made possible through the knowledge accumulated by a succession of distinguished scientists who, during the seventeenth and eighteenth centuries, combined the study of pneumatic chemistry with that of the physiology of respiration.

The history of the interrelation of these two subjects during this period has been fully dealt with by Professor J. R. Partington, Professor Charles Singer, Sir Michael Foster, and others, and for detailed studies of the work of particular men there are the papers of Dr. T. S. Patterson on John Mayow ; [1] of Sir Philip Hartog on Priestley and Lavoisier,[2] and the latter's contribution on ' Priestley's scientific work ', in the *Dictionary of national biography* ; Dr. E. Ashworth Underwood's paper on ' Lavoisier and the history of respiration ' (referred to in detail later) ; and Dr. Douglas McKie's book on Lavoisier.

The unrelated although nearly contemporaneous observations of the Belgian, Jean Baptiste van Helmont (1577–1644), and the Englishman, William Harvey (1578–1657), were largely responsible for kindling interest in these two fields of research, the more so, perhaps, because these particular observations—

---

[1] *Isis*, 1931, **15**, 47–96, 504–43.　　　　[2] *Ann. Sci.*, 1941, **5**, 1–56.

van Helmont's upon gases and Harvey's upon the state of blood in the lungs—ended abruptly in speculation.

Van Helmont first recognized a class of gaseous substances distinct from atmospheric air and attempted, with indifferent success, to collect and classify specimens.[1] Harvey, in the course of his work upon the circulation,[2] drew attention to the fact that the dark venous blood is sent through the lungs, and while there becomes more intensely florid in colour than it was in the arteries themselves. This, Harvey thought, was due to the blood being strained through the pulmonary tissue, but he would not make any definite statement as to the function of the lungs in relation to the circulation—whether or not, for instance, their principal function was to draw in air to cool the blood—maintaining that to do so would be to wander too wide of his immediate purpose, which was to describe the use and motion of the heart and blood.[3]

In 1667 Robert Hooke (1635–1703) repeated, before a meeting of the Royal Society, the Vesalian experiment of widely opening the thorax of a dog and keeping the animal alive by pumping air into the lungs with bellows attached to the end of the trachea severed just below the epiglottis.

Hooke further demonstrated that even when the lungs were immobilized by making punctures all over their surface with a sharp pen-knife, so long as insufflation was continuous the heart beat regularly and the blood circulated. From this Hooke concluded that the importance of the respiratory process must lie not in the intrinsic motion of the lungs (then generally supposed necessary to promote the circulation of the blood) but in the adequate supply of fresh air to the lung tissue.[4]

Richard Lower (1631–91), in repeating Hooke's experiment, made the further deduction that the change in the colour of venous blood, injected into the insufflated lungs, from dark to bright red, must be due to the absorption of air.[5]

In 1672 Robert Boyle (1627–91) published an account of experiments in which he showed that if a small bird and a lighted

[1] Cf. Helmont, J. B. van. 1682. *Opera omnia.* Frankfurt. 102 *et seq.*
[2] Harvey, W. 1628. *Exercitatio anatomica de motu cordis et sanguinis in animalibus.* Frankfurt.
[3] Harvey, W. 1847. *The works of William Harvey,* translated by Robert Willis. (Sydenham Society.) London. 39–40 ; 114–15.
[4] *Philos. Trans.*, 1667, **2**, 539–40.
[5] Lower, R. 1669. *Tractatus de Corde.* London. 168–70. (Translated by K. J. Franklin. 1932. *Early science in Oxford.* Oxford. **9**, 168–70.)

taper were confined together in a vessel from which the air was then pumped out, both the ' common flame ' of the taper and the ' vital flame ' of the bird became extinct, although the bird outlived the flame. ' Whether ', Boyle commented, '. . . this survival proceed from this, that the common flame and the vital flame are maintained by distinct substances or parts of the air ; or, that common flame making a great waste of the aërial substance they both need to keep them alive, cannot so easily as the other find matter to prey upon, and so expires, whilst there yet remains enough to keep alive the more temperate vital flame ; or, that both these causes, and perhaps some other, concur to the phaenomenon, I leave to be considered '.[1]

It has been suggested that an answer to Boyle's speculation is to be found in the works of John Mayow (1643–79), and that this enthusiastic young chemist had both conceived the idea that a particular gaseous portion of the air enters into respiration and combustion and had demonstrated the fact by experiments which he described in his *Tractatus quinque medico-physici* (Oxford, 1674). Patterson, however, has marshalled a great deal of carefully sifted evidence to show that Mayow was not in fact clearly aware of the existence of a particular gaseous constituent of air essential to both respiration and combustion, and that such sound ideas as he entertained in this connexion he derived in great part from the researches of his contemporaries, in particular Boyle, Hooke,[2] and Lower.

That progress in elucidating the true nature of the processes of respiration and combustion should temporarily have ceased during the last quarter of the seventeenth century was no doubt due in some measure to the fact that the plausible but erroneous *phlogiston theory* evolved by Joachim Becher (1632–82), and elaborated by his pupil Georg Ernst Stahl (1660–1734), was beginning to monopolize the attention of physiologists and chemists. The theory postulated the existence of a mysterious element, ' the material of fire ', called by Stahl *phlogiston*, and this was believed to be an essential constituent of all combustible bodies and to take part in respiration. The fact that both life and combustion

[1] Boyle, R. 1772. *The works of the Honourable Robert Boyle.* London. **3,** 586.
[2] For example, in referring to the part which he supposed air to play in the processes of respiration and combustion, Mayow used the term *nitro-aërial particles.* The identity of an active principle occurring in both nitre and air had been postulated by Robert Hooke in 1665. (Hooke, R. 1665. *Micrographia.* London. 103 ; *see also* R. T. Gunther's edition, 1938, *Early science in Oxford.* Oxford. **13,** 103.)

eventually became extinct in a confined space was held to be due to the air becoming completely saturated with phlogiston. To account for the gain in weight [1] of calcined metals (from which phlogiston was supposed to be liberated) it was found necessary to attribute negative weight to phlogiston.

In August 1774, Joseph Priestley, who was then a believer in the phlogiston theory, liberated the gas to which Lavoisier afterwards gave the name oxygen.[2] At the time, and indeed until March of the following year, Priestley was very much perplexed as to the nature of this ' air ' which he had obtained by focussing a burning-lens on to a sample of ' *mercurius calcinatus per se* ' (mercuric oxide) enclosed in a glass vessel inverted over mercury.

' By means of this lens ', wrote Priestley, ' air [oxygen] was expelled from it [the mercuric oxide] very readily. Having got about three or four times as much as the bulk of my materials, I admitted water to it, and found that it was not imbibed by it. But what surprized me more than I can well express, was, that a candle burned in this air with a remarkably vigorous flame, very much like that enlarged flame with which a candle burns in nitrous air [3], exposed to iron or liver of sulphur ; but as I . . . knew no nitrous acid was used in the preparation of *mercurius calcinatus*, I was utterly at a loss how to account for it.' [4]

At first Priestley suspected the purity of his sample of mercuric oxide ' but ', he said, ' being at Paris in the October following, and knowing that there were several very eminent chymists in that place, I did not omit the opportunity . . . to get an ounce of *mercurius calcinatus* prepared . . . of the genuineness of which there could not possibly be any suspicion ; and, at the same time, I frequently mentioned my surprize at the kind of air which I had got from this preparation to Mr. Lavoisier, Mr. le Roy, and several other philosophers, who honoured me with their notice in that city. . . .

' At the same time that I had got the air above mentioned

---

[1] The gain in weight of calcined metals had been demonstrated by Jean Rey in 1630.

[2] Hartog draws attention to Priestley's subsequent statement that he had, ' before the month of November 1771 ', liberated this gas from saltpetre without recognizing the fact. (*Nature*, 1933, **132**, 25–6.)

[3] Nitric oxide, first liberated by Priestley in 1772, and from which he obtained nitrous oxide. (Priestley, J. 1774. *Experiments and observations on different kinds of air*. London. **1**, 108–28.)

[4] *Ibid.* 1775. **2**, 34.

from *mercurius calcinatus* and the red precipitate, I had got the same kind from *red lead* or *minium*. . . .

' This experiment with *red lead* confirmed me more in my suspicion that the *mercurius calcinatus* must get the property of yielding this kind of air from the atmosphere, the process by which that preparation and this of red lead is made, being similar.' [1]

During November 1774, Priestley made further tests with his new ' air ' and came to the conclusion that it certainly was not nitrous oxide, as in August he had supposed it might be. Nevertheless it was not until March 1, 1775, that Priestley was led to investigate its respirability. This he did by first applying his usual test for the ' goodness ' of common air—he added two measures of his new ' air ' to one of nitric oxide and noted the reduction in volume. ' I found ', he said, ' not only that it was diminished, but that it was diminished quite as much as common air.' [2] Hartog emphasizes that Priestley himself regarded March 1, 1775 (not August 1774), ' as the date on which he discovered the gas which we now call oxygen '.[3]

During the second week of March, Priestley discovered not only that a mouse would live longer in the new ' air ' than in an equal volume of common air, but that on applying the nitric oxide test to the residual air which the mouse had breathed, there was ' a diminution of 2/9 in a short time, whereas in a long time common air was never reduced more than 1/5 of its bulk '.[4] These observations led Priestley to conclude that this air was *better* than common air. He concluded that this superiority lay in a greater capacity for absorbing phlogiston, and he reasoned that the gas originally contained less phlogiston than common air. Accordingly he named it *dephlogisticated air*.[5] A letter from Priestley about dephlogisticated air was read to the Royal Society on March 23, 1775.

His preoccupation with phlogiston led Priestley badly astray in attempting to assess the part played by dephlogisticated air in respiration.[6]

In September 1772, Antoine Lavoisier carried out an experi-

[1] Priestley, J. 1775. *Experiments and observations on different kinds of air.* London. **2**, 36–8.
[2] *Ibid.* **2**, 41.   [3] *Ann. Sci.*, 1941, **5**, 30.
[4] McKie, D. 1935. *Antoine Lavoisier.* London. 169.
[5] Priestley, J. 1775. *Experiments and observations on different kinds of air.* London. **2**, 40–9.   [6] *Ibid.* **2**, 70–84.

ment on the combustion of phosphorus, and this was the starting-point from which 'slowly and with great difficulty . . . he arrived at a clear idea of the composition of air'.[1] He was already working on the hypothesis that when phosphorus and sulphur burn their gain in weight is due to their combination with atmospheric air. Moreover an entry in his laboratory note-book for the first part of the year 1773 shows that Lavoisier was aware that his researches on combustion must be complemented by a study of the respiratory process.[2] The subsequent researches of Lavoisier, considered particularly from the physiologist's point of view, have been carefully investigated by Dr. E. Ashworth Underwood,[3] and it is to his work in particular (and to Dr. McKie's book on Lavoisier) that I am indebted for the following account. Lavoisier's various papers will be found in the *Mémoires de l'Académie Royale des Sciences* and in the *Œuvres* (Paris, 1864–93).

In a report on further experiments on the combustion of phosphorus, carried out during 1773, Lavoisier stated that ' either air itself, or another elastic fluid contained, in a certain propor-tion, in the air which we breathe ' combines with the phosphorus. But as yet he had formed no clear idea of the identity of this elastic fluid.

When in the autumn of 1774 Lavoisier learned from Priestley of the latter's new ' air ', he realized that therein lay the key to the problem of combustion and of respiration. After repeating Priestley's experiments Lavoisier, in April 1775, read a memoir to the Académie des Sciences, ' On the nature of the principle which combines with metals during calcination, and which in-creases their weight.' McKie considers, however, that Lavoisier still did not recognize this principle as being a distinct constituent of air. But in 1777, no doubt having revised his views in the light of Priestley's later researches on the respirability of dephlogisti-cated air, Lavoisier was able to show that if to the *mofette* or vitiated air remaining after the complete combustion of phos-phorus, the correct amount of dephlogisticated air was added (and Lavoisier found this amount to be constant) then the residual air again became respirable and capable of supporting combustion. Common air he now knew to consist of two elastic fluids, one (the smaller portion) necessary for respiration and

[1] McKie, D. 1935. *Antoine Lavoisier.* London. 93.
[2] Meldrum, A. N. 1932. *Archeion,* **14,** 14–30.
[3] *Proc. R. Soc. Med.,* 1943–4, **37,** 246–62.

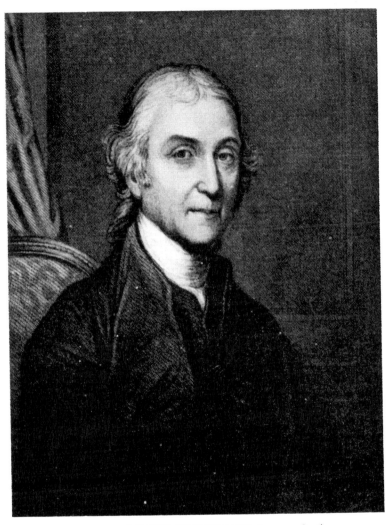

FIG. 2.—JOSEPH PRIESTLEY (1733–1804)

Theologian and scientist. He liberated oxygen in 1771 and again in August 1774, but it was not until March 1775 that he identified the gas under the name of *dephlogisticated air*. He first made nitrous oxide in 1772.

combustion, the other non-respirable and incapable of supporting combustion.

This new conception was elaborated in a revised version of the memoir of April 1775, on calcination, which was once more read to the Académie in 1778. What in 1775 had been referred to merely as the ' purest part of the air ' which combines with metals during calcination, had now become ' the most salubrious part of the air '—' none other than the purest part of the air itself which surrounds us, which we breathe '. Furthermore Lavoisier recognized ' fixed air '[1] as a compound of charcoal and ' eminently respirable air '. It is, then, from these two years, 1777 and 1778, that the modern theory of combustion and of calcination dates.

During the autumn of 1776, Lavoisier had been making experiments on the respiration of birds in dephlogisticated air. In 1777 he completed and read a memoir on ' Experiments on the respiration of animals ', in which he generously acknowledged Priestley's work but disagreed with his conclusions about respiration.

He himself noted that exhaled air precipitated lime water (which the air remaining after calcination did not), and he demonstrated that about one-sixth of the volume of respired air consists of chalky-acid air (Lavoisier's new name for carbon dioxide). To re-create common air from exhaled air not only had the correct amount of ' eminently respirable air ' to be added (as after calcination), but carbon dioxide had also to be removed.

In view of these findings Lavoisier advanced alternative explanations of the respiratory process : either eminently respirable air is changed in the lungs to chalky-acid air, or an exchange takes place, the eminently respirable air being absorbed, and another almost equal volume of chalky-acid air being given up to the residual air from the lungs. Underwood thinks that ' while Lavoisier obviously favoured the change of eminently respirable air into chalky-acid gas, he had to admit that there were strong grounds for believing that eminently respirable air did combine with the blood to produce the red colour '. Underwood emphasizes the point that Lavoisier's further progress was considerably retarded by the fact that he failed to appreciate that it was not necessary that the chalky-acid which left the lung

[1] Carbon dioxide had been identified under the name ' fixed air ', by Joseph Black, in 1757.

during one expiration should have been derived from the eminently respirable air which entered the lung *during the inspiration
immediately preceding.*[1]

In another memoir on combustion in general, written in 1777,
Lavoisier drew an analogy between the 'decomposition' of
eminently respirable air passing through the lungs and the combustion of charcoal ; and he attributed the body temperature to
heat liberated in the former process.

Although Lavoisier considered respiration to be a process
analogous to slow combustion, taking place in the lung, he was
puzzled as to exactly what was reacting with the eminently
respirable air and so liberating heat.

Lavoisier continued to ponder this problem, and meanwhile
he had begun but not completed a series of experiments on
specific heat. In the winter of 1782–3 Lavoisier, with the collaboration of the mathematician P. S. Laplace, continued these
researches and in the course of them made a number of quantitative experiments on respiration, using guinea-pigs in a confined
atmosphere. These experiments went far towards providing
Lavoisier with a complete answer to his problem. The experiments showed, Lavoisier and Laplace concluded, that the
changing of oxygen into carbonic acid [2] 'is the *only* effect of respiration on air'. They further stated that it was to this process
that animal heat was due. In giving what is very nearly an accurate explanation of the facts Lavoisier and Laplace were chiefly
led astray by Lavoisier's belief that caloric, 'the matter of fire',
was an element : ' Respiration is then a combustion, admittedly
very slow, but nevertheless completely analogous to that of
charcoal ; it takes place in the interior of the lungs, without
liberation of perceptible light, because this matter of fire is no
sooner liberated than it is absorbed by the humidity of these
organs. The heat which is produced in this combustion is transmitted to the blood which passes through the lungs and from
thence it courses through the whole animal system.'

Lavoisier continued working on these lines, and in 1785 he
made an important amendment to his previous theory that
respiration consisted wholly in the interaction of carbon and
oxygen. New quantitative experiments had shown him that the

[1] *Proc. R. Soc. Med.*, 1943–4, **37**, 255.
[2] The names *oxygen* (and the synonym 'vital air') and *carbonic acid* were first used
by Lavoisier in 1781.

whole of the oxygen entering the lung was not converted in the formation of carbonic acid ; a part combined with hydrogen to form water.[1] Lavoisier also recorded that air which can be breathed easily must consist of a mixture of about 25 parts of vital air to 75 of azote (nitrogen).

Lavoisier's greatest contribution to the study of respiration, made with the collaboration of his young assistant, Armand Seguin, was contained in a memoir read in 1789. By experiments carried out partly on guinea-pigs confined with vessels of caustic alkali to absorb carbon dioxide, partly upon Seguin himself, Lavoisier showed that while respiration is the same in any concentration of oxygen, provided carbon dioxide is removed, the amount of oxygen absorbed depends upon three factors, temperature, food, and work. In all circumstances the temperature of the blood remains approximately constant. The average oxygen consumption for a man, Lavoisier gave as 3·40 litres per hour, and he also gave provisional figures for the carbonic acid liberated and the amount of carbon and hydrogen taken from the blood.

The latest extant records of Lavoisier's researches on respiration (he was guillotined in 1794), are contained in two memoirs on transpiration, and these were read in 1790 and 1792. Lavoisier attempted to solve the problem of the disposal of the water generated during respiration through the pores of the body, by investigating loss of weight. The experiments were made upon Seguin, who was equipped with a special, close-fitting suit of impermeable material, from inside which samples of air were withdrawn and analysed.

Pneumatic Medicine

An outcome of the researches of Priestley and Lavoisier on the chemistry and physiology of respiration, and one which had an important influence in preparing the way for inhalation anaesthesia was the empirical method of therapeutics adopted towards the close of the eighteenth century under the name ' pneumatic medicine '. During the last ten or so years of the century, a few medical men, emboldened by their newly acquired, although still scanty, knowledge of the function of the lungs and the parts played by oxygen and carbon dioxide in the respiratory process, attempted to treat certain bodily ailments,

---

[1] Henry Cavendish had demonstrated the composition of water in 1783.

and even abnormal states of mind, by causing their patients to inhale certain of the newly identified gases in small quantities.

Priestley himself seems to have been the principal founder of this method, and as early as 1772, before oxygen was discovered or the process of respiration properly understood, he suggested ' fixed air ' (carbon dioxide) as an inhalant.

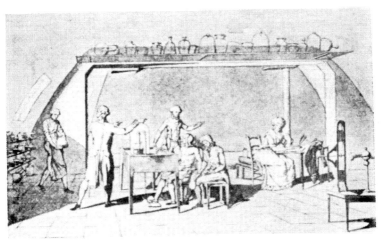

Fig. 3.—ANTOINE LAURENT LAVOISIER (1742-94)

in his laboratory. He is said to be directing an experiment on the respiratory exchange during muscular exertion. The subject sits with the inhaling tube in his mouth and appears to be working some kind of mechanism with his right foot. His pulse rate is being taken by an assistant. Madame Lavoisier makes notes. (From a drawing by Mme. Lavoisier.)

Priestley had made a special study of this gas—indeed his interest in chemistry is said to have dated from the time when he lived next door to a brewery and amused himself by collecting and examining samples of carbon dioxide—and he was fully in agreement with a theory current in his day, that carbon dioxide was capable of checking putrefaction :

' Sir John Pringle [1] first observed, that putrefaction was checked by fermentation, and Dr. Macbride discovered that this effect was produced by the fixed air which is generated in that process.' [2]

---

[1] Sir John Pringle, P.R.S. (1707-82), military surgeon.
[2] Priestley, J. 1772. *Directions for impregnating water with fixed air.* London. 2.

In addition to recommending that sufferers from ' diseases
. . . of a putrid nature ' should drink water artificially aerated
with carbon dioxide, Priestley suggested introducing carbon
dioxide into the body ' in the form of clysters ', a single trial of
such a procedure having proved ' perfectly easy and safe '.

Priestley further suggested introducing the gas into the lungs :

' Being satisfied that fixed air is not noxious *per se* . . . I
hinted to some physicians of eminence among my acquaintance,
that it may possibly be of use in the case of *ulcerated lungs*, if
persons in that most deplorable situation would breathe as much
as they found they could do of it, by holding their heads over
vessels containing fermenting mixtures. . . . Those gentlemen
were pleased to think favourably of the proposal, and I am
informed by Dr. Percival that the same ideas had occurred to
other persons, and that in three cases in which the breathing of
fixed air had been tried, it appeared to have been of great service.
One patient intirely recovered. The method in which it was
applied was putting chalk into oil of vitriol diluted with water,
and breathing the fumes as they issued from the orifice of a
funnel, which covered the vessel that contained the mixture. . . .

' Being no physician, I run no risque by throwing out these
random hints and conjectures. . . . My friend Dr. Percival has
for some time past been employed in making experiments on
fixed air, and he is particularly attentive to the medicinal uses
of it. . . .' [1]

In 1775 Priestley inhaled oxygen, though not yet with any
therapeutic end in view.

' My reader will not wonder, that, after having ascertained
the superior goodness of dephlogisticated air [oxygen] by mice
living in it . . . I should have the curiosity to taste it myself.
I have gratified that curiosity by breathing it, drawing it through
a glass-syphon, and, by this means, I reduced a large jar full of
it to the standard of common air. The feeling of it to my lungs
was not sensibly different from that of common air ; but I
fancied that my breast felt peculiarly light and easy for some time
afterwards. Who can tell but that, in time, this pure air may
become a fashionable article in luxury. Hitherto only two mice
and myself have had the privilege of breathing it.' [2]

After Lavoisier had made clear the nature of oxygen and had
defined its function in the respiratory process, the therapeutic

[1] Priestley, J. 1772. *Directions for impregnating water with fixed air*. London. 18–21.
[2] Priestley, J. 1775. *Experiments and observations on different kinds of air*. London.
2, 102.

inhalation of it began to be extensively practised on the Continent as well as in England.

Abroad it was particularly applied as a resuscitative. Macquer is said to have proposed its use in cases of asphyxia from noxious gases, in 1778 ; Chaussier applied it in phthisical dyspnoea (1780) and in asphyxia of the new born, devising a laryngeal tube for its administration.[1]

In England the first headquarters of pneumatic medicine was Birmingham, among that brilliant circle of which Priestley, James Watt, Josiah Wedgwood, Richard Pearson, and by ties of friendship, Thomas Beddoes, were members.

Richard Pearson was reputed to be the original advocate for the inhalation of the vapour of sulphuric ether, although the use of ether drops given by mouth, in wine or on a lump of sugar, as a palliative and expectorant, particularly in chest complaints where much thick, purulent, phlegm was present and coughing was unproductive, was old-established. Such a use had, indeed, been suggested about 1540, by Valerius Cordus (1515–44) who first gave a clearly recognizable description of sulphuric ether and its preparation, calling it *sweet oil of vitriol*.[2]

The name ' Aether ' was applied to this liquid by August Siegmund Frobenius, F.R.S., in 1730.[3]

A report of Pearson's activities appeared in 1796 in the first volume of a new medical periodical, the *Annals of Medicine* : [4]

' Dr. Pearson, of Birmingham, has transmitted to many of his friends the following circular letter, dated July 1, 1796, respecting a particular practice in phthisis pulmonalis, which he thinks, he has employed with great benefit.' The letter ran as follows :

' Having, for the last two years, prescribed the vapour of vitriolic (sulphuric) aether to patients labouring under phthisis pulmonalis, and having, both in hospital and private practice, experienced the best effects from its use . . . I am preparing a report of the cases. . . .

' My method of using this application . . . is simply this : I direct the patient to pour one or two teaspoonsful of pure vitriolic aether or of aether impregnated with cicuta [*i.e.* ether

[1] See Hahn, L. 1899. 'L'oxygène et son emploi médical.' *Janus*, **4**, 6.
[2] Cordus, V. 1561. *Annotationes in Pedacii Dioscoridis Anazarbei de medica materia libros quinque*. Strasbourg. ff. 228v, 229r. (Translated by G. K. Tallmadge. *Isis*, 1925, **7**, 409–10.)
[3] *Philos. Trans.*, 1729–30, **36**, 283–9.
[4] *Annals of medicine*, 1796, **I**, 401.

containing extract of hemlock, a drug then popular as an anti-spasmodic] . . . into a tea-cup, or wine-glass, and afterwards to hold the same up to the mouth, and draw in the vapour that arises from it with the breath, until the aether is evaporated. This is repeated three, four, or five times in the course of a day, for a month or six weeks. . . . The first effects of this application are an agreeable sensation of coolness in the chest, an abatement of the dyspnoea and cough, and, after ten minutes or a quarter of an hour, easier expectoration. . . . The only unpleasant circumstance attending the inhalation of this aethereal tincture of cicuta is a slight degree of sickness and giddiness, which, however, soon go off. . . .'

In order to avoid wasting the ether vapour, Pearson directed that a funnel should be inverted over the cup through the tube-end of which the patient was to inhale. In cold weather the cup was to be placed in a small basin of warm water and a larger funnel placed.over both cup and basin to rest on the table. The edge of the funnel was to be raised slightly by the thickness of a quill or a folded slip of paper to allow the ingress of air. For children and even infants ether was to be administered sprinkled on a folded handkerchief.[1]

Another method of inhaling ether was devised by the botanist and physician, R. J. Thornton, about 1795 :

' Two teaspoonfuls of aether are put into a teapot. This is held near a candle, and the thumb is put over the spout. When the vapour begins to press upon the thumb it is transferred to the mouth, and the air is drawn into the lungs. This is repeated until the whole be consumed, or ease acquired.'

A warning that ether is inflammable was given.[2]

The most important contribution to the study of therapeutic inhalation in general was made by Thomas Beddoes. No doubt through his friendship with various members of the Birmingham circle Beddoes became deeply interested in pneumatic medicine. About 1791 he published two small works on the subject, *A letter to Erasmus Darwin, M.D., on a new method of treating pulmonary consumption and some other diseases hitherto found incurable* and *Observations on the nature and cure of calculus, sea scurvy, consumption, catarrh and fever.* These attracted so much attention among scientific men that Beddoes was persuaded to embark on the

---

[1] *Med. Repository*, 1804, **I**, 142–4.
[2] Beddoes, T., and Watt, J. 1796. *Considerations on the medicinal use of factitious airs.* Bristol (iii), 143.

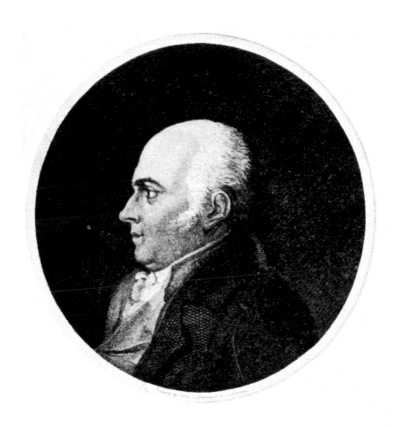

FIG. 4.—THOMAS BEDDOES (1760–1808)

Born at Shifnal, Shropshire. Took his D.M. at Oxford and became
Reader in Chemistry, 1788–92. In 1793 he left Oxford for Clifton,
Bristol, where he founded an institution for research on pneumatic
medicine, called the Pneumatic Institution.

ambitious project of founding a research institution for the study of inhalation therapy.

'At the close of the year 1792', wrote Beddoes, ' three of my friends conceived that some good might arise from an experimental investigation of those physiological conjectures which I had lately published. They accordingly offered to bear a part of the expense attending the construction of a pneumatic apparatus, and the salary of a person to construct and superintend it. Without their co-operation, I should probably have attempted nothing of this kind.' [1]

These three friends contributed £200 each, but another friend and patron was Josiah Wedgwood, the potter, who contributed £1000, and public subscriptions were also canvassed during 1794. [2]

'I . . . make no pretensions to discovery', wrote Beddoes, ' and have merely endeavoured to promote investigation in cases where either uniform failure, or frequent want of success, proves how much we need something better than we possess. . . .

'This object, I conceive, may be much more effectually accomplished in two years, by means of a small appropriated *Institution*, than in twenty years of private practice. . . .

'Such an Institution should be conducted with a view to the attainment of two objects.—1. To ascertain the effects of these powerful agents [gases] in various diseases ; and 2. To discover the best method of procuring and applying them.' [3]

Clifton, Bristol, was the place chosen for the Institution. James Watt (1736–1819), the engineer, designed the apparatus.

Watt, in addition to his Birmingham associations and his personal inclination towards the study of chemistry, had a poignant reason for his interest in pneumatic medicine. His brilliant son by a late second marriage was, in his teens, dying of consumption. [4]

The designs for the apparatus were prepared by the summer of 1794, and Watt wrote to Beddoes :

'I send you with this, drawings of my apparatus for producing and receiving the various airs which may be supposed to be useful in Medicine. . . .

[1] Beddoes, T., and Watt, J. 1796. *Considerations on the medicinal use of factitious airs.* Bristol. 3.

[2] *Med. commentaries*, 1794, **9,** 409.

[3] Beddoes, T., and Watt, J. 1796. *Considerations on the medicinal use of factitious airs.* Bristol. 4.

[4] *Dictionary of national biography*, London, 1909. **20,** 971 ; Beddoes, T., and Watt, J. 1796. *Considerations on the medicinal use of factitious airs.* Bristol. (ii), 15.

' The apparatus consists of an alembic, or pot, and its capital. The latter is connected by a pipe with the refrigeratory or washing vessel which again communicates by a pipe with the Hydraulic Bellows which receives the air as it is generated or produced, and transfers it into oiled silk bags, or other vessels from which it may be conveniently inhaled by the patient. . . .

' The oiled silk bags should be made in the form of a common sack, and have a wooden nozzle fitted to them in the shape of a common faucet, with the smaller end outwards, that it may fit into the tube of the bellows ; and this faucet should be provided with a spiggot to keep in the air when required. . . . When the silk is made into a bag, anoint the seams with japanners' gold size, diluted with some oil of turpentine. . . .

' In chusing oiled silk . . . that which is green should be avoided as it is coloured with verdegris, which adds to the bad smell, and rots the silk. The yellow, or yellowish, is the best. . . .

' As it is troublesome to empty the hydraulic bellows of the artificial air every time we want to measure common air into the oiled silk bags, it will be found convenient to have an additional bellows for that use. . . .' [1]

In a subsequent letter Watt wrote :

' As silk bags are costly and not very durable, it is thought that the larger bellows may be used to breathe the mixed airs out of ; for this purpose a flexible tube with a mouth-piece should be inserted into one of the pipes at bottom of the bellows ; so that the patient may not be confined to one posture while inspiring the air. These tubes may either be made of caoutchouc . . . or they may be made of the new water-proof leather for boots and shoes . . . if the tube be more than half an inch diameter, it should be sowed together upon a spiral of brass wire, to prevent it crushing in bending. . . .' [2]

Watt paid particular attention to the form of the mouth-piece :

' Many patients with difficulty acquire the habit of inhaling air from a bag and returning the air from their lungs through the nose . . . a mouth-piece has therefore been constructed with two valves of silk. . . . With this mouth-piece a person may breathe perfectly in their natural manner without straining the muscles of the breast, and without any other subjection than the holding of a small pipe in their mouth, the end of which is, for the greater ease, made in an oval form.' [3]

[1] Beddoes, T., and Watt, J. 1796. *Considerations on the medicinal use of factitious airs.* Bristol. (ii), 1–11.

[2] *Ibid.* (ii), 26.   [3] *Ibid.* (v), 11.

For those cases in which the shape of the patient's mouth prevented the lips fitting snugly round the tube, Watt invented ' a tin plate conical mouthpiece fixed to the cheeks and accurately adapted to the lips '.[1] He also devised ' a cap in the form of a beehive, about a foot diameter at the base ' to envelop the head down to the level of the chin. The tube of the breathing bag was introduced beneath this cap in the region of the mouth and the bag gently pressed. This device was intended for administering hydrogen to patients too weak to hold a mouth-tube between the lips. ' As inflammable air [hydrogen] is lighter than atmospheric, the cap will be filled with it, and they most infallibly breathe it, and at the same time will be under no teazing constraint.' [2]

By 1796 pneumatic medicine was at the zenith of popularity and it was possible for the public to purchase its own apparatus in a ' simplified and portable ' form. In a large size the cost of the generating apparatus was £6. 16s. 6d., with an additional £3. 6s. for ' auxiliary articles '.[3]

The principal ' factitious airs ' which, after carrying out a series of tests on animals, Beddoes recommended for clinical use were carbon dioxide, hydrogen, ' hydro-carbonate ' [4] and

---

[1] Davy, H. 1800. *Researches, chemical and philosophical, chiefly concerning nitrous oxide.* London. 537.

[2] Beddoes, T., and Watt, J. 1796. *Considerations on the medicinal use of factitious airs.* Bristol. (ii), 9.

[3] *Ibid.* (v), 24.

[4] ' Heavy Inflammable Air, Carbonated Hydrogene, or Hydro-Carbonate ' was prepared by strongly heating the charcoal of some soft, non-resinous wood (*e.g.* willow) in a tubular retort or crucible and then allowing water to drop sparingly on to it. ' No water should be admitted ', wrote Watt, who particularly recommended the gas, ' until the fire tube has been for some time red-hot . . . otherwise air will be produced which has not the power of causing vertigo '—this power being considered therapeutically important. Such a process would produce what is to-day called *water gas*, a mixture of hydrogen, some carbon dioxide, and carbon monoxide, the proportion of the latter being greater the higher the temperature in the crucible. That fatalities from the inhalation of ' hydro-carbonate ' do not seem to have occurred (although Davy had a narrow escape from death when experimenting with it, cf. Davy, H. 1800. *Researches . . . chiefly concerning nitrous oxide.* London. 468) was probably due to the care with which Watt's advice was followed :

' The hydro-carbonate having powerful effects in causing vertigo, ought always to be administered cautiously : where there is much debility, it may be prudent to begin with half a pint of this air, diluted with 10 or 20 pints of common air, to be increased in the subsequent doses, till each dose shall cause vertigo : how far this latter effect should be pushed, must depend upon the situation of the patient, and the nature of the disease. It is also proper, especially in the use of the hydro-carbonate, for the patient to rest a little at every five or six inhalations, to observe whether any vertigo takes place.' (Beddoes, T., and Watt, J. 1794 ed. *Considerations on . . . factitious airs.* Bristol. (v), 38–9.)

oxygen. The diseases to which each was considered applicable were many. Pneumatic treatment was not, perhaps, quite so drastic as it appears, because the gases were cautiously inhaled greatly diluted with atmospheric air. Even in the case of oxygen ' where symptoms do not decidedly indicate larger doses, it is prudent to begin with a pint of oxygene air in a bagful of common air, that is to say, diluted with from 20 to 40 times its bulk of common air, and gradually to increase the dose as symptoms direct ; observing always to dilute with at least 20 times the quantity of common air '.[1]

Davy's Researches on Nitrous Oxide

In the summer of 1798 Thomas Beddoes and his friend Professor Hailstone found themselves deep in geological controversy over the Plutonic and Neptunian theories. To help them decide the points at issue they took a holiday along the Cornish coast, and with them went a contemporary of Beddoes's at Pembroke College, Oxford, the Cornishman Davies Giddy, who later adopted the name Gilbert and achieved the distinction of becoming President of the Royal Society.

A year or so before, in Penzance, Giddy had accidentally made the acquaintance of Humphry Davy, who was idly swinging on the half gate ' at the house of the surgeon Borlase to whom he was apprenticed '. He struck Giddy as an exceptional boy, with his enthusiastic talk about chemistry and physics. Afterwards Davy met the Wedgwoods, wintering in Penzance, and became friendly with poor consumptive Gregory Watt, who had also come there for his health's sake and lodged at Mrs. Davy's.

Taking into consideration young Davy's friends, his obvious brilliance of intellect, his charm of person and manner (and even the fact that he was only nineteen years old), it is understandable why the shrewd but impulsive Beddoes, when he met him during that summer holiday in 1798, should immediately offer him the post of Superintendent of the Institution at Clifton. There Davy was to undertake an extensive series of chemical and physiological experiments on factitious airs. By the middle of October 1798 the matter was finally settled and Davy, released from his apprenticeship, began his new duties with characteristic energy.

---

[1] Beddoes, T., and Watt, J. 1796. *Considerations on the medicinal use of factitious airs.* Bristol (v), 38.

Already in the spring of 1798 Davy, on his own initiative, had disproved the curious theory put forward by the American, Samuel Latham Mitchill,[1] that nitrous oxide ' was the principle of contagion, and capable of producing the most terrible effects when respired by animals in the minutest quantities or even when applied to the skin or muscular fibre '. This he did by preparing nitrous oxide from ' zinc and diluted nitrous acid ' and exposing wounds to its action, immersing animals in it without injury and himself breathing it ' mingled in small quantities with common air ' without remarkable effects.[2] Now, with all the resources of Beddoes's newly equipped laboratory at his disposal, Davy returned to the investigation of nitrous oxide with renewed enthusiasm.   He first succeeded in obtaining it in a pure state in April 1799 and proceeded to inhale it :

' It passed through the bronchia without stimulating the glottis ', Davy wrote, ' and produced no uneasy feeling in the lungs. . . . I made many experiments to ascertain the length of time for which it might be breathed with safety, its effects on the pulse, and its general effects on the health when often respired. . . .
' I found that I could breathe nine quarts of nitrous oxide for three minutes [from and into a silk bag, the lungs being previously exhausted and the nostrils closed] and twelve quarts for rather more than four.   I could never breathe it in any quantity so long as five minutes.' [3]

Always, when breathing nitrous oxide, Davy experienced an apparent intensification of visual and auditory perception and a ' sensation analogous to gentle pressure on all the muscles, attended by an highly pleasurable thrilling, particularly in the chest and the extremities. . . . The sense of muscular power became greater, and at last an irresistible propensity to action was indulged in '.   But ' whenever its operation was carried to the highest extent, the pleasurable thrilling . . . gradually diminished, the sense of pressure on the muscles was lost ; impressions ceased to be perceived ;   vivid ideas passed rapidly

[1] See Beddoes, T., and Watt, J. 1796. *Considerations on the medicinal use of factitious airs.* Bristol. Appendix No. 1.
[2] Davy, H. 1800. *Researches, chemical and philosophical, chiefly concerning nitrous oxide.* London. 453.
[3] That Davy was able to breathe nitrous oxide for ' rather more than four ' minutes without becoming completely unconscious, indicates that the gas must have been considerably diluted with air. (Davy, H. 1800. *Researches . . . chiefly concerning nitrous oxide.* London. 456, 459, 460.)

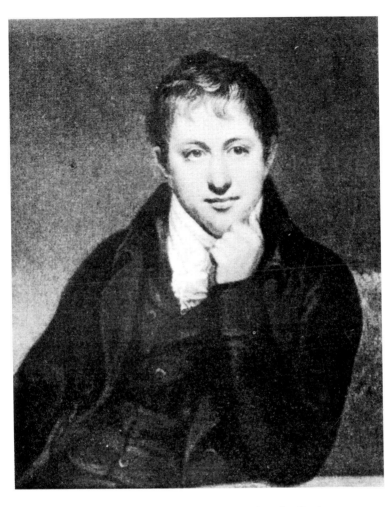

FIG. 5.—HUMPHRY DAVY (1778–1829)

Natural philosopher. Became Superintendent of Beddoes's Pneumatic Institution (1798) and carried out a series of researches upon the physiological effects of nitrous oxide. Having himself experienced the analgesic effects of the gas he suggested that this property might be utilized in certain types of surgical operation.

through the mind, and voluntary power was altogether destroyed,
so that the mouthpiece generally dropt from my unclosed lips '.[1]

On several occasions, as a result of breathing nitrous oxide,
Davy experienced an analgesic state, that is to say, a state in
which without completely losing consciousness he lost the faculty
of feeling pain. These occasions he recorded as follows :

' In one instance, when I had head-ache from indigestion, it
was immediately removed by the effects of a large dose of gas ;
though it afterwards returned, but with much less violence. In
a second instance, a slighter degree of head-ache was wholly
removed by two doses of gas.

' The power of the immediate operation of the gas in removing
intense physical pain, I had a very good opportunity of ascertaining.

' In cutting one of the unlucky teeth called dentes sapientiae,
I experienced an extensive inflammation of the gum, accompanied
with great pain which equally destroyed the power of repose,
and of consistent action.

' On the day when the inflammation was most troublesome,
I breathed three large doses of nitrous oxide. The pain always
diminished after the first four or five inspirations ; the thrilling
came on as usual, and uneasiness was for a few minutes, swallowed
up in pleasure. As the former state of mind however returned,
the state of organ returned with it ; and I once imagined that
the pain was more severe after the experiment than before.' [2]

Although Davy did not test the degree of that immunity
from pain which he had observed in himself during the inhalation
of nitrous oxide by submitting while under the influence of the
gas to pain-provoking stimuli inflicted by another person, he
nevertheless suggested that nitrous oxide might be used as an
anodyne in surgery. This suggestion occurs among the *Conclusions*
which he drew from his researches on nitrous oxide :

' As nitrous oxide in its extensive operation appears capable
of destroying physical pain, it may probably be used with advantage during surgical operations in which no great effusion of blood
takes place.' [3]

Davy did not explain why he considered that nitrous oxide
might be found useful only ' during surgical operations in which
no great effusion of blood takes place ' ; but as he believed that
nitrous oxide increased the force with which the blood circulates [4]

[1] Davy, H. 1800. *Researches, chemical and philosophical, chiefly concerning nitrous oxide.*
London. 458, 460.
[2] *Ibid.* 464, 465.   [3] *Ibid.* 556.   [4] *Ibid.* 548.

he may, on that account, have anticipated increased difficulty in controlling haemorrhage.

To the modern mind, primed with the knowledge that nitrous oxide is in fact an excellent anaesthetic for minor surgery, this often quoted passage is apt to assume a significance greater than that which it appears to have when read in its context ; it occurs unstressed among various conclusions drawn by Davy from the results of his experiments relating to nitrous oxide. Although less than two years earlier Davy had been serving his apprenticeship to the surgeon, Borlase, and must then have assisted at painful if minor operations, his imagination was not fired by the potentialities of his own suggestion that the inhalation of nitrous oxide might in certain cases obviate such pain. Moreover, after the publication, in 1800, of Davy's carefully recorded researches, anyone who had read through the book could then have attempted to put this suggestion to the test ; the fact remains that, so far as is known, no such attempt was made. Davy had no direct influence in shaping the course of anaesthetic history ; nevertheless, he was the first to associate the inhalation of a gas with the idea of destroying the patient's sense of pain during a surgical operation.

Early in 1801 Davy, not yet twenty-three years old, resigned his superintendency of the Pneumatic Institution to become Assistant Lecturer in Chemistry and Director of the Chemical Laboratory of the recently founded Royal Institution. Thenceforward his interest in things medical, never dominant, gave place to his enthusiasm for physics and chemistry. Indeed, he lived to regret the publication of his researches on nitrous oxide, describing them as ' the dreams of misemployed genius which the light of experiment and observation has never conducted to truth '.[1]

By 1800 Davy realized, and there is small doubt that Beddoes, also, had come to realize, that the immediate progress of pneumatic medicine was insuperably impeded by the lack of exact fundamental knowledge. In the *Researches* Davy wrote :

' Whenever we attempt to combine our scattered physiological facts we are stopped by want of numerous intermediate analogies and so loosely connected or so independent of each other, are the different series of phaenomena, that we are rarely able to make probable conjectures, much less certain predictions concerning the results of new experiments. An immense mass of

[1] *Dictionary of national biography.* 1908. London. **5**, 638.

3*

pneumatological, chemical, and medical information must be collected, before we shall be able to operate with certainty on the human constitution.

'Pneumatic chemistry in its application to medicine, is an art in infancy, weak, almost useless, but apparently possessed of capabilities of improvement. To be rendered strong and mature, she must be nourished by facts, strengthened by exercise, and cautiously directed in the application of her powers by rational scepticism.'[1]

The two-year period of research of which Beddoes had predicted so much had more than doubled itself, and pneumatic medicine was still only 'an art in infancy, weak, almost useless'. Realizing the futility of continuing in these circumstances, once Davy had left, Beddoes closed the Institution.

Long after Beddoes himself was dead, however, the theories which he had supported continued to find both advocates and opponents, not only in England but on the Continent and in America. Oxygen therapy, for instance, was firmly established although the circumstances of its application underwent many changes. Silliman, in his *Journal* for 1824, noticed the following opinion of Berzelius on the inhalation of hydrogen :

'When Hydrogen gas is substituted for azotic air [nitrogen] in the mixture which constitutes atmospheric air, and this mixture is respired by men or other animals, it very soon throws them into a profound sleep, without appearing to have any injurious effect, especially if a little common air is admitted to the mixture.'[2]

Belief in the antiseptic powers of carbon dioxide also persisted,[3] and the fact that it acts as a respiratory stimulant was referred to by Pereira, in 1839, in his handbook on materia medica :

'The impression produced on the pulmonary extremities of the par vagum, by the carbonic acid in the lungs, is supposed by some physiologists to be the ordinary stimulus to inspiration.'

Describing the effects of its inhalation in man, Pereira, paraphrasing a finding of Davy's,[4] stated :

'If an attempt be made to *inhale* pure carbonic acid gas, the glottis spasmodically closes, so as to prevent the smallest portions from entering the lungs. . . . When mixed with more than twice its volume of air, the gas ceases to provoke spasm of the glottis,

[1] Davy, H. 1800. *Researches, chemical and philosophical, chiefly concerning nitrous oxide.* London. 558, 559.
[2] *Amer. J. Sci.*, 1824, **8**, 372.   [3] Cf. *Lond. med. surg. J.*, 1831, **7**, 45.
[4] *Researches . . . chiefly concerning nitrous oxide.* 472–3.

and may be taken into the lungs. In this case it gives rise to symptoms resembling those of apoplexy. It usually causes a sensation of tightness at the chest, uneasiness, giddiness, loss of muscular power, insensibility, and stertorous breathing, sometimes accompanied by convulsions or delirium. These symptoms are succeeded by asphyxia and death.' [1]

Between the years 1829 and 1833 there was a considerable revival of interest in pneumatic medicine, due to a series of clinical experiments carried out by Albers, of Bonn, in hospital and private practice, on the use of chlorine [2] in diseases of the respiratory tract. His method was to immure the patient for intermittent periods in ' a chamber filled with a very weak chlorine vapour '.[3] Albers's work attracted sufficient attention for researches on the inhalation of chlorine to be undertaken by others, both in Great Britain and in the United States.

The Inhalation of Nitrous Oxide and of Ether Vapour as a form of Entertainment

Pneumatic medicine had a curious collateral development which played an important part in the events which began to take place in America during the early eighteen-forties, and which culminated in the establishment of the use of inhalation anaesthesia in 1846.

Davy's demonstration of the respirability of nitrous oxide and his description of the sensations experienced while under its influence had caught the popular fancy, perversely enough not because of any potential value to medicine which the gas might have, but because its inhalation provided a novel and apparently harmless form of entertainment. At the Pneumatic Institution both Beddoes and Davy with scientific zeal had pressed those who visited the Institution, both celebrities and nonentities, to breathe the gas and subsequently to give an account of the experience. Robert Southey, the poet, for instance, on taking the tube of the breathing bag from his mouth laughed involuntarily and felt a tingling in his toes and fingers, ' a sensation perfectly new and delightful '. S. T. Coleridge also felt ' an highly pleasurable sensation of warmth over my whole frame ' and noted that ' the only motion which I felt inclined to make was that of laughing at those who were looking at me '.

---

[1] Pereira, J. 1839. *Elements of materia medica.* London. **1**, 191, 192.
[2] Discovered by Scheele in 1774.   [3] *Brit. foreign med. Rev.*, 1837, **4**, 212.

On another occasion he could not ' avoid, nor indeed felt any wish to avoid, beating the ground with my feet '. A less distinguished visitor, after breathing the gas, exclaimed ' I felt like the sound of a harp '. Dr. Peter Mark Roget, afterwards famous as the author of the *Thesaurus of words*, was less enthusiastic. His reactions were violent but he recorded, ' I cannot remember that I experienced the least pleasure from any of these sensations '. The majority, however, agreed with Southey, Coleridge and the anonymous visitor, ' compared the effects to champagne ', laughed and by their ridiculous antics made others laugh. Soon nitrous oxide became known as laughing gas.

During his first year at the Royal Institution Davy still occasionally invited visitors to inhale the gas—an experience half scientific, half amusing—very much as he might have invited them to pull a penny out of electrified water. Such demonstrations were afterwards undertaken by others and achieved a lasting popularity both in England and, more particularly, in America. They became the fashion not only among undergraduate chemistry students [1] but at popular lectures and social gatherings.

In 1818 an annotation, attributed to Michael Faraday, appeared under the heading *Miscellanea*, in the official organ of the Royal Institution, the *Journal of Science*.[2] In it the writer pointed out the similarity between the effects of inhaling nitrous oxide and ether vapour. He also recorded that ' it is necessary to use caution in making experiments of this kind. By the imprudent inspiration of ether, a gentleman was thrown into a very lethargic state, which continued with occasional periods of intermission for more than 30 hours, and a great depression of spirits ; for many days the pulse was so much lowered that considerable fears were entertained for his life '.

Despite this discouraging anecdote, ' ether frolics ', conducted on similar lines to the nitrous oxide parties, became remarkably popular, especially in certain of the American States. This popularity was no doubt due to the greater simplicity of obtaining, storing and administering ether.

The direct bearing of these frolics upon the establishment of inhalation anaesthesia is referred to in Chapter II.

[1] Davy, H. 1800. *Researches, chemical and philosophical, chiefly concerning nitrous oxide.* London. 497–548.
[2] *Lancet*, 1827–8, **13**, 455 ; *Amer. J. Sci.*, 1822, **5**, 194.

PIONEERS OF INHALATION ANAESTHESIA

Hickman—Long—Wells

Hickman. In the same year, 1800, in which Davy published his suggestion that ' nitrous oxide . . . may probably be used with advantage during surgical operations in which no great effusion of blood takes place', to destroy physical pain (see p. 72), Henry Hill Hickman was born in a Shropshire village. In 1824 Hickman unequivocally formulated the principle oı general surgical anaesthesia by the inhalation of a gas.

Little is known about Hickman's boyhood, but in 1820 he was admitted a member of both the Royal College of Surgeons of England and the Royal Medical Society of Edinburgh. Thereafter he set up in general practice in Shropshire, first in Ludlow, then at Shifnal (Beddoes's birthplace) and finally at Tenbury.

In February 1824 Hickman addressed the following letter to T. A. Knight, of Downton Castle, near Ludlow, who was a Fellow of the Royal Society : [1]

' DEAR SIR,—The object of the operating Surgeon is generally considered to be the relief of his patient by cutting some portion of the human body whereby parts are severed from each other altogether or relieving Cavities of the aggravating cause of disease. There is not an individual who does not shudder at the idea of an operation, however skilful the surgeon or urgent the case, knowing the great pain that the patient must endure, and I have frequently lamented, when performing my own duties as a Surgeon, that something has not been thought of whereby the fears may be tranquilized and suffering relieved. Above all, from the many experiments on suspended Animation I have wondered that some hint has not been thrown out, of its probable utility, and noticed by Surgeons, and, consequently, I have been induced to make experiments on Animals, endeavouring to ascertain the practicability of such treatment on the human subject and by particular attention to each individual experiment, I have witnessed results which show that it may be applied to the animal world, and ultimately I think will be found used with perfect safety and success in Surgical operations. I have never

[1] Hickman, H. H. MS. now in the possession of the Wellcome Historical Medical Museum, London.

known a Case of a person dying after inhaling Carbonic Acid Gas, if proper means were taken to restore the animal powers, and I have no hesitation in saying that suspended animation may be continued a sufficient time for any surgical operation providing the Surgeon acts with skill and promptitude ; and I think it would be found particularly advisable in Cases where hemorrhage would be dangerous or the Surgeon is apprehensive of Gangrene taking place after the operation, as it is well known that carbon has a most powerful antiputrescent quality. It will be found, if the means for suspending animation are slow and gradual, the return of the powers of life will be in the same proportion ; if the means of suspension are sudden, it generally happens by the application of certain agents that the return of life is equally so ; and I think it very probable, if the Galvanic Fluid could have been applied in Cases that have proved fatal, the persons may have been saved. From a number of others I have selected the experiments now sent ; each is correctly noted in as few words as possible, which I think will prove a vast object. With great respect.—I am Dr. Sir, Your Obt. St.

'H. H. HICKMAN.'

The experiments selected by Hickman numbered seven :

'Experiment 1st [see Fig. 6]

'March 20th. I took a puppy a month old and placed it on a piece of wood surrounded by water over which I put a glass cover so as to prevent the access of atmospheric Air ; in ten Minutes he showed great marks of uneasiness, in 12 respiration became difficult, and in 17 Minutes ceased altogether, at 18 Minutes I took off one of the Ears, which was not followed by hemorrhage, respiration soon returned and the animal did not appear to be the least sensible of pain, in three days the Ear was perfectly healed.

'2nd

'Four days after the same puppy was exposed to a decomposition of the carbonate of lime by sulphuric Acid. In 1 Minute respiration ceased. I cut off the other Ear which was followed by very trifling hemorrhage, and as before did not appear to suffer any pain, in four days the wound healed. The day after the operation he seemed to require an additional quantity of food, which induced me to weigh him, and I found he gained 9 Oz. 1 Dr. & 24 grains in 9 days.'

The third experiment was similar to the first. The puppy was again confined in a bell jar over water and became insensible through reinhaling his own breath. His tail was then docked

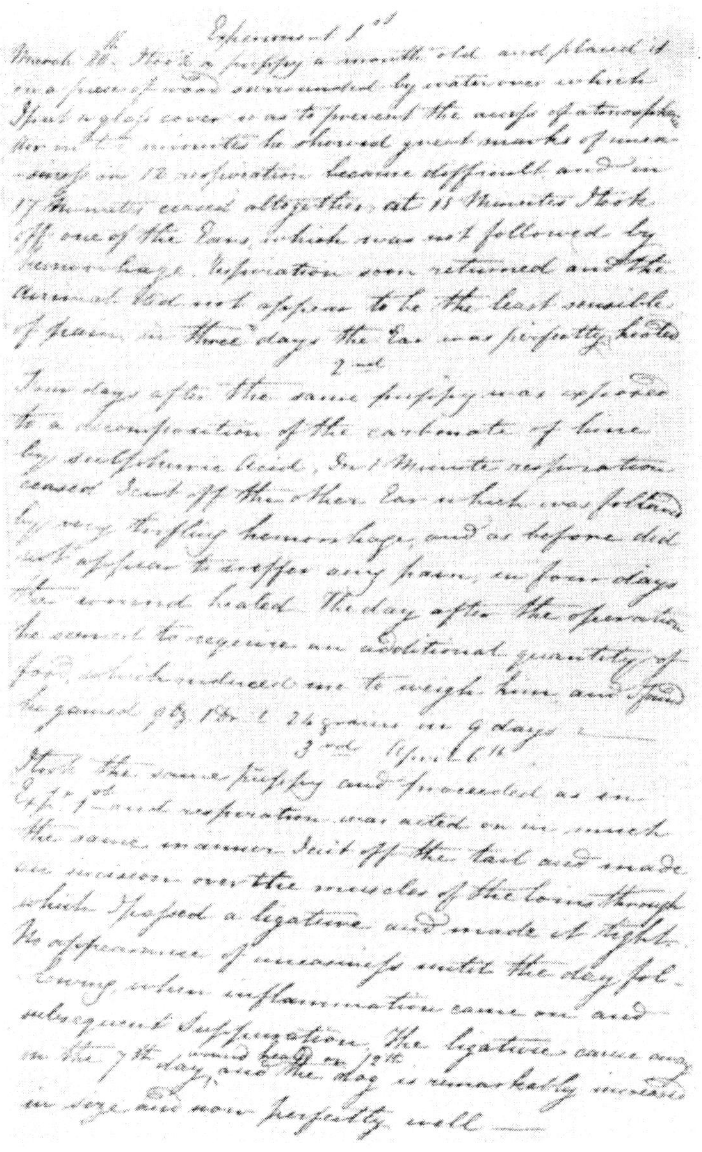

FIG. 6

Hickman's MS. notes on surgical anaesthesia recording experiments (made during the spring of 1823) on animals by making them inhale carbon dioxide.

(From the original MS. in the Wellcome Historical Medical Museum.)

and an incision made over ' the muscles of the loins ' through which a ligature was passed and made tight. Hickman remarked ' no appearance of uneasiness until the day following, when inflammation came on and subsequent Suppuration. The ligature came away on the seventh day, wound healed on twelfth and the dog is remarkably increased in size and now perfectly well '. In the fourth experiment a mouse was confined under a glass surrounded by water and carbonic acid gas was passed slowly in :

' Respiration ceased in three minutes, I cut all its legs off at the first joint, and plunged it into a basin of cold water, the Animal immediately recovered and ran about the table apparently without pain ; the stumps soon healed and I kept it a fortnight, after which I gave it liberty.'

In the fifth experiment an adult dog was

' exposed . . . to carbonic acid gas quickly prepared and in large quantity ; life appeared to be extinct in about 12 seconds. Animation was suspended for 17 minutes, allowing respiration occasionally to intervene by the application of inflating instruments. I amputated a leg without the slightest appearance of pain to the animal. There was no hemorrhage from the smaller vessels. The ligature that secured the main Artery came away on the fourth day and the dog recovered without expressing any material uneasiness.'

In the sixth experiment a rabbit was made insensible by the method used in experiment five and both ears were cut off. In the seventh experiment Hickman collected his own exhalations in a globe, into which he then introduced a kitten :

' In 20 seconds I took off its Ears and tail ; there was very little hemorrhage, and no appearance of pain to the Animal.'

In August 1824, Hickman, again addressing himself to Knight, published a pamphlet in which he set out in more detail his proposal that the inhalation of carbonic acid gas to procure insensibility to surgical pain should be applied in clinical practice. In a foreword ' To the Public ', Hickman wrote :

' At the particular request of gentlemen of the first rate talent, and who rank high in the scientific world, it is, that the author of the following letter is induced to lay it before the public generally, but more particularly his medical brethren ; in the hope that some one or other may be more fortunate in reducing the object of it beyond a possibility of doubt. It may be said, and with truth, that publications are too frequently the vehicles of self-adulation, and as such, suffer greatly from the lash of severe criticism ; but the author begs to assure his readers, that his views are totally different, merely considering it a duty incumbent on him (as a medical practitioner, and servant to the public), to make known any thing which has not been tried, and which ultimately may add something towards the relief of human suffering, arising from acute disease. The only method of obtaining this end is, in the author's opinion, candid discussion, and liberality of sentiment, which, too commonly is a deficient ingredient in the welfare of so important a profession, productive of serious consequences, not only to the parties themselves, but to the patient whose life is entrusted to their care. . . .'

This foreword was followed by a modified version of the original letter to Knight :

' SIR,—The facility of suspending animation by carbonic acid gas, and other means, without permanent injury to the subject, having been long known, it appears to me rather singular that no experiments have hitherto been made with the object of ascertaining whether operations could be successfully performed upon animals whilst in a torpid state ; and whether wounds inflicted upon them in such a state would be found to heal with greater or less facility than similar wounds inflicted on the same animals whilst in possession of all their powers of feeling and suffering. Several circumstances led me to suspect that wounds made on animals whilst in a torpid state, would be found, in many cases, to heal most readily ; and the results of some experiments which I have made lead me to think that these conjectures are well founded, and to hope that you will think the results sufficiently interesting to induce you to do me the honour to lay them before the Royal Society. The experiments were necessarily made upon living animals, but they were confined to animals previously condemned to death ; and as their lives were preserved, and their suffering very slight, (certainly not so great as they would have sustained if their lives had been taken away by any of the ordinary methods of killing such animals) I venture to hope that they, in the aggregate, rather received benefit than injury. Subjects of different species were employed, chiefly puppies of a few weeks or months old, and the experiments were often repeated, but as the results were all uniform, and as my chief object is to attract the attention of other medical men to the subject, I wish to do little more than state the general results.' [1]

[1] Hickman, H. H. 1824. *A letter on suspended animation, containing experiments showing that it may be safely employed during operations on animals, with the view of ascertaining its probable utility in surgical operations on the human subject, addressed to T. A. Knight, Esq., of Downton Castle, Herefordshire, one of the Presidents of the Royal Society.* Ironbridge.

After describing six experiments similar to those described in the original letter to Knight, Hickman continued :

' As the recital of such experiments as those preceding must be as little agreeable to you, as the repetition of them has been to myself, I shall not give a detail of any others, but shall only state the opinions which the aggregate results have led me to entertain. I feel perfectly satisfied that any surgical operation might be performed with quite as much safety upon a subject in an insensible state as in a sensible state, and that a patient might be kept with perfect safety long enough in an insensible state, for the performance of the most tedious operation. My own experience has also satisfied me that in very many cases the best effects would be produced by the patient's mind being relieved from the anticipation of suffering, and his body from the actual suffering of a severe operation ; and I believe that there are few, if any Surgeons, who could not operate more skilfully when they were conscious they were not inflicting pain.

' There are also many cases in which it would be important to prevent any considerable hemorrhage, and in which the surgeon would feel the advantages of a diminished flow of blood during an operation. I have reason to believe that no injurious consequence would follow if the necessity of the case should call for more than one suspension of animation ; for a young growing dog was several times rendered insensible by carbonic acid gas, with intervals of about twenty-four or forty-eight hours, without sustaining, apparently, the slightest injury. . . . I am not, at present, aware of any source of danger to a patient, from an operation performed during a state of insensibility, which would not operate to the same extent upon a patient in full possession of his powers of suffering, particularly if he were rendered insensible by being simply subjected to respire confined air. I used inflating instruments in one experiment only, and therefore am not prepared to say to what extent such may be used with advantage ; but I think it probable that those and the Galvanic fluid would operate in restoring animation in some cases. I was prepared to employ the Galvanic fluid if any case had occurred to render the operation of any stimulant necessary, but all the subjects recovered by being simply exposed to the open air ; and I feel so confident that animation in the human subject could be safely suspended by proper means, carefully employed, that, (although I could not conscientiously recommend a patient to risk his life in the experiment) I certainly should not hesitate a moment to become the subject of it, if I were under the necessity of suffering any long or severe operation.' [1]

It was unfortunate that Hickman should have hit upon a

[1] Hickman, H. H. 1824. *A letter on suspended animation.* . . . Ironbridge.

A

LETTER

ON

SUSPENDED ANIMATION,

CONTAINING

EXPERIMENTS

Shewing that it may be safely employed during

OPERATIONS ON ANIMALS,

With the View of ascertaining

ITS PROBABLE UTILITY IN SURGICAL OPERATIONS ON THE

𝕳uman 𝕾ubject,

Addressed to

T. A. KNIGHT, ESQ. OF DOWNTON CASTLE,
Herefordshire,

ONE OF THE PRESIDENTS OF THE ROYAL SOCIETY,

⸻

BY DR. H. HICKMAN,

OF SHIFFNAL;

Member of the Royal Medical Societies of Edinburgh, and of
the Royal College of Surgeons, London.

⸻

IRONBRIDGE: Printed at the Office of W. Smith.

1824.

Fig. 7

Title-page of Henry Hill Hickman's pamphlet on surgical anaesthesia produced in animals by causing them to inhale carbonic acid gas and his proposal that the principle should be applied in man.

83

method of obviating surgical pain which necessitated partially asphyxiating the subject. Nevertheless, judged by contemporary standards, the reasons which he gave for choosing carbonic acid gas as his stupefying agent [1] were sound, particularly his main reason : that he had ' never known a case of a person dying after inhaling carbonic acid gas '. That Hickman realized at least the most obvious asphyxial dangers of the prolonged inhalation of carbon dioxide and made some attempt to avoid them is shown in experiment five (recorded in both the original letter to Knight and the published pamphlet), in which animation in an adult dog ' was suspended during seventeen minutes, allowing respiration occasionally to intervene by means of inflating instruments '.

Hickman was convinced by his experiments that he had made a discovery which was potentially of the utmost importance to humanity ; but although he was thus far confident he, a young and unknown general practitioner in a small provincial town, was diffident of undertaking alone the formidable task of testing his theory clinically. He decided, therefore, that he must gain the co-operation of medical men of recognized standing and ability who, having themselves confirmed the results of suspended animation combined with surgical intervention in animals, would cautiously proceed to apply the principle to man. Although Knight seems to have encouraged Hickman to publish the pamphlet on suspended animation he was, on the whole, an indifferent patron (being chiefly interested, as it appears from the indexes of the *Philosophical Transactions*, in the growth of trees) and either did not attempt to interest his fellow members of the Royal Society in Hickman's proposal or did not succeed in doing so.

After waiting more than three years for some sign of practical help or encouragement from his fellow-countrymen, and finding none, Hickman went, in the spring of 1828, to Paris, then the recognized centre of scientific research. There he addressed himself to Charles X of France, once more setting out his proposal for suspending animation during surgical operations, and appealing for collaboration.

' SIRE,—In addressing Your Majesty upon a scientific subject of great importance to mankind, I feel a properly humble, but a

[1] One hundred years later, in 1925, Lundy ' suggested in a guarded way that . . . carbon dioxide might assist in producing anaesthesia ' and ' in 1929 Leake and Waters undertook a study of the anaesthetic properties of carbon dioxide.' (Beecher, H. K. 1938. *The physiology of anesthesia.* New York. 133, 134.) Cf. also pp. 223-4.

firm confidence in Your Majesty's universally known disposition to countenance valuable discoveries : this relieves me from all apprehension of being considered presumptuous.

' Permit me, Sire, to state that I am a British Physician, Member of the Royal College of Surgeons, London, who has visited Paris in part for the purpose of bringing to completion a discovery to which I have been led by a course of observations and experiments on suspended animation.

' This object has engaged my practical attention during several years : It appears demonstrable that the hitherto most agonizing, dangerous and delicate surgical operations may now be performed with perfect safety, and exemption from pain, on brute animals in a state of suspended animation. Hence it is to be strongly inferred, by analogy, that the same salutary effects may be produced on the human frame, when rendered insensible by means of the introduction of certain gases into the lungs : I have discovered a number of facts connected with this important subject, and I wish to bestow them on society.

' Paris, the great Metropolis of Continental Europe, is the place above all others where the profound studies of Humanity are, with the utmost facility, carried to their highest extent and perfection : and, Sire, I feel confident that I do not say too much, with a due regard for the scientific distinctions of my own Country, in avowing that these facilities, no where else to be found, and their most admirable results, have deservedly conferred on Your Majesty's Chief City, and its illustrious Schools of practical Philosophy, the eminent title of the Centre of Science to the Civilized World.

' Presuming thus, Sire, to attract Your Majesty's thoughts to this interesting subject, I have resorted to the French Capital for the completion of my discovery, hoping to have the honour of placing it under Your Majesty's Royal and gracious auspices. . . .

' . . . I have ventured on the liberty of praying Your Majesty to be pleased, by an express intimation, or command, on the subject, to permit me to develop my ideas on operations in a state of suspended animation, in the presence of Your Majesty's Medical and Surgical schools, that I may have the benefit of their eminent and assembled talent, and emulous co-operation.

' It is also my desire, at a fit opportunity, to solicit the honour of presenting to Your Majesty . . . a Book containing an account of my discovery which, as far as I know or can learn, has entirely originated with myself ; and should my labours meet with the approbation of Charles the Tenth, I shall ever enjoy the grateful satisfaction of believing that I have devoted myself to my profession to a distinguished and to a happy end. . . .' [1]

[1] Hickman, H. H.   MS. now in the possession of the Wellcome Historical Medical Museum, London.

At the end of August 1828 Hickman's letter to Charles X was passed on to the Académie Royale de Médecine for consideration, and Monsieur Géradin was asked to report upon its contents to the Section of Medicine. This he did on September 28, and a committee of investigation consisting of five members was appointed. Of these five the most distinguished was Anthelme Richerand.[1]

What attempt the members of this committee made to investigate Hickman's claim or what report of it they gave, if indeed they gave any, cannot be traced in the archives of the Académie, but it is certain that Hickman received little more help or encouragement in France than he had received in England. His contemporaries, unable to grasp the significance of what this young man so plainly and so insistently laid before their notice, were content to dismiss the possibility of surgical anaesthesia as illusory.[2]

After this second rebuff Hickman returned to England. Early in 1830 he died. He had tried hard to gain recognition for the principle of surgical anaesthesia by the inhalation of gases, but he failed. Hickman no doubt lacked both the force of character to compel the interest of others and the self-assurance which would have led him unhesitatingly to risk human life in order to prove his theory; but he also lacked the spirit of self-seeking which, had he been a man of less integrity, might have led him to exploit his discovery for personal gain.

One point in connection with the letter addressed to Charles X is noteworthy. Hickman no longer specified carbonic acid gas as the agent to be used for procuring insensibility to surgical pain ; he wrote, ' the . . . effects may be produced on the human frame, when rendered insensible by means of the introduction of certain gases into the lungs '. Unfortunately he gave no indication of which gases he had in mind. Some years later,

---

[1] It has been stated that Richerand himself ' adopted the plan of intoxicating'his patients before applying the knife'. (Buxton, D. W. 1920. *Anaesthetics, their uses and administration.* London. 6.) In fact, Richerand, referring not to surgical pain but to the necessity for muscular relaxation in treating dislocations, wrote : ' Opium administered with a view to provoking sleep, or at least a state approaching intoxication, induces such an enfeeblement in the strength of the muscles that they cease to oppose reduction. One knows how easy it is to operate upon intoxicated persons : finally, success has been achieved by tiring the muscles by prolonged traction and repeated attempts . . . because a sustained action exhausts the contractility of the organs. . . .' (Richerand, A. 1812. *Nosographie chirurgicale.* Paris. **3,** 181.)

[2] Cf. Velpeau, L. 1839. *Nouveaux éléments de médecine opératoire.* Paris. ' To obviate pain in operations is a chimera which it is to-day no longer permissible to seek after.'

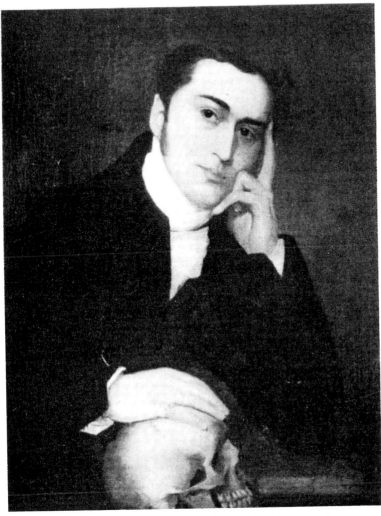

FIG. 8.—HENRY HILL HICKMAN (1800–30)

Physician and surgeon, practised in Shropshire. He spent his adult life trying to persuade his contemporaries to apply the principle that surgical operations could be safely and painlessly performed upon patients in a state of suspended animation induced by the inhalation of a gas.

(From a portrait in the Wellcome Historical Medical Museum.)

87

in 1847, when each of the three Americans, Jackson, Morton, and Wells (see pp. 122–4, 125), was separately importuning French scientific circles to recognize his particular claim to be considered the discoverer of the principle of surgical anaesthesia, a letter from Wells about his use of nitrous oxide gas was read at a meeting of the Académie de Médecine. Géradin was present and during the discussion which followed the reading of the letter he said :

'Seventeen or eighteen years ago, when the Académie was divided into three sections, the Minister of the King's Household sent to the Académie a letter from an English physician in which were set out various means of deadening sensibility during surgical operations : among other means, nitrous oxide was mentioned. The Section nominated, according to custom, a commission of which I had the honour to be the reporter. I need hardly say that this proposition met with much incredulity. Only one member, Baron Larrey [1], said that it merited the attention of surgeons. The matter went no further, but references to it may be found in the minutes.' [2]

At a subsequent meeting of the Académie Géradin produced the minutes of the meeting of September 28, 1828, where a brief résumé of Hickman's letter addressed to Charles X was recorded, but he produced no documentary evidence supporting his previous assertion that nitrous oxide had been specifically mentioned by Hickman.[3] Géradin relied, therefore, upon a remembrance which was in fact more than eighteen years old, when he associated Hickman's name with the use of nitrous oxide as an anaesthetic. Perhaps his memory was accurate ; perhaps after being for so long uncalled to mind it had become confused by the mention of nitrous oxide in Wells's letter. Whether or not Hickman made use of nitrous oxide in his later experimental work must therefore remain in doubt.

No less doubtful is the answer to another question which arises in considering Hickman's work : to what extent was he familiar with Davy's suggestion that the gas might be applied in surgery to obviate pain ? In addressing himself to Knight, Hickman implied that before beginning his experiments he had studied at least some part of the literature relating to therapeutic inhalation and pneumatic chemistry and this, coupled with the

---

[1] The military surgeon, Dominique Jean Larrey (1766–1842).
[2] *Bull. Acad. Méd. Paris*, 1847, **12**, 396.   [3] *Ibid.* **12**, 418.

fact that in 1824 he was living in Beddoes's birthplace, Shifnal, makes it hard to believe that he was entirely unaware of the work carried out at the Pneumatic Institution only twenty-five years earlier (see p. 70 *et seq.*). It is quite possible, however, that up to the time when his pamphlet was published, and even to the end of his short life, Hickman had neither had an opportunity of examining a copy of Davy's *Researches* nor heard any definite account of the latter's suggestion, which indeed had made little if any impression upon Davy's immediate contemporaries. If this were so it would explain why Hickman, who appears to have been so candid in all his actions, should have made no reference to Davy's researches in writing of his own.

Long. Within a few years of Hickman's death the possibility of producing adequate and controllable surgical anaesthesia by inducing in the patient a state of hypnotic trance, or as it was called ' mesmeric sleep ', was claimed by John Elliotson [1] and others in England, on the Continent and in America, and by James Esdaile [2] working in India. The claim was supported by case histories and by a considerable body of circumstantial evidence but it was received with ridicule although, at the same time, it was given wide publicity. Whereas, during the late eighteen-thirties and early forties few people had heard of Hickman's ' suspended animation ' almost everyone had heard of ' mesmeric sleep ' in connection with obviating surgical pain.[3]

Although the inhalation of a gas or of a vapour to produce surgical anaesthesia was still unrealized, at this period the inhalation of nitrous oxide or of ether vapour as an amusing pastime had lost none of its attraction and in America, where the system of popular lecture tours—entertainment combined with edification—had already taken a firm hold, nitrous oxide and the demonstration of its properties when inhaled was a favourite subject with both lecturer and audience.

In 1840 Crawford W. Long, newly qualified in medicine, set up in general practice in the small town of Jefferson in the State of Georgia. Long was a likable fellow and his surgery soon became a kind of clubroom where the town's more intelligent

---

[1] Elliotson, J. 1843. *Numerous cases of operations without pain.* London.
[2] Esdaile, J. 1846. *Mesmerism in India.* London.
[3] Cf. *e.g. Lond. med. Gaz.*, 1837–46, *passim.*

youths met of an evening and discussed current topics. Long himself described how

' In the month of Dec. 1841, or in Jan. 1842, the subject of the inhalation of nitrous oxide gas was introduced in a company of young men assembled at night in the village of Jefferson, Ga., and the party requested me to prepare them some. I informed them I had not the requisite apparatus for preparing or preserving the gas, but that I had an article (sul. ether) which would produce equally exhilarating effects and was as safe. The company were anxious to witness its effects, the ether was introduced and all present in turn inhaled. They were so much pleased with its effects that they afterwards frequently used it and induced others to do the same, and the practice soon became quite fashionable in the county and some of the contiguous counties.

' On numerous occasions I inhaled ether for its exhilarating properties, and would frequently, at some short time subsequent to its inhalation, discover bruised or painful spots on my person which I had no recollection of causing and which I felt satisfied were received while under the influence of ether. I noticed my friends while etherized received falls and blows which I believed were sufficient to produce pain on a person not in a state of anaesthesia, and on questioning them they uniformly assured me that they did not feel the least pain from these accidents. Observing these facts I was led to believe that anaesthesia was produced by the inhalation of ether, and that its use would be applicable in surgical operations.' [1]

On March 30, 1842, Long put his observations on the effects of ether to practical use. A boy named James Venable, who was often in and out of Long's surgery, several times asked whether two small tumours could not be removed from the back of his neck, but on each occasion the operation had to be postponed because of the lad's dread of pain. ' At length,' said Long, ' I mentioned to him the fact of my receiving bruises while under the influence of the vapor of ether without suffering, and as I knew him to be fond of and accustomed to inhale ether, I suggested to him the probability that the operations might be performed without pain, and proposed operating on him while under its influence. He consented to have one tumor removed, and the operation was performed the same evening. The ether was given to Mr. Venable on a

---

[1] Paper read by Long before the Georgia State Medical Society, in 1852. Reprinted by H. H. Young in ' Long, the discoverer of anaesthesia.' *Johns Hopk. Hosp. Bull.*, 1897, **8**, 182.

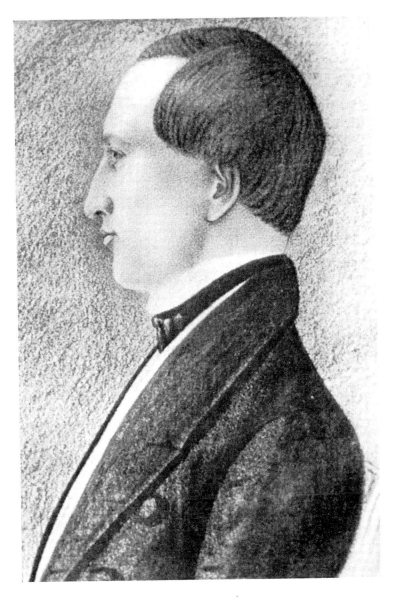

FIG. 9.—CRAWFORD WILLIAMSON LONG (1815-78)

Physician and surgeon, practised in the State of Georgia, U.S.A.
He was the first to perform a surgical operation upon a patient
anaesthetized by the inhalation of a volatile agent (sulphuric ether).

towel, and when fully under its influence I extirpated the tumor.

' It was encysted and about half an inch in diameter. The patient continued to inhale ether during the time of the operation, and when informed it was over, seemed incredulous until the tumor was shown to him.

' He gave no evidence of suffering during the operation, and assured me, after it was over, that he did not experience the least degree of pain from its performance.' This, the first surgical operation on a patient made insensible to pain by the inhalation of a vapour, took place in the presence of four witnesses.

Long was delighted by the success of the experiment and proceeded to look about him for other cases suitable for a similar procedure. In June 1842, he removed the second tumor from the back of Venable's neck and in July he amputated the toe of a negro boy. ' These,' Long stated in 1852, ' were all the surgical operations performed by me during the year 1842 upon patients etherized, no other case occurring in which I believed the inhalation of ether applicable. Since '42 I have performed one or more surgical operations annually on patients in a state of etherization.

' I procured some certificates in regard to these operations, but not with the same particularity as [I did] in regard the first operations, from the fact of my sole object in the publication being to establish my claim to priority of discovery of power of ether to produce anaesthesia. . . .

' The reasons which influenced me in not publishing earlier are as follows :

' I was anxious, before making my publication, to try etheriza-tion in a sufficient number of cases to fully satisfy my mind that anaesthesia was produced by the ether, and was not the effect of the imagination or owing to any peculiar insusceptibility to pain in the persons experimented on.

' At the time I was experimenting with ether there were physicians high in authority . . . who were advocates of mes-merism, and recommended the induction of the *mesmeric state* as adequate to prevent pain in surgical operations. Notwithstanding thus sanctioned I was an unbeliever in the science, and of the opinion that if the mesmeric state could be produced at all it was only on those of strong imaginations and weak minds. . . . En-tertaining this opinion, I was the more particular in my experi-ments on etherization.

'Surgical operations are not of frequent occurrence in a country practice, and especially in the practice of a young physician, yet I was fortunate enough to meet with two cases in which I could satisfactorily test the anaesthetic power of ether. From one of these patients I removed three tumors the same day ; the inhalation of ether was used only in the second operation, and was effectual in preventing pain, while the patient suffered severely from the extirpation of the other tumors. In the other case I amputated two fingers of a negro boy ; the boy was etherized during one amputation and not during the other ; he suffered from one operation and was insensible during the other. . . . In my practice, prior to the published account of the use of ether as an anaesthetic [by Morton] I had no opportunity of experimenting with it in a capital operation, my cases being confined . . . to the extirpation of small tumors and the amputation of fingers and toes.

'While [I was] cautiously experimenting with ether, as cases occurred . . . others more favorably situated engaged in similar experiments, and consequently the publication of etherization did not " bide my time ".' [1]

In spite of these statements made by Long himself in 1852, it has been suggested by his daughter, Mrs. Frances Long Taylor among others, that ' owing to the prejudice and ignorance of the populace, Dr. Long was prevented from using ether in as many cases as he might have. He was considered reckless, perhaps mad. It was rumored throughout the country that he had a strange medicine by which he could put people to sleep and carve them to pieces without their knowledge. His friends pleaded with him to abandon its use as in case of a fatality he would be mobbed or . . . lynched.' [2]

Ill-natured gossip possibly occurred, but one doubts whether such gossip was not given a dramatic twist and an exaggerated importance by friends who, after Morton's success in establishing the use of ether inhalation in surgery, in 1846, were anxious to justify Long's failure to achieve as much. The fact that Long gave no hint that any such opposition had existed and that he, whose livelihood depended upon his good reputation in the community, was able to continue from 1842 onwards to etherize patients when he considered such a procedure suitable to the case, goes far to discredit so highly coloured a description of events.

[1] *Johns Hopk. Hosp. Bull.*, 1897, **8**, 182–4.
[2] Taylor, F. Long. 1928. *Crawford W. Long*. New York. 41.

Wells. At the beginning of December 1844, the following advertisement was circulated in the town of Hartford, Connecticut :

' A Grand Exhibition of the effects produced by inhaling Nitrous Oxid, Exhilarating or Laughing Gas ! will be given at Union Hall this (Tuesday) Evening, Dec. 10th, 1844.

' Forty Gallons of Gas will be prepared and administered to all in the audience who desire to inhale it.

' Twelve Young Men have volunteered to inhale the Gas, to commence the entertainment.

' Eight Strong Men are engaged to occupy the front seats to protect those under the influence of the Gas from injuring themselves or others. This course is adopted that no apprehension of danger may be entertained. Probably no one will attempt to fight.

' The effect of the Gas is to make those who inhale it either Laugh, Sing, Dance, Speak or Fight, and so forth, according to the leading trait of their character. They seem to retain consciousness enough not to say or do that which they would have occasion to regret.

' *N.B.*—The Gas will be administered only to gentlemen of the first respectability. The object is to make the entertainment in every respect a genteel affair.'

The advertisement added : ' The entertainment is scientific to those who make it scientific. . . . The History and properties of the Gas will be explained at the commencement of the entertainment.'[1]

The lecturer, Gardner Quincy Colton (1814–98), had studied medicine but without taking a degree, and he now made his living by travelling up and down the States delivering popular scientific lectures, each of which ended with a demonstration in which his audience could take part. Colton's favourite subjects were electrical phenomena and nitrous oxide gas, no doubt because both provided the opportunity for hilarious yet ' genteel ' demonstrations.

The story of what came of that particular evening's entertainment, Tuesday, December 10, 1844, has been so often told as scarcely to bear repetition ; but the following sworn account, given subsequently in support of Wells's claim to be the discoverer of anaesthesia, by a young man named Cooley, is interesting because he took a leading part in the events :

' I, Samuel A. Cooley, a citizen of Hartford . . . Connecticut, depose and say, that on the evening of the 10th day of December, in the year 1844, that one G. Q. Colton gave a public exhibition in the Union Hall, in the said city of Hartford, to show the effect

[1] Quoted in *Anesth. & Analges.*, 1935, **14,** 181.

produced upon the human system by the inhaling of nitrous oxide, or laughing gas ; and in accordance with the request of several gentlemen, the said Colton gave a private exhibition on the morning of December 11th, 1844, at the said hall ; and that the deponent then inhaled a portion of said nitrous oxide gas, to ascertain its peculiar effect upon his system ; and that there were present at that time, the said Colton, Horace Wells, C. F. Colton, Benjamin Moulton, and several other gentlemen ; . . . and that the said deponent, while under the influence of the gas did run against and throw down several of the settees in the said hall and thereby throwing himself down, and causing several severe bruises upon his knees and other parts of his person ; and that after the peculiar influence of said gas had subsided, his friends then present asked if he had not injured himself, and then directed his attention to the acts which he had committed unconsciously while under the operation of said gas. He then found by examination that his knees were severely injured, and he then exposed his knees to those present, and found that the skin was severely abraised and broken ; and that the deponent then remarked, " that he believed that a person might get into a fight with several persons and not know when he was hurt, so unconscious was a person of pain while under the influence of the said gas " and the said deponent further remarked, " that he believed that if a person could be restrained, that he could undergo a severe surgical operation without feeling any pain at the time ". Dr. Wells then remarked, " that he believed that a person could have a tooth extracted while under its influence and not feel any pain " ; and the said Wells further remarked, " that he had a wisdom tooth that troubled him exceedingly, and that if the said G. C. Colton would fill his bag with some of the gas, he would go up to his office and try the experiment ", which the said Colton did ; and the said Wells, C. F. Colton, and G. Q. Colton, and your deponent, and others . . . proceeded to the office of said Wells ; and that said Wells there inhaled the gas and a tooth was extracted by Dr. Riggs, a dentist then present ; and that the said Wells, after the effect of the gas had subsided, exclaimed, " A new era in tooth-pulling ! " ' [1]

Horace Wells was himself a dentist by profession, and he immediately realized that if his patients could be prepared for dental extraction by breathing nitrous oxide gas the greatest deterrent from submitting to the operation—pain—would be removed. He therefore learned from Colton how to make the gas and, assisted by Riggs, proceeded to put the idea into practice.

[1] United States : 32 Congress, 2d Session in Senate of the United States, Feb. 19, 1853 : *Walker Report*, 16, 17.

By the middle of January 1845, Wells had fifteen successful cases of painless extraction to his credit. Wishing then to gain a wider publicity for his method Wells went to Boston, the centre of medical life in the Eastern States, and approached a former dental partner of his who, he hoped, might be able to give him an introduction to the surgeons of the Massachusetts General Hospital. This man was William Thomas Green Morton.[1]

Morton was slightly acquainted with several members of the hospital staff and introduced Wells to two of the surgeons, George Hayward and J. C. Warren. ' I . . . made known to them the result of the experiments I had made ', Wells afterwards wrote. ' They appeared to be interested in the matter, and treated me with much kindness and attention. I was invited by Dr. Warren to address the medical class upon the subject. . . . I was then invited to administer it [nitrous oxide] to one of the patients, who was expected to have a limb amputated.

' I remained some two or three days in Boston for this purpose, but the patient decided not to have the operation performed at that time. It was then proposed that I should administer it to an individual for the purpose of extracting a tooth. Accordingly, a large number of students, with several physicians, met to see the operation performed—one of their number to be the patient. Unfortunately for the experiment, the gas bag was by mistake withdrawn much too soon, and he was but partially under its influence when the tooth was extracted. He testified that he experienced some pain, but not as much as usually attends the operation ; and there was no other patient present, that the experiment might be repeated, and as several expressed their opinion that it was a humbug affair (which, in fact, was all the thanks I got for this gratuitous service), I accordingly left next morning for home.' [2]

Unfortunately no detailed and impartial contemporary account of this demonstration exists ; but many years later, in 1876, H. J. Bigelow, who in 1845 was a junior surgeon on the staff of the Massachusetts General Hospital, stated :

' Wells's want of success can now be satisfactorily explained. He had, through Colton, in following Davy's instructions, made

[1] Wells, H., 1847. *A history of the discovery of the application of nitrous oxide gas, ether, and other vapours to surgical operations.* Hartford. 6.
[2] United States: 32 Congress, 2d Session in Senate of the U.S., Feb. 19, 1853. *Walker Report*, 14, 15, quoted from the *Hartforc' Courant*, letter dated December 7, 1846.

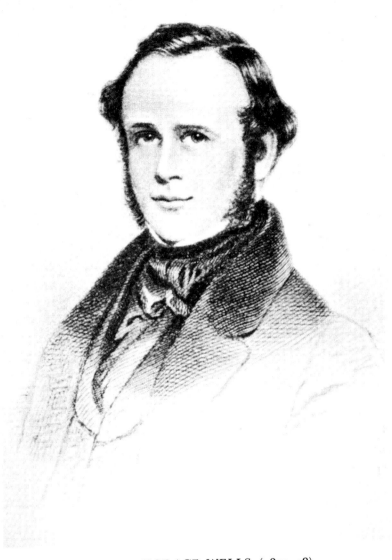

FIG. 10.—HORACE WELLS (1815–48)

Dentist, of Hartford, Connecticut. Between December 1844 and February 1845 he successfully anaesthetized a number of patients for dental extractions, with nitrous oxide gas ; but a demonstration of nitrous oxide anaesthesia which he gave at the Massachusetts General Hospital was so decidedly a failure that his method was discredited.

use of the traditional exhilarating gas bag, and of Davy's ex- hilarating dose. This volume of gas is inadequate to produce anaesthesia with any certainty ; and Wells failed to suggest a larger dose. This small omission closed his chances. . . .'[1]

Judged by the standards of 1876 (cf. pp. 290, 307) Wells's apparatus was indeed inadequate as a means of producing ' anaesthesia '—the state of complete insensibility. Nevertheless, with this apparatus Wells, on a number of occasions, had produced in his patients a sufficient degree of insensibility to the pain of a dental extraction. It is probable, however, that he never deliberately achieved complete insensibility but was satisfied with analgesia, a state in which the patient is semi-conscious yet oblivious to pain—such a state as Davy himself had experienced in 1779 (see p. 72).

Wells's own explanation of his failure at the Massachusetts General Hospital to demonstrate insensibility to pain is probably the true one : that the inhalation was interrupted when the gas had barely begun to take effect on the patient—an error of judgment on Wells's part probably due to his being flustered by the presence of a highly critical audience. A contributory cause of failure has been suggested by R. R. Macintosh :

' It may be surmised that the patient was of the robust type now described as " anaesthetic resistant ", for under nitrous oxide such a patient becomes cyanosed before anaesthesia has been attained. To this day it is sometimes impossible to produce perfectly tranquil narcosis, even for dental extractions, if nitrous oxide is used to anaesthetise a robust male, particularly if he is nervous and unpremedicated.' [2]

Whatever the reason for the fiasco, the surgeons of the Massachusetts General Hospital took no further interest in Wells and his method and he returned home discouraged, although he seems to have continued for a time to administer nitrous oxide in his own practice. Not long after his return to Hartford, however, his health broke down, and when at last he became well again he decided to abandon dentistry and everything connected with it.

[1] Bigelow, H. J. 1876. *The discovery of modern anaesthesia.* Philadelphia. 142.
[2] Macintosh, R. R., and Bannister, F. B., 1943. *Essentials of general anaesthesia.* Oxford. 5.

Chapter III

MORTON AND ETHERIZATION

The Establishment of Etherization in America and the Controversy
with Jackson

TOWARDS the middle of the year 1846 William Thomas Green Morton began to give serious thought to the problem of obtunding surgical pain. Morton, who was ambitious, enterprising and persevering, had studied dentistry for a short time in the newly founded Baltimore College of Dental Surgery. Afterwards, in order to acquire some slight knowledge of chemistry, he became a pupil-boarder in the house of the chemist and geologist, Charles T. Jackson, in Boston. He attended, also, two courses of medical lectures at the Massachusetts Medical College. There he encountered J. C. Warren and others of the staff of the Massachusetts General Hospital, who were later to play an important part in his affairs.

After a brief and unsuccessful partnership with Horace Wells during 1842 and 1843, Morton set up in practice on his own account in Boston. He specialized in prosthetic dentistry, building up a flourishing business. Contrary to the usual custom among his contemporaries, Morton considered it necessary to extract all broken tooth stumps from the jaws of his patients before attempting to fit dental plates—a laborious and painful procedure which deterred many possible clients. ' Thus,' wrote Richard H. Dana, Morton's legal adviser, ' Dr. Morton had a direct pecuniary motive, bearing almost daily upon him, to alleviate or annihilate pain under his operations.' [1]

Wells's recent use of nitrous oxide as an inhalant to prevent or lessen the pain of dental extractions had shown Morton that this agent was unreliable in its action, but an alternative agent was obvious—ether vapour. Already, during 1844, at C. T. Jackson's suggestion, Morton had used liquid ether as a local application to deaden pain while filling a sensitive tooth ; and that the vapour of ether mixed with atmospheric air was respirable, ' producing a succession of effects analogous to those caused by

[1] *Littell's Living Age*, 1848, **16**, 532.

the protoxide of nitrogen ' and would, if inhaled in sufficient concentration, cause stupefaction, was not only widely known but was known to Morton in particular, for he himself stated that he read the section dealing with sulphuric ether in Jonathan Pereira's *Elements of materia medica*,[1] where these facts were clearly stated.

Having decided to try the use of ether vapour all that Morton need have done to test its efficiency was to inhale it from a handkerchief (the method commonly used at ether frolics) in the presence of one or more witnesses who, when he became stupefied, could prick him with pins, pull his hair, kick him on the shins or apply any other reasonably painful but innocuous stimuli to test his responses. Such a simple procedure did not recommend itself to Morton, who was already fearful that unless he acted with great secrecy someone might steal his idea and forestall him in applying etherization to obtund pain.

Morton began his researches in earnest in the summer of 1846, with a few inconclusive experiments on his household pets. ' The most marked and satisfactory ', wrote Nathan P. Rice, Morton's biographer, ' was upon a water spaniel. The ether was poured upon some cotton wool in the bottom of a tin pan, and the dog's head was held directly over it. In a short time " the dog wilted completely away in his hands and remained insensible to all his efforts to arouse him by moving or pinching him ; yet after the removal of the pan he became in two or three minutes as lively and conscious as ever ".' [2] By the end of June Morton was so occupied with various problems connected with ether that he felt obliged to take a partner to supervise his dental business. He chose Grenville G. Hayden, who gave the following account of the forming of the partnership :

' About the last of June, 1846, Dr. William T. G. Morton called upon me . . . and stated . . . that he wished to make arrangements with me that would relieve him from all care as to the superintendence of those employed by him in making teeth, and all other matters in his office. He stated . . . he had an idea in his head . . . which he thought " would be one of the greatest things ever known ". . . . Being extremely urgent in the matter, I made an engagement with him the same day. . . . I then asked him what his " secret " was . . . and he finally told me the same night . . . that " it was something he had discovered which would enable him to extract teeth without pain ".

[1] London, 1839, **1,** 210, 211.
[2] Rice, N. P. 1859. *Trials of a public benefactor.* New York. 55.

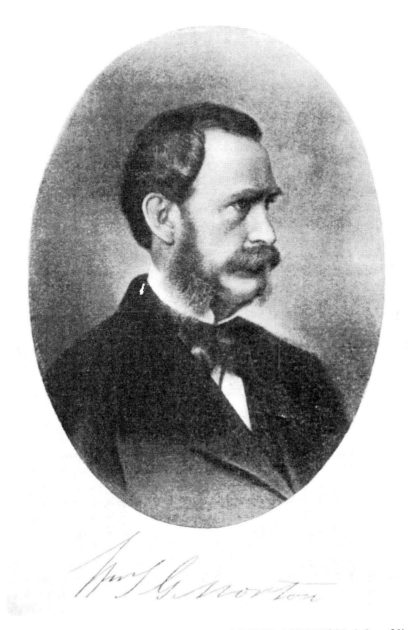

FIG. 11.—WILLIAM THOMAS GREEN MORTON (1819–68)

Dentist, of Boston, Massachusetts. By a successful demonstration (on October 16, 1846) he convinced the surgeons of the Massachusetts General Hospital, and through their influence the rest of the world, that the inhalation of ether vapour could produce satisfactory surgical anaesthesia.

I then asked him if it was not what Dr. Wells, his former partner, had used ; and he replied " No ! nothing like it ", and further-more " that it was something that neither he, nor any one else, had ever used ". He then told me he had already tried it upon a dog, and described its effects upon him which (from his descrip-tion) exactly correspond with the effects of ether upon persons who have subjected themselves to its influence, under my observa-tion. . . . He then requested me not to mention what he had communicated to me.' [1]

Among Morton's student apprentices were two lads, William P. Leavitt and Thomas R. Spear who, in March 1847, described, under oath, certain events which took place during the summer and autumn of 1846. Leavitt, in his statement, said :

' About one week after Dr. Hayden came to practise dentistry in connection with Dr. Morton, with whom I was then a student . . . about the first of July 1846, Dr. Morton stepped into his back office, much excited, and exclaimed, with great animation (as nearly as I can recollect his language), " I have got it now. I shall take my patients into the front room and extract their teeth, and then take them into the back office and put in a new set, and send them off without their knowing anything about the operation ".' [2]

During the week that followed, Morton called Leavitt aside and, enjoining him to keep everything to himself, sent him to buy some ' pure ether '. He also sent the boy to Gay, a chemist, to ask if ether would affect india-rubber as he wanted to put some into an india-rubber bag (no doubt remembering Wells's nitrous oxide inhaler). Morton was now prepared for the crucial experiment.

' About a week after this,' Leavitt continued, ' Dr. Morton told me that, if I would find a man who would have a tooth extracted, and have an experiment tried upon him, which was perfectly harmless, he would give me five dollars, and he sent me out with Thos. R. Spear, Jr., for that purpose. We went down to the wharves and spoke to a number of persons ; but they declined coming. . . . Dr. Morton then asked me to try it ; but I refused. He then said that he had taken it, and that it was perfectly harmless and that he wanted some one else to take it, that he might SEE how it operated.

[1] *Littell's Living Age*, 1848, **16**, 535.   [2] *Ibid.* **16**, 534.

Dr. Hayden said, " Tom will take it " ; but he said no, he had no teeth he wished extracted. But he finally said, " I will take some, won't you ? " We both took it the same evening, inhaling it from a handkerchief.'

Spear then continued the narrative :

' About the first of August 1846, at request of Dr. Morton, I inhaled a portion of ether . . . in Dr. Morton's office. The rest of the young men in the office were afraid to take it ; but having taken what I supposed to be the same before, at the Lexington Academy, I did not hesitate. . . .' [1]

Although he had now tried ether upon the dog, himself and two of his assistants, Morton told Hayden, ' towards the last of September . . . that in some particulars, his discovery did not work exactly right, and, in my presence,' said Hayden, ' was consulting his books to ascertain something further about ether. Upon this I recommended him to consult some chemist on the subject. Dr. Morton then sent . . . to see if Dr. Jackson was at home . . . but Dr. J. was not at home '.[2]

Morton, who seems to have been acutely conscious of a lack of intellectual attainment in himself, was in the habit of turning to his former tutor in chemistry, C. T. Jackson, for advice on all manner of technical points. The next day Morton himself called and found Jackson in.

' . . . About the last of September, 1846 ', said Hayden, ' Dr. M. said he had that day seen Dr. Jackson, and derived from him a hint by which Dr. M. thought he could remove the only remaining difficulty. Dr. M. said that, in his interview with Jackson, the subject of nitrous oxide gas and of ether gas, and atmospheric air, was freely talked of, as having an effect on the imagination of the patient, and various experiments which had been tried with these gases on students at Cambridge college ; also, the experiments of Dr. Wells and himself together, with the nitrous oxide gas ; but that he withheld from Dr. Jackson the fact that he had been experimenting on ether gas before.' [2]

Upon this last point Morton probably overestimated his powers of concealment and underestimated Jackson's perspicacity. In any case it was an irony of fate that Morton, with his fear of being forestalled and his subterfuges to prevent such a

[1] *Littell's Living Age,* 1848, **16**, 534.   [2] *Ibid.* **16**, 535.

happening, should have turned to Jackson for information. For although Jackson was undoubtedly a distinguished scholar, particularly in the science of geology, he had a deplorable tendency, upon the most slender grounds, to try to father other people's inventions which gave promise of being outstandingly successful—especially from a financial point of view.[1] Within three months Jackson claimed that at this very interview *he* had suggested to Morton the use of ether vapour as an inhalant to obviate surgical pain. Almost immediately after Morton's successful demonstration of etherization at the Massachusetts General Hospital Jackson gave his version of the circumstances of the interview between himself and Morton to his friend Caleb Eddy, who reported them as follows :

' On the evening of Friday, October 23, 1846, Dr. Charles T. Jackson visited my house. During the evening, I requested him to relate to me the particulars of the new discovery for prevention of pain in surgical operations. He stated to me, that Dr. W. T. G. Morton called on him near the latter part of last month to obtain the loan of a gas-bag, which he said it was his intention to use for the purpose of administering atmospheric air, or something else, to a patient to quiet her fears in order that he might extract one of her teeth ; that he informed Dr. Morton that his gas-bags were in the attic story of his house, and it would be attended with some trouble to procure them ; that Dr. Morton stated that he was desirous of operating on the imagination of the person in some such way as was said to have been practised on a criminal condemned to death, viz.—by suffering warm water to trickle upon and from some wound or lanced part of the body while the eyes of the person were bandaged. Dr. Jackson stated, that he told Dr. Morton that such an experiment would prove a failure, and he would be ridiculed for making it ; that he had better let her breathe some ether (if he could induce her to inhale it), which would put her to sleep, and then he could pull her tooth, and she could not help herself, or could not prevent him by any resistance ; that Dr. Morton inquired of him as to the danger

---

[1] Between 1837 and 1842 Jackson held the appointments of State geologist to Maine, Rhode Island, and New Hampshire and carried out official surveys.

When, in 1840, S. F. B. Morse patented the electric telegraph Jackson claimed that *he* had pointed out its underlying principles to Morse in 1836. ' It was known that Jackson had previously perfected a working model of such a device, but he thought lightly of the instrument and failed to realize its commercial value.' After Schönbein announced the discovery of gun-cotton in 1846, Jackson made a claim of priority in respect to this also.

Jackson's mind became completely unbalanced in 1873 and he died in an asylum in 1880. (*Dictionary of American biography.* New York. 1930.)

and mode of using it. He replied to him, that he might saturate a sponge or cloth with it, and apply it to her mouth or nose. After Dr. Jackson had related the above ', added Caleb Eddy, ' I said to him, " Dr. Jackson, did you know at such time, that, after a person had inhaled ether, and was asleep, his flesh could be cut with a knife without his experiencing any pain ? " He replied, " No ! nor Morton either ; he is a reckless man for using it as he has ; the chance is, he will kill somebody yet ".' [1]

Referring to this claim of Jackson's the trustees of the Massachusetts General Hospital, to whom he was well-known, in 1847, described him as a man ' honestly self-deceived in this matter '.

When Morton returned to his office after the interview with Jackson at the end of September 1846, he immediately proceeded to apply the information he had gleaned. ' The same day ', Hayden said, ' Dr. Morton told me that he had just tried ether again—in accordance with Jackson's hint—on himself, and that he had remained insensible seven or eight minutes by the watch.' Morton did not say what the hint was, but it was evidently valuable.

That evening, September 30, a willing patient, Eben H. Frost, made an opportune call at Morton's surgery. After allowing himself to be etherized for the extraction of a tooth he made and signed a statement :

' I applied to Dr. Morton, at 9 o'clock this evening, suffering under the most violent toothache ; that Dr. Morton took out his pocket-handkerchief, saturated it with a preparation of his, from which I breathed about half a minute, and then was lost in sleep. In an instant more I awoke, and saw my tooth lying upon the floor. I did not experience the slightest pain whatever. I remained twenty minutes in his office afterward, and felt no unpleasant effects from the operation.' [1]

' We tried repeated experiments with the same means subsequently,' wrote Hayden, ' and they all resulted in total failures. Dr. M. said that Dr. Jackson recommended a certain apparatus, which he lent Dr. Morton from his laboratory, consisting of a glass tube of equal size throughout, having a neck, and being about three feet long. This was likewise a total failure. So far, all our experiments, with one exception, proving abortive, we

[1] *Littell's Living Age*, 1848, **16**, 541.

4*

found that a different apparatus must be obtained, and it was at this time that Dr. M. procured from Mr. Wightman . . . a conical glass tube, with which, by inserting a sponge saturated with ether in the larger end, we had better success, and our experiments began to assume a more promising aspect.'[1] Wightman was an instrument maker and he himself described this container as being ' a tubulated glass globe receiver into which he [Morton] proposed to put a piece of sponge, to be kept saturated with ether, and have the opening through which the retort usually enters placed over the mouth, and the air admitted through the *tubulure*, or hole for the stopper '. Wightman suggested that if this apparatus answered the purpose ' an appropriate vessel ' could then be made.[2]

Immediately after the painless extraction of Eben Frost's tooth Morton took two important steps. First, he decided to try to patent etherization, and he called at the office of R. H. Eddy, son of Jackson's friend Caleb Eddy, a commissioner of patents, and enquired what the possibility of success might be. Eddy was doubtful but said that he would ' consult the law '. There, for a time, the matter rested. Secondly, Morton called upon Dr. John Collins Warren, Senior Surgeon of the Massachusetts General Hospital. Warren was interested in this new possibility of producing insensibility to surgical pain and promised that a demonstration should be arranged. Morton, with his usual secretiveness and, moreover, hoping to patent etherization, did not disclose to Warren the exact nature of the agent by which he proposed to produce insensibility.

On Wednesday, October 14, 1846, Warren sent a note to Morton inviting him to be present on the following Friday ' at 10 o'clock, at the hospital, to administer to a patient who is then to be operated upon the preparation which you have invented to diminish the sensibility to pain '. This gave Morton one clear day in which to improve the still imperfect apparatus made by Wightman. On Thursday afternoon he once more called on Wightman, in great haste, and begged him to ' assist him to prepare an apparatus with which he could administer the ether to a patient at the hospital the next day. . . . I consented,' said Wightman, ' to arrange a temporary apparatus under these circumstances. This apparatus was composed of a quart tubulated globe receiver, having a cork fitted into it

[1] *Littell's Living Age*, 1848, **16**, 535.   [2] *Ibid.* **16**, 537.

instead of a glass stopper, through which cork a pipette or dropping tube was inserted to supply the ether as it was evaporated. *I then cut several large grooves around the cork to admit the air freely into the globe to mix with the vapour,* and delivered it to Dr. Morton '.[1] Still the inhaler was far from perfect and Morton was hard pressed for time. He called to his assistance Augustus A. Gould, a Boston physician and natural scientist of some distinction, and ' sat up very late ' with him, ' contriving the most proper apparatus '. It was Gould, according to R. H. Dana, who that night suggested to Morton ' the valvular system instead of that which Dr. Morton had previously used ' (*i.e.* in which the patient breathed to and fro into a valveless although not entirely closed flask). Dana was probably right in attributing to Gould the suggestion of introducing valves into the flask, though Hayden stated that Morton himself suggested it.[2]

During the few hours which still remained before the demonstration ' a diagram was drawn and the next morning Dr. Morton was early at Mr. Chamberlain's [an instrument maker] and remained there, superintending the making of the apparatus until the hour of the experiment '. This apparatus (see Fig. 12) and its method of use were described by H. J. Bigelow :

' A small two-necked glass globe contains the prepared vapour with sponges to enlarge the evaporating surface. One aperture admits the air to the interior of the globe, whence, charged with vapour, it is drawn through the second into the lungs. The inspired air passes through the bottle, but the expiration is diverted by a valve in the mouthpiece, and escaping into the apartment is thus prevented from vitiating the medicated vapour.'[3]

The mouthpiece itself consisted of a tube which the patient held between his lips ; a flange encircling the tube cupped the outside of the mouth, rather as an eyebath cups the eye, and so helped to exclude additional atmospheric air. Breathing was entirely oral, for the patient's nostrils were pinched shut by the fingers of the administrator or his assistant. An accidental feature of this inhaler, which weighed in its favour, was its small size (the diameter of the base was about 10 centimetres) so that during administration it was held in the hand and the warmth of the palm automatically aided vaporization.

[1] *Littell's Living Age,* 1848, **16,** 537.   [2] *Ibid.* **16,** 535.
[3] *Brit. foreign med. Rev.,* 1847, **13,** 310.

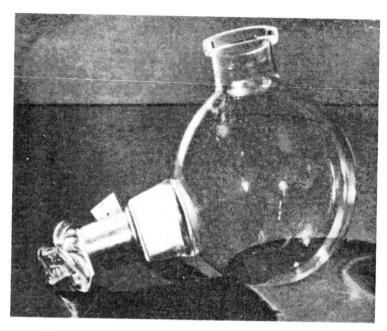

FIG. 12.—MORTON'S ETHER INHALER (1846)

This example is in the possession of the Massachusetts General Hospital, Boston, Massachusetts, and is believed to be the inhaler actually used by Morton at the demonstration on October 16, 1846. It is described by the hospital authorities as follows : ' A sea sponge inside the globe held the ether. While we still have the sponge it is not practical to place it inside the apparatus now. The subject held the mouthpiece, which is shaped for the purpose, in his lips. The brass cylinder which connects the globe with the mouthpiece contained a leather flap valve hung in such a way as to open during inspiration and close at the beginning of expiration. The expiratory breath passed forth through the protrusion at the side of the cylinder. This side port, which is approximately square and has a sloped cover of appropriate shape, was fitted with a leather flap hung so as to open during expiration and close at the beginning of inspiration. Thus a unidirectional flow was obtained through the ether chamber to the patient and out at the side '.

A lively account of the events of the morning of October 16 was given by Nathan P. Rice. He described the scene in Chamberlain's workshop and later at the hospital :

' Morton, becoming nervous and impatient, hurried him on in his work until at last, fearing lest he should be too late, he seized the instrument directly from his hands, and started in haste for the hospital, almost breathless with apprehension and the celerity of his movements.

' He had taken the precaution to request Mr. Frost to accompany him, to conduce in some way to his relief, in case of failure, and act as a voucher as regards his statements of what he had already accomplished. At this moment his mind was in one great whirl of doubts and conflicting emotions. Mixed with fear that his new and untried instrument might not work, and perhaps render the issue abortive, was his own vague doubt of a successful exhibition. . . .

' Luckily for Morton was it that he arrived at the precise moment at which he did. For previous to the operation, Dr. Warren, having waited ten or fifteen minutes, again turned to those present, and said : " As Dr. Morton has not arrived, I presume he is otherwise engaged " ; apparently conveying the idea that Dr. Morton did not intend to appear. The remark of Dr. Warren brought out a great laugh. Dr. Warren then sat down to his patient. Just as he raised his knife Dr. Morton appeared. . . . Dr. Warren . . . turning first to the patient and then to himself, said, ' Well, sir ! your patient is ready ". . . . Dr. Morton stepped to the bedside of the patient. Taking the man by the hand he spoke a few encouraging words to him, assuring him that he would partially relieve if he did not entirely prevent all pain during the operation and pointing to Mr. Frost, told him there was a man who had taken it and could testify to its success. " Are you afraid ? " he asked. " No ! " replied the man. . . .' [1]

J. C. Warren himself described the performance of the operation :

' The patient was a young man, about twenty years old, having a tumor on the left side of the neck, lying parallel to and just below the left portion of the lower jaw. This tumor, which had probably existed from birth, seemed to be composed of tortuous, indurated veins extending from the surface quite deeply under the tongue. My plan was to expose these veins by dissection sufficiently to enable me to pass a ligature around

[1] Rice, N. P. 1859. *Trials of a public benefactor.* New York. 92.

them. The patient was arranged for the operation in a sitting posture, and everything made ready. . . . The patient was then made to inhale a fluid from a tube connected with a glass globe. After four or five minutes he appeared to be asleep, and was thought by Dr. Morton to be in a condition for the operation. I made an incision between two and three inches long in the direction of the tumor, and to my great surprise without any starting, crying, or other indication of pain. The fascia was then divided, the patient still appearing wholly insensible. Then followed the insulation of the veins, during which he began to move his limbs, cry out, and utter extraordinary expressions. These phenomena led to a doubt of the success of the application ; and in truth I was not satisfied myself, until I had, soon after the operation and on various other occasions, asked the question whether he had suffered pain. To this he always replied in the negative, adding, however, that he knew of the operation, and comparing the stroke of the knife to that of a blunt instrument passed roughly across his neck.' [1]   Finally, Warren is said to have turned to the onlookers and made his famous remark, ' Gentlemen, this is no humbug '.

' On the following day a woman requiring the removal of an adipose tumor from the arm was rendered insensible by ether given by Dr. Morton ; and Dr. Warren requested Dr. Hayward, one of the visiting surgeons who was present, to perform the operation. This was successful ; the ether being continued through the whole operation, which was a short one, and the patient being entirely insensible.' [2]

Morton was greatly excited by his success. The newspapers were giving prominence to accounts of the painless operations. Boston scientific circles were eager for information and letters to Morton about the discovery were pouring in, so that ' he was obliged to employ a secretary to answer these communications '. This was Morton's heyday. So far his luck had been exceptional. Circumstance had suggested to him the use of sulphuric ether vapour where to Wells it had suggested nitrous oxide. Warren, at once willing to believe in, yet sceptical of, the possibility of painless operations, had arranged a demonstration. For this Morton arrived late, flustered and with an unfamiliar and untested piece of apparatus snatched barely finished from the

---

[1] Quoted in *Trans. Amer. surg. Ass.*, 1897, **15,** 16.
[2] *Trans. Amer. surg. Ass.*, 1897, **15,** 17.

maker's hands. Ignorant of the precise nature of the physiological processes he was setting in motion he nevertheless succeeded in rendering his patient sufficiently insensible to pain to convince a critical audience that his claim was genuine. In not very dissimilar circumstances Wells had failed to substantiate his claim ; he failed primarily because he was not using ether but the weaker (and with the apparatus at his disposal) far less manageable agent, nitrous oxide. Warren and his colleagues, who had been apathetic in Wells's case, now lent Morton their enthusiastic support, endorsing the value of etherization with their own names.

Elated by the patronage of the hospital authorities, Morton was full of grandiose schemes for the future. ' From the day of the first experiment forward, it is safe to say,' wrote Dana, ' that Dr. Morton hardly knew a full night's rest, or a regular meal, for three months. . . . His dental business was neglected '. He began to publish numbers of pamphlets recording successful cases and elaborating fresh ideas about the use of his still secret ' preparation '. He planned a world-wide advertising scheme and ' had great numbers of the inhaling apparatus made and presented to various surgeons and charitable institutions, at home and abroad ; and . . . sent several very costly ones to the chief sovereigns of Europe '.[1] Confident that his patent would be granted he set about appointing agents to sell the rights.

On October 19, 1846, Morton wrote to Horace Wells :

' FRIEND WELLS. DEAR SIR,—I write to inform you that I have discovered a preparation, by inhaling which a person is thrown into a sound sleep. The time required to produce sleep is only a few moments, and the time in which persons remain asleep can be regulated at pleasure. While in this state, the severest surgical or dental operations may be performed, the patient not experiencing the slightest pain. I have perfected it, and am now about sending out agents to dispose of the right to use it. I will dispose of a right to an individual to use it in his own practice alone, or for a town, county or state. My object in writing to you is to know if you would not like to visit New York and the other cities, and dispose of rights upon shares. I have used the compound in more than a hundred and sixty cases in extracting teeth ; and I have been invited to administer to patients in the Massachusetts General Hospital, and have succeeded in every case.

' The professors, Warren and Hayward, have given me certificates to this effect. . . . For further particulars, I will refer you to extracts from the daily journals of this city, which I forward to you.'

[1] *Littell's Living Age*, 1848, **16**, 543.

Wells replied on October 20 :

'DR. MORTON. DEAR SIR,—Your letter dated yesterday is just received ; and I hasten to answer it, for I fear you will adopt a method in disposing of your rights which will defeat your object. Before you make any arrangements whatever, I wish to see you. I think I will be in Boston the first of next week—probably Monday night. If the operation of administering the gas is not attended with too much trouble, and will produce the effect you state, it will undoubtedly be a fortune to you, provided it is rightly managed.' [1]

Events were soon to prove that Wells's forebodings were not groundless.

The next day, October 21, Eddy informed Morton that he had come to the conclusion that etherization could be patented. He added, however, that Dr. C. T. Jackson had been to see him and that what he learned from Jackson led him to consider the discovery a joint one. If a patent were applied for then Jackson's name ought to be associated with Morton's. Two days later Jackson called at Morton's office. Morton described the interview :

' He said he thought he would just look in, that he heard I was doing well with the ether, and learned from Mr. Eddy that I intended to take out a patent. . . . He said . . . he believed he must make me a professional charge for advice. I asked him why in this case, more than in any other case of his advice. . . . He said that his advice had been useful to me, that I should make a good deal out of the patent, and that I ought to make him a compensation. I told him I would do so if I made much by the patent. . . . He then said he should charge me $500. I told him I would pay him that, if ten per cent. on the net profits of the patent amounted to so much . . .' [2]

After this encounter Morton again visited Eddy. Unfortunately for Morton, Eddy was one of Jackson's many friends and admirers in Boston and he afterwards admitted that in all his early dealings with Morton in connection with the patent he was prejudiced in Jackson's favour. This attitude becomes understandable, if not excusable, when the circumstances of the two men, as they were known to Eddy, are contrasted : Jackson

[1] United States : 32 Congress, 2d Session in Senate of the United States, Feb. 19, 1853 : *Walker Report*, 22.
[2] *Littell's Living Age*, 1848, **16**, 545.

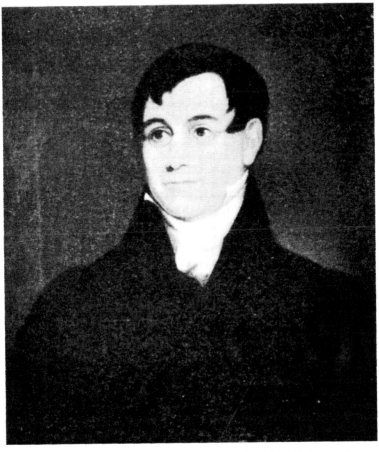

FIG. 13.—CHARLES THOMAS JACKSON (1805–80)

Chemist and geologist, of Boston, Massachusetts, who claimed that it was he who first made known to W. T. G. Morton the anaesthetic properties of sulphuric ether and recommended Morton to make a trial of it in preference to any other drug.

was a scientist, an established and a respected figure in Boston's intellectual circle ; Morton, on the other hand, was 'not a man of much cultivation or science ',[1] who had come to Eddy as a client obviously hoping to make money and a reputation for himself from etherization.

At this second interview between Eddy and Morton, Eddy, who in the meantime had heard Jackson's own account of his visit to Morton on October 23, suggested that instead of paying Jackson a fee Morton should ' interest him in the patent ' and give him 10 per cent. of the net profits. Not only would the patent then have the benefit of Jackson's name but his knowledge would the more readily be at Morton's disposal in developing the technique of etherization.

Eddy could not have used more persuasive arguments. The dentists of Boston, each jealous of Morton's success and apprehensive of its effects upon his own practice, had lately ' entered into a systematic and organized opposition. They appointed a committee of vigilance to ascertain and publish every instance in which experiments had failed, or had produced ill-effects '. Such instances were neither hard to find nor difficult to embellish and the outcry against Morton was beginning to spread so that ' all the medical magazines in the Union, except Boston [where the influence of Warren and his colleagues was strong] were arrayed against it [etherization] '.[2] ' If a suit was brought ', Eddy pointed out to Morton, ' and Dr. Jackson should be a witness, as he doubtless would be, the aid he had given [Morton] . . . might be made a handle of by persons impeaching the patent, to invalidate . . . [his] claim as the discoverer '.[3] ' My views,' wrote Eddy, ' seemed to strike Dr. Morton very favourably and he acquiesced in them. . . . Had Dr. Morton, during this time, stated to me what I have since read in the affidavit of Dr. G. G. Hayden, Messrs. Leavitt, Spear and Whiteman, I am confident I never should have advised him to associate Dr. Jackson in the discovery or patent '.[4]

Morton's own explanation of his acquiescence was this : ' I felt the need of all the aid I could get and was conscious of

---

[1] These words are Jacob Bigelow's (*Boston med. surg. J.*, 1870, N.S. **5**, 187). Bigelow was well qualified to express such an opinion for he was on terms of professional friendship with the senior members of the staff of the Massachusetts General Hospital, had watched Morton demonstrate at the hospital and had been the first to send the news of etherization to England (see p. 130).

[2] *Littell's Living Age*, 1848, **16**, 545.   [3] *Ibid.* **16**, 570   [4] *Ibid.* **16**, 547.

want of thorough scientific education myself. I was induced by these motives to accede to Mr. Eddy's request, but did not then understand that Dr. Jackson claimed to be a discoverer at all.' [1] ' I am ready to acknowledge my indebtedness to men and to books for all my information upon this subject [etherization]. I have got here a little and there a little. I learned from Dr. Jackson, in 1844, the effect of ether directly applied to a sensitive tooth, and proved by experiment that it would gradually render the nerve insensible. I learned from Dr. Jackson, also in 1844, the effect of ether when inhaled by students at college, which was corroborated by Spear's account and by what I read. I further acknowledge that I was subsequently indebted to Dr. Jackson for valuable information as to the kinds and preparations of ether, and for the recommendation of the highly rectified [ether] from Burnett's [a Boston druggist], as the most safe and efficient. But my obligations to him hath this extent, no further.' [2]

This is almost certainly a true valuation of Morton's indebtedness to Jackson. But in attempting to silence adverse criticism by securing Jackson's name on the patent (at the cost of 10 per cent. of possible profits) Morton had, therefore, only the slender justification of advice from Jackson which, although helpful, had not been essential to the establishment of etherization. His behaviour towards Jackson, in this matter, appears disingenuous, and he certainly placed himself in a vulnerable position of which Jackson was not slow to take advantage.

Jackson at first refused to be associated in the patent and insisted on his fee of $500. His enemies later said that this was because he feared Morton's success might not be lasting and, indeed, might end disastrously in the death of a patient. Jackson himself, at the time,[3] said that it was because he believed such an undertaking to be against the laws of the Massachusetts

[1] *Littell's Living Age*, 1848, **16**, 570.
[2] Letter addressed to the Académie des Sciences (cf. p. 125), quoted by N. P. Rice in *Trials of a public benefactor*, p. 194.
[3] Some five months later, Martin Gay, M.D., a supporter of Jackson, with a witness, ' called at Dr. Morton's office . . . and dramatically cancelled the bond . . . that secured to Dr. Jackson ten per cent. on the net profits of the American patent. On the same day, the anniversary of the Massachusetts Medical Society took place, and at the dinner . . . Dr. Jackson made a speech, in which he claimed to have been entirely disinterested in his connection with the discovery, and said he had destroyed the bond. He did not say that he had destroyed it that morning '. (*Littell's Living Age*, 1848, **16**, 551.)

Medical Society, of which he was a respected member.[1] But whatever the reason, Eddy finally succeeded in convincing him that his reputation could in no way be injured. It was then agreed that the patent, which claimed as original inventions both the use of ether to produce insensibility to surgical pain and the inhaler for administering it, should be taken out jointly in the names of Morton and Jackson ; but Jackson, at the same time, further agreed to assign all his rights in the patent to Morton.[2] On account of this concession Jackson was to receive 10 per cent. of the profits accruing from the American sales of the patent and an agreement accordingly was drawn up. The application for the patent was signed by the patentees on October 27, 1846, and the Letter Patent, No. 4848, was issued by the United States Patent Office on November 12, 1846.[3] Subsequently another patent was taken out to cover sales abroad and this too was issued in the names of Morton and Jackson jointly, because Eddy believed that it would not otherwise be valid in France.

As Eddy had feared, the issuing of the patent immediately gave a handle to Morton's brother dentists and they published a manifesto in which they protested ' against holding the right to use [ether] on such tenure, or as a secret medicine '. More damaging still to Morton, the surgeons of the Massachusetts General Hospital suddenly adopted a similar attitude and totally suspended the use of Morton's ' preparation ' in the hospital. They banned it partly because it was a ' secret remedy ' (for although it obviously consisted principally of sulphuric ether, Morton in fact had never made known what, if any, were the other constituents of his ' preparation '), partly because it was now protected under patent.

' Anxious to extend the benefits of the inhalation to as many patients as possible ', wrote J. C. Warren, and ' believing a particular apparatus necessary, and having the use of none excepting that in the hands of Dr. Morton, I requested Dr. Charles Heywood, the house surgeon of the hospital (who took an early and active interest in the matter), to procure a glass globe and add to it the tube necessary for its application.   At this period, however, I was checked by the information that an exclusive patent had been taken out, and that no application could be made without the

[1] *Littell's Living Age*, 1848, **16**, 546–7.   [2] See Appendix A.
[3] For the patent specification see Appendix A.

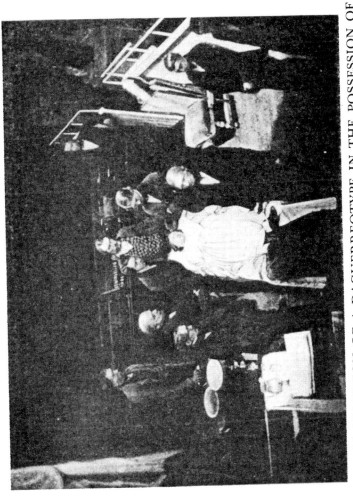

FIG. 14.—REPRODUCTION OF A DAGUERREOTYPE IN THE POSSESSION OF THE WARREN FAMILY (1897).

'The illustration represents the operating-theatre of the Massachusetts General Hospital in the winter of 1847. The sponge used here is known as the first sponge with which ether was given. . . . The surgeons whose portraits appear in this picture are, on the patient's left, Dr. John C. Warren, Dr. Samuel Parkman ; on the patient's right, Dr. J. Mason Warren and Dr. Townsend. The etherizer is probably Dr. Heywood.'

This illustration forms an interesting comparison with Fig. 15 (p. 119).

permission of the proprietor. The knowledge of this patent decided me not to use nor encourage the use of the inhalation until a more liberal arrangement could be made.' [1]

On November 5 Morton hastily agreed to relax the patent in favour of the hospital ; he presented the surgeons with an inhaler and promised to give any information that should be required regarding the exact nature and use of his ' preparation '. Nevertheless, he stipulated that such information must be considered confidential. The hospital authorities accepted these terms and etherization was resumed on November 7, 1846, for an amputation, the first to be performed under its influence. On November 21, the identity of ether was officially cloaked by the name ' Letheon ' (suggested by Gould) at a meeting between Morton and two representatives of the hospital, H. J. Bigelow and Oliver Wendell Holmes. [2]

Meanwhile the first paper on etherization had been read ; it was delivered by H. J. Bigelow on November 9, 1846, at a meeting of the Boston Society of Medical Improvement.

After asserting the importance of the discovery, Bigelow described the first operation at the hospital on October 16. He also said that he himself had carried out a few experiments to discover ' the nature of the new agent '. After testing sulphuric ether against ethereal oil and chloric ether he concluded from his unsatisfactory results with these latter substances that the agent was in fact sulphuric ether. Case histories followed.

' I have been unable to learn that any serious consequences have ensued ', said Bigelow. ' One or two robust patients have failed to be affected . . . very young subjects are affected with nausea and vomiting and for this reason Dr. Morton has refused to administer it to children.

' It is natural to inquire ', Bigelow continued, ' with whom this invention originated. Without entering into details I learn that the patent bears the name of Dr. Charles T. Jackson, a distinguished chemist, and of Dr. Morton, a skilful dentist of this city, as inventors. . . . It has been considered desirable by the interested parties that the character of the agent employed by them should not be at this time announced, but it may be stated that it has been made known to those gentlemen who have had occasion to avail themselves of it.'

[1] *Trans. Amer. surg. Ass.*, 1897, **15,** 17.
[2] Holmes soon afterwards suggested that the noun *anaesthesia*, and the adjective *anaesthetic* which he derived from it, should be substituted for the name *Letheon* (see Appendix B).

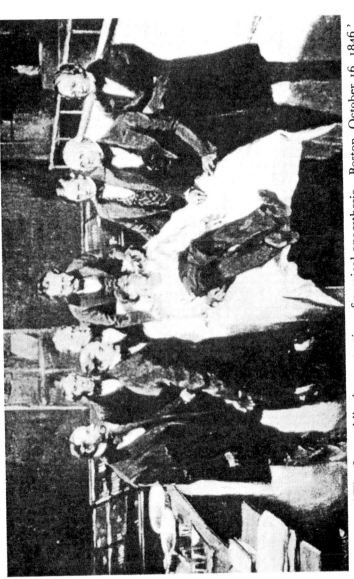

FIG. 15.—' The first public demonstration of surgical anaesthesia—Boston, October 16, 1846 '
—a scene obviously reconstructed from the daguerreotype shown in Fig. 14 (q.v.).

For the original figures have been substituted :
(*On the left, in front*) H. J. Bigelow, J. Mason Warren.   (*Behind*) A. A. Gould, J. C. Warren.
(*In the middle*) W. T. G. Morton applying his inhaler (not clearly shown) to the patient's mouth.
(*On the right, in front*) S. D. Townsend, George Hayward.   (*Behind*) Samuel Parkman.

This illustration appeared in *The semi-centennial of anaesthesia, October 16, 1846, October 16, 1896*, published by
the Trustees of the Massachusetts General Hospital, Boston, 1897.   Another variant of it had appeared in N. P.
Rice's *Trials of a public benefactor* (New York, 1859), facing p. 92.

119

In spite of the fact that his colleagues at the hospital were not bound by the patent, Bigelow seems to have felt that some justification for it was necessary :

' No one will deny ', he explained, ' that he who benefits the world should receive from it an equivalent. The only question is . . . shall it be voluntarily ceded by the world or levied upon it ? . . . Many will assent with reluctance to the propriety of restricting by letters patent the use of an agent capable of mitigating human suffering. There are various reasons, however, which apologise for the arrangement which I understand to have been made with regard to the application of the new agent. 1. It is capable of abuse and can readily be applied to nefarious ends. 2. Its action is not yet thoroughly understood, and its use should be restricted to responsible persons. 3. . . . In the mechanical art of dentistry many processes are by convention, secret. It is especially with reference to this art that the patent has been secured. . . . [The patentees'] intentions are extremely liberal with regard to the medical profession generally ; and so soon as necessary arrangements can be made for publicity of the process, great facilities will be offered to those who are disposed to avail themselves of what now promises to be one of the important discoveries of the age.' [1]

An abstract of this paper had already, on November 3, been submitted to a meeting of the American Society of Arts and Sciences. Both this institution and the Boston Society of Medical Improvement received the paper well and the text was reprinted in the current medical journals and in the daily press. A copy of the *Boston Daily Advertiser* containing H. J. Bigelow's paper was sent, on November 28, 1846, by his father Jacob Bigelow, Professor of Materia Medica in the Harvard Medical School, to an old friend in England, the American-born and Harvard-educated Dr. Boott of Gower Street, London (see p. 130).

Jackson, returning to Boston after a week's absence, found that the attitude of the general public towards etherization had changed from growing hostility to cordial interest ; and it appeared likely that scientific opinion also would be favourable, certainly in America and probably abroad. At all events the good reception given to Bigelow's paper in Boston clearly showed which way the wind was blowing there, and Jackson trimmed his sails accordingly.

[1] *Lancet*, 1847, i, 6–8.

On November 15, at an informal meeting between Eddy and Jackson, Jackson for the first time claimed not merely that he had given Morton advice but that the entire discovery that ether could be used to produce insensibility to surgical pain was his, Morton having acted in every particular merely upon his instructions. ' Mr. Eddy was astonished beyond measure at this ', affirmed R. H. Dana, ' and reasoned with Dr. Jackson upon it, but to no purpose '.[1]

The next day Jackson called at Eddy's office with his solicitor and demanded a percentage of the profits on the European patents (cf. p. 116). This was at first refused by Eddy, who now seriously began to doubt Jackson's good faith, whereupon Jackson threatened to send an already-prepared communication to Europe by that day's mail boat, claiming the whole discovery as his alone, ' which would defeat the European patents alto- gether '. Finally Eddy agreed that Jackson should receive a percentage on the European patents on condition that no com- munication was despatched to Europe.[1]

Directly the fact that Morton had obtained a patent for etherization became publicly known, friends of Horace Wells began urging him to assert his prior claim to the discovery of surgical anaesthesia.

Wells, soon after his rebuff at the Massachusetts General Hospital (see p. 96), became ill, no doubt through worry and disappointment, as he himself claimed.[2] On his recovery, finding his neglected dental practice gone and his hopes of success in the use of nitrous oxide uncertain, he took other employment which promised to bring in the ready money which he needed. During 1845 and 1846 he drifted from one unsatisfactory occu- pation to another, and in December 1846 he was about to sail for France on a new enterprise, art dealing in a small way. Before he left America he so far acted upon his friends' advice as to address a long letter to the editor of the *Hartford Courant*, giving a somewhat modified account of how he came to use nitrous oxide. He also claimed that ' when I was deciding what exhilarating agent to use . . . it immediately occurred to me that it would be best to use [either] nitrous oxide or sulphuric ether. I advised with Dr. Marcy, of this city, and by his advice

[1] *Littell's Living Age*, 1848, **16**, 548.
[2] Well, H.   1847.   *A history of the discovery of the application of nitrous oxide gas . . . to surgical operations*.   Hartford.   7.

I continued to use the former, as being the least likely to do injury, although it was attended with some trouble in its preparation '. Wells ended this letter with the pertinent statement :

' If Drs. Jackson and Morton claim that they use something else, I reply that it is the same in principle, if not in name, and they can not use anything which will produce more satisfactory results, and I made these results known to both these individuals, more than a year since. After making the above statement of facts, I leave it for the public to decide to whom belongs the honor of discovery.'

Later, Wells addressed a letter to the members of the Académie des Sciences in Paris, an extract from which appeared in the *Comptes Rendus* (March 8, 1847). In this letter he described his use of nitrous oxide during December 1844, and the unfortunate demonstration at the Massachusetts General Hospital in 1845, and again claimed that he had experimented with the inhalation of ether vapour (during November 1844, *i.e. prior* to Colton's lecture), but had rejected it in favour of nitrous oxide gas.[1]

Soon after the beginning of the year 1847 news reached Morton that letters dated from Boston, November 13 and December 1, 1846, had, contrary to the undertaking given to Eddy, been despatched by Jackson to Europe, addressed to his friend Élie de Beaumont, in Paris. The letter dated November 13 claimed for Jackson the discovery of the anaesthetic use of sulphuric ether and the responsibility for its introduction into surgical practice through his agent, whom he did not mention by name but described merely as ' a dentist of this city '. The letter, dated December 1, stated briefly that the use of ether vapour had been thoroughly tested in America and introduced with great success at the Massachusetts General Hospital. These letters, in a sealed packet, were deposited in the Archives of the Académie des Sciences[2] by Élie de Beaumont on December 28, 1846.[3] They remained there until January 18, 1847, when— the subject of etherization having been raised by other members of the Académie in the course of a meeting—Élie de Beaumont considered the time opportune for advancing Jackson's claims.

[1] *C.R. Acad. Sci.*, Paris, 1847, **24**, 372.　　[2] *Ibid.* 1846, **23**, 1159.
[3] Scientists wishing to establish priority in a discovery were in the habit of stating the facts of the case in a letter which remained sealed, in the archives of the institution concerned, until further research had either confirmed or disproved the value of the ' discovery '. Then at the request of the depositor or his agent the letter could be opened and read before the members of the institution or destroyed unopened.

He therefore asked that the sealed packet should be opened and the contents read, which was accordingly done (cf. p. 136).

A translation of Jackson's letter of November 13, addressed to Élie de Beaumont, which was in French, reads as follows :

' I ask your permission to communicate to the Académie des Sciences through you, a discovery which I have made and which I believe to be important to the relief of suffering humanity, and of great value in the art of surgery.

' Five or six years ago I recognized the peculiar state of insensibility into which the system is plunged by the inhalation of the vapour of pure sulphuric ether, which I breathed in great quantity, at first as an experiment and later at a moment when I had a severe cold caused by the inhalation of chlorine. I lately turned this fact to useful account by persuading a dentist of this city to administer the vapour of ether to persons from whom he had to extract teeth. It was observed that these persons showed no sign of pain during the operation, and that no inconvenience resulted from the administration of ether vapour.

' I then requested this dentist to go to the Massachusetts General Hospital and administer ether vapour to a patient about to undergo a painful surgical operation. The result was that the patient showed not the least sign of pain during the operation and subsequently did well. An operation on the jaw, the amputation of a leg and the dissection of a tumour have been the subjects of the initial surgical tests. Since then numerous surgical operations have been performed on different patients with the same success and always without pain. The patients have had remarkably easy convalescences, showing no signs of nervous shock. . . .

' I desire that the Académie des Sciences will have the goodness to nominate a commission entrusted with the task of making the necessary experiments to prove the correctness of the assertions which I have made to you on the marvellous effects of the inhalation of ether vapour.

' One can breathe this vapour very comfortably by dipping a large sponge in the ether, placing it in a short, conical tube or in a funnel and drawing atmospheric air into the lungs through the ether-saturated sponge. The air may then be exhaled through the nostrils or else valves may be added to the tube or funnel, so that the breath does not escape through the sponge, where it dilutes the ether with the water vapour it contains.

' At the end of a few minutes the patient falls into a peculiar state of sleep and may be submitted to any surgical operation without evincing any pain. His pulse generally becomes a little more rapid and his eyes shine as though through the effects of some special state of excitement. On coming to himself, at the end of a few minutes, he will tell you that he has both *slept* and *dreamed*.

' If the ether is weak it does not produce its proper effect. The patient will be inebriated only, and will subsequently experience a dull headache.

' One must not, consequently, make use of any but the most highly rectified ether.

' If a dentist is to extract teeth at night, it is advisable to have a Davy safety lamp to contain the light, in order to prevent the danger of explosions caused by the ether vapour, which would explode if a naked flame were approached to the mouth.

' In order to administer ether vapour it is important to have a large volume of it, so that it can be respired freely and produce its effect promptly, because in this way all disagreeable sensation is avoided ; but no danger is to be feared from a prolonged inhalation of ether vapour, so long as atmospheric air shall itself be adequately admitted. In prolonged operations one may reapply the ether vapour several times at convenient intervals so as to keep the patient asleep.' [1]

Directly Morton learned the contents of this letter he began collecting evidence to prove the falsity of Jackson's statements. This evidence consisted chiefly of sworn statements made by Morton's employees and by fellow-citizens who, in various ways, had rendered Morton professional services in connection with etherization.

At about this time it was suggested to Jackson by J. C. Warren and Edward Everett, both distinguished members of the American Academy of Sciences, that he should describe from the scientist's point of view, at the next meeting of the Academy, the anaesthetic properties of sulphuric ether and how these came to be applied. On March 1, 1847, just before the meeting, Jackson published in the Press the text of the paper which he proposed to read and several copies were despatched to Europe by the steamer which left Boston on the day of publication. The text submitted to the Press was so worded as to imply not only that it had been read before the American Academy, but that claims and opinions expressed in it by Jackson had received the approval of the Academy and of Warren and Everett in particular. Jackson, rating nothing so high as his scientific reputation among the members of the Académie des Sciences, had been particularly anxious to get his speech into print in time to catch the mail for Paris. He apparently overlooked the possible consequences of this action in Boston.

[1] *C.R. Acad. Sci.*, Paris, 1847, **24**, 74.

The effect produced by this paper in Paris was all that Jackson hoped and for a time his name alone was associated with the discovery.[1] But at home Jackson was immediately censured for what was considered a piece of sharp practice. The American Academy refused to publish the unauthorized text in its *Transactions* and many men of importance began for the first time seriously to doubt the truth of Jackson's assertion that, but for his knowledge and the advice which he had given to Morton, the discovery and application of ether anaesthesia could not have been possible.

Since no boat again left for Europe until April 1, 1847, it was a month before Morton could himself address a letter to the Académie des Sciences, refuting Jackson's claims and asserting his own. The receipt of this letter was recorded in the *Comptes Rendus* of the Académie on May 17, 1847, but the text was not published.[2]

Morton, meanwhile, had published a pamphlet entitled *Some account of the Letheon*. Its appearance was seized upon by Jackson as an excuse finally to reject a suggestion made more than once by Morton and Eddy since Jackson's first despatch of letters to Europe, that their rival claims should be submitted to the decision of an impartial judge or judges.[3]

It was now daily becoming more evident that the patent could not be enforced either in America or abroad. Even at the Massachusetts General Hospital, John Mason Warren, son of John Collins Warren, in February 1847, had finally abandoned Morton's inhaling apparatus in favour of a bell-shaped sponge[4] which, after being saturated with ether, was applied directly over the patient's nose and mouth[5] (see Fig. 14).

[1] In 1850 the Académie des Sciences decided to award one of the prizes (amounting to 2500 francs) for medicine and surgery for the years 1847 and 1848, to Jackson, ' for his observations and experiments on the anaesthetic effects produced by the inhalation of ether ', and a similar prize to Morton, ' for having introduced this method into surgical practice according to the directions of M. Jackson '. (*C.R. Acad. Sci.*, Paris, 1850, **30**, 244.)
During 1852 Jackson twice questioned the grounds on which the prize had been awarded to Morton ; his aim was to make the Académie state definitely that it recognized Jackson himself as the ' inventor ' and Morton merely as his ' agent '. The Académie refused, referring Jackson to the wording of the original announcement of the two prizes in the *Comptes Rendus*. (*C.R. Acad. Sci.*, Paris, 1852, **34**, 774, 922.)
[2] *C.R. Acad. Sci.*, Paris, 1847, **24**, 878.   [3] *Littell's Living Age*, 1848, **16**, 551.
[4] *Trans. Amer. surg. Ass.*, 1897, **15**, 25.
[5] The use of an ether-soaked sponge, at first alone, later enclosed in a cone improvised from a folded towel or cut out from cardboard, felt, leather, or even from metal, quickly spread in the States and remained in general use there from the early months of the year 1847 until the end of the nineteenth century (see, *e.g.*, pp. 313, 319 and footnote).

Morton, instead of making a fortune, found himself falling deeply in debt and, since he had neglected his dental business past retrieving, he was without ready means of recuperating his losses. He addressed letters to both the United States Navy and the Surgeon-General of the Army, drawing attention to his discovery and suggesting the use of ether ' for the relief of the suffering soldiers and sailors engaged in the Mexican war '. He offered ' to send agents to Mexico at once, whose expenses to the Government would be but a few hundred dollars, while the apparatus would be furnished at wholesale price, and the ether would cost but one or two cents to each patient '.[1] Both Services declined his offer, the Navy on April 17, the Army on May 3, 1847 ; both proceeded to make use of etherization, the patent notwithstanding.   Here was a curious anomaly : the United States Government first issued a patent, then refused to subscribe to it and finally infringed it.

On April 20, 1847, Eddy wrote to Jackson :

' I am required as often as once in six months, to render you an account of the net profits resulting from sales of certain patents, etc. . . . I have now to inform you . . . that, up to this date, April 2d, 1847, I have received no net profits on account of any and therefore can render you no further account than this, nor pay to you any moneys resulting from any net profits received.'

The result of this communication, according to Nathan P. Rice,[2] was that :

' On the 26th of May, Dr. Gay, attended by a witness, called at the office of Dr. Morton, and . . . informed him that he was present at the request of Dr. Jackson. He said that the tender conscience of Dr. Jackson was troubled . . . that he was unwilling to receive ten per cent. on the profits which he had before bargained for, as he could not but feel that it would burn in his pockets as so much blood money, etc. After which long peroration, Dr. Gay, in the presence of Dr. Morton, destroyed the bond by which Dr. Jackson was enabled to show that he ever owned any rights under the patent.' [3]

In November 1847, Morton, jointly with Augustus A. Gould, took out a patent for a new ether inhaler[4] which, although considerably elaborated, was nevertheless similar in

[1] Rice, N. P. 1859. *Trials of a public benefactor.* New York. 121.
[2] Cf. footnote, p. 115.
[3] Rice, N. P. 1859. *Trials of a public benefactor.* New York. 231, 233.
[4] See Appendix A.

principle to the inhaler patented by Morton and Jackson in 1846. This was Morton's last achievement as a practical anaesthetist. Thenceforward his energies were directed not to the development of etherization but towards gaining recognition as its sole discoverer, and to securing some substantial financial reward on that account, to recompense him for the failure of the patents as well as for the loss of his formerly prosperous dental business.

Already, on December 28, 1846, Morton, supported by his friends, had presented a memorial to Congress claiming a monetary reward for his discovery. The application was promptly opposed by the friends of Horace Wells, on the grounds that Wells had, in principle, a prior right to be considered the discoverer of anaesthesia. Neither Morton nor Wells gained anything by their petitions ; but this further failure to achieve recognition as the pioneer of anaesthesia seriously disturbed the balance of Wells's mind and in 1848, in sad and sordid circumstances, he killed himself.

In January 1849, Morton visited Washington and—supported by a resolution passed in his favour by the Governors of the Massachusetts General Hospital and others—again petitioned Congress. On this occasion a committee of investigation was set up and the chairman ' addressed a letter to the opponents of Dr. Morton, requesting them to put in before the committee any documents against his claim and in support of their own '. On this occasion the committee reported in Morton's favour, but still the matter did not progress.[1]

Morton retired to the country and took up farming, at which he proved successful ; but the urge to seek recognition would not leave him, and in 1851 he made a third and last application to Congress. The Select Committee of the House of Representatives then recommended that the sum of one thousand dollars should be paid to Morton on condition that he surrendered his patent to the United States Government. This recommendation was bitterly opposed by the widow and friends of Wells and also, of course, by Jackson. The official proceedings moved slowly.

In 1852 Crawford W. Long was persuaded by his friends to come forward as the original discoverer of etherization. Jackson

---

[1] Morton, W. T. G. 1850. *Remarks on the comparative value of ether and chloroform.* Boston. 15.

himself supported Long's claim, seeing in it an opportunity to weaken Morton's case. Subsequently the names of other claimants were added to those of Long, Wells, Morton and Jackson, although their pretensions were too flimsy to merit the Committee's serious consideration.[1]

A Bill ' to recompense the discoverer of practical anaesthesia ', after many amendments, passed the Senate on April 19, 1854. Two days later it came up for consideration before the House of Representatives. On the grounds of ' the multiplicity of claimants ' the Bill was summarily rejected and Morton was advised to enforce his patent.[2] Backed by a number of influential men Morton organized a protest against this decision. After months of waiting he was granted an interview with the President of the United States.

At this interview he was told that ' before paying any sum for the patent, the government wished a legal decision on the case ; it had decided that a judgment should be procured against it, so that it should be compelled to make restitution '. The President himself ' proposed that a suit should be commenced against some surgeon of the government service who had at some period used the discovery, and who should be instructed by the Executive to admit the use of any agent covered by his patent, and consequently Dr. Morton would be put to no trouble or expense to prove it ; that the suit when brought should be considered as brought against the government . . . and that the government [which could not itself be sued] should shoulder all the responsibility '.[3]

Despite the President's advice and assurances Morton was reluctant to begin this undertaking. In 1853 his farm stock had been sold up or seized by his creditors and the farm itself mortgaged, and he was now practically without means and heavily in debt. He hesitated until 1858 and then instigated a suit against the Superintendent of the United States Marine Hospital at Chelsea, near Boston. Fresh delays occurred and Morton's misgivings proved to be well founded. The Government failed to support him either morally or financially and in 1862 the case was dismissed on the grounds that the patent was not, after all, valid.

[1] Cf. United States : 32 Congress, 2d Session in Congress of the United States, Feb. 19, 1853.
[2] Rice, N. P. 1859. *Trials of a public benefactor.* New York. 282–373.
[3] *Ibid.* 415, 416.

These proceedings finally ended any hope Morton still had of gaining a reward from the State. Although many men of standing in America and abroad now acknowledged the importance of Morton's part in the establishment of anaesthesia, and estimated Jackson's contribution at its true value, their recognition came too late. When Morton returned to his farm in 1862 he was a broken man. He lived there with his family in aimless, squalid poverty until 1868, when a new pamphlet of Jackson's on ' his discovery ' goaded Morton into action. He journeyed to New York, intending to file a suit against Jackson, and arrived during a heat wave. Not many days later, while out driving with his wife, he had an apoplectic seizure and within a few hours was dead.

PART TWO

THE USE OF ANAESTHESIA ESTABLISHED

CHAPTER IV

ADOPTION OF ETHER ; PHYSIOLOGY OF ANAESTHESIA

Introduction of Etherization into Europe and Early Methods of Administration—Early Work on the Physiology of Anaesthesia—Flourens and Snow and their Establishment of Basic Principles in connection with Anaesthesia.

Etherization Introduced into Europe and Early Methods of Administration

' MY DEAR BOOTT ', wrote Professor Jacob Bigelow on November 28, 1846, from Boston, to his friend in London, ' I send you an account of a new anodyne process lately introduced here, which promises to be one of the important discoveries of the present age. . . .

' The inventor is Dr. Morton, a dentist of this city, and the process consists of the inhalation of the vapour of ether to the point of intoxication. I send you the *Boston Daily Advertiser*, which contains an article written by my son Henry . . . relating to the discovery. . . . The newspaper will give you the details up to its date, since which other operations have been performed with uniform success.' [1]

The letter was three weeks in transit, but on receiving it Boott immediately appreciated the importance of this news from America and set about broadcasting it. He wrote to the *Lancet*, enclosing the elder Bigelow's letter and the copy of the son's article. He wrote to Robert Liston, Professor of Clinical Surgery in the University of London, famous for his dexterity. When Liston amputated ' the gleam of his knife was followed so instantaneously by the sound of sawing as to make the two actions appear almost simultaneous '.[2] Such speed had always been

[1] *Lancet*, 1847, i, 5.
[2] *Dictionary of national biography*, London, 1909, **11**, 1236.

highly prized in a surgeon, but now its intrinsic value—the shortening of the duration of agony for the patient—had become a thing of the past.

A few days later Boott again wrote to the *Lancet*, reporting the first anaesthetic use of ether in this country. ' On Saturday, the 19th, a firmly fixed molar tooth was extracted in my study

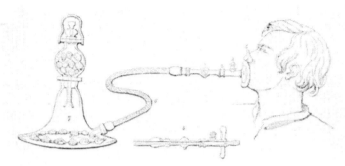

THE APPARATUS FOR RENDERING SURGICAL OPERATIONS PAINLESS.

Fig. 16.—HOOPER'S INHALER

Made to the specification of Boott and Robinson, during December 1846.

1. Pad for mouth, to be held by the operator.
2. Horizontal valve for the escape of expired air.
3. Vertical flap valve
4. Stop-cock.
5. Nasal spring.
6. Elastic tube.
7. Glass vessel, with a smaller one having pieces of sponge saturated with ether, and having a small perforated stopper, to be opened when the apparatus is in use.
8. Sectional view of the pad, showing the mouthpiece.

from Miss Lonsdale, by Mr. Robinson . . . without the least sense of pain, or the movement of a muscle. The whole process of inhalation, extracting and waking was over in three minutes.' It was stated in the *Illustrated London News* for January 9, 1847, that on this occasion an apparatus made by Hooper, of Pall Mall, to the specification of Boott and Robinson (see Fig. 16), was used ; but Boott himself, in his communication to the *Lancet*, made no reference to the nature of the apparatus.

On Monday, December 21, 1846, Liston wrote to Boott :

' My Dear Sir,—I tried the ether inhalation to-day in a case of amputation of the thigh, and in another requiring evulsion of both sides of the great toe-nail, one of the most painful operations in surgery, and with the most perfect and satisfactory results.

' It is a very great matter to be able thus to destroy sensibility to such an extent, and without, apparently, any bad result. It is a fine thing for operating surgeons, and I thank you most sincerely for the early information you were so kind as to give me of it.' [1]

Liston's first two operations on etherized patients, to which he referred, were performed at University College Hospital and many notable men, including Joseph Lister, were present ; and among the nonentities was a young surgeon, Joseph Thomas Clover, who in later years became famous as an anaesthetist.

The scene in the operating theatre was described by an eye-witness, a certain Dr. Forbes :

' Shortly after being placed on the operating table, the patient began to inhale, and became apparently insensible in the course of two or three minutes. The operation was then commenced, and the limb was removed in what seemed to us a marvellously short space of time—certainly less than a minute ; the patient remaining, during the incisions and the tying of the arteries, perfectly still and motionless. While the vessels were being secured, on being spoken to he rose partially up (still showing no signs of pain) and answered questions put to him in a slow drowsy manner. He declared to us that at no part of the operation had he felt pain, though he seemed partially conscious ; he had heard some words, and felt that something was being done to his limb. He was not aware, till told that the limb was off, and when he knew it, expressed great gratification at having been saved from pain. . . . Mr. Liston afterwards performed one of the minor but most painful operations of surgery—the partial removal of the nail in onychia—on a man similarly narcotized. . . . The patient seemed to feel no pain, and, upon rousing up after the operation, declared that he had felt none.

' In these cases the ether vapour was administered by means of an ingenious apparatus extemporaneously contrived by Mr. Squire of Oxford Street [Fig. 17]. It consisted of the bottom part

[1] *Lancet*, 1847, i, 8.

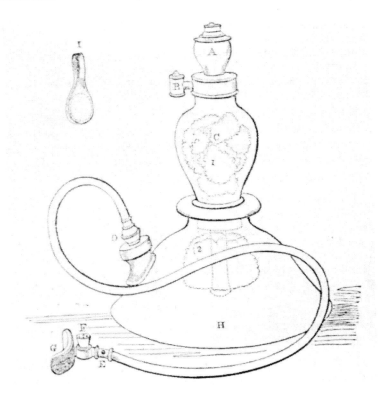

FIG. 17.—SQUIRE'S INHALER

for ether, first used by Robert Liston on December 21, 1846, at
University College Hospital, London.

A. The urn with its stopper, into which the ether is poured.
B. Valve which admits the air.
C. Contains sponge saturated with ether.
D. Valve which opens at each inspiration, and closes at each expiration.
E. Ferrule for regulating the quantity of atmospheric air admitted.
F. Valve for the escape of expired air.
G. Mouthpiece
H. Lower vase.
I. Spring for closing the nose.

of a Nooth's Apparatus [1], having a glass funnel filled with sponge
soaked in pure washed ether, in the upper orifice, and one of

[1] Dr. Nooth was a contemporary of Joseph Priestley, who described and illustrated
Nooth's apparatus. It was intended for impregnating water with carbon dioxide and
the ' bottom part ' held marble chips and sulphuric acid. The water to be impregnated was contained in an upper vessel. (Cf. Priestley, J. 1775. *Experiments and
observations on different kinds of air.* London, **2,** 302, pl. 3.)

43434343

Read's flexible inhaling tubes in the lower. [This tube was fitted with an expiratory valve and a mouthpiece. By turning a ferrule placed behind the mouthpiece the supply of fresh air which the patient received could be regulated.[1]] As the ether fell through the neck of the funnel it became vaporized, and the vapour being heavy descended to the bottom of the vase, and was thence inspired through the flexible tube. No heat was applied to the apparatus or the ether.'[2]

Hard upon the batch of letters which Boott sent to the editor of the *Lancet* there followed one from Morton's newly appointed agent, James A. Dorr, of Duke Street, St. James's, dated December 28, 1846.

'Having noticed, in several periodicals and newspapers', he wrote, 'reports of two operations recently performed by Mr. Liston . . . upon patients under the anodyne influence of inhaled vapour of ether . . . I take this earliest opportunity of giving notice, through the medium of your columns, to the medical profession, and to the public in general, that the process for procuring insensibility to pain by the administration of the vapour of ether to the lungs, employed by Mr. Liston, is patented for England and the Colonies, and that no person can use that process, or any similar one, without infringing upon rights legally secured to others.'[3]

Having successfully launched etherization in this country Boott was not prepared to see its progress checked in this manner. 'I beg to ask your insertion of the following letter', he wrote to the editor of the *Lancet*, 'which I have received from one of her Majesty's council "learned in the law".

' " MY DEAR DR. BOOTT,—In answer to your question with respect to the patent . . . I beg to say, that I am clearly of the opinion no patent can be valid, giving the patentee the exclusive privilege of *administering the vapour of ether to the lungs.* . . .

' " Upon the whole, I am satisfied you may safely advise your professional friends to continue the use of ether in their operations, without the slightest fear of legal consequences. Whether the instruments which are manufactured for the purpose are an infringement of any valid patent will be a question between the patentee and the manufacturers ; but the operators can have nothing to do with this ; and it would be most deplorable to have any interruption to such a mitigation of human suffering ".'[4]

[1] *Pharm. J.*, 1846–7, **6**, 350.   [2] *Lond. med. Gaz.*, 1847, **4,** 38.
[3] *Lancet*, 1847, i, 8.   [4] *Ibid.* 1847, i, 49.

The *Lancet* [1] commented : ' This question of patent is a stain upon the whole matter. We trust it will speedily be relinquished.' The editor of the *London Medical Gazette* made a similar comment on January 29 : [2] ' We do not believe that the patent could be sustained. The English agent for the patentees appears to be of the same opinion, as the ether vapour is now almost universally employed, and no notice is taken of the alleged infringement '.

Although news of the successful use of etherization at the Massachusetts General Hospital reached several distinguished men in France at about the same time that it reached Boott in England, no one immediately took the initiative in spreading it, as Boott had done. In fact it was January 12, 1847, before the surgeon, Joseph François Malgaigne, prompted not by first-hand information but by enthusiastic reports in American and British journals, thought it time that France took notice of the discovery, and at a meeting of the Académie de Médecine, in Paris, attempted to rouse general interest. At that meeting Malgaigne described five anaesthetics which he himself had recently given, three successfully, one incompletely and one without result. He also described his apparatus and how he came to use it.

' In America and in England ', he said, ' they use a flask with two tubular openings. Inside is a sponge moistened with sulphuric ether. One of these tubes is introduced into the patient's mouth, the other communicates with the air. Having no such apparatus at my disposal I made use of a simple tube into which I put a certain amount of ether and which I introduced into one nostril, the other being plugged. I took care ', he added, ' that inspiration took place with the mouth closed, expiration with the mouth open. After a short while the patients grasped this little manœuvre very well '.

Malgaigne's five experiments with etherization emboldened even the most sceptical among his colleagues—with the exception of François Magendie—to make similar trials.

' I have heard of the procedure about which M. Malgaigne has just told us ', said Louis Velpeau, Professor of Clinical Surgery in the University of Paris, '. . . I heard of it from Boston. Nevertheless, I made no use of it because I was deterred by a fear that, although wishing to spare my patients pain, which possibly has its uses, I might do them some injury. Who knows whether the prolonged inhalation of ether is absolutely without

[1] *Lancet*, 1847, i, 75.　　　　　　[2] *Lond. med. Gaz.*, 1847, **4**, 214.

danger ? However, after M. Malgaigne's experiments I am prone to believe in it and I shall walk with more assurance now he has shown us the way '.[1]

Many who followed Malgaigne's example also copied his method of administration by the nasal route (indeed this route retained its popularity in France for some years). Landouzy, of Rheims, among others, used two tubes, one in each nostril, the free ends hanging down over the surface of ether in a flask warmed to 32° C. But his results, though 'agreeable' to the patient, cannot be considered satisfactory. After twenty minutes' inhalation one patient, a nervous woman of thirty, said that she felt light-headed, just as she would after three *flutes* of champagne. At the end of forty-five minutes the lady felt drowsy but was still answering questions ; nevertheless a molar tooth was extracted, and though she ' gave a little cry of surprise rather than pain ', she assured Landouzy that she had suffered ' *incomparably* less than when, a little time back, the same dentist pulled out the corresponding tooth on the opposite side '.[2]

The surgeon Philibert Joseph Roux was among those who preferred to follow the American and English method of using a flask filled with ether-soaked sponge, through which air was drawn to a valved mouthpiece.[3] Of this conventional type of flask, that devised by the surgical instrument maker Charrière, during January 1847, quickly became popular. This instrument (Fig. 18) consisted of a broad-based flask, sometimes containing small pieces of ether-soaked sponge, sometimes merely a small quantity of liquid ether. Air was drawn through the apparatus and the ether-air mixture passed, by a length of leather tubing, to a mouthpiece. The apparatus was fitted with two ball valves, one inspiratory the other expiratory.[4]

Intensive experiment in the field of anaesthesia was barely a week old in France when Élie de Beaumont requested, on January 18, 1847, that Jackson's sealed letter to the Académie des Sciences should be opened (see pp. 122–4). Its contents fell rather flat. ' The secret referred to in the note which has just been read ', remarked Velpeau, ' has been no secret for some time past ; the medical journals have been giving it publicity in America and England since November. A letter from Dr.

---

[1] *Bull. Acad. Méd. Paris*, 1846–7, **12**, 263, 264.
[2] *Ibid.* **12**, 299.   [3] *Ibid.* **12**, 306.
[4] Cf. *J. Chim. méd.*, 1847, **3**, 169.

War[r]en, of Boston, told me all about it more than a month ago and Dr. Willis Fisher of the same city proposed, about the middle of last December, that I should try it at the Charité. . . .

' And now ', he continued, ' must we accept at their face value all the marvels which have been attributed to the subject in the . . . journals ? Assuredly not. . . . One finds in the

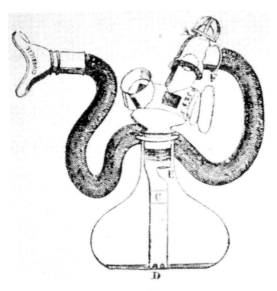

FIG. 18.—CHARRIÈRE'S INHALER
for ether, in use in Paris during 1847.

A. Ball valve, expiratory (inspiratory valve below shown by dotted line).
CD. Tube down which air passed from the entry port above the flask, into the liquid ether in the flask.
E. Tube (presumed to be unconnected with CD) through which the ether-air mixture was drawn, through the flexible tubing, to the mouthpiece.
F. Tap simultaneously closing the air entry port and the passage of the anaesthetic mixture to the mouthpiece, thus throwing the inhaler out of action when the administrator so desired.

observations of English surgeons the same uncertainty and the same inconsistency as in our own. . . .

' It is possible, moreover, that the unreliableness of the effects of ether is due as much to the imperfections of our apparatus as to the nature of the drug itself or to the various idiosyncracies of patients. We should be wrong, after all, to pass any judgment on the value of this procedure at present.' [1]

[1] *C.R. Acad. Sci.*, Paris, 1847, **24**, 76.

5*

Among the first in Germany to use ether was the surgeon Johann Friedrich Dieffenbach, of Berlin. He gave it from an inhaler somewhat resembling Morton's, except that into the wider of the two necks of Dieffenbach's flask was fitted a long glass tube bearing a valveless gum-elastic mouthpiece, so that in fact there was a large dead-space in this inhaler (see Fig. 19, cf. Fig. 12).

Shortly before his death, in 1847, Dieffenbach wrote a small monograph, *Der Aether gegen den Schmerz* (Berlin, 1847), in which he recorded the results of his experience of etherization. Dieffenbach expressed the opinion that since ether was able to

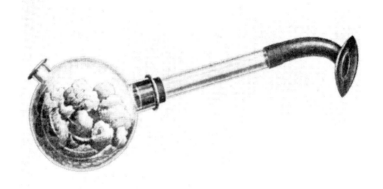

FIG. 19.—DIEFFENBACH'S INHALER

for ether, in use in Berlin during 1847.

obviate completely even the most intense pain during capital operations it afforded the greatest possible relief to the patient ; but for the surgeon (except in dealing with dislocations) it merely made matters more difficult. He stressed the dangers of etherization : its liability to produce apoplexy and haemorrhage, the possibility of instantaneous death through overdosage, the tendency to increased post-operative bleeding, the slow healing of wounds where much tissue had been lost ; he alleged, also, that a heightened sense of pain and even maniacal excitement might result from etherization. He found, indeed, that the post-operative condition of patients who had been etherized was in general less favourable than that of patients operated upon without ether.

' If one takes into account, over a large number of patients, all the small disadvantages bound up with etherization ', wrote Dieffenbach, ' the sum total of illness is found to be raised, so that out of a thousand etherized and a thousand unetherized cases a few more deaths occur among the former than among the latter '.

Although he considered that from the point of view of suffering humanity the value of the agent was very great, he advised that its use should be restricted to extremely painful operations and that it should be administered with the utmost care.[1]

During the early months of 1847, indeed, both the Council of Health of Zürich and the Grand Duke of Hesse-Darmstadt found it necessary to prohibit the use of ether anaesthesia by ' those who practice dentistry, bleeding and other minor surgical operations . . . in consequence of certain accidents having arisen from the use of ether by inexperienced persons '.   In Hesse-Darmstadt, midwives also were forbidden to use it.[2]

In the course of the year 1847, both the English and the French devoted much time and thought to improving methods of etherization, but it was to France, and particularly to Paris, then the generally acknowledged centre of scientific activity, that other countries on the European Continent turned for guidance.[3]

Commenting on early types of inhaler (with descriptions and illustrations of which the pages of the medical journals were full during the spring of 1847), John Snow, the man who changed anaesthesia from a craft to a science, some years later summed up their common failings :

' When the inhalation of ether was first commenced, the inhalers employed consisted generally of glass vases containing sponge, to afford a surface for the evaporation of the ether.   Both glass and sponge being very indifferent conductors of caloric, the interior of the inhalers became much reduced in temperature, the evaporation of ether was very much checked, and the patient breathed air much colder than the freezing point of water, and containing very little of the vapour of ether.   On this account, and through other defects in the inhalers, the patient was often very long in becoming insensible, and, in not a few cases, he did not become affected beyond a degree of excitement and inebriety.'[4]

[1] Dieffenbach, J. F. 1847. *Der Aether gegen den Schmerz.* Berlin.   227.
[2] *Lond. med. Gaz.*, 1847, **4**, 525 ; *ibid.*, **5**, 85.
[3] In Russia the great military surgeon, Pirogoff, broke new ground when he successfully gave ether by the rectal route. (*C.R. Acad. Sci.*, Paris, 1847, **24**, 789.)
[4] Snow, J. 1858. *On chloroform and other anaesthetics.* London.   348.

Elsewhere he wrote upon the same subject :

'Many of the apparatuses at first invented did not allow of easy respiration, but offered obstructions to it—by sponges, by the ether itself, by valves of insufficient size, but more particularly by tubes of too narrow calibre : and there is reason to believe that, in many instances, this was the cause of failure, and that in others the insensibility, when produced, was partly due to asphyxia.' [1]

Apparatuses designed to overcome these very defects were indeed produced, but until the teaching of Snow himself made its impression, efforts in this direction were more often remarkable

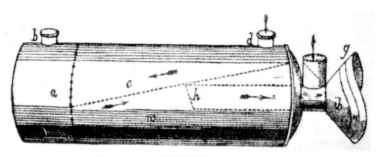

FIG. 20.—SMEE'S INHALER
for ether, February 1847.

a. Hot water chamber. b. Aperture with screw. c. Ether chamber.
d. Aperture to admit air and ether, with a screw to be employed when
  the inhaler is not in use. e. Diaphragm.
f. Mouthpiece. g. Expiratory valve. h. Inspiratory valve.

for ingenuity than for insight into the true nature of the problems of ether vaporization.

Attempts to assist vaporization by the application of heat were frequently made. In February 1847, Alfred Smee invented a valved ether container to which a flanged mouthpiece was fitted without tubing (Fig. 20). The container was cylindrical and made of tin. The bottom third was partitioned off and could be filled with hot water. A diaphragm placed diagonally across the interior of the vaporizer forced the air drawn in by the patient to pass over the surface of the ether before reaching the mouthpiece. Immediately behind the mouthpiece was an expiratory valve.[2]

[1] Snow, J. 1847. *On the inhalation of ether in surgical operations.* London. 21.
[2] *Pharm. J.*, 1846–7, **6**, 425.

During March, Hoffman, of Margate, described an inhaler (Fig. 21) which consisted simply of an ordinary glass flask partly filled with ether.   In the neck was inserted a glass tube for the ingress of air, its end dipping below the surface of the liquid ether.   Into a hole cut in the side of the flask, well above the level of the ether, was inserted a second glass tube and this was connected by a length of flexible tubing to a mouthpiece. Behind the mouthpiece was an inspiratory flap valve and an expiratory valve which, when necessary, could be held open by

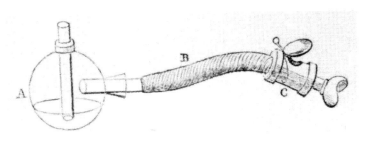

FIG. 21.—HOFFMAN'S INHALER

for ether, March 1847.

A. Glass flask. Air entered through the tube dipping into the liquid ether.
    The ether-air mixture passed through the second tube to
B. flexible inhaling tube and through
C. which contained an inspiratory flap valve and the expiratory valve, held
    open by the small lever, when necessary to dilute the anaesthetic mixture
    with additional air. Beyond C was the flanged mouth-tube.
Immediately before administration the flask was warmed in hot water or over
    a spirit lamp to facilitate vaporization.

a small lever to allow the anaesthetic mixture to be diluted by additional air.   Hoffman intended the flask, just before use, to be warmed either by dipping it into hot water or over a spirit lamp.[1]

An interesting inhaler which both warmed the ether and made provision not merely for diluting but for regulating the amount of vapour taken up by the stream of air drawn over the liquid,[2] was described in the *Illustrated London News*, February 6, 1847, p. 91, by a correspondent who signed himself with the

[1] *Pharm. J.*, 1846-7, **6**, 472.
[2] The actual concentration of ether vapour in the mixture was not, however, known, cf. p. 152 *et seq.*

pseudonym ' Inhaler '. This apparatus (Fig. 22), called the ' graduated-dose inhaler ',

' is constructed in metal, and is divided into two chambers ; the upper one to contain the Ether, and the lower one to contain warm water. The Æther chamber is divided by diaphragms

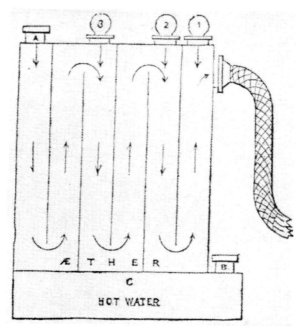

FIG. 22.—THE GRADUATED-DOSE INHALER

Ether inhaler described in the *Illustrated London News*, February 6, 1847.

Air entered through A, but the anaesthetic mixture, before passing along the flexible tubing to the mouthpiece (not shown), could be increasingly diluted by opening the supplementary air ports 3, 2 and 1, in that order.

into several [6] cells : the intention of these divisions is to cause the air, which enters at A, to perform the long route indicated by the arrows, that it may be perfectly saturated with Ether before it leaves the Inhaler.

' The figures 1, 2, 3, on the top of the Inhaler, indicate several openings for the entrance of air ; it is by these openings that the strength of the dose is graduated. For example, if No. 1 is open, the air, entering at that point, will be in contact with only a small portion of the Ether vapour ; No. 2, being opened, will produce a stronger mixture ; No. 3, still stronger, etc. ; until, all being closed with the exception of A, we then have the most powerful dose that can be had, without the assistance of heat.

' In addition to this arrangement, a stop-cock is so constructed, and adapted to the tube, that the Æther can, at any time, be turned off, and the air turned on, or any proportion of each. This is a most valuable addition, since it gives the operator a perfect command over the power of the instrument, without, in any degree, disturbing the patient.'

In Paris a member of the Académie de Médecine deprecated the warming of ether :

' One ought not to imitate ', he said, ' those who advise that, in order to facilitate the vaporization of ether, it should be heated. It is a useless and a dangerous practice. The heat of the hand is sufficient to bring about vaporization.' [1]

On January 13, 1847, Jacob Bell, the editor of the *Pharmaceutical Journal*, is reported to have observed ' that most of the instruments hitherto recommended had been constructed without reference to expense. He thought it was also desirable to contrive a means of attaining the result as economically as possible '. The apparatus which he designed to fulfil this condition (see Fig. 23) was on the lines of Squire's, but simplified, and instead of sponge he introduced a little water into the flask with the ether and drew air through. Set behind the mouthpiece, which was made of glass to allow it to be readily cleansed after each administration, were alternately acting inspiratory and expiratory non-return valves formed from disks of glass, each resting on a short length of tubing.[2]

In December 1846, the *Pharmaceutical Journal* had stated that ' the old plan of introducing a teaspoonful of ether into a bladder or silk bag, and inhaling it in the same manner as nitrous oxide gas ' was far less effective than the use of Squire's inhaler because ' the same air is inhaled repeatedly, either with small additions, which dilute the ethereal vapour, or in a vitiated state, without the requisite oxygen '.[3] Nevertheless, during January 1847, a number of people in England,[4] and soon afterwards on the Continent, adopted the use of bladders, no doubt because it was easier to obtain one than to have made even the simplest piece

[1] *Bull. Acad. Méd. Paris*, 1846–7, **12**, 301.   [2] *Pharm. J.*, 1846–7, **6**, 355.
[3] *Ibid.* **6**, 338.   [4] Cf. *Ibid.* **6**, 356.

of apparatus. The significance of rebreathing—the condensation of the patient's exhalations within the bladder, which restored heat lost by the evaporation of the ether and the inevitable

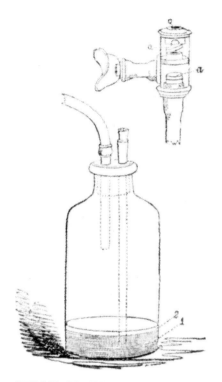

FIG. 23.—BELL'S SIMPLIFIED ETHER INHALER
January 1847.

The glass flask contained 1. water, and 2. ether. A flexible tube joined the flask to a valve box and glass mouthpiece. As air was drawn through the inhaler by the patient the glass disk valve *a* rose on its seating. The exhaled mixture raised *a*** and passed out of the inhaler at *c*.

accumulation of carbon dioxide, which acted as a respiratory stimulant and so lessened the duration of induction—was, however, not yet clearly appreciated.

The bladder was sometimes partly inflated with air before adding ether, sometimes ' merely washed out with hot water previous to placing the ether in it '. Occasionally the bladder

containing ether was floated in warm water before being applied
to the patient's mouth.[1]

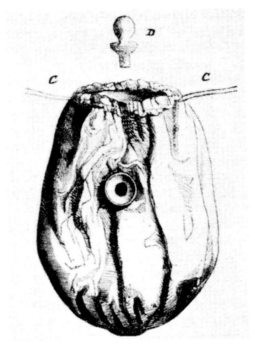

FIG. 24.—JULES ROUX'S *SAC*

for the administration of ether, used at Lyons from 1847
until the close of the nineteenth century.

CC. Draw-strings to pull the mouth of the bag to fit round the
patient's nose and mouth.
D. Peg used for closing the air hole in the side of the bag.

The bag could be held in position on the patient's face
by knotting the draw-strings behind his head. While the
bag was in position a certain amount of fresh air filtered
in through the puckers round its mouth. Additional air
was allowed to enter, when necessary, by temporarily
removing the peg from the hole in the side of the bag.

Herapath, at the Bristol General Hospital, perhaps calling
to mind the technique for nitrous oxide inhalation formerly
used at the Pneumatic Institution at Clifton, was among the
first to anaesthetize a patient with a bladder of ether vapour.

[1] *Lond. med. Gaz.*, 1847, **4,** 261, 282.

His successful experiment took place on January 4, 1847.[1] It was Herapath's example which the Swiss surgeon Demme copied when, on January 23, 1847, at the Inselspital at Berne, he gave the first anaesthetic in Switzerland.[2]

Ormsby's inhaler (see Fig. 95) was foreshadowed in France by the inhalers of Jules Roux and of Munaret. Roux's inhaler (Fig. 24) consisted of ' a bag, made like a lady's reticule, its opening being dilated or contracted by the drawing or loosing of the strings around it, and lined by a pig's bladder. . . . In using this apparatus, the mouth and nostrils are both placed in the sac drawn over them, and inhalation goes on with the ether vapour given off from sponges soaked in ether, and placed in the bladder '.[3]

Munaret's apparatus was simpler, being ' a bladder, the aperture of which is made sufficiently large to be adapted to the face, and to cover the mouth and nose. A flexible iron (or copper) wire is secured to the margin so as to allow of its enlargement or contraction . . . and to prevent injury to the lips the edge is surrounded with several layers of cotton or velvet '. Munaret's apparatus contained no sponge ; the ether was poured straight into the bladder immediately before administration.[4]

At about the same time, February 1847, that John Mason Warren, in Boston, gave up the use of Morton's inhaler in favour of a bell-shaped sponge (see p. 125), Thomas Smith of Cheltenham wrote to the *London Medical Gazette* :

' Experience has taught me that the most simple contrivance for the effectual and safe administration of ether by inhalation is to saturate a sponge with . . . ethereal solution, and apply it to the mouth and nostrils, so that the patient may breathe easily through it.' [5]

In Edinburgh, Professor James Miller, abandoning the ' very beautiful yet simple apparatus made by Squire ' (which Liston, whose pupil he had been, presented to him at the end of December 1846), also adopted the use of an ether-soaked sponge. His example was followed by his Edinburgh colleague, James Young Simpson, and by S. J. Tracy, of St. Bartholomew's Hospital in London.[6]

[1] *Lond. med. Gaz.*, 1847, **4**, 81.
[2] Fueter, F. 1888. *Klinische und experimentelle Beobachtungen über die Aethernarkose.* Leipzig. 1.   [3] *Lancet*, 1847, ii, 102 ; see also, pp. 206–7, 424.
[4] *Lond. med. Gaz.*, 1847, **5**, 474.   [5] *Ibid.* 1847, **4**, 395.
[6] Miller, J. 1850. *The principles of surgery.* Edinburgh. 755 ; *Lond. med. Gaz.* 1847, **5**, 349.

Earlier in 1847 Tracy had invented a quaint inhaler shaped like a hookah pipe (Fig. 25), the bowl being filled by an ether-soaked sponge.[1]

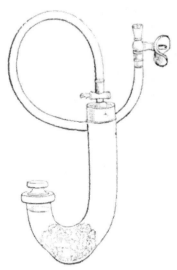

FIG. 25.—TRACY'S INHALER (1847)

shaped like a hookah pipe and containing ether-soaked sponge.

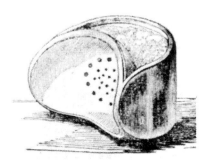

FIG. 26.—SMEE'S " PORTABLE " INHALER (1847)

A crescent-shaped metal trough containing sponge to receive the liquid ether.   The perforated concave side fitted over the patient's mouth.

Among other early types of inhaler were two inspired by the design of the small respirators worn over the mouth to filter foggy air.   One of these, ' Smee's portable inhaler ' (Fig. 26).

[1] *Pharm. J.*, 1846–7, **6**, 357.

consisted of a little crescent-shaped trough in which ether-soaked sponge or wadding was placed and the patient breathed in and out through the perforated concave side. The *Pharmaceutical Journal* suggested to Smee that the inhaler needed ' a division, so placed as to prevent the possibility of the liquid ether running into the mouth '.[1] A slightly more elaborate version of the respirator type of inhaler was that of N. S. Heineken, of Sidmouth (Figs. 27A and 27B). It consisted of a crescent-shaped tin box, $5\frac{1}{4}$ inches in diameter, 2 inches in width and $1\frac{1}{4}$ inches deep. To the convex side was attached a small rectangular box, its outermost wall being of perforated zinc. Within was a leather flap which acted as an inspiratory valve. The main box contained sponge, confined between two perforated zinc diaphragms, and on to this ether was dropped through an aperture which, after filling, was closed with a cork. An oval area on the concave side of the box was dotted with perforations and padded round the edge to act as the mouthpiece. Between the mouthpiece and the nearer of the two diaphragms confining the sponge was a small space to prevent liquid ether being inhaled and in the lid of the box, immediately above this space and to the right and left of the mouthpiece, were two expiratory valves. Each valve could be raised by a lever to admit air as required.[2]

The practice of pinching shut the nostrils and forcing the patient to breathe entirely by mouth through a small tube, either with or without a flange to cup the lips, was early recognized as inexpedient. So much was obvious, although the fact that ' when the stage of surgical anaesthesia is reached, respiration is entirely nasal '[3] was not appreciated. Malgaigne discovered administration through the nose alone to be feasible, although he spoilt its effect by painstakingly coaching his patients to inspire nasally but to expire orally (see p. 135). J. M. Warren and his colleagues in Boston, the Londoners Smith and Tracy, and Miller and Simpson in Edinburgh, allowed the patient to breathe in and out as he chose, through a conical sponge covering both nose and mouth. Jules Roux, of Toulon, adopted his wide-mouthed bladder chiefly because it allowed inhalation ' to go on by the mouth and nose at the same time '.

---

[1] *Pharm. J.*, 1846–7, **6**, 424.   [2] *Ibid.* **6**, 471,
[3] Macintosh, R. R., and Bannister, F. B. 1943. *Essentials of general anaesthesia.* Oxford. 201.

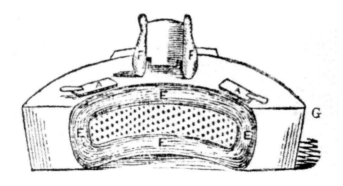

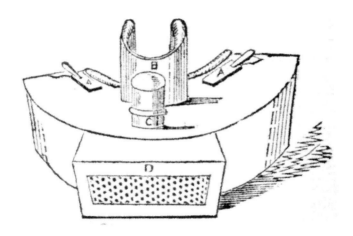

HEINEKEN'S INHALER (1847)

Front view (27A), back view (27B)

AA. Expiratory valves with small levers to raise them and allow the entry of additional air.
B. Spring band to close nostrils.
C. Stoppered hole through which ether was poured into the inhaler.
D. Rectangular box with perforated wall behind which was a leather flap acting as an inspiratory valve.
E. Concave, perforated zinc mouthpiece with padded edging.
F. Padding round nose clip.
G. Main box containing ether soaked sponge.

Dr. Andrew Ure, at a meeting of the Pharmaceutical Society in London, went to the extreme of suggesting ' instead of a mouthpiece, a hood to enclose the head, and having a glass window in front, as the labour of " wire-drawing " the air and vapour through a small tube was likely to interfere with the result '.[1] This method was adopted, apparently with success, by Matthias Mayor, of Lausanne.[2] He enclosed the head and chest in a towelling tent with a window over the face, and into this tent he introduced an evaporating dish containing ether.[3]

In Paris, Cloquet, who believed ' that the inhalation of ether took effect more rapidly when made through the nose rather than the mouth ', devised during February 1847 an ingenious apparatus which, if it left something to be desired as an ether vaporizer, made a positive contribution to the technique of nasal inhalation. This apparatus was described as ' a kind of large pipe made of metal, or better still, glass. The bowl is closed by a grid and is fitted with a large elastic tube, the area of which must be greater than that of the trachea, that is, at least 2 cm. in diameter. This tube ends in a metal cap with a rubber-covered rim, which fits over the nose and upper lip in such a way that the nostrils remain perfectly free. . . . Tube and cap are furnished each with a large easily-movable valve, one an inlet valve for the ether vapour, the other expiratory. . . . By enlarging the dimensions of the cap it may be applied to the mouth and nose simultaneously, and the patient can breathe as he chooses . . . without having to take lessons '.[4]

Meanwhile Francis Sibson, Resident Surgical Officer at the Nottingham General Hospital, was independently evolving first a nose-piece then a combined nose-and-mouthpiece (Fig. 28). At the time he was experimenting with the inhalation of ether in

[1] *Pharm. J.*, 1846–7, **6,** 359 ; cf. p. 68.
[2] Fueter, F. 1888. *Klinische und experimentelle Beobachtungen über die Aethernarkose.* Leipzig. 1.
[3] Snow stated that J. T. Clover introduced a similar method for administering chloroform at University College Hospital. ' The head and face of the patient were covered by a towel, under which the lint wetted with chloroform was held. The countenance and state of respiration could not be observed in this mode of giving the chloroform ; the person administering it had to depend almost entirely on the pulse. . . . This plan of administering chloroform . . . was introduced by Mr. Clover, who was for several years a resident officer of the institution [1848–53] ; and it is but right to state that it led to no accident in his hands ; in those of his successors it was, however, less successful ; three accidents having occurred in a little more than a year and a half.' (Snow, J. 1858. *On chloroform and other anaesthetics.* London. 184.)
[4] *Bull. Acad. Méd. Paris,* 1846–7, **12,** 348.

the treatment of facial neuralgia. In addition to the manifest difficulties of ' ensuring the inhalations when the patient is on the verge of unconsciousness, or when there are convulsive or intoxicated strugglings and resistance to the inhalation ' Sibson had to deal with cases of tic, in particular, one in which there were constant convulsive movements of the jaw.

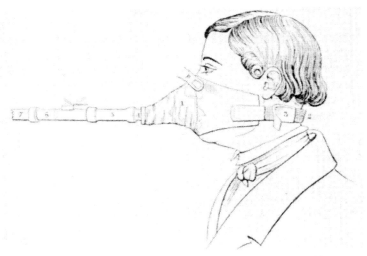

FIG. 28.—SIBSON'S FACEPIECE (February 1847)

1. Nose- and mouthpiece—a funnel fitting, as closely as possible, over the nose and mouth, made of mackintosh, lined with oiled silk. The thumb compresses it over the nose, the fingers, if needful, over the chin.
2. Vulcanized india-rubber strap to keep the nose- and mouthpiece in its place by means of
3. A buckle.
4, 5. Two inches of vulcanized india-rubber tube attached to the mouthpiece.
6. Brass tube with valves. The outer valve is almost poised by a lever ; the inner valve is closed by a weak spring.
7. Eighteen inches of flexible tube connecting the facepiece to a modified ' Snow's spiral ether-chamber ' (cf. Figs. 29 and 30).

' I first constructed a nasal inhaler ', wrote Sibson, '. . . it answered very well. . . . I afterwards tried to combine a nasal and an oral inhaler in one instrument : at length I bought a common sixpenny mask, lined it within with oiled silk, cut away the septum of the nose, the lips, and the whole circumference of the mask to within an inch of the nose and mouth. I then pasted a funnel of mackintosh cloth over the nose and mouth, and over this a piece of mackintosh to go over the cheeks ; to these I attached a vulcanized India-rubber strap and buckle. When this is fastened, the nose and mouthpiece fit delightfully. Usually all that is needed is to compress the nose-piece with the finger and thumb against the sides of the nose and in the most difficult subjects it is only needful to bring both hands together, the fingers under the chin, the thumbs to each side of the nose, and the head pressed back against one's own body '. [1]

John Snow, who had been experiencing the usual difficulties of inhalation with a mouth-tube, ' was therefore ready to adopt ' Sibson's facepiece. But Snow seldom touched a piece of apparatus without improving it and after using Sibson's rather clumsy mask for a few weeks he set to work and himself designed one, introducing valves into the facepiece itself and allowing for ' greater adaptation to faces of different dimensions '. He described this new facepiece, which he began to use in May 1847, as follows :

' . . . The central part, containing the valves, is made of metal—brass, tinned iron, or plated copper ; all the rest of thin sheet-lead, the pliability of which admits of its being easily adapted to the peculiar form of the features. The lead is covered with silk or glove-leather externally [2], and is lined with oil-silk where it comes in contact with the face. The valves are made of vulcanised India-rubber ; they are light, are attached so as to rise with the least appreciable force, and they close again, of themselves, in any posture in which the patient can be required to be placed. I have contrived the expiratory valve to turn on a pivot, so as to allow of the admission of external air, and to supersede the use of a ferrule or two-way tap, at the same time that it is performing the office of a valve.' [3]

All the advances so far made in the technique of anaesthesia—attempts to facilitate the vaporization of ether by applying heat, attempts to control the admixture of atmospheric air with the vapour, the abandoning of the mouth-tube in favour of some device for administration through the nose or through both nose and mouth—were based not upon scientific reasoning but upon empiricism. They did not touch upon the more important problem—a fundamental requirement of successful inhalation anaesthesia—how to control the depth of anaesthesia by regulating

[1] *Lond. med. Gaz.*, 1847. **4,** 363.
[2] The typical Snow's facepiece of the eighteen-fifties and early 'sixties had leather outside the lead rim, velveteen inside.
[3] Snow, J. 1847. *On the inhalation of the vapour of ether in surgical operations.* London. 22.

the concentration of ether in the mixture delivered to the patient. This consideration, however, early began to worry a few men.

'The new application of ether to surgery which has just been made', said a certain Monsieur Boullay, at a meeting of the Académie de Médecine in Paris, on January 26, 1847, 'is one of the most fortunate we could have hoped for. The public is quite preoccupied with it, and rightly so ; but it must be remarked with regret that Science should not so far hold the process in check that the same result should always be obtained. No one has yet determined even the proper dose of ether to be given '.[1]

Ten days before Boullay spoke, John Snow had in fact described a practical method for controlling anaesthetic dosage and was busily working upon an apparatus for its clinical application.

He took advantage of the known fact that at different temperatures air will take up different amounts of ether vapour. In the *London Medical Gazette*,[2] Snow is reported to have said at a meeting of the Westminster Medical Society, on January 16, 1847 :

'The great effect of temperature over the relations of atmo-spheric air with the vapour of ether, had apparently been over-looked in the construction and application of the instruments hitherto used. This circumstance would explain in some measure the variety of the results, and account for some of the failures. The operators did not at present know the quantity of vapour they were exhibiting with the air ; it would vary immensely according to the temperature of the apartment, as would be seen by some calculations he had made. . . . One hundred cubic inches of air, saturated with the vapour of ether, at a temperature of—

44°	would contain	27	cubic inches of vapour	
54°	,,	34·3	,,	,,
64°	,,	43·3	,,	::
74°	,,	53·6	,,	,,
84°	,,	66.6	,,	,,

being doubled by a rise of only thirty degrees [F.].

'He (Dr. Snow) was getting an instrument made which would enable the surgeon, merely by placing it in a bason of water, warmed or cooled to a given temperature, to administer an

[1] *Bull. Acad. Méd. Paris*, 1846–7, **12**, 301.   [2] *Lond. med. Gaz.*, 1847, **4**, 156.

atmosphere of any strength he wished, and by this means to gain correct experience to guide him in future. The instrument . . . was on the plan of the inhaler of Mr. Jeffreys [for therapeutic, not anaesthetic, inhalation], with some alterations and additions. The air would meet with no obstruction from having to pass through sponge or ether, and the instrument, which would be of metal, as a good conductor of caloric, would be cheap and portable.'

A week later, on January 23, Snow showed his inhaler at the Westminster Medical Society. Subsequently he modified both it and his table for calculating the concentration of ether vapour in the mixture to be administered. The modified version of the inhaler was described by Snow in his monograph, *On the inhalation of the vapour of ether in surgical operations*, London, 1847 (see Figs. 29 and 30).

It consisted of a japanned tin or plated copper box ' of the size and form of a thick octavo volume '. This box served a dual purpose ; it was a case for carrying the dismantled apparatus and was also, during administration, a water-bath of 100 cubic inches capacity.

The ether chamber itself was circular, made of thin tinned brass or plated copper. It was nearly 6 inches in diameter and $1\frac{1}{4}$ inches in depth and was filled with a spirally-coiled baffle-plate soldered to its lid and reaching to within one-sixteenth of an inch of its bottom. The space between each volute was five-eighths of an inch. There was one small aperture, with a cap, in the lid of the chamber for filling and emptying ether, and a second aperture, near the circumference, into which could be screwed a length of brass tubing five-eighths of an inch in internal diameter. Through this air was drawn into the apparatus by the patient inspiring. ' The tube ', explained Snow, ' is merely for preventing a trifling loss of ether which would arise from evaporation of it into the apartment . . . and it effects this object in a more simple manner than a valve would, and offers less resistance to the ingress of air than the most delicately-balanced valve. The vapour of ether, being heavier than air, will not diffuse itself, in opposition to gravity, through the air in the tube, in the short space of time between the inspirations of the patient.' To a third opening was attached a three-foot length of flexible tubing the other end of which joined with Snow's facepiece. Each of the various dimensions of the inhaler

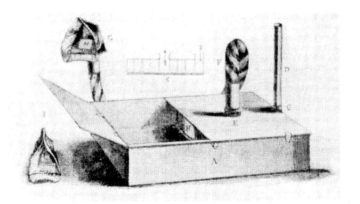

FIG. 29.—SNOW'S ETHER INHALER

A. Japanned metal box, acting as a water-bath, in which was placed
B. Vaporizing chamber (part of the circumference only, showing).
C. Aperture with thread into which screwed
D. Tube through which the patient drew air into the vaporizing chamber.
E. Aperture over which fitted
F. Wide calibre flexible inhaling tube.
G. Facepiece with
H. Inspiratory valve.
I. Facepiece removed, showing inspiratory valve, and expiratory valve in back wall.
S. Diagram of the vaporizing chamber, in section.

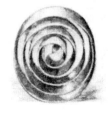

FIG. 30

The interior of the vaporizing chamber, showing the spiral baffle-plate and the central aperture (E in Fig. 29).

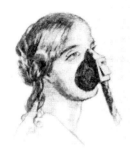

(*Below*). The facepiece applied. The dotted line indicates the position of the expiratory valve when turned aside on its pivot to admit air to dilute the anaesthetic mixture.

was significant and had been decided upon by Snow only after careful experiment.

The inspired air was forced to pass round four times over the surface of the ether. ' It is desirable to have the chamber as shallow as practicable ', wrote Snow, ' in order that all the air passing through it may be brought successively in contact with the surface of the ether ; and, on the other hand, it is necessary to leave a considerable space above the ether for the air ; otherwise, when a patient draws vigorous and deep in-spirations . . . the ether will be agitated into waves, and splashed into the elastic [flexible] tube '. This tube was three feet in length ' in order to leave as much room as possible for the operator and his assistants. It ought to be so capacious as to offer no impediment to the most rapid inspiration ; and to meet this requirement it must be wider than the trachea, to compensate for the resistance arising from friction of air against the interior of the tube. It is, therefore, three-quarters of an inch in internal diameter.'

The water-bath was made to contain not less than 100 cubic inches, because ' a small quantity of water would be cooled by the conversion of ether into vapour during the process of in-halation, and the intention of accurately regulating the pro-portion of vapour to the air would not be efficiently fulfilled : 100 cubic inches of water will, however, supply the caloric necessary to the conversion of one or two ounces of ether into vapour, without being much reduced in temperature ; and, as the heat of the water employed differs little from that of the air of the patient's room, it is not much altered during an operation, by radiation or other causes '.[1]

' It must not be supposed ', Snow warned his readers, ' that because the air of the apartment is of a suitable temperature, the use of the water-bath may be dispensed with ; for the vaporiza-tion of the ether in the inhaler would cool the apparatus and the air passing through it : less and less ether would be taken up, and at the time when the full strength of the vapour is most required, the patient would probably be breathing air of a freezing temperature, with very little vapour in it '.[2]

The temperature of the water in the bath which Snow at first advocated was about 60° F. (cf. p. 164). ' I did not think

[1] Snow, J. 1847. *On the inhalation of the vapour of ether in surgical operations.* London. 16–21.   [2] *Ibid.* 29.

it ever necessary to raise it above 65°.[1] In winter a little hot
water requires to be added . . . but in hot weather the water
is often 70° or upwards, and its temperature requires to be
lowered, which may be done by mixing spring water with
it. Or, to save time and trouble, the operator may be provided with some sal-ammoniac and nitrate of potash, powdered,
and mixed together in equal parts ; three or four ounces of
which mixture being dissolved in the water in the apparatus will
depress its temperature about ten degrees. At the heat I have
mentioned, the air will exceed in quantity the vapour, in the
mixture the patient breathes ; and although it is desirable
to induce insensibility as rapidly as possible, this is better than
giving the vapour stronger, for a greater quantity will generally
be inhaled in a given time than if it were more concentrated,
since, when it is too strong, it excites coughing, or causes the
patient to hold his breath. The indication is to give as much
vapour in the air as the patient can be got freely to breathe ;
and 90 parts of vapour to 100 of air—nearly 47 per cent. is
usually about this limit.' [2] By turning aside on its pivot the
expiratory valve of his facepiece, Snow could further dilute
the mixture with air just as it reached the patient. Induction,
in fact, was begun with the valve fully open ' so that the patient
may breathe scarcely anything but air at first ; and then the
valve should be turned a little at each inspiration, gradually to
cover the opening, and by this means to cause the etherized air
from the apparatus to be admitted by degrees, to the exclusion
of the external air. . . . The external aperture can generally
be quite closed by the valve, in from a quarter to half a minute.' [3]

   Two to two-and-a-half ounces was the amount of ether which
Snow generally introduced into the inhaler. ' I always measure
it ', he stated, ' and again measure what is left at the end of the
operation. The quantity of ether required to produce complete
insensibility, is, usually, from six drachms to one ounce in the
adult.' [4]

Early Work on the Physiology of Anaesthesia

   Although questions relating to practical administration tended
to monopolize attention during the first few weeks of etheriza-

[1] Elsewhere Snow gave a definite warning against the use of ' hot or even warm
water . . . as by it a risk was incurred that the patient might get all vapour and
no air.' (Lancet, 1847, i, 259.)
[2] Snow, J. 1847. On the inhalation of the vapour of ether in surgical operations. London.
28, 29.   [3] Ibid. 31, 32.   [4] Ibid. 29.

158 THE USE OF ANAESTHESIA ESTABLISHED

tion, the physiology of anaesthetic action and its bearing upon the patient's reactions to inhalation soon began to be investigated. In this connection a noteworthy, but more or less isolated, piece of research was carried out in Germany by Ernst von Bibra and Emil Harless, who made chemical and physiological tests on animals of the effects of sulphuric ether and also of ethyl chloride—first mentioned as an anaesthetic by Flourens in February 1847 (see p. 170)—and by their clinical collaborator J. F. Heyfelder, working at the hospital at Erlangen (see p. 170).

Von Bibra and Harless chiefly concerned themselves with the effects of sulphuric ether upon what, since 1876, have been termed the lipoids of the body, but which they termed simply ' fat ' (*Fett*). Comparing normal with etherized animals, they stated that in the latter, in a large majority of cases, the fats of the brain and spinal cord showed a reduction in quantity which was both positive and relative. Almost always, however, part of these fats was found again in the liver, so that the fatty content of the liver of etherized animals was greater than that of non-etherized animals. It appeared, they thought, that the effect of the ether vapour was to draw fats from the central nervous system, part of which fats was conveyed to the liver.

An investigation of the blood of etherized animals did not succeed in demonstrating any constantly greater fatty content than was found in that of non-etherized animals. Similarly, von Bibra and Harless found no fats in the urine of etherized animals, or only such traces as might also be found in the urine of the control animals. They were unable, also, from their experiments, to reach any conclusion as to the relatively greater or smaller content of fibrin and blood corpuscles in the blood of etherized animals.[1]

In France physiologists at once concerned themselves in the development of anaesthesia (cf. also pp. 356-74, 379-80, 397-8), although François Magendie shook his head over what he considered to be the too hasty clinical application of the new discovery.

' The intoxication caused by sulphuric ether ', he said, ' is still little understood ; it is, then, useful to study it, not only

[1] Bibra, E. v., and Harless, E. 1847. *Die Wirkung des Schwefeläthers in chemischer und physiologischer Beziehung.* Erlangen. 183. The modern lipoid theory of narcosis was formulated independently by H. Meyer (*Arch. exp. Path. Pharmak.,* 1899, **42,** 109) and E. Overton (*Studien über die Narkose zugleich ein Beitrag zur allgemeinen Pharmakologie.* Jena. 1901). (Cf. pp. 218-9 and footnote, p. 219.)

from the point of view of surgical operations, but by itself and for its own sake. . . . Here indeed is a fine and important study to be made ! But this study, like all serious studies, should be silent, calm and sufficiently prolonged to lead to certain results ; only thus could one safely, and with a clear conscience, apply it to man.

' But if one continues to experiment without due caution, if one makes over to the public the same night what one has begun but not finished in the morning, then it may, finally, have disastrous consequences. And one runs the risk of jeopardising a procedure which may, perhaps, be useful one day when it is thoroughly studied, thoroughly understood and suitably applied. If, on the contrary, it is exploited as it is to-day, it may soon be reduced to the level of one of those pretended discoveries—to one of those scientific *puffs* which come periodically to amuse the curiosity of the public and satisfy its irrational passion for all things erroneous and untruthful.' [1]

In 1822 Magendie [2] had amended Charles Bell's classification of the spinal nerve roots as ' sensible and insensible ', by demonstrating that the function of the posterior nerve roots is sensory while that of the anterior is motor.[3] Magendie had also investigated and demonstrated the circulation of the cerebro-spinal fluid.[4] Nevertheless, the nature of this previous work did not prompt Magendie, as his colleague Pierre Flourens was prompted, to undertake researches upon the physiology of anaesthesia.

Flourens, repeating J. J. C. Legallois's experiments, which demonstrated that the respiratory centre could be localized in the medulla oblongata,[5] succeeded in isolating the respiratory centre.[6] Upon the introduction of anaesthesia into practice Flourens hastened to widen the scope of his previous researches by investigating the effects not only of sulphuric ether but of other vapours (among them chloroform and ethyl chloride) which he presumed would act similarly upon the sensory and motor spinal nerve endings and upon the respiratory centre.

[1] *C.R. Acad. Sci.*, Paris, 1847, **24,** 137.
[2] See also footnote, p. 376.
[3] *Journal de Physiologie expérimentale et pathologique*, Paris, 1822, **2,** 276–9. (Reference quoted by Garrison, F. H. 1929. *Introduction to the history of medicine*. London and Philadelphia. 466.)
[4] Magendie, F. 1833. *Précis élémentaire de physiologie*, Paris. **I,** 223.
[5] Legallois, J. J. C. 1812. *Expériences sur le principe de la vie*. Paris. 37.
[6] Flourens, P. 1842. *Recherches expérimentales sur les propriétés et les fonctions du système nerveux dans les animaux vertébrés*. Paris. 198, 204.

Flourens and Snow, their Establishment of Basic Principles in Connection with Anaesthesia

During February and March, 1847, Flourens carried out an important series of experiments on dogs to ascertain the action of ether upon the nervous system. From his observations he concluded that the action of the anaesthetic follows a set course, acting first upon the cerebrum—affecting the intellectual functions ; secondly upon the cerebellum—deranging the equilibrium of movements ; then upon the spinal cord—successively inhibiting sensibility and motility ; finally upon the medulla oblongata, and when this phase is reached life becomes extinct.[1]

At this time, as might perhaps be expected, a great deal of specious reasoning was being done about the physiological action of ether. A favourite analogy was that between etherization and asphyxia.[2] Flourens in France and Snow in England both rightly distinguished between the two states.

' In ordinary asphyxia ', said Flourens at a meeting of the Académie des Sciences, ' the nervous system becomes paralyzed through the action of . . . blood *deprived of oxygen* ; during etherization the nervous system becomes paralyzed primarily through the direct action upon it of this singular agent. . . . And to express my full opinion ', he added, ' this death by successive stages in the nervous system is the real point and the great point brought out by the new experiments. . . . This isolation of *life*, of the point, the *vital knot (noeud vital)* in the nervous system, is certainly the most striking feature. In the etherized animal a single spot survives, and so long as it survives all the other living parts have at least a *latent life* and can resume full life : that single spot being dead, all dies.' [3]

Flourens had not succeeded, however, in working out the rationale of this ultimate cessation of life. It was for him simply a phenomenon of ether anaesthesia. Flourens's colleague Longet, however, from observations made while carrying out a series of researches on the effects of anaesthesia, stated that, in his experimental animals, death from overdosage

---

[1] *C.R. Acad. Sci., Paris,* 1847, **24,** 161, 253, 340.
[2] Cf. *e.g. Retrosp. practical Med.,* 1847, **16,** 408.
[3] *C.R. Acad. Sci., Paris,* 1847, **24,** 343.

appeared to be due to a kind of asphyxia undoubtedly connected with the etherization of the medulla oblongata (*bulbe*) itself.[1]

It was Snow who first began to appreciate the significance of oxygen-lack in anaesthesia as well as in asphyxia. A paper on

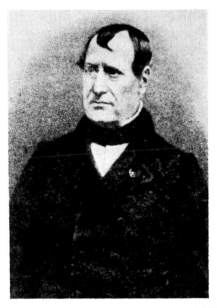

FIG. 31.—PIERRE JEAN MARIE FLOURENS
(1794–1867)

Physiologist. He was among the first to undertake experiments upon the physiological effects of anaesthetics. He preceded J. Y. Simpson in making a trial of chloroform (upon an animal).

the subject, read by him at the Westminster Medical Society during February 1847, was reported as follows :

' He said, that as the vapour [of ether] occupied space when mixed with air, it might be supposed that its action was partly due to its excluding a great deal of the oxygen of the air and causing a kind of asphyxia ; such, however, was not the case, for he [Snow] found that supplying the displaced oxygen did not counteract the effects of the vapour. Mixed with oxygen gas it affected mice as powerfully as when mixed with the air, as he had

[1] *Bull. Acad. Méd. Paris*, 1846–7, **12**, 368.

6

found in several experiments. Asphyxia was a very different state from that produced by ether. Although an animal in a state of asphyxia from breathing air deficient in oxygen, was insensible to pain, as he had ascertained, yet the insensibility was of but short duration, ending soon either in return to sensibility or in death. . . . [Ether] allowed the blood to be changed from venous to arterial in the lungs, but probably interfered with the changes which take place in the capillaries of the system. He had ascertained that a little vapour of ether mixed with air would prevent the oxidation of phosphorus placed in it, and considered that it had a similar effect over the oxygen in the blood, and reduced to a minimum the oxidation of nervous and other tissues. . . .'¹

At the next meeting of the Society Snow supplemented his paper :

' He had completed some experiments, by which he had ascertained that the vapour of ether was given out again from the lungs unchanged, and that the amount of carbonic acid gas produced during the inhalation of ether was less than at other times : these circumstances he considered confirmed the explanation of the *modus operandi* of ether [*i.e.* that it reduced to a minimum the oxidation of nervous and other tissues] which he had previously given.'²

For the guidance of clinicians Snow divided the progress of anaesthesia into five stages :

' The point requiring most skill and care in the administration of the vapour of ether is, undoubtedly, to determine when it has been carried far enough ', he wrote. ' In order to communicate, with some degree of clearness, what I have been able to observe by close attention to the subject, I shall divide the effects of ether into five stages or degrees ; premising, however, that the division is, in some measure, arbitrary—that the different degrees run gradually into each other, and are not always clearly to be distinguished—and that the language I have used has been chosen with the sole object that my meaning might not be mistaken.

' In the first degree of etherization I shall include the various changes of feeling that a person may experience, whilst he still retains a correct consciousness of where he is, and what is occurring around him, and a capacity to direct his voluntary movements. In what I call the second degree, mental functions may

¹ *Lancet*, 1847, i, 227.   ² *Ibid.* i, 228.

be exercised, and voluntary actions performed, but in a disordered manner.   In the third degree, there is no evidence of any mental function being exercised, and consequently no voluntary motions occur ; but muscular contractions, in addition to those concerned

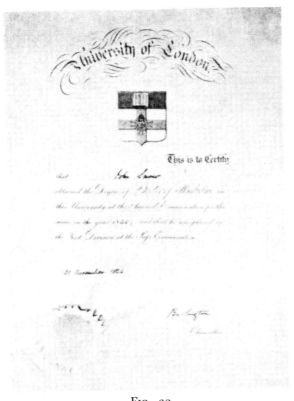

FIG. 32

Certificate issued to John Snow by the University of London upon his receiving the degree of Doctor of Medicine, on December 20, 1844.

in respiration, may sometimes take place as the effect of ether, or of external impressions.   In the fourth degree, no movements are seen except those of respiration, and they are incapable of being influenced by external impressions.   In the fifth degree (not witnessed in the human being), the respiratory movements are more or less paralysed, and become difficult, feeble or irregular.'[1]

[1] Snow, J. 1847. *On the inhalation of the vapour of ether in surgical operations.* London. 1, 2.

Snow reckoned that the fourth degree of anaesthesia was reached, in an average middle-aged man, after four minutes' inhalation of air containing 45 per cent. ether vapour. ' When the ether is administered in the method that I recommend ', wrote Snow, ' the patient usually passes quietly and quickly through the second degree of etherization without its being manifested in any way.' [1]   In the third degree, Snow pointed out, ' persons in a full state of health, and more particularly those in a state of plethora, are more liable to struggling and rigidity . . . than those whose strength is reduced by illness.' [2]

Describing further indications by which the depth of anaesthesia might be gauged, Snow admitted that ' in the earlier cases I had to raise the eyelid to look at the pupil. I was not able to learn much from it, as generally it is not much altered from its natural state, and remains more or less sensible to light in all stages of etherization ; but I soon found that the eyelids furnished very good information with regard to the state of the patient.' [3]

As Snow's experience of ether anaesthesia increased he found it feasible to reduce the heat of the water-bath of his inhaler to 50° F. and generally administered a 30 per cent. mixture of ether in air to his patients. He noted that, as a rule, satisfactory surgical anaesthesia was established in children in from two to three minutes, in adults in from four to five minutes.[4] This time factor—exactly how long the patient had been inhaling—was, in Snow's opinion, a fairly safe indication of the degree of etherization ; but ' if there is any doubt about the patient's condition ', he advised, ' it is preferable to wait a little longer till the excito-motory action of the eyelids diminishes, or till the breathing is decidedly automatic, or accompanied with a tendency to snoring, or till the countenance is somewhat altered, which is sometimes the case before the eyelids are quite passive '. If cyanosis should at any stage appear, Snow advised discontinuing administration by removing the facepiece for half a minute.[5]

In spite of Snow's timely and excellent advice and the almost daily example of his successful methods in the theatres of St. George's and University College Hospital (where Snow was now anaesthetist), very many of his contemporaries were beset with technical difficulties and conscientious doubts. During March

[1] Snow, J. 1847. *On the inhalation of the vapour of ether in surgical operations.* London 3.   [2] *Ibid.* 6.   [3] *Ibid.* 34.
[4] Snow, J. 1858. *On chloroform and other anaesthetics.* London. 356, 357.
[5] Snow, J. 1847. *On the inhalation of the vapour of ether* . . . London. 35, 36.

1847 two so-called ether fatalities—one at Grantham, the other at the Essex and Colchester Hospital—shook public confidence. An inquest was held on the body of the Grantham victim, a young woman. Despite the fact that the patient did not die under the anaesthetic (given from a Squire's type of apparatus) and that the post-mortem findings were entirely negative, indeed because of this, a verdict was returned—

'That the deceased . . . died from the effects of the vapour of ether, inhaled by her for the purpose of alleviating pain during the removal of a tumour from her left thigh, and not from the effect of the operation, or from any other cause.' [1]

In the second case also, at the Essex and Colchester Hospital, the patient, a man of fifty-two, survived the operation, lithotomy, and died in a state of collapse many hours afterwards. Again post-mortem findings were vague. Nunn, the surgeon involved, made the following statement, however :

'It may be said that the ether fulfilled its intended offices. But I think another question is involved, viz. whether the artificial means thus employed may not produce very serious depressing effects upon the nervous system, depriving a patient of that reactive power so necessary to the reparative process ? . . . Pain is doubtless our great safeguard under ordinary circumstances ; but for it we should hourly be running into danger ; and I am inclined to believe that pain should be considered as a healthy indication, and an essential concomitant with surgical operations, and that it is amply compensated for by the effects it produces on the system as the natural incentive to reparative action.' [2]

This theory of the usefulness of pain gained many adherents among unsuccessful anaesthetists and sceptical laymen, but fortunately their influence over general opinion was slight. More thoughtful men, nevertheless, began to look about them for an alternative to ether easier to administer and more reliable in action than this agent had so far proved. A prime mover in this field of research was James Young Simpson, Professor of Midwifery in the University of Edinburgh.

[1] *Lancet*, 1847, i, 342.   [2] *Ibid.* i, 343

CHAPTER V

SIMPSON AND CHLOROFORM

Waldie's Part in the Discovery—The Use of Anaesthesia in Childbirth and the ' Religious ' Controversy arising therefrom—Chloroform Supersedes Ether in Practice.

Waldie's Part in the Discovery

' FROM the time at which I first saw Ether-Inhalation successfully practised in January last ', wrote Simpson at the beginning of November 1847, ' I have had the conviction impressed upon my mind, that we would ultimately find that other therapeutic agents were capable of being introduced with equal rapidity and success into the system, through the same extensive and powerful channel of pulmonary absorption. . . .

' With various professional friends, more conversant with chemistry than I am, I have, since that time, taken opportunities of talking over the idea . . . and I have had, during the summer and autumn, ethereal tinctures, etc., of several potent drugs, manufactured for me for experiment. . . .

' Latterly, in order to avoid, if possible, some of the inconveniences and objections pertaining to sulphuric ether (particularly its disagreeable and very persistent smell, its occasional tendency to irritation of the bronchi during its first inspirations, and the large quantity of it occasionally required to be used [ether was given on a sponge at Edinburgh] more especially in protracted cases of labour), I have tried upon myself and others the inhalation of different other volatile fluids, with the hope that some one of them might be found to possess the advantages of ether without its disadvantages. For this purpose, I selected for experiment and have inhaled . . . the chloride of hydro-carbon (or Dutch liquid) [= 1,2-dichloroethane, $C_2H_4Cl_2$], acetone, nitrate of oxide of ethyle (nitric ether) [= ethyl nitrate, C_2H_5 ONO_2], benzin [= benzene, C_6H_6], the vapour of iodoform, etc.' [1]

[1] Simpson here added a footnote acknowledging the help of various chemists and of his two assistants, Keith and Duncan. He also mentioned that ' Mr. Waldie first named to me the Perchloride of Formyle [Chloroform] as worthy among others of a trial.' These few words later gave rise to disputation (see p. 173 *et seq.*).

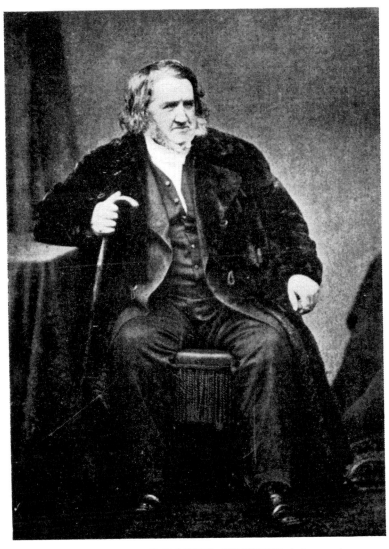

FIG. 33.—JAMES YOUNG SIMPSON (1811–70)

Created first baronet, 1866 ; physician ; appointed Professor of Midwifery at Edinburgh, 1839. Introduced the use of chloroform anaesthesia into practice in November 1847.

167

' I have found, however ', Simpson continued, ' one infinitely more efficacious than any of the others, viz. Chloroform, or the Perchloride of Formyle, and I am enabled to speak most confidently of its superior anaesthetic properties, having now tried it upon upwards of thirty individuals. . . .

' As an inhaled anaesthetic agent, it possesses over Sulphuric Ether the following advantages :

' 1. A greatly less quantity of Chloroform . . . is requisite to produce the anaesthetic effect. . . .

' 2. Its action is much more rapid and complete, and generally more persistent. . . .

' 3. Most of those who know . . . the sensations produced by ether inhalation, and who have subsequently breathed the Chloroform, have strongly declared the inhalation and influence of Chloroform to be far more agreeable and pleasant than those of Ether.

' 4. I believe that, considering the small quantity requisite, as compared with Ether, the use of Chloroform will be less expensive. . . .

' No special kind of inhaler or instrument is necessary for its exhibition. A little of the liquid diffused upon the interior of a hollow-shaped sponge, or a pocket-handkerchief, or a piece of linen or paper, and held over the mouth and nostrils, so as to be fully inhaled, generally suffices in about a minute or two to produce the desired effect.' Simpson added, in a footnote, ' when used for surgical purposes, perhaps it will be found to be most easily given upon a handkerchief, gathered up into a cup-like form in the hand of the exhibitor, and with the open end of the cup placed over the nose and mouth of the patient. For the first inspiration or two, it should be held at the distance of half an inch or so from the face, and then more and more closely applied to it. To insure a rapid and perfect anaesthetic effect . . . one or two teaspoonfuls of the Chloroform should be at once placed upon the hollow of the handkerchief, and immediately held to the face of the patient. Generally a snoring sleep speedily supervenes ; and when it does so, it is a perfect test of the superinduction of complete insensibility. But a patient may be quite anaesthetic without this symptom supervening.'

At the time of writing this report Simpson admitted, ' I have not yet had an opportunity of using Chloroform in any capital surgical operation, but have exhibited it with perfect success in tooth-drawing, opening abscesses, for annulling the pain of dysmenorrhoea and of neuralgia, . . . etc. I have employed it also in obstetric practice with entire success.' He was able to add a postscript on November 15 :

'I have—through the great kindness of Professor Miller and Mr. Duncan—had an opportunity of trying the effects of the inhalation of Chloroform to-day in three cases of operation in the Royal Infirmary of Edinburgh.' [1]

On November 20, 1847, ' several operations were performed at St. Bartholomew's Hospital, upon patients rendered insensible to pain by the administration of chloroform, after the manner described in a recently-published pamphlet, by Professor Simpson. . . . The chloroform . . . was administered by Mr. Tracy, by means of a thin, flat piece of sponge, impregnated with the fluid, and of sufficient size to cover the mouth and the apertures of the nose.' [2]

Tracy closely followed Edinburgh methods (cf. p. 146), but there was possibly a further reason for this rapid adoption of chloroform at St. Bartholomew's. During the summer of 1847, William (later Sir William) Lawrence, one of the hospital's leading surgeons, had already been experimenting both in private and hospital practice, with a new anaesthetic agent which went by the name of chloric ether. This was, in fact, a solution of chloroform in alcohol, a mixture which in pre-anaesthetic days had, as an antispasmodic, a similar although lesser reputation to that of sulphuric ether.

Lawrence published no account of his experiments with chloric ether as an anaesthetic, but his colleague, Holmes Coote, who regularly reported on work at St. Bartholomew's for the *Lancet*, stated that in November 1847 Lawrence was ' in the habit of directing its administration ' and found it in many ways more satisfactory than sulphuric ether. It was less irritating to the lungs, pleasanter to the taste, provided more tranquil induction and was followed by milder after-effects.[3]

A still earlier use of chloric ether, in February 1847, was briefly noticed in a footnote by Jacob Bell in the *Pharmaceutical*

---

[1] Simpson, J. Y. 1847. *Account of a new anaesthetic agent as a substitute for sulphuric ether in surgery and midwifery.* Edinburgh. 5–18.

[2] *Lancet*, 1847, ii, 571.

[3] *Ibid.* ii, 571, 572 ; Channing, W. 1848. *On etherization.* Boston. 61 ; *Pharm. J.,* 1870–1, N.S. **1**, 467.

6*

Journal : ' Chloric ether has been tried in some cases with success, it is more pleasant to the taste, but appears to be rather less powerful in its effects than sulphuric ether.' [1]   This trial is believed to have been made at the Middlesex Hospital and to have been abandoned on account of ' the great expense of it compared with ether.' [2]

During February 1847, Flourens, in the course of his physiological experiments on animals, used chloroform alone and also ethyl chloride.

' *Hydrochloric ether* ' (*l'éther chlorhydrique*, ethyl chloride), he said at a meeting of the Académie des Sciences, ' gave me the same results as *sulphuric ether*. The use of *hydrochloric ether* has led me to test the new compound known under the name of *chloroform*. At the end of a very few minutes (six in the first case, four in the second and one in a third) an animal forced to breathe the vapour of chloroform has been completely etherized[3]. The spinal cord was then laid bare : . . . the posterior roots were insensible ; out of five anterior roots successively tested, only two still retained their motricity ; the other three had lost it.' [4]

This short series of researches on chloroform attracted no immediate attention. But Flourens's statement that the action of ethyl chloride was similar to that of sulphuric ether was followed up by von Bibra and Harless in the laboratory (see pp. 157–8) and by J. F. Heyfelder clinically, although in three cases only (the insertion of a seton in a twenty-three-year-old man ; Chopart's amputation in a thirty-year-old spinster ; and the excision of a condyloma in a forty-four-year-old matron). Heyfelder noted the rapid but transient action of ethyl chloride, as compared with that of ether, the pleasantness of induction and the absence of coughing and of all respiratory embarrassment and the absence, also, of increased mucous secretion and of any after-effect of anaesthesia. In spite of these satisfactory results, Heyfelder stated that in his opinion the extreme volatility of the drug combined with its high price and the difficulty of obtaining it pure, precluded its frequent use.

Heyfelder tested chloroform also, but after its introduction into practice by Simpson. He was immediately convinced of its superiority. By comparison with ether he found chloroform

[1] *Pharm. J.*, 1846–7, **6**, 357.
[2] *Lond. med. Gaz.*, 1847, **5**, 939, footnote ; 1153, footnote.
[3] The term *éthérisé* was afterwards commonly used in France to describe the anaesthetic state produced by chloroform. (See Appendix B.)
[4] *C.R. Acad. Sci., Paris*, 1847, **24**, 342, 457.

pleasanter to inhale, less likely to produce coughing, headache, nausea and vomiting, and he was favourably impressed by the speed with which the effects of anaesthesia passed off post-operatively.[1]

When Flourens, in February 1847, spoke of chloroform as a ' new agent ' it was, in fact, just over fifteen years old, having been discovered in 1831 by the French chemist, Soubeiran and independently by the American, Samuel Guthrie of Sackett's Harbour in the State of New York.

By distilling a mixture of chloride of lime and alcohol Soubeiran obtained impure chloroform which he provisionally called ' bichloric ether ' (*éther bichlorique*).[2] A purer chloroform was obtained by a similar process by Liebig in the following year. He called it ' liquid chloride of carbon ' (*chlorure de carbone liquide*), but made an error in the analysis.[3] It was not until 1834 that Dumas succeeded in obtaining and correctly analysing pure chloroform, and it was he who first gave it that name.[4]

Guthrie was less interested in the chemical than in the therapeutic significance of the new agent which he accidentally discovered. The term *chloric ether* had been applied by the English chemist Thomson, in 1820, to the Dutch liquid or chloride of olefiant gas (cf. p. 166). An alcoholic solution of this agent was, in 1831, esteemed ' a grateful and diffusible stimulant '[5] and it was in attempting to prepare Thomson's *chloric ether* for solution in alcohol by a cheap and simple process that Guthrie obtained chloroform. He continued to believe, however, that the properties of this new drug were identical with those of the Dutch liquid.

' As the usual process for obtaining chloric ether for solution in alcohol is both troublesome and expensive, and as from its lively and invigorating effects it may become an article of some value in the Materia Medica ',

wrote Guthrie, in a letter to Benjamin Silliman, editor of the *American Journal of Science and Arts*,

' I have thought a portion of your readers might be gratified with the communication of a cheap and easy process for preparing it. . . .

[1] Heyfelder, F. 1848. *Die Versuche mit dem Schwefeläther, Salzäther und Chloroform, und die daraus gewonnenen Resultate in der chirurgischen Klinik zu Erlangen.* Erlangen. 83–5.
[2] *Ann. Chim. (Phys.)*, 1831, **48**, 131 *et seq.*   [3] *Ibid.* 1832, **49**, 163 *et seq.*
[4] *Ibid.* 1834, **56**, 115–20.   [5] *Pharm. J.*, 1845–6, **5**, 112.

'Into a clean copper still put three pounds of chloride of lime and two gallons of well flavored alcohol . . . and distil. Watch the process, and when the product ceases to come highly sweet and aromatic, remove and cork it up closely in glass vessels. . . . By redistilling the product from a great excess of chloride of lime, in a glass retort, in a water bath, a greatly concentrated solution will be obtained. This new product is caustic, and intensely sweet and aromatic. . . .

'During the last six months', Guthrie added, 'a great number of persons have drunk of the solution of chloric ether [*i.e.* the 'new product', chloroform, in alcohol] in my laboratory, not only very freely, but frequently to the point of intoxication.'

Upon this last assertion Silliman commented : 'We ought to discountenance any other than a medicinal use of this singular solution. . . . He would be no benefactor to his species who should add a new attraction to intoxicating spirit.'[1]

During 1832 Eli Ives, Professor of the Theory and Practice of Medicine in the Medical Institution at Yale, applied the 'solution of chloric ether' both in small doses by mouth and as a therapeutic inhalant in various diseases involving the respiratory tract.[2]

From 1832 onwards it was no longer the Dutch liquid but Guthrie's preparation, chloroform in alcoholic solution, which was commonly known as 'chloric ether'; nevertheless, confusion as to the identity of 'chloric ether' occurred from time to time.

According to David Waldie, Chemist to the Apothecaries' Company of Liverpool, who made many inquiries on the subject, American 'chloric ether' was introduced into British practice 'as a medical agent, first in Liverpool, where, indeed, in the form of a spirituous solution, it has been more known than in any other part of the country, and from which, I believe, the knowledge of its therapeutic properties has extended. About the year 1838 or 1839, a prescription was brought to the Apothecaries' Hall [Liverpool] . . . one ingredient of which was chloric ether. No substance being known there of that name having the properties of that with which the mixture had been previously prepared . . . the company's chemist, in investigating the subject, found in the United States Dispensatory, the formula for its preparation . . . and prepared some. Its properties pleased some of the medical men, particularly Dr. Formby, by whom it

[1] *Amer. J. Sci.*, 1832, **21**, 64–5.   [2] *Ibid.* **21**, 406.

was introduced into practice in this town. After coming to take charge of the company's laboratories ', Waldie stated, ' I . . . altered the process [of preparation] by separating and purifying the chloroform, and dissolving it in pure spirit, by which a product of uniform strength and sweet flavour was always obtained.' [1]

Describing how, while in Scotland in October 1847, he directed the attention of Simpson to chloroform, Waldie said :

' Dr. Simpson introduced the subject to me, inquiring if I knew of any thing likely to answer [for anaesthetic purposes]. Chloric ether was mentioned during the conversation, and being well acquainted with its composition, and with the volatility, agreeable flavour, and medicinal properties of Chloroform, I recommended him to try *it*, promising to prepare some after my return to Liverpool, and send it to him.   Other engagements, and various impediments prevented me from doing this so soon as I should have wished, and in the meantime Dr. Simpson having procured some in Edinburgh, obtained the results which he com-municated to the Medico-Chirurgical Society of Edinburgh on the 10th November, and which he published in a pamphlet . . .' [2]

When Waldie read the paper, from which the passages just quoted have been taken, before a meeting of the Liverpool Literary and Philosophical Society on November 29, 1847, he appeared to have no grievance. But time passed and Simpson made no acknowledgement to Waldie beyond the single mention of him in the footnote to the published account of chloroform anaesthesia (see p. 166, footnote). As months stretched into years Waldie, and perhaps more particularly his friends and relations, came to believe that he had been the prime mover in establishing the anaesthetic use of chloroform and that, as such, he had been unjustly neglected.

Soon after Simpson's death in 1870, Waldie once more publicly drew attention to his share in the application of chloro-form in anaesthesia, by publishing a ' Re-statement ' in which he wrote :

' The recognition which my share in the discovery has met with has been considered by many as inadequate ; nor was it altogether satisfactory to myself. . . .'

[1] Waldie, D. 1870. *The true story of the introduction of chloroform into anaesthetics.* Linlithgow and Edinburgh. 7.
[2] *Ibid.* 88.

After describing his recommendation of chloroform to Simpson and his own unavoidably unfulfilled promise to prepare and send a sample to Edinburgh, Waldie continued :

' When the news [of Simpson's anaesthetic use of chloroform] came . . . I felt pleased at the success of my recommendation, but was also mortified that from . . . unfortunate circumstances [the destruction of his laboratory by fire just previous to his interview with Simpson] I had not been able to do something in carrying it out. I had inhaled both nitrous oxide gas and ether vapours before, and felt interested in the enquiry ; and have no doubt but that if I had been in a position to prepare the Chloroform, I should at once have discovered its properties on my own person. But when the small pamphlet announcing the discovery was introduced to my notice, I was further disappointed, for all the acknowledgement made by Dr. Simpson of my suggestion was, that amongst chemists with whom he had conversed on the subject, Mr. Waldie first mentioned Chloroform as likely to answer, and this too was given not in the text, but in a footnote. I at once saw that this was well adapted, even if not intended, to lead to my share in the matter being altogether lost sight of ; and the account of my recommendation as merely a matter *mentioned*, was a parsimony of acknowledgement for which I was not prepared. . . . As I did not wish to quarrel ', Waldie added, ' and did not feel inclined to go a-begging for more credit than those concerned were willing to give spontaneously, I made no remark on the subject.

' Some of my friends have considerably over-rated the importance of my share in the discovery [1], but this I have uniformly discountenanced. Willingly do I acknowledge that the discovery was Dr. Simpson's, and the honour his due. All that I looked for was a distinct and honest acknowledgement that I had recommended or even suggested to him to try Chloroform. . . . His reputation cannot suffer by my getting credit for what I am justly entitled to, and that is all I ask ; and I would willingly entertain the hope, that had he been still living amongst us, and my claim been placed before him as it now is before the public, he himself would have admitted its justice.' [2]

In fact, the credit which Waldie so much desired had already been freely given to him, if not by Simpson at least by others of

[1] Cf. *e.g.* O'Leary, A. J. 'Who was the person who discovered chloroform for anaesthesia : was it Simpson or Waldie ? ' *Brit. J. Anaesth.*, 1934–5, **12**, 41–5.
[2] Waldie, D. 1870. *The true story of the introduction of chloroform into anaesthetics.* Linlithgow and Edinburgh. 21–5.

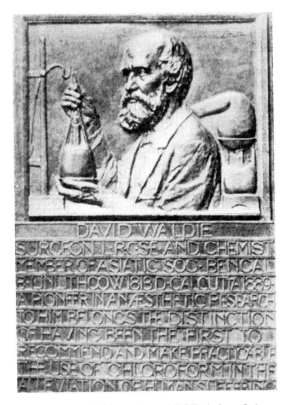

Fig. 34.—DAVID WALDIE (1813–89)

who, in October 1847, directed the attention of
Simpson to the probability that chloroform would
prove a satisfactory anaesthetic agent.

equal reputation in the anaesthetic world, but because he had
been working in India for many years he was possibly unaware of
acknowledgements such as Snow's :

'Mr. Waldie, of Liverpool, had a greater share in the introduction of chloroform than Dr. Jackson had in the introduction
of ether . . . for when he informed Dr. Simpson of the existence and nature of chloroform, he was able to give him, not
merely an opinion, but an almost certain knowledge of its
effects.' [1]

[1] Snow, J. 1858. *On chloroform and other anaesthetics.* London. 17.

The Use of Anaesthesia in Childbirth and the 'Religious' Controversy

Towards the end of January 1847, Simpson began to use ether anaesthesia as a routine measure to relieve the pains of childbirth in his obstetrical practice. In this particular application Simpson was the pioneer, although in February Baron P. Dubois, in Paris, also began to use ether in labour. Their example was quickly followed by other medical men.

The attitude of the Scot and of the Frenchman differed, however, for Simpson used ether with full confidence, Dubois with misgiving.

'Since the latter part of January', wrote Simpson, 'I have employed etherization, with few and rare exceptions, in every case of labour which has been under my care. And the results . . . have been, indeed, most happy and gratifying. I never had the pleasure of watching over a series of more perfect or more rapid recoveries ; nor have I once witnessed any disagreeable result to either mother or child.' [1]

Dubois, after his first five cases, was also able to say, 'None of the women who inhaled ether have experienced any bad effects attributable to ether.' But he hastened to qualify this statement :

'However, two of these women died of metroperitonitis . . . those two who underwent the application of the forceps. I have put to myself the question, whether the adhibition of ether did in any way contribute to the fatal result in these two cases.'

Dubois admitted :

'That the delivery of the two women . . . did take place under circumstances that may easily account for death . . . one of these patients had been in labour during 40 and the other during 38 hours ; such, we are well aware, are very unfavourable preliminaries to delivery, and in these cases they proved the more unfavourable still, from the circumstances of the Maternité being at that period under the influence of a slight epidemic of puerperal fever.'

Nevertheless Dubois continued to doubt :

'My profound feeling on the subject is, that inhalation of ether in midwifery should be restrained to a very limited number of cases, the nature of which ulterior experience will better allow us to determine.' [2]

[1] Simpson, J. Y. 1847. *Remarks on the superinduction of anaesthesia in natural and morbid parturition.* Edinburgh. 12.   [2] *Lancet,* 1847, i, 246–9.

In America, Walter Channing, of Harvard, adopted the use of ether in childbirth after news of Simpson's and Dubois's cases had crossed the Atlantic.

In spite of the gratitude and enthusiasm expressed by Simpson's patients for the blessing of ether during labour, he was soon attacked in Scotland and elsewhere, on the grounds that he was contravening the Divine Will. Had not God, setting his primeval curse upon woman, decreed ' *In sorrow* thou shalt bring forth children ' ?

When, in November 1847, Simpson began to use chloroform in place of ether in childbirth, the publicity accorded to the new agent caused this argument to be repeated with fresh vehemence.

Simpson replied to his critics with an erudite article in which he showed, with a great deal of counter-quotation, ' that the Hebrew term which, in our English translation of the primeval curse, is rendered " sorrow " (Genesis, iii, 16), principally signifies the severe muscular *efforts* and *struggles* of which parturition— and more particularly human parturition—essentially consists ; and does not specially signify the *feelings* or *sensations* of pain to which these muscular efforts or contractions give rise.' [1]

Many pamphlets were written in support of Simpson's views and the obstetrician, E. W. Murphy, pointed out, ' that man who was destined " to eat bread *in sorrow* all the days of his life " contrived to dine as comfortably as his means permitted, notwithstanding the curse.' [2]

Fortunately common sense won. ' Medical men may oppose for a time the superinduction of anaesthesia in parturition ', wrote Simpson, ' but they will oppose it in vain ; for certainly our patients themselves will force the use of it upon the profession. The whole question is, even now, one merely of time.' [3]

By the middle of the year 1848 the practice of administering an anaesthetic during labour was well established. In 1850, discreet inquiries on behalf of Queen Victoria herself about chloroform anaesthesia were made of John Snow, before the birth of Prince Arthur. Three years later, in April 1853, the seal of perfect propriety was set upon it when Snow was summoned

[1] Simpson, J. Y. 1848. *Answer to the religious objections advanced against the employment of anaesthetic agents in midwifery and surgery.* Edinburgh. 13.
[2] Murphy, E. W. 1855. *Chloroform in childbirth.* London. 3.
[3] Simpson, J. Y. 1847. *Remarks on the superinduction of anaesthesia in natural and morbid parturition.* Edinburgh. 13.

to give chloroform to Her Majesty during the birth of Prince Leopold.

Ether superseded by Chloroform in Practice

Within a few months of Simpson's demonstration of the anaesthetic properties of chloroform, ether was almost universally discarded in favour of the new agent. ' The introduction of chloroform produced an excitement scarcely less than that of the discovery of the narcotic effect of ether ', wrote John Collins Warren.[1]

Snow, referring in 1858 to the early days of chloroform anaesthesia, wrote :

' Chloroform was immediately used everywhere to a greater extent than ether had been. An impression became very prevalent that chloroform was safer than ether. This impression arose rather from the general tenour of Dr. Simpson's essay than from any direct statement, for he had not treated on this point.

' The great strength of chloroform as compared with ether, and the extreme care required in its use, were indeed soon pointed out ; [2] these precautions, however, attracted but little attention till the first death from chloroform occurred near Newcastle on the 28th January, 1848 [see pp. 195–7]. Ether was exhibited by inhalation during eleven months in Europe, and about sixteen months in America, before chloroform was introduced. During all this time no death was occasioned by its use, if we except one at Auxerre in France, which appeared to be occasioned by want of air, owing to an imperfect inhaler, and not to the effect of ether. Chloroform had only been employed between two and three months when the above mentioned death occurred, and this was soon followed by others in nearly all parts of the world. These accidents have prevented many persons from inhaling chloroform, and they have prevented a still greater number from enjoying that freedom from anxiety and apprehension before an operation, which ought to be one of the greatest advantages of any plan for preventing pain.' [3]

The fear—shared equally by administrator and patient— that, skill and care notwithstanding, the action of chloroform was unpredictable and uncontrollable, and that as a result of its

[1] Warren, J. C. 1849. *Effects of chloroform and of strong chloric ether.* Boston. 5.
[2] *E.g.* by Snow himself : *Lond. med. Gaz.*, 1847, **5,** 1031.
[3] Snow, J. 1858. *On chloroform and other anaesthetics.* London. 22–3.

application the patient might die, was a serious deterrent from its continued use.

What was to be done ? One possible course of action was to return to the use of sulphuric ether. This was the course adopted by Pétrequin, of Lyons, during 1848, after the occurrence of two deaths from chloroform ; by the surgeons of Naples, following Pétrequin's example (see p. 204) ; by Cantu, of Turin, and at the Massachusetts General Hospital, where the use of chloroform was prohibited not long after its introduction there. The readoption of ether soon became general throughout the Northern States of America.[1]

An alternative course was to try to discover some anaesthetic agent which would combine the safety of ether with the potency, pleasantness and simplicity of application afforded by chloroform. In Vienna and in certain parts of the Austrian Empire, notably Northern Italy, mixtures of chloroform and ether were used in the belief that each drug would counteract the disadvantages of the other. The famous ' Vienna anaesthetic ', for example, was said, during the eighteen-fifties, to consist of one part of chloroform to six or eight parts of ether.[2]

A third course was to persevere in the use of chloroform, trusting that greater experience would teach how its inherent dangers could be avoided or completely overcome. This was the course chosen by the vast majority of the medical profession in the Old World.

Snow himself readily admitted the greater safety of ether :

' I believe that ether is altogether incapable of causing the sudden death by paralysis of the heart, which has caused the accidents which have happened during the administration of chloroform. I have not been able to kill an animal in that manner with ether, even when I have made it boil, and administered the vapour almost pure. The heart has continued to beat after the natural breathing has ceased, even when the vapour has been exhibited without air. . . . Even in cases where the natural breathing had ceased, if the animal made a gasping inspiration after its removal from the ether it recovered.

' I hold it, therefore, to be almost impossible that a death from this agent can occur in the hands of a medical man who is applying it with ordinary intelligence and attention.' [3]

[1] *Lond. med. Gaz.*, 1849, **8,** 758.
[2] Cf. Kidd, C. 1859. *A manual of anaesthetics.* London. 14, 42.
[3] Snow, J. 1858. *On chloroform and other anaesthetics.* London. 362.

Snow also expressed a preference for ' the flavour of ether vapour to that of chloroform ; and the sensations I experience from the inhalation of ether are more pleasurable than those from chloroform '. He added : ' The quantity of ether expended in causing insensibility is eight or ten times as great as that of chloroform, but the quantity used in a protracted operation is not so disproportionate ; for, owing to the great solubility of ether and the large quantity of it which is absorbed, it is much longer in exhaling by the breath, and when the patient is once fairly insensible, it does not require to be repeated so frequently as chloroform. . . . On account of this longer duration of the effects of ether, it is better adapted than chloroform for certain operations on the face, as removal of tumours of the jaws, the operation for hare-lip, and making a new nose. The relaxation of the muscular system from the effects of ether seems greater in general than from chloroform, and ether therefore seems to be the better agent to employ in the reduction of old dislocations, and strangulated hernia '.[1]

In spite of all these advantages Snow preferred to use chloroform. His biographer, Benjamin Ward Richardson, tells the story that Snow was once challenged to give his reasons for thus persisting in its use if, as on his own showing it appeared, ether were so much safer. He is said to have replied : ' I use chloroform for the same reason that you use phosphorus matches instead of the tinder box. An occasional risk never stands in the way of ready applicability '.[2]

A tendency to be strongly influenced by expediency is apparent more than once in Snow's writings. Nevertheless, to satisfy him, expediency had to be based upon scientific reasoning and careful experiment. He disapproved, for instance, of the kind of haphazard expediency resorted to in the early days of chloroform administration at Edinburgh—methods such as those reported by Simpson's colleague, Professor Miller :

' The apparatus for inhaling need be of the simplest kind ; anything that will admit of chloroform in vapour being brought fully into contact with the mouth and nostrils, a handkerchief, a

---

[1] In suggesting the use of ether as preferable to that of chloroform in these particular types of case Snow expressed an opinion which was exactly the opposite of that which came generally to be held during the latter part of the nineteenth century (see pp. 340–2). (Snow, J. 1858. *On chloroform and other anaesthetics*. London. 357, 361.)
[2] B. W. Richardson, in Snow, J. 1858. *On chloroform . . .* London. xxxv.

towel, a piece of lint, a worsted glove, a nightcap, a sponge. . .
In the winter season, the glove of a clerk, dresser, or onlooker,
has been not unfrequently pressed into service.' [1]

Snow, in quoting the above passage, scornfully italicised
worsted glove and *nightcap* and commented that the method was
' somewhat slovenly, and not very cleanly '.[2]

Nevertheless the method of anaesthetizing by boldly pouring
an unmeasured quantity of a volatile anaesthetic on to a sponge
or cloth held over the patient's nose and mouth was found, by
those who used it, to be both simple and effective ; they held,
moreover, that by such means the dangers of overdosage and
asphyxia were potentially less than when any kind of mechanical
apparatus was used. Both the Americans, returning to the use
of ether poured on to a bell-shaped sponge, and the Scots giving
chloroform from a cloth, believed their own procedure to be as
nearly foolproof as could be hoped for, and to a considerable
extent results appear to have justified them. For almost half a
century in America, and for a longer period in Scotland, few
medical men saw the need for change or presumed to make any.

During the early eighteen-fifties Continental administrators
adopted methods of chloroform anaesthesia akin to the Scottish
(see pp. 228, 233).

For the remainder of the nineteenth century the design of
apparatus for inhalation anaesthesia was studied and developed
chiefly in England. The very facts that apparatuses were far
from perfect and that as a result of chloroform anaesthesia patients
were liable unpredictably to die, acted as a constant stimulus to
English anaesthetists. Many became deeply interested in the
physiological action of anaesthetics, attempting always to relate
experimental research to clinical needs. Although the death-
rate from chloroform anaesthesia continued to be high in
England, it was, for the most part, from this country that ad-
vancement in the science and art of inhalation anaesthesia came.

---

[1] Miller, J. 1848. *Surgical experience of chloroform.* Edinburgh and London. 16.
[2] Snow, J. 1858. *On chloroform and other anaesthetics.* London. 79.

CHAPTER VI

EARLY EXPERIENCES WITH CHLOROFORM

Methods of Administration—Snow's Researches—The first Chloroform
Fatality—Scottish and Continental Methods.

Methods of Administration

THE simplicity and cheapness of Simpson's method of pouring
chloroform on to a folded cloth recommended it to a great
number of medical men in England, particularly in hospitals
and in provincial practice. But although its use was widespread,
it was never, as in Scotland and very generally on the Continent
of Europe, exclusive of other methods.

In England, in 1848, there was a spring flush of inhalers,
as there had been just a year earlier after the introduction of
etherization. This time, however, the number was smaller and
the inhalers showed much less variety and much greater economy
of design.

A popular type of inhaler consisted of a small metal box,
circular or semicircular in shape, containing sponge. Some
were fitted with a facepiece for oral and nasal breathing, others
had only a mouthpiece and depended for success on the patient's
nostrils being closed (see *e.g.* Fig. 35).[1]

Several chloroform inhalers were made simply by adopting a
facepiece alone, adding wires to the inside to hold a sponge
(see *e.g.* Fig. 36), or attaching to the back a small metal cylinder
with a wire mesh cap for the same purpose (see *e.g.* Fig. 37).[2]

Francis Sibson designed an inhaler (Fig. 38) which he
described as follows :

' The basis of this inhaler is the mask that I invented for the
inhalation of ether, which mask Dr. Snow employed in May
last [cf. Figs. 28, 29].

'This inhaler is made of copper, brass, or white metal. It
has a border or face-piece of thin flexible lead lined with oiled
silk, covering the nose and mouth, and from its ductility easily
adapted to any face. The lower or inspiring valve, as seen in

[1] *Pharm. J.*, 1847–8, **7**, 313–14.
[2] *Ibid.* **7**, 313, 393 ; *Lancet*, 1847, ii, 655 ; *ibid.*, 1848, i, 154, 179.

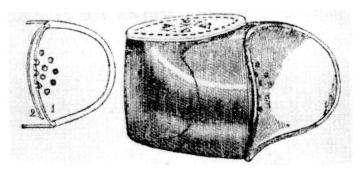

FIG. 35.—CHLOROFORM INHALER MADE BY COXETER
(December 1847)

The body of the inhaler contained sponge. Air entered through the perforations above. The diagram of the mouthpiece in section shows :

1. Front plate with perforations.
2. The second plate to prevent the fluid being drawn into the mouth (cf. Fig. 26).

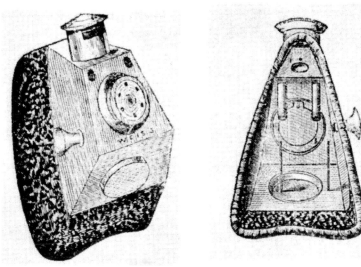

FIG. 36.—CHLOROFORM INHALER ADAPTED FROM A
" SNOW'S FACEPIECE "

(*Left.*) Exterior view. In the back wall, the perforated cap of the inspiratory valve ; above, the orifices of two air-inlet tubes. In the roof, the expiratory valve. On the side wall, a funnel for replenishing the sponge within with chloroform.

(*Right.*) Interior view. In the back wall, the flap of the inspiratory valve ; above, the two air-inlet tubes. In the roof, the orifice of the expiratory valve. From the floor rise two wires to support a sponge. The circular depression in the floor presumably caught surplus liquid chloroform (so long as administration was made with the patient in the sitting position).

the cut [see Fig. 38], is constructed on the principle of Arnott's ventilators, having a counterpoise weight which keeps it shut, unless acted on by pressure from without. The upper, or expiring valve, is a plain metallic lid always closed unless acted on by pressure from within. The tube to which this valve is attached may be drawn out so as to expose an aperture for the admission of air when desired.'

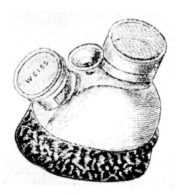

FIG. 37

Modification, made by Weiss *c.* 1865, of a chloroform inhaler designed by Coxeter in 1847. The patient drew air through the wire-mesh of the cylinder attached to the back of the inhaler, which contained chloroform-saturated sponge. Below the cylinder is the expiratory valve. The presence of the small filling funnel in this example suggests that part of the sponge entered the body of the inhaler ; in the original it was confined within the cylinder and there was no funnel.

Sibson also gave directions for using this mask in resuscitation :

' To perform artificial respiration with this inhaler, draw out the expiratory tube : imbed the mask firmly on the face—press back the larynx against the oesophagus and spine—inspire deeply, and distend the chest by blowing through the upper tube. Renew the artificial respirations in rhythmical succession, about sixteen in each minute.' [1]

Whitelock, of Salisbury, devised ' a small mask enclosing the mouth and nose ' made of ' porous cloth or silk lined with lint ', and having a thin piece of sponge sandwiched between the outer and inner covers. Another mask, recommended at the time for

[1] *Lond. med. Gaz.*, 1848, **6**, 270–1.

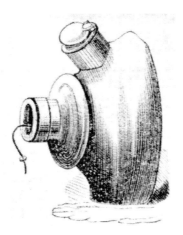

FIG. 38.—SIBSON'S CHLOROFORM INHALER

showing the counterpoise which kept the inspiratory
valve closed except during inspiration.   Above, the
expiratory valve attached to a tube which drew out
' to expose an aperture for the admission of air
when desired.'   Presumably the mask contained a
chloroform-saturated sponge.

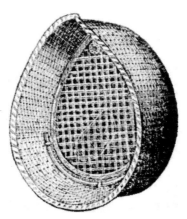

FIG. 39.—CHLOROFORM MASK (1848)

Made of wickerwork.   Between the double walls at the
back of the inhaler was a small piece of sponge.

its cheapness, was of wickerwork (Fig. 39). It was oval and contained a small sponge held behind a frame.[1]

In Paris, Charrière designed an inhaler for chloroform (Fig. 40) to which, ten years later, in 1858, Snow referred as 'the apparatus which is in most reputation on the Continent'.[2]

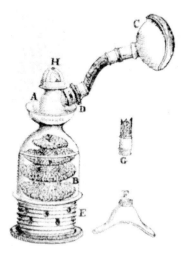

FIG. 40.—CHARRIÈRE'S CHLOROFORM INHALER
In use in Paris, 1848.

A. Trough with perforations (made patent by a screw movement) in the floor, to receive and disperse the chloroform on to B. Spiral framework covered with absorbent material. C. Facepiece (an alternative to F. mouthpiece). D. Ferrule with a hole in it and turning to uncover a similar hole in the tube within, to admit additional air when desired. E. Tin base perforated by two rows of holes (made patent by a screw movement) through which air entered the flask containing B. H. Expiratory ball-valve of cork. The inhaler also contained an inspiratory valve, possibly in the neck of the flask containing B, but said to be at G ; its exact situation in relation to H is, however, doubtful.

Snow stated that he himself, for some weeks after the introduction of chloroform anaesthesia, 'employed the same apparatus in the exhibition of chloroform which [he] . . . had used for ether ; but afterwards ', he continued, ' I contrived a more portable one, still employing this face-piece, which I have used with ether since June last '.[3]

[1] *Pharm. J.*, 1847–8, **7**, 314, 442.
[2] Snow, J. 1858. *On chloroform and other anaesthetics.* London. 85.
[3] *Lancet*, 1848, i, 179.

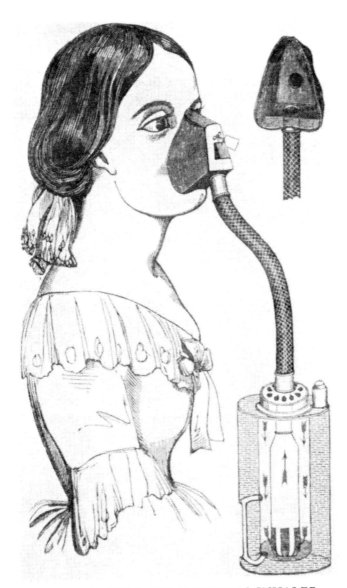

FIG. 41.—SNOW'S CHLOROFORM INHALER

Sectional view of the vaporizing chamber, showing the surrounding water-jacket, chloroform level gauge (bottom left), and, in the inner cylinder, the roll of blotting paper supported on wires and dipping into the liquid chloroform. Arrows indicate the direction of the current of air drawn into the inhaler, through the ring of holes, by the patient's inspiration.

187

The new apparatus (Fig. 41), designed upon the same principle as the ether inhaler (see p. 153), consisted of two metal cylinders, one within the other, the space between them being filled with cold water, which adequately compensated for the heat lost during vaporization, and so prevented the apparatus from freezing up. Snow emphasized that the temperature of the water should not exceed 60° F.

The inner cylinder formed the evaporating chamber and into it was screwed ' a frame, having numerous openings for the admission of air, and four stout wires which descend nearly to the bottom of the space, and are intended to support two coils of stout bibulous paper, which are tied round them, and reach to the bottom of the inhaler. In the lower part of this paper four notches are cut, to allow the air to pass. . . . As the quantity of chloroform which is put in [usually about two to two-and-a-half fluid drachms] should never fill the apertures or notches, the air which passes through the inhaler meets with no obstruction whatever. There is a glass tube communicating with the interior of the inhaler, and passing to the outside, to enable the operator to see when the chloroform requires to be renewed '.

Inhaler and facepiece were connected by a short length of tubing ' three-quarters of an inch in internal diameter, to allow of the passage of as much air as the patient can possibly breathe '.[1] The sole object of the tubing was to allow the inhaler to be applied ' in all positions of the patient '.[2]

When the water-bath of his vaporizer was at a temperature of 60° F. Snow obtained a chloroform-air mixture containing 5 per cent. chloroform. This he diluted with air, by turning aside the expiratory valve on the facepiece, to give him ' about four cubic inches of vapour, or rather more than five grains of chloroform to each hundred cubic inches of air . . . the proportion which . . . [he] found most suitable in practice for causing insensibility to surgical operations '. He advised that ' in medical and obstetric cases, it should be inhaled in a more diluted form '.[3]

Snow decided upon the 4 per cent. mixture of chloroform vapour in air after carrying out, on small animals, an extensive

[1] Snow, J. 1858. On chloroform and other anaesthetics. London. 81, 84.
[2] Lancet, 1848, i, 179.
[3] Snow, J. 1858. On chloroform . . . London. 78, 84.

series of experiments to ascertain the 'amount of vapour of chloroform absorbed to cause the various degrees of narcotism '.[1] ' The experiments were based ', he stated, ' on the following circumstance :

' When air containing vapour is brought in contact with a liquid, as water or serum of blood, absorption of the vapour takes place, and continues till an equilibrium is established ; when the quantity of vapour in both the liquid and air bears the same relative proportion to the quantity which would be required to saturate them at the temperature and pressure to which they are exposed.'

This fact Snow verified ' by numerous experiments in graduated jars over mercury '.

Snow continued :

' The intervention of a thin animal membrane may alter the rapidity of absorption, but cannot cause more vapour to be transmitted than the liquid with which it is imbued can dissolve. The temperature of the air in the cells of the lungs and that of the blood circulating over their parietes is the same ; and, therefore, when the vapour is too dilute to cause death, and is breathed till no increased effect is produced, the following formula will express the quantity of any substance absorbed : As the proportion of vapour in the air breathed is to the proportion that the air, or the space occupied by it, would contain if saturated at the temperature of the blood, so is the proportion of vapour absorbed into the blood to the proportion the blood would dissolve.' [2]

From the results of the series of experiments on animals, Snow deduced ' that two grains of chloroform to each hundred cubic inches of the inspired air cause a state of very complete insensibility, corresponding with what I have designated the fourth degree of narcotism. . . . In experiments . . . in which quantities of chloroform were employed intermediate between one and two grains to each hundred cubic inches of air, a moderate amount of insensibility was induced, corresponding very much with the state of patients during operations under chloroform '. In Snow's opinion, however, although his experiments proved that ' rather less than two grains of chloroform, in one hundred cubic inches [of air], is capable of causing a state of insensibility, sufficiently deep for surgical operations : . . . in a creature the size of the human being, an inconvenient

[1] *Lond. med. Gaz.*, 1848, **6,** 819, 850.
[2] Snow, J. 1858. *On chloroform and other anaesthetics.* London. 59.

length of time would be occupied in causing insensibility with vapour so much diluted '.[1]

Snow was not able satisfactorily to determine from his experiments ' the exact proportion of chloroform which requires to be absorbed to arrest the respiration of animals of warm blood ', although he believed that such a definite proportion existed. He gave two reasons ' why it is not so easy to ascertain it. . . . In the first place, the breathing often becomes very feeble before it ceases, so that the animal inhales and absorbs but very little chloroform, and remains on the brink of dying for some time. In the next place, the temperature of the body falls in a deep state of narcotism . . . and, as the temperature falls, the amount of chloroform which the blood can dissolve from any given mixture of air and vapour increases '.[2]

For clinical purposes Snow estimated that :

' To induce the third degree of narcotism, or the condition in which surgical operations are usually commenced, would require that about 18 minims should be absorbed by an adult of average size and health ; . . . and to induce the deep state of insensi-bility, which I have termed the fourth degree of narcotism, would require 24 minims ; whilst to arrest the function of respiration would require that about 36 minims should be absorbed.' [3]

At one of the Lumlian lectures, held at the Royal College of Physicians on March 29, 1848, Snow neatly demonstrated ' how entirely the effects of a narcotic vapour depend on the quantity of air with which it is mixed, and on other physical conditions '.

' I introduced a chaffinch . . . into a glass jar holding nearly 1000 cubic inches ', said Snow, ' and put a frog into the same jar, covered it with a plate of glass, and dropped five grains of chloro-form on a piece of blotting paper suspended within. In less than ten minutes the frog was insensible, but the bird was not affected. . . . I then placed another frog and another small bird in a jar containing but 200 cubic inches, with exactly the same quantity of chloroform. In about a minute and a half, they were both taken out—the bird totally insensible, but the frog not appreci-ably affected, as from its less active respiration it had not had time to absorb much of the vapour.' [4]

Snow constantly stressed the fact that ' insensibility is not caused so much by giving a dose as by performing a process '.

[1] Snow, J. 1858. *On chloroform and other anaesthetics.* London. 69, 78.
[2] *Ibid.* 69, 70.   [3] *Ibid.* 74.   [4] *Ibid.* 73.

' The great point to be observed in causing insensibility by any narcotic vapour ', he stated, ' is to present to the patient such a mixture of vapour and air as will produce its effects gradually, and enable the medical man to stop at the right moment. . . . If a proper mixture of air and vapour is supplied, each patient will gradually inhale the requisite quantity of the latter to cause insensibility, according to his size and strength. It is indeed desirable to vary the proportions of vapour and air, but rather according to the purpose one has in view, whether medicinal, obstetric, or surgical, than on account of the age or strength of the patient ; for the respiratory process bears such a relation to the latter circumstances, as to cause each person to draw his own proper dose from a similar atmosphere in a suitable time '.[1]

The great fault which Snow found with the Scottish method of administering chloroform—an initial dose of ' two or three drachms spilt on the handkerchief or lint ', and more chloroform added ' from time to time, as circumstances require ' [2]—was : ' that the proportions of vapour and of air which the patient breathes cannot be properly regulated. Indeed ', Snow added, ' the advocates of this plan proceed on the supposition that there is no occasion to regulate these proportions, and that it is only requisite that the patient should have sufficient air for the purposes of respiration, and sufficient chloroform to induce insensibility, and all will be right. The truth is, however, that if there be too much vapour of chloroform in the air the patient breathes, it may cause sudden death, even without previous insensibility, and whilst the blood in the lungs is of a florid colour '.[3] Snow maintained that dangerously high percentages, in the order of 9·5 per cent. of chloroform, might be inhaled from a cloth at 70° F.[4] In this opinion he was supported by A. E. Sansom, who thought that at 60° to 64° F. ' when a drachm of chloroform is sprinkled upon lint ' it was possible for the patient ' to inspire an atmosphere containing more than thirteen per cent. of the vapour '.[5]

Joseph Lister, however, after carrying out a series of experiments by which he attempted to estimate the percentage of vapour given off from the underside of a cloth under conditions similar to those obtaining in clinical practice, came to the

[1] Snow, J. 1858. *On chloroform and other anaesthetics.* London. 80, 81.
[2] Miller, J. 1848. *Surgical experiences of chloroform.* Edinburgh. 17.
[3] Snow, J. 1858. *On chloroform . . .* London, 78, 79.
[4] *Ibid.* 34.   [5] *Med. Times, Lond.,* 1870, i, 436.

conclusion that the percentage inhaled by the patient was below
4·5 per cent.

In 1882 Lister began to administer chloroform by dropping
it sparingly on the corner of a towel pinched together between
finger and thumb or drawn through a safety-pin and fanned out
to from a roughly triangular, concave face-mask to reach from
the root of the nose to the chin (see Fig. 42 ; see also p. 540).
He claimed that by this method the patient inhaled only about
1·2 per cent. of chloroform vapour, a much smaller percentage
than that obtained by the use of Snow's inhaler.[1]

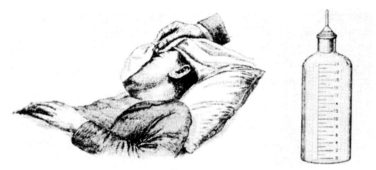

FIG. 42

Method of administering chloroform by dropping it from a drop-
bottle on to a single layer of cloth held so as to form a mask over
the patient's face.   Such a method was originally introduced by
J. Y. Simpson, c. 1860.   It was adopted by Joseph Lister in 1882.

Many years earlier than Lister, J. Y. Simpson himself had
modified his own technique of administration in this way :

' For some time past ', he wrote on November 14, 1860, ' I
have administered chloroform in a manner somewhat different
from that in which it was formerly used ; and I believe that by
the new method the patient is more rapidly anaesthetised, whilst
a great saving is effected in the amount of the drug employed.
The difference of the two modes consists in this, that according
to the old plan the fluid is poured upon a cloth folded into several
layers, and the hand of the administrator has to be kept between
the cloth and the patient's face in order to secure the due access
and admixture of air ; while in following out the new method,
one single layer of towel or handkerchief is laid over the patient's
nose and mouth, care being taken not to cover the eyes, and on

[1] Lister, Joseph, Baron. 1909.   *The collected papers of Joseph, Baron Lister.*   Oxford.
1, 168.

this single fold the chloroform is poured, drop by drop, until complete anaesthesia is induced. There is little or none of the drug lost by evaporation when it is administered in this manner, for the patient inhales it at the moment when it is poured on the cloth, and inhales it mixed with a sufficient quantity of air, which is easily inspired through a single layer of an ordinary napkin. . . . I believe that this manner of using chloroform will add to the safety of its employment. I have often feared lest the lives of patients should be sacrificed by the careless manner in which, in particular, students and young practitioners sometimes employ the damp folded cloth over the patient's face without admitting a sufficient supply of air ; and no doubt many of the deaths attributed to chloroform are due only to the improper administration of it, and are consequently no more chargeable on the drug itself than are the many deaths resulting from overdoses of opium, etc. etc. But the dangers from carelessness and improper administration would be diminished were there never placed over the patient's nose and mouth more than one single layer of cloth moistened with a few drops of fluid. The first patient to whom I administered it in this manner had been chloroformed several times previously, and had never gone to sleep till an ounce and a half or two ounces of the fluid had been used ; but when administered drop by drop on a single layer of thin towel one drachm sufficed to induce the most profound sleep. . . . There is only one precaution to be attended to in employing chloroform in this manner, viz. care must be taken to anoint the lips and nose of the patient beforehand with oil or ointment, to prevent the skin being injured by the contact of the fluid with the patient's face, resulting from the close application of the wetted towel.' [1]

Strongly as John Snow condemned pouring chloroform on to a cloth in the original Edinburgh manner as a means of producing surgical anaesthesia, he occasionally used this method to produce analgesia [2] in childbirth. ' There is not ', he explained,

[1] Simpson, J. Y.   1871.   *Anaesthesia, hospitalism and other papers.*   (Ed. by W. G. Simpson).   Edinburgh.   179.

[2] ' It may be remarked ', wrote Snow, ' that complete anaesthesia is never induced in midwifery, unless in some cases of operative delivery. The diminution of common sensibility to a certain extent, together with the diminution or removal of consciousness, suffice to prevent the suffering of the patient during labour ; and she never requires to be rendered so insensible as in a surgical operation, when the knife may be used without causing a flinch or a cry. The nerves of common sensation must be allowed to retain their functions to a certain extent during labour ; otherwise the assistance of the respiratory muscles, which consists of reflex action . . . would not take place, even if the contractions of the uterus should still continue.' Snow also noted : ' Drs. Murphy and Rigby were, I believe, amongst the first to state, that relief from pain may often be afforded in obstetric cases without removing the consciousness of the patient.' (Snow, J. 1858. *On chloroform and other anaesthetics.* London. 318, 321.)

7

' the same necessity for an accurate means of regulating the proportion of vapour in the air which the patient is breathing during labour, where but a trifling amount of narcotism requires to be induced, as in surgical operations, where a deeper effect is necessary ; still I find the inhaler much more convenient of application than a handkerchief, and it contains a supply of chloroform which lasts for some time, thereby saving the trouble of constantly pouring out more. When I do administer chloroform on a handkerchief during parturition, I follow the plan of putting only ten or fifteen minims of chloroform on the handkerchief at one time.' [1]

According to B. W. Richardson, it was on a handkerchief, not with his inhaler, that Snow gave chloroform in fifteen-minim doses to Queen Victoria for fifty-three minutes during the birth of Prince Leopold.[2]

Another circumstance in which Snow permitted himself to lay aside the inhaler was in maintaining anaesthesia during prolonged plastic operations (*e.g.* ' for the remedy or mitigation of deformity caused by burns') involving the head and face. He ' made the patients insensible with the inhaler before the operation was commenced, and afterwards kept up the insensibility by means of chloroform, diluted with spirit, on a hollow sponge '.[3]

Snow admitted that there was one method of administration which gave an even greater margin of safety than his own regulating inhaler. ' The most exact way in which it is practicable to exhibit chloroform to a patient . . . is to introduce a measured quantity into a bag or balloon of known size, then fill it up by means of the bellows, and allow the patient to inhale from it ; the expired air being prevented from returning into the balloon, by one of the valves of the face-piece to which it is attached. I tried this plan in a few cases, in 1849, with so much chloroform in the balloon as produced four per cent. of vapour in proportion to the air. The effects were extremely uniform, the patients becoming insensible in three or four minutes, according to the greater or less freedom of respiration ; and the vapour was easily breathed, owing to its being so equally mixed with the air. I did not try, however, to introduce this plan into general use, as the balloon would sometimes have been in the way of the

[1] Snow, J. 1858. *On chloroform and other anaesthetics.* London. 322–3.
[2] Richardson, B. W., in Snow, J. 1858. *On chloroform* . . . London. xxxi.
[3] Snow, J. 1858. *On chloroform* . . . London. 300.

surgeon, and filling it with the bellows would have occasioned a little trouble.   It seemed necessary to sacrifice a little of absolute perfection to convenience.' [1]

In 1862 J. T. Clover successfully designed an inhaler upon this principle, and ingeniously overcame the difficulties of filling and stowing the balloon out of the way (see p. 241 *et. seq.*).

Snow recorded that in the first fifty cases of death from chloroform anaesthesia, inhalers were used in twelve cases only ; in all the other cases (except four in which the method of administration was not certainly known) some form of folded cloth or a sponge saturated with chloroform was used.[2]

The First Chloroform Fatality

The first death under chloroform anaesthesia occurred near Newcastle, on January 28, 1848.   The patient, Hannah Greener, was a healthy girl of fifteen, who was to have a toe-nail removed. The corresponding nail on the other foot had been removed successfully under ether anaesthesia three months before.

T. M. Meggison, the surgeon who gave the anaesthetic on the fatal occasion, described events as follows :

' She appeared to dread the operation, and fretted a good deal. . . . The inhalation [undertaken with the patient seated in a chair] . . . was done from a handkerchief on which a teaspoonful of chloroform had been poured.   After drawing her breath twice, she pulled my hand from her mouth.   I told her to put her hands on her knees, and breathe quietly, which she did. In about half a minute, seeing no change in breathing, or alteration of pulse, I lifted her arm, which I found rigid.   I looked at the pupil and pinched her cheek, and, finding her insensible, requested Mr. Lloyd to begin the operation.   At the termination of the semi-lunar incision she gave a kick or twitch, which caused me to think the chloroform had not sufficient effect.   I was proceeding to apply more to the handkerchief, when her lips, which had been previously of a good colour, became suddenly blanched, and she spluttered at the mouth, as if in epilepsy.   I threw down the handkerchief, dashed cold water in her face, and gave her some internally, followed by brandy, without, however, the least effect, not the slightest attempt at a rally being made.   We laid her on the floor, opened a vein in her arm, and the jugular vein, but no blood flowed.   The whole process of inhalation, operation, venesection, and death, could not, I should say, have occupied more than two minutes.' [3]

[1] Snow, J.   1858.   *On chloroform and other anaesthetics.*   London.   8o.
[2] *Ibid.* 233.   [3] *Lond. med. Gaz.*, 1848, **6,** 255.

This tragic and apparently unaccountable death created a great deal of interest and speculation in medical circles. A post-mortem on the girl was carried out by the distinguished Newcastle surgeon, Sir John Fife, assisted by Dr. Mortimer Glover, Lecturer in Materia Medica in the Newcastle Medical School, who in 1842 had made a series of experiments on the physiological, though not, of course, the anaesthetic, effects of chloroform.

Fife and Glover found that the lungs were not collapsed but ' in a very high state of congestion. . . . They were everywhere crepitant. . . . The stomach was distended with food. . . . The heart contained dark fluid blood in both cavities : very little in the left. Its structure, and that of the great vessels near it, quite healthy. The brain, externally and internally, was more congested than usual '.[1]

At the inquest Fife stated that ' in his opinion, the cause of death was the *congestion of the lungs* ; and this congestion he was compelled to ascribe to the inhalation of chloroform. . . . He attributed the fatal result in this young woman's case to *some peculiarity in her constitution*—not to be detected beforehand—either in the lungs or in the nervous system '.[2]

This latter opinion was strenuously contradicted by Snow. Such an opinion, he thought, ' would necessarily invest the inhalation with some degree of danger, however small, and would entail some anxiety on both the operator and the patient. My view of the matter ', he stated, ' holds out more hope for the future. I look on the result as only what was to be apprehended from the over-rapid action of chloroform when administered on a handkerchief . . . and consider that danger may be avoided by adopting another method. I have observed that the effects of the vapour may accumulate for about twenty seconds after the inhalation is discontinued,[3] and this accumulation will be the more formidable in proportion to the quantity of vapour that is being inhaled at the moment, and the velocity with which the symptoms were being induced. . . . Now, in the case under consideration, when the girl had inhaled for about half a minute, there was rigidity of the arm ; this would indicate that she was in the third degree [according to Snow's assessment of the stages of anaesthesia, see p. 162], and supposing that the cloth was

[1] *Lond. med. Gaz.*, 1848, **6**, 253.   [2] *Ibid.* **6**, 253.
[3] Cf. *Ibid.* **6**, 75.

removed at that very instant . . . if the vapour was inhaled of the same strength during the thirty seconds, its effects might increase at the same pace for twenty seconds longer ; and at the end of fifty seconds from the commencement she would be in the fifth degree of narcotism, in which " the respiratory movements are more or less paralyzed, and become difficult, feeble, or irregular " '. [1] Snow, at this time, concluded that Hannah Greener's death was due to overdosage resulting in paralysis of the respiratory muscles (cf. p. 200).

This first fatal case served to exemplify not only the peculiar dangers of chloroform anaesthesia, which so mystified the early, and indeed later, anaesthetists, but also many of the pitfalls which, through bitter experience, they eventually learned to avoid (cf. pp. 455–6). Hannah Greener was young and healthy and the operation to which she submitted was a minor one. At the same time she was extremely apprehensive and her stomach was full of food. A moderate amount of chloroform (about one teaspoonful) was poured on to the handkerchief, but this was possibly held in such a way that air was excluded. Furthermore, the girl was in the sitting position. Although Meggison seems to have been a careful administrator and to have been watching his patient closely, she died suddenly and without giving any warning signs which he could recognize, within two minutes of the beginning of induction.

Within the next four months three more deaths occurred : two in the United States and one in France. Francis Sibson, after studying the available information about these first four fatalities, made several very perspicacious deductions ; the danger points of chloroform anaesthesia which he indicated and the steps which he advised for avoiding them had a lasting influence upon anaesthetic practice. A considerable reciprocal influence between Sibson and Snow may also be traced, and the two men actually collaborated on several series of experiments.

Writing of the four fatalities in question, Sibson observed :

' In the three later . . . cases the heart was quite flaccid. In the case of Greener the state of the heart is not specified, but the countenance became suddenly blanched. In all the four cases it is manifest the immediate cause of the instantaneous death lay in the heart. The heart, influenced by the poison, ceased to

[1] *Lond. med. Gaz.*, 1848, **6**, 277.

contract, not from the cessation of respiration, for the heart in asphyxia will beat from one to three minutes after respiration has ceased, but from immediate death of the heart.

' There is no doubt a combination of causes operating to destroy the heart's contractile power : the mental influence, the congestion in the systemic, and that in the pulmonic capillaries, will all have a material influence. . . .

' But besides these three causes, all co-operating to arrest the heart's action, there is indisputably the direct action of the poison on the muscular tissue of the heart. The poison penetrates to the heart from the lungs in a single pulsation ; and at the beginning of the next systole, the blood is sent through the coronary artery to the whole muscular tissue of the heart. The blood passing into the coronary artery is . . . more strongly impregnated with chloroform . . . than is the blood in any other part of the system, except the lungs. . . .

' I fear, from the experience of these fatal cases, that we must regard chloroform as one of the most uncontrollable narcotic poisons when its action is pushed so far as to suspend *circulation* and *respiration*. . . .

' We are obliged, then, from the experience of these cases, to conclude, that in man the death is usually instantaneous, and due, as every instantaneous death is, to paralysis of the heart. In animals, the death is usually due to paralysis of the muscles of respiration. . . .

' These cases ', Sibson continued, ' suggest some important considerations on the *mode of chloroformization*. In three out of the four fatal cases the chloroform was given in the sitting posture. This posture requires much greater power in the heart to carry on the circulation than the recumbent. Chloroform should not, if possible, be administered in the sitting posture.

' In three out of the four fatal cases, the chloroform was administered by the operator : this should never be. Chloroformization is the exhibition of a subtle poison, and ought to be watched by the administrator with undivided attention during the whole of its operation.

' During chloroformization, the state of the eyes, the lips, the pulse, and respiration should be continually watched. . . .

' As soon as the eye turns up, and the eyelids cease to quiver and resist, draw up one eyelid, and keep the eye constantly open ; watch the pupil closely—it is usually contracted, and ought never to proceed to dilatation excepting, perhaps, in the reduction of dislocation and in the reduction of hernia. If the eyeballs begin to move, and the eyelids to quiver, apply the inhaling mask again for a few seconds until they again become fixed : thus, with the inhalation of very little chloroform, a person may, at will, be kept long under its influence, and yet not a minute longer than

is needful, as you have the patient just on the margin of unconsciousness.

' The inhaler should be so constructed that every inspiration
be made palpable by it.   The tell-tale valve of my inhaler [see
Fig. 38] does this perfectly, and may be, and indeed has been,
adapted to other inhalers.   Without some such precaution, the
patient might cease to breathe unnoticed.

' The chloroform should be administered gradually, much
diluted with air at first, and less so afterwards.   The effects
should neither be produced too quickly nor too slowly : in either
case, the accumulative effect pointed out by Dr. Snow [see p. 196]
may endanger the patient after the chloroform has been withdrawn.

' If the respiration ceases before the pulse, artificial respiration
must be immediately resorted to ; it may be performed instantly,
by breathing into the lungs through the inhaling mask [see p.
184]. . . .

' If the heart has ceased to beat, the case is almost hope-
less. . . .

' In each of the four cases the operation, though painful,
was not serious.   In such cases, the mind usually fears the chloroform more almost than the operation.   It is otherwise when the
operation is serious.

' In dental surgery (except in extreme cases) and in trivial
operations, the use of chloroform is not justifiable.

' As the heart is subject to paralysis from the action of chloroform, its use should not be lightly resorted to when there is
affection of the heart.   I do not speak so much of organic disease
of the heart as of those cases where palpitation and dyspnoea are
easily excited, either from abdominal distension or from mental
emotion.   To such persons chloroform is, I conceive, more likely
to prove destructive than to those with organic disease of the
heart, when they do not suffer from palpitation. . . .' [1]

Ten years after Sibson's observations on the causes of death
under chloroform anaesthesia, Snow, basing his deductions both
on wide clinical experience and on careful animal experiment,
wrote :

' If it were possible for a medical man to mistake or disregard
the symptoms of approaching danger, and to go on exhibiting
vapour of chloroform, diluted to a proper strength [i.e. not more
than 4 per cent. chloroform vapour] till the death of the patient,
this event would take place slowly and gradually. . . . The
action of the heart would survive the respiration ; there would
be a great tendency to spontaneous recovery, and the patient

[1] *Lond. med. Gaz.*, 1848, **7**, 108.

would be easily restored by artificial respiration, if it were performed whilst the heart was still acting ; as I have always found
it to be successful in animals under these circumstances.

' In examining the recorded cases of fatal inhalation of
chloroform [at the time of writing, 1858, 50 cases were definitely
attributed to chloroform and still others were alleged to be due to
it, cf. Appendix C] we . . . find, however, that they have
none of them taken place in this gradual manner ; but that in
all cases the fatal symptoms, if not the actual death, have come
on very suddenly.' [1]

Snow now agreed with Sibson in believing this sudden death
to be due solely to the paralyzing effect of strong chloroform
vapour on the heart. ' In all the cases in which the symptoms
which occurred at the time of death are reported ', he wrote,
' there is every reason to conclude . . . that death took place
by cardiac syncope, or arrest of the action of the heart '.[2]

' There is in a great number of cases ', Snow stated, ' an
evident connection between the accident and the probable
strength of the mixture of vapour and air. In six cases the
accident occurred just after the commencement of the inhalation ;
in two . . . the fatal symptoms occurred just after fresh chloroform had been applied on the handkerchief and sponge ; and in
several cases, in which the circulation was suddenly arrested just
after the patient had been rendered insensible, the insensibility
had been induced so quickly as to prove that the vapour must
have been inhaled in a very insufficient state of dilution.' [3]

Snow disagreed with Sibson and others who thought that
fear was an important factor in chloroform anaesthesia :

' It has been said that chloroform ought not to be administered
if the patient is very much afraid, on the supposition that fear
makes the chloroform dangerous. This is, however, a mistake ;
the danger, if any, lies in the fear itself. . . . Fear and chloroform
are each of them capable of causing death, just as infancy and old
age both predispose to bronchitis, but it seems impossible that
fear should combine with the effects of chloroform to cause
danger, when that agent is administered with the usual precautions. Fear is an affection of the mind, and can no longer exist
when the patient is unconscious ; but the action of that amount
of chloroform which is consistent even with disordered consciousness is stimulating, and increases the force and frequency of the
pulse, in the same way as alcohol. I believe that no one would

[1] Snow, J. 1858. *On chloroform and other anaesthetics.* London. 120–1.
[2] *Ibid.* 217.   [3] *Ibid.* 222.

assert that a person would die the sooner of fright for having taken a few glasses of wine, or a small amount of distilled spirits, whatever might be the state of his health. When chloroform has been absorbed in sufficient quantity to cause unconsciousness, fear subsides, and with the fear its effects on the circulation.' [1]

When the patient was in an apprehensive state, however, ' either about that agent [chloroform] itself or the operation which calls for its use ', Snow believed it to be ' desirable to allay the patient's fears, if possible, before he begins to inhale, as he will then be able to breathe in a more regular and tranquil manner '.[2]

Snow, again differing from Sibson, maintained that the sitting posture held no inherent danger. ' There is no objection ', he asserted, ' when that is most convenient to the operator. In that case, however, the patient should be placed in a large easy chair with a high back, so that the head as well as the trunk may be supported without any effort, otherwise he would have a tendency to slide or fall when insensible. It has been said that it is unsafe to give chloroform in the sitting posture, on the supposition that it would in some cases so weaken the power of the heart as to render it unable to send the blood to the brain. Observation has proved, however, that chloroform usually increases the force of the circulation ; and although the horizontal position is certainly the best for the patient under an operation in all circumstances, I consider that the sitting posture is by no means a source of danger, when chloroform is given, if the ordinary precaution be used . . . of placing the patient horizontally if symptoms of faintness come on. I have preserved notes of nine hundred and forty-nine cases in which I have given chloroform to patients in the sitting posture, and no ill effects have arisen in any of these cases.' [3]

A still further point of disagreement between Snow and others, including Sibson, was on the question of chloroform in dentistry.

' It is the custom in the medical journals and medical societies ', wrote Snow, ' to object occasionally to the use of chloroform in tooth-drawing, as if the operation were not sufficiently severe to require it. . . . I have notes of 867 cases in which I have administered chloroform during the extraction of teeth. . . .

[1] Snow, J. 1858. *On chloroform and other anaesthetics*. London. 76, 77.
[2] *Ibid*. 76.   [3] *Ibid*. 75–6.

7*

The number of teeth extracted at an operation has varied from one to nineteen . . . but [both dentists and Snow himself] . . . have thought it better, as a general rule, to make more than one operation when the number of teeth to be drawn exceeded ten, in order that the mouth might not contain too many wounds at one time, and that the loss of blood might not be very great. . . .

' The patients have been seated in an easy chair in all the operations on the teeth, except in a very few cases where a female patient was too ill to sit up. . . . I am not aware of any inconvenience from the chloroform in any of the cases of tooth-drawing, excepting sickness and vomiting, which in a very few of the cases have been troublesome for some time.' [1]

To the end of his life Snow continued to deny that death from chloroform could be due to idiosyncrasy of the patient. This view, first put forward by Fife after Hannah Greener's death (see p. 196), had become popular with some administrators because it appeared to provide a ready explanation of otherwise inexplicable death in healthy subjects. Neither did Snow believe that organic disease, even fatty degeneration of the heart, for instance, was necessarily a contra-indication to the use of chloroform, nor that the age of the patient was in itself important.

' I arrived at the conclusion, after much careful observation ', wrote Snow, ' that chloroform might be given with safety and advantage in every case in which the patient requires, and is in a condition to undergo, a surgical operation ; and having acted on this conclusion for several years, I have found no reason to change it.'

At the same time he stressed his belief, on general grounds, that ' it is desirable . . . to pay attention to every circumstance connected with the health and constitution of the patient before exhibiting chloroform, as many of these circumstances influence its effect '.[2]

In 1858, the year of his death, Snow was able to state : ' I have not myself declined to give chloroform in any case in which a patient required to undergo a painful operation, whatever evidence of organic disease I have met with on careful examination ; and although I have memoranda of upwards of four thousand cases in which I have administered this agent, I have not, as I believe, lost a patient from its use ; the only person

---

[1] Snow, J. 1858. *On chloroform and other anaesthetics.* London. 313–15.
[2] *Ibid.* 48, 49.

who died whilst under its influence [a man of seventy-three, during lithotrity, in September 1852 [1]], having, in my opinion, succumbed from other causes ' [2]—viz. fatty degeneration of the heart.

Snow was undoubtedly an extremely skilful anaesthetist, but in certain respects, where chloroform was concerned, he ignored or brushed aside evidence which ran counter to his theory (proved to his own satisfaction by experiments on animals in the laboratory), that if the vapour were sufficiently diluted with air then it could not cause death without warning. In the case cited above, for example, his reason for declaring that chloroform was not a contributory factor to the patient's death was that ' the air he was breathing just before he died did not contain more than three or four per cent. of vapour of chloroform at the utmost, and he had previously breathed quite as much, both during the same operation and on previous occasions '.[3]

' The first rule . . . in giving chloroform is to take care that the vapour is so far diluted that it cannot cause sudden death, without timely warning of the approaching danger ; and the next rule is to watch the symptoms as they arise.' [4] These were the rules which Snow repeatedly stressed in his writings, and upon which he himself acted as scrupulously as he knew how, throughout his career as an anaesthetist.

The fallacy of Snow's reasoning was not satisfactorily explained until 1911, when A. Goodman Levy demonstrated that although chloroform vapour could not, without timely warning of the approaching danger, cause sudden death through *over-dosage*, it could and did cause sudden death without readily obvious warning signs, from ventricular fibrillations of the heart ; for the occurrence of these a state of *light* anaesthesia in the patient was the essential predisposing factor (see p. 452 *et seq.*).

Although Levy's explanation of the cause of sudden death under chloroform anaesthesia was not given until 1911, many people during the nineteenth century perceived that a state of light chloroform anaesthesia was more dangerous to the patient than deep anaesthesia. The danger was erroneously attributed to a variety of causes.[5]

[1] Snow, J. 1858. *On chloroform and other anaesthetics.* London. 205.
[2] *Ibid.* 249.   [3] *Ibid.* 208.   [4] *Ibid.* 251.
[5] Cf. *e.g.* Hewitt, F. W. 1893. *Anaesthetics and their administration.* London. 227 *et seq.*

Scottish and Continental Methods

In contrast to Snow's cautious methods of administration were the bold Scottish methods. At Edinburgh the rules were : give chloroform powerfully and speedily, and look after the respiration ; the pulse and the pupil will look after themselves. James Syme, Professor of Clinical Surgery at Edinburgh, who particularly insisted upon the observance of these rules, was, like Snow (but with no possible exception among the 5000 administrations for which he bore the responsibility), able to say towards the end of his life that he had never had a death under chloroform.[1]

From 1848 onwards chloroformists in England tended to follow Snow's rules for safe administration ; Scottish and Continental administrators followed the Edinburgh rules. Both persuasions were agreed, however, during the eighteen-fifties and sixties, that chloroform was the most important anaesthetic agent yet to be discovered.

In Europe J. E. Pétrequin, Senior Surgeon of the Hôtel-Dieu at Lyons, and a few of his colleagues, were the first to dissociate themselves from this opinion. Petrequin himself returned to the exclusive use of sulphuric ether in 1849, but it was 1855 before the majority of surgeons in Lyons likewise returned to its use.

Pétrequin's example was followed in 1851 by the surgeons of Naples, who first heard of the Lyonnais methods of etherization through a fellow-citizen, Palasciano, at that time engaged upon surgical and anatomical researches in Lyons. Armédée Bonnet, a colleague of Pétrequin's, was, in 1851, invited to Naples to demonstrate ether anaesthesia.

Many years later Pétrequin described the events which led him to return to the use of ether :

' A year had scarcely passed ', he wrote, referring to the events of the autumn of 1847, ' when chloroform, proposed by M. Simpson . . . brought about a revolution which gave rise to considerable perturbation. . . . The new anaesthetic agent was represented as producing more rapid and more complete effects than ether without, like the latter, occasioning nervous agitation. Paris adopted chloroform ; at Lyons we too hastened to make a trial of it ; but, alas ! fatal accidents speedily occurred with us,

[1] Cf. *The collected papers of Joseph, Baron Lister.* Oxford. **I,** 137.

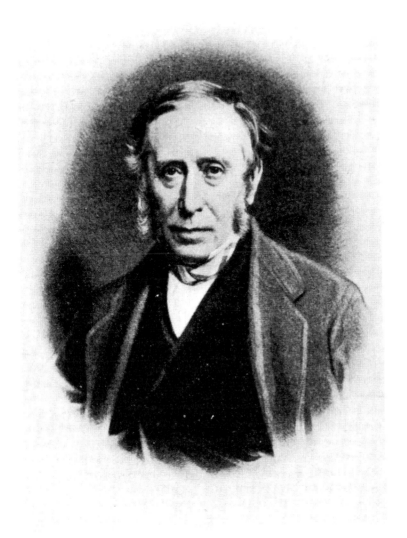

FIG. 43.—JAMES SYME (1799–1870)

Surgeon ; appointed Professor of Clinical Surgery at Edinburgh, 1833. His teaching that death during chloroform anaesthesia was due primarily to respiratory failure, not to heart failure and that, consequently, if the respiration were carefully watched the pulse could be ignored, was the predominant influence in Scottish anaesthetic practice during the nineteenth century.

as elsewhere. When I saw patients, in the able hands of my colleagues, suddenly succumb to the action of chloroform, so that nothing could recall them to life and without the least warning of this catastrophe, I made up my mind as humanity dictated that I should. I abandoned the use of so dangerous an agent, which gave no security to the operator and constantly exposed patients to the risk of a death always unpredictable and almost always irrevocable, and which must sooner or later occasion the operator remorse. I had always found ether innocuous ; it continued to give me good results without ever placing the patient's life in peril. . . .

'We, M. Diday and I, started a campaign in favour of ether ; he published a notable series of articles and I undertook propaganda in my teaching, in my hospital practice and on the medical committees, in my clinical lectures, etc. . . . We led M. Gensoul to share our preference for ether ; but all our other colleagues were in favour of chloroform, as in Paris.

'In 1850, I ascertained in Paris that ether was almost forgotten ; there was an exaggerated admiration for chloroform. . . . Nothing, in fact, could disillusion their minds.' [1]

By 1864, however, Pétrequin found that the Parisian admiration for chloroform was no longer excessive ; conviction had been shaken and he observed that several surgeons then no longer operated without a certain apprehension. As the chloroform fatalities mounted, from year to year, so the number of dissenters grew also ; 'it seemed to me', said Petrequin, 'that the moment was not far off when ear would at last be given to all these accounts of deaths, so sadly reported'.[2] Petrequin was mistaken. No widespread revival of the use of ether took place in France before 1895 (see pp. 423-5).

Pétrequin expressed the opinion that the three principal reasons which prevented ether becoming popular were : (1) the imperfections of the inhalers used ; (2) the impurity of the ether ; (3) the inexperience of the administrators.

The first of these difficulties Pétrequin overcame by using the 'sac à éthériser' invented by Munaret and popularized by Roux' (see p. 146 ; Fig. 24). As for the second difficulty, he stated that in 1847 the only ether obtainable from the druggists was impure to a varying degree and too weak for anaesthetic purposes, so that 'instead of the desired sleep a kind of intoxication' resulted from its use. 'Lyonnais surgery exerted a

[1] Pétrequin, J. E. 1869. L'Éthérisation et la chirurgie Lyonnaise. Lyons. 1-5.
[2] Ibid. 14.

considerable influence in modifying the drug trade in this respect. Between 1849 and 1850 it became possible to procure rectified ether at every reliable druggist's in Lyons.' The third difficulty, the inexperience of the administrators, was one which Pétrequin particularly stressed. ' One remembers ', he wrote, ' how it was successively proposed that the administration of ether should be graduated, intermittent, limited—all defective methods likely to prolong its operation, to exaggerate its inconveniences, and give rise to intoxication.'

Pétrequin's own method of administration, tested by long experience, was as follows :

' The patient is laid with the head slightly raised, so that ether cannot be swallowed. I begin by pouring 20 to 25 grams of ether on to the sponges [in Roux's sac] and then cover the patient's chin, mouth and nose quickly with the mouth of the sac, pulling on the draw-strings to keep out air. I advise the patient to breathe deeply, and when everything is well under way I gradually close the inlet hole in the sac with the plug. Then I double the dose of ether. It is necessary to proceed in silence, without addressing or replying to the patient ; and it is a good thing to cover his eyes with a handkerchief, to isolate him more completely from the outside world. Generally, anaesthesia is established quickly and peacefully enough. If any signs of nervous agitation appear I have the limbs held and add a fresh dose of ether ; the patient in struggling breathes more deeply and is soon asleep [cf. p. 313]. Once anaesthesia is completely established I have the sac raised to allow free respiration, reapplying the apparatus whenever the least sign of returning consciousness is perceived. With these precautions I have been able, without the least inconvenience, to prolong anaesthesia for forty and fifty minutes. I have never had either a death or any serious accident to regret, and I am deeply convinced that they are practically impossible with rectified ether if one proceeds with care. Four to six minutes at the least and seven at the most, suffice to establish sleep. . . . It is to be noted that accidents are easily foreseen if both the circulation and the respiration are carefully watched.' [1]

The maintenance of anaesthesia was entrusted entirely to an assistant who had been so thoroughly trained in all the details of the fixed routine of administration which had been evolved by Pétrequin, that the latter was able to devote his undivided attention to the surgery in hand.[2]

[1] Pétrequin, J. E. 1869. L'Éthérisation et la chirurgie Lyonnaise. Lyons. 5.
[2] Ibid. 186.

PART THREE

THE PERIOD OF THE PREDOMINANT USE OF CHLOROFORM

CHAPTER VII

SEARCH FOR THE 'PERFECT' ANAESTHETIC

Nunneley's Researches—Snow's Researches

Nunneley's Researches

THE hunt for new anaesthetic agents, which began almost as soon as the use of sulphuric ether was well-established in Europe, covered a wide field. Simpson himself, before he discovered what seemed the perfect alternative, chloroform, had tried a number of substances (see p. 166).

One of the most zealous of the early researchers was Thomas Nunneley, of Leeds, and, although he chose the dangerous course of reasoning from particular cases to general conclusions, the inductions he made from his painstaking experiments were, in many respects, remarkably astute.

'The practical application of these agents', he wrote in 1849, of anaesthetics in general, 'is a most important question, and one that deserves to be well and thoroughly investigated. . . . But I must confess it appears to me that as yet the information which has been before the profession is neither sufficiently extensive, nor of that precise character which is absolutely necessary to enable us to arrive at an accurate and certain conclusion as to their practical value, and the circumstances in which, and under which, they . . . should be employed or not : in fact, hitherto their use has been mainly, if not altogether empirical. . . . The intention of the present inquiry is to assist in affording that information, and to furnish evidence from which such inferences and deductions may be fairly drawn. . . .

'Nearly all of the substances which hitherto have been mentioned as anaesthetics, are compounds of the hypothetical radical ethyle . . . substances which are formed of hydrogen and carbon united with oxygen, as an oxide of ethyle. . . .

' From reflecting upon this circumstance, I was, some time ago, led to the supposition that not improbably many other bodies might be found to possess similar powers, possibly even in a more advantageous form than some already known, since the use of these appears, so to speak, to have been rather accidental and fortuitous, than the consequence of any reasoning upon their nature and mode of operating.' [1]

Nunneley began to work upon the hypothesis that ' hydrogen and carbon . . . might be combined with another . . . element the properties of the compound remaining, to a great extent, the same '. Later he ' ascertained that in order to possess anaesthetic powers, it was not necessary for a body to have a triple composition '.[2]

Nunneley recorded the testing of more than thirty different substances upon dogs and cats. He administered these agents not only by brief and prolonged inhalation but in some instances locally, applied directly to the skin, intravenously, rectally and by mouth. He concluded that inhalation gave, on the whole, the best results. In a few cases, where experimental findings seemed to justify him, Nunneley proceeded to test new anaesthetics clinically.[3]

' By far the greater number of the substances which have been tried,' he stated, ' even of those which have been shown to be capable of producing anaesthesia, may be dismissed without much comment ; for though valuable in a scientific point of view . . . they are . . . not likely to be employed while we are in possession of much better. The substances which appear to possess the greatest power, and the effects of which are the least objectionable, are the oxide of ethyl (sulphuric ether), the gaseous carburetted hydrogens (of which common coal gas is perhaps the best), chloric ether, hydrobromic ether [ethyl bromide, C_2H_5Br], chloroform, the chloride of olefiant gas [i.e. Dutch liquid, see p. 166] and the chloride of carbon [tetrachloroethylene, $CCl_2 : CCl_2$].' [4]

To the use of sulphuric ether Nunneley raised the usual objections of his day :

' In power, it certainly is much inferior to several of the other bodies ; its action is not uniform and certain ; more excitement is frequently manifested in its use ; it produces more irritation while being inhaled, and afterwards headache and feverishness are more liable to follow. These are objections so

[1] Trans. provincial med. surg. Ass., 1849, N.S. 4, 167–9.
[2] Ibid. 4, 170.   [3] Ibid. 4, 172 et seq.   [4] Ibid. 4, 370.

weighty,' Nunneley added, 'although in some degree counter-
balanced by its general safety and the less liability to collapse
supervening, that . . . it will hereafter, I apprehend, be rarely
used.'[1]

Coal gas, Nunneley described as 'a safe and effective agent.
Its cheapness is also an important recommendation. On the
other hand, the disagreeableness of its odour . . . and its
gaseous form, especially the latter, are serious impediments to
its general employment. Under any circumstances, the inhalation of a gas is not of so easy and convenient accomplishment
as that of the vapour of an easy evaporable fluid, more complicated apparatus being requisite '.[2]

Chloric ether (see p. 172) Nunneley recommended as 'a
pleasant substance . . . and in a very young or feeble person,
I should feel disposed to employ it in preference to chloroform'.
Chloroform itself he considered to be 'undoubtedly one of the
pleasantest and most powerful anaesthetic substances known.
. . . That it is the safest can by no means be maintained with
equal certainty ; on the contrary, in safety I believe it to be
inferior to all the other substances mentioned just now '.

Ethyl bromide, called by Nunneley hydrobromic ether, he
found both safe and pleasant, but 'the very great cost of it will,
unless this can be materially reduced, entirely prevent its general
use. One manufacturer ', he stated, 'would not prepare it for
me under one guinea an ounce '.[3]

Nunneley appears to have been the first to test 'chloride
of carbon ' (cf. p. 209). 'I am not aware that any one has tried
the effects . . . besides myself', he wrote. He found it 'a safe
and not unpleasant anaesthetic ' and, at the same time, 'the
cheapest of all fluids which have yet been proposed '. Although
he suspected that the samples he obtained were impure, containing traces of hydrogen and alcohol, he reported :

'A few days ago I gave the fluid sent to me as chloride of
carbon to a person under amputation of the leg. The action
was pleasant and satisfactory, but a considerable quantity was
required, nearly four drachms.'[4]

Among all the agents investigated by him, Nunneley believed
the chloride of olefiant gas (Dutch liquid) to be 'one of the most

[1] *Trans. provincial med. surg. Ass.*, 1849, N.S. **4**, 370.
[2] *Ibid.* **4**, 371.   [3] *Ibid.* **4**, 371.   [4] *Ibid.* **4**, 341, 342 footnote.

valuable anaesthetics yet tried '. He mentioned seven cases
' in which it was given to patients during operations with perfect
success ', and added, ' I have . . . given it, in several other
serious and important operations '. He observed, in particular,
that ' it appears to be unattended with the troublesome excitement produced by ether, on the one hand, and on the other with
less of the tendency to collapse, which is so objectionable in
chloroform '.[1]

The effects of olefiant gas itself (C_2H_4), used in modern
anaesthetic practice under the name ethylene, were tested by
Nunneley on cats and dogs in eight experiments. He concluded
that :

' not only would there be the difficulty and trouble in preparing
and preserving it, but it is not a safe and manageable agent ;
since, when employed in innocuous doses, the anaesthesia is not
complete : when used in larger, death may not improbably be
caused. 10 per cent. of the gas does not appear to produce such
a degree of insensibility of any permanence as could be depended
upon in a painful operation of even moderate length ; 15 per cent.,
though causing total insensibility, also induces a dangerous condition, while life is speedily destroyed by from 20 to 25 per cent.'[2]

Nunneley made a trial in the laboratory of nitrous oxide also,
largely because of Davy's suggestion of its possible anaesthetic
use (see p. 72) ; he was disappointed with its effects.

' The gas was pure and well washed, and the experiments
were conducted with every care. . . . They are quite sufficient
to show that nitrous oxide never could be employed as an
anaesthetic, and that the inhalation of it is not altogether so
harmless as is generally stated.'

His experiments, he thought, ' clearly prove that with animals
the state of insensibility, when safe, passes off so quickly as to be
practically useless, while if it be rendered more profound or
more prolonged, it is highly dangerous '. The occurrence of
cyanosis perplexed him :

' It is curious to remark, that with a gas so rich in oxygen the
blood should be dark, while with some of the pure hydrocarbons,
where there is no oxygen, it is perfectly florid, a fact which it is
very difficult to account for in accordance with the received
notions of physiology.'[3]

[1] *Trans. provincial med. surg. Ass.*, 1849, N.S. **4,** 325, 372.
[2] *Ibid.* **4,** 228–9, 331.   [3] *Ibid.* **4,** 344–6.

Summing up the results of these researches Nunneley wrote :

' I think, we may legitimately arrive at the conclusion, that to constitute an anaesthetic agent, carbon must be present, and that by the combination of it with hydrogen (or perhaps chlorine) we have the basis of the most effective anaesthetic agents.' [1]

Of the substances investigated by Nunneley few were tested as anaesthetics by others. The chloride of olefiant gas, about which he was enthusiastic, had already been tried by Simpson and by Snow and condemned by both as dangerous—but that, Nunneley believed, was because each had used an impure preparation.

Ethyl bromide, on the other hand, eventually gained a recognized place among anaesthetic agents. Nunneley again drew attention to it in 1865,[2] and in 1876 A. Rabuteau, in France, made a laboratory investigation of its physiological effects ; in particular, the way in which it was eliminated from the system.[3] In the following year, 1877, Laurence Turnbull, J. Marion Sims and other Americans began to use it clinically, with various degrees of success.[4]

The anaesthetic use of ethyl bromide in America was noticed in the *British Medical Journal* during 1880, but J. T. Clover, whose opinion carried a great deal of weight, wrote to say that he was not in favour of its adoption.[5]

In the same year, 1880, Terrillon, in France, used ethyl bromide with Richardson's spray (see also p. 265) to obtain refrigeration of the skin for minor surgery.[6]

During 1888 and 1889 a number of German dentists began to use ethyl bromide for general anaesthesia and the sudden vogue for it in dental practice spread to England where J. F. W. Silk, in particular, recommended it.[7]

Snow's Researches

When Nunneley, in 1849, complained that information relating to anaesthetic agents was ' neither sufficiently extensive

---

[1] *Trans. provincial med. surg. Ass.*, 1849, N.S. **4,** 355.

[2] *Brit. med. J.*, 1865, ii, 192.

[3] *C.R. Acad. Sci.*, Paris, 1876, **83,** 1294.

[4] Cf. *e.g.* Turnbull, L. 1896. *Artificial anaesthesia.* Philadelphia. 228.

[5] *Brit. med. J.*, 1880, i, 586.

[6] *Bull. Soc. Chirurgie Paris*, 1880, **6,** 198.

[7] *Jber. Leist. ges. Med.*, 1888, **23** (ii), 604 ; *ibid.*, 1889, **24** (ii), 595 ; *Trans. odont. Soc., Lond.*, 1891, N.S. **23,** 120.

nor of that precise character which is absolutely necessary ', he ignored, for some reason, the experiments which Snow was then making. In fact Snow began to publish his results in the *London Medical Gazette* in 1848.

Snow was primarily concerned with establishing the principles of anaesthetic action. The investigation of the action of individual drugs served always as a means to this end, never as an end in itself. Nevertheless Snow dreamed of finding the perfect anaesthetic, as did most of his contemporaries, except, perhaps, those at Edinburgh who believed they already had it in chloroform.

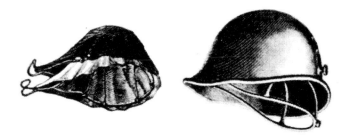

FIG. 44.—MASKS FOR ADMINISTERING ETHYL BROMIDE

Designed by Gilles, of Cologne (1892). That on the left consisted of a stout, hinged, double frame enclosing a layer of surgical gauze and overlaid with an impermeable felt or rubber cover. The upper frame bearing the cover could readily be lifted during administration, to allow the patient to breathe fresh air and to replenish the gauze with ethyl bromide. The drug was at first dropped on, then, as induction proceeded, poured on in a large dose. In the mask figured on the right, a metal hood took the place of the upper frame and impermeable cover.

' His grand search ', wrote Richardson of Snow, ' was for a narcotic vapour which, having the physical properties and practicability of chloroform, should, in its physiological effects, resemble ether in not producing, by any accident of administration, paralysis of the heart.' According to Richardson, Snow furthermore believed that there must ultimately be discovered ' an anaesthetic which might be inhaled with absolute safety, and which would destroy common sensation without destroying consciousness '.[1]

[1] Richardson, B. W., in Snow, J. 1858. *On chloroform and other anaesthetics.* London. xxviii, xxx.

Snow's most important contribution to the literature of anaesthetics, apart from his book *On chloroform and other anaesthetics* upon which he was actually working when he ' was seized by his fatal illness ', was the series of articles ' On narcotism by the inhalation of vapours ' which he wrote for the *London Medical Gazette* at intervals between 1848 and 1851 when the journal ceased to exist.

In those articles Snow recorded his current experiments made in the laboratory and clinically, and there he propounded his completed theory of anaesthesia. Richardson said of the articles :

' I infer that they have been more talked about than read for few people seem to be aware of the enlarged and positive physiological arguments which they contain. Chloroform and ether are not alone discussed but all narcotics. Narcotics are not alone considered, but various of the functions of life.' [1]

During 1848 Snow undertook an ' experimental inquiry into the action of eight volatile substances : chloroform ; ether ; nitrate of oxide of ethyle [nitric ether (ethyl nitrate, $C_2H_5ONO_2$)] ; bisulphuret of carbon [carbon disulphide, CS_2] ; benzin [benzene, C_6H_6] ; bromoform [tribromomethane, $HCBr_3$] ; bromide of ethyle [ethyl bromide, see p. 209] and Dutch liquid ' (see p. 166).[2]

Snow's views upon chloroform and ether have already been described (see pp. 179–80).

His opinion of nitric ether was favourable, after two preliminary experiments on mice and one clinical administration, using his chloroform inhaler at St. George's Hospital for a tooth extraction from a middle-aged man. ' The . . . case, I think, affords encouragement for further trials of this medicine ', he wrote, but he himself made no more.[3]

After experimenting on animals with bisulphuret of carbon, Snow found himself in agreement with Simpson who had used the drug ' in a surgical operation and an obstetric case '. Simpson, according to Snow, did not recommend it because ' its effects were so powerful and so transient, that it was very unmanageable '.[4]

' Benzin or benzole ' Snow used ' in some cases of toothdrawing, and in one amputation. . . . Its action in the minor

[1] Richardson, B. W., in Snow, J. 1858. *On chloroform and other anaesthetics.* London. xvi.

[2] *Lond. med. Gaz.*, 1848, **6**, 893, 1074 ; *ibid.* 1848, **7**, 330.
[3] *Ibid.* **6**, 1075.   [4] *Ibid.* **6**, 1076.

operations ', he found, ' was very nearly the same as that of nitric ether . . . ; but in the amputation, where its effects were carried further, the patient had violent convulsive tremors for about a minute, which, although not followed by any ill consequences, were sufficiently disagreeable to deter me from using it again.' [1]

Snow's tests with both bromoform and ethyl bromide were confined to animals, and he failed to recognize the advantages which were claimed for the latter agent by Nunneley and by later anaesthetists.[2]

Of Dutch liquid Snow's first opinion, based on laboratory experiments, coincided with Simpson's, which was ' that its vapour, when inhaled, causes so great irritation of the throat that few persons can persevere in inhaling it long enough to produce anaesthesia.' [3] But after Nunneley's suggestion in the following year, 1849, that the irritating qualities experienced by both Simpson and Snow were due to impurity in the drug, Snow made a fresh trial. He gave it clinically in five cases of tooth-drawing, in three obstetrical cases and to one cholera patient to give temporary relief from sickness and spasm. In four of the five dental cases Snow used his chloroform inhaler for administration, in the fifth he used the method which he first advocated in connection with chloroform anaesthesia (see p. 194), that is to say, he introduced into a balloon of known capacity 4 minims of the liquid drug for every 100 cubic inches of air. This gave him a mixture containing ' a small fraction over ' 4 per cent. of the vapour of Dutch liquid.

Even after this fresh trial of Dutch liquid Snow's opinion of it was not favourable :

' I cannot unite with Mr. Nunnelly [sic] in his general praises of Dutch liquid. The only advantages which it possesses over chloroform, in any case, are such as are connected with its slower action and more persistent effects—properties that Mr. Nunnelly failed to recognize. In all other respects its effects appear to be the same as those of chloroform. It is undoubtedly a very safe anaesthetic ; but I doubt very much whether practitioners would be content to wait for its slower action, after they have been accustomed to use chloroform, even if it could be obtained at the same cost, of which there is no prospect.' [4]

[1] *Lond. med. Gaz.*, 1848, **6**, 1078.   [2] *Ibid.* 1848, **7**, 330, 331.
[3] *Ibid.* **7**, 332.   [4] *Ibid.* 1849, **9**, 272 *et seq.*

In spite of his rejection of Dutch liquid [1,2-dichloroethane, $C_2H_4Cl_2$] as a suitable anaesthetic, Snow, in the same year, 1849, and in the following year, ' tried several times to make the mono-chlorurretted chloride of ethyle [ethidene dichloride = 1,1-di-chloroethane, CH_3CHCl_2] . . . but did not succeed in pro-curing more than a drachm or two at once, owing to the constant over-action of the chlorine.'

Snow described this substance as having the same composition and the same specific gravity as Dutch liquid, and a similar taste and smell ; the difference between the two lay in the boiling point and in the fact that ethidene dichloride was not decomposed ' by an alcoholic solution of potassa '.[1]

In 1851 Snow learned that an impure form of ethidene dichloride was being ' recommended in Paris as [a] local applica-tion in rheumatism and other painful affections ', and a friend was commissioned to send a sample to England. In due course a pint of reasonably pure liquid arrived, but subsequent samples were found to consist ' chiefly of chloride of carbon ' (see p. 209).[2]

Using his chloroform inhaler, Snow began making a series of clinical tests with his pint of ethidene dichloride. The tests were begun in June 1851, at King's College Hospital, and the results seem to have compared favourably with his chloroform results.[3] It was in June 1858, while engaged on recording these ethidene dichloride cases for his book, *On chloroform and other anaesthetics*, that Snow was taken ill. He died without stating his final opinion of the drug.[4]

[1] Snow, J. 1858. *On chloroform and other anaesthetics*. London. 420.
[2] *Ibid*. 421.   [3] *Ibid*. 421-3.
[4] The use of ethidene dichloride was revived about 1870 by Liebreich and Langen-beck, in Berlin. Nine years later the Glasgow Committee, then investigating the physiological effects of anaesthetics, independently recommended ethidene dichloride (see p. 428). The decision to experiment with it was based on its chemical com-position which seemed to promise well, and the results of the initial experiments were so encouraging that the Committee was ' led to enter on a special investigation of its action as compared with chloroform '.
The Committee's results led Clover to use ethidene dichloride, and by May 1880 he was able to record 1877 cases (287 in major surgery) without a fatality. Although he thought highly of the drug, Clover pointed out that its action on the heart was depressing, but less so than that of chloroform.
Clover's method of administration was to induce anaesthesia with nitrous oxide and continue with ethidene dichloride. He himself used his ' small sized gas and ether inhaler ' (cf. Fig. 83), but he thought that his portable ether inhaler (see Fig. 88) ' would do equally well '. (*Brit. med. J.*, 1880, i, 641, 797 ; *ibid*. 1880, ii, 957.)

Summarising the results of his experiments on animals with the eight volatile substances, Snow wrote :

' We find that the quantity of each substance in the blood, in corresponding degrees of narcotism, bears a certain proportion to what the blood would dissolve—a proportion that is almost exactly the same for all of them. . . . The actual quantity of the different substances in the blood, however, differs widely ; being influenced by their solubility. When the amount of saturation of the blood is the same, then it follows that the quantity of vapour required to produce the effect must increase with the solubility, and the effect produced by a given quantity must be in the inverse ratio of solubility. . . . This rule holds good with respect to all the substances of this kind that I have examined ; including, in addition to those enumerated . . . bichloride of carbon [dichloromethane], iodide of ethyle, acetate of oxide of ethyle, nitrate of oxide of methyle . . . pyroxilic spirit [methyl alcohol], acetone, and alcohol. . . .

' This general law, of course, does not apply to all narcotics . . . but only to those producing effects analogous to what are produced by ether, and having, I presume, a similar mode of action. I am not able at present to define them better than by calling them, that group of narcotics whose strength is inversely as their solubility in water (and consequently in the blood). In estimating their strength, when inhaled in the ordinary way, another element has to be taken into account, *viz.*, their volatility ; for that influences the quantity that would be inhaled.' [1]

Upon this question of volatility Snow wrote in 1850 :

' I have assumed from the first that the speedy subsidence of the narcotism caused by chloroform and ether, in comparison with that from alcohol and other narcotics, depends on the volatility of the former substances, which allows of their ready exit by the expired air. . . . Children recover from the effects of chloroform more rapidly, on account of their quicker circulation and respiration. Old people . . . more slowly, for the opposite reason. . . .

' Ether is more volatile than chloroform ; but being also much more soluble, the relative quantity absorbed into the system is so much greater, as to more than compensate for the superior volatility ; and consequently the effects of ether subside somewhat more slowly than those of chloroform, the ether taking rather longer to pass off in the expired air.

' It follows as a necessary consequence of this mode of excretion of vapour, that, if its exhalation by the breath could in any way be stopped, its narcotic effects ought to be much prolonged.' [2]

. . [1] *Lond. med. Gaz.*, 1848, **7,** 332.   [2] *Ibid.* 1850, **11,** 753.

Snow proceeded to demonstrate this point upon himself by rigging up a primitive closed-circuit apparatus, which included an absorber for carbon dioxide.

' About 750 cubic inches of oxygen gas were introduced into a balloon of thin membrane, varnished with solution of Indian rubber in turpentine. The balloon was attached to one of the apertures of the spiral box which forms part of the ether inhaler I employ [see Figs. 29 and 30] . . . Four ounces of solution of potassa were put into the inhaler, and to its other opening was attached a tube, connected with a face-piece without valves. After inhaling as much chloroform as I could without being rendered unconscious, I immediately began to breathe the oxygen from and to the balloon, and over the solution of potassa. In this way the vapour exhaled in the breath had, the greater part of it, to be re-inspired. This process was continued for ten minutes, during which time the feeling of narcotism subsided very little, and it passed off very slowly afterwards. . . . The solution of caustic potash was employed for the purpose of absorbing the carbonic acid gas generated by respiration as the air passed to and fro over a large extent of its surface. . . .

' . . . On another day the same quantity of oxygen and solution of potassa were employed, and fifteen minims of chloroform were placed in the spiral inhaler, in a small glass vessel. . . . I then began to breathe as in the former experiment, and continued to do so for fifteen minutes. The effects of the chloroform were gradually induced during the first three minutes, causing a considerable feeling of narcotism, but not producing unconsciousness. After the end of three minutes, the feeling of narcotism remained stationary till twelve minutes had elapsed, and during the last three minutes it very slightly diminished. The experiment was discontinued on account of a feeling of want of breath.'

Snow repeated this latter experiment substituting $2\frac{1}{2}$ fluid drachms of ether for the 15 minims of chloroform and breathing to and fro for twenty minutes, with very similar results. In both cases the recovery period was slow, half an hour or longer elapsing between the discontinuance of inhalation and the return to complete normality. ' The effects of the small quantity of chloroform and ether inhaled in these experiments ', said Snow in his summary, ' would have passed off in three or four minutes, if the exhaled vapour had been allowed to diffuse itself in the air in the usual way.' [1]

From these and further experiments, on animals, Snow was able ' to determine the amount of carbonic acid gas excreted

[1] *Lond. med. Gaz.*, 1850, **II,** 753-4.

under the influence of chloroform and ether' and he found that this amount was smaller than that normally excreted. This finding confirmed his belief in his original theory of anaesthesia by volatile narcotics.

'The diminution of the amount of carbonic acid formed in the system under the influence of chloroform, ether, and alcohol, taken in conjunction with [the] . . . circumstance . . . that the chloroform and ether are exhaled unchanged from the blood, assist to prove a view of their *modus operandi* which I suggested with respect to ether, early in 1847. That view may be stated as follows :

'Chloroform, ether, and similar substances, when present in the blood in certain quantities, have the effect of limiting those combinations between the oxygen of the arterial blood and the tissues of the body which are essential to sensation, volition, and, in short, all animal functions. The substances modify, and in larger quantities arrest, the animal functions, in the same way, and by the same power, that they modify and arrest combustion, the slow oxidation of phosphorus, and other kinds of oxidation unconnected with the living body, when they are mixed in certain quantities with the atmospheric air.

'This explanation', Snow added, 'is probably applicable to the action of all narcotics whatever, but is here applied only to the class considered in these papers, namely, the volatile narcotic substances not containing nitrogen, or those substances whose power was found to be in the inverse ratio of their solubility in water and the serum of the blood.' [1]

Richardson, writing of Snow and his theory of anaesthesia,[2] recorded : 'In his modest way, he often spoke to me with

[1] *Lond. med. Gaz.*, 1851, **12**, 626.
[2] Another theory of the physiological action of anaesthetics put forward during the nineteenth century was that of Claude Bernard.
'We think ', wrote Bernard, ' that certain arguments derived from the accurate analysis of facts may permit us to form a clear enough conception of the physico-chemical action which . . . [anaesthetics] exercise on the nerves. In our view this action should consist in a semi-coagulation of the substance of the nerve-cell itself— a coagulation which would not be final ; that is to say, the cell substance would be able to return to its original, normal state upon the elimination of the toxic agent. . . .
'Anaesthesia, however, is not a poison to the nervous system only ; it anaesthetises all the cells, all the tissues, paralyzing and momentarily arresting their metabolic irritability.' (Bernard, C. 1875. *Leçons sur les anesthésiques et sur l'asphyxie*. Paris. 149.)
According to H. K. Beecher, ' As early as 1860, Binz had made observations which foreshadowed the modern colloid theory of narcosis [*Arch. exp. Path. Pharmak.*, 1887, **6**, 310]. He stated that, when brain tissue was exposed to 1 per cent. morphine hydrochloride solution, it would coagulate the cells, and early states of this process were reversible. . .
'Claude Bernard continued this line of study. . . . It was mainly due to his observations that the colloid theory was formulated.' (Beecher, H. K. 1938. *The physiology of anesthesia*. New York. 30.) (Cf. p. 158—the origin of the lipoid theory of narcosis.)

honest pride on this observation. He himself thought it the best observation he had ever made and believed that it would not be lost as an historical truth. Placing a taper, during one of our experiments, in a bottle through which chloroform vapour was diffused, and watching the declining flame, he once said, " there, now, is all that occurs in narcotism ; but to submit the candle to the action of the narcotic without extinguishing it altogether, you must neither expose it to much vapour at once, nor subject it to the vapour too long ; and this is all you can provide against in submitting a man to the same influence. I could illustrate all the meaning of this great practical discovery on a farthing candle, but I fear the experiment would be thought rather commonplace ".' [1]

Snow's quest for the perfect anaesthetic led him at last to amylene (C_5H_{10}), which seemed at first to fulfil many of his requirements, particularly that of destroying ' common sensation without destroying consciousness '.

Amylene was discovered by Balard in 1844, but Snow ' was not aware of . . . [its] existence till 1856, or ', he wrote, ' I should have tried it sooner. . . . I believe that amylene had but rarely been made, and only in very small quantity, until I requested Mr. Bullock to make it for me. . . .

' As soon as Mr. Bullock succeeded. . . . I proceeded to perform some experiments with it on small animals.'

Snow then tested the vapour upon himself. He found that it had ' more odour than chloroform, but much less than ether ', and that, unlike both chloroform and ether, it was almost entirely without pungency, so that ' after two or three inspirations, one cannot tell whether the air one is breathing contains any of the vapour or not '. Snow further concluded that ' viewed in the light of the small quantity which requires to be absorbed into the system to cause insensibility, amylene is a very powerful agent ; but when considered in relation to the quantity which is consumed during inhalation in the ordinary way, it is very far from being powerful. This arises from the great tension and the small solubility of the vapour, in consequence of which it is, with the exception of a small fraction, expelled from the lungs again without being absorbed. . . . It takes from three to four fluid drachms of amylene to cause insensibility in the adult. . . . In

---

[1] Richardson, B. W., in Snow, J. 1858. *On chloroform and other anaesthetics.* London. xvii.

administering amylene for surgical operations, it is desirable that the patient should take in 15 per cent. of the vapour with the air he breathes.'[1]

In the course of his experiments on animals Snow found 'that amylene is, like chloroform and some other agents, capable of causing sudden death by over-narcotism of the heart, and paralysis of that organ ', but whereas the ' vapour of chloroform, when inhaled of twice the proper strength, *i.e.* 8 or 10 per cent., is capable of causing sudden death . . . amylene is required to be of nearly 40 per cent., or more than twice its proper strength, before it could produce this result '.[2]

Snow's first clinical administrations, in November 1856, were ' to two boys, about fourteen years old, previous to . . . extracting some teeth. . . . The effects . . . as far as they extended were so favourable as to encourage a further trial '.

' From November 1856 to July 1857, I exhibited amylene in 238 cases. . . .
' The greater number of the operations under amylene were performed while the patient was . . . apparently awake, although not really conscious of surrounding objects. This usual absence of coma in the employment of amylene cannot be looked on otherwise than as an advantage. It must conduce to the safety of the agent when the proportion of vapour in the air is properly regulated. . . . During the inhalation of amylene the patient is often entirely regardless of the surgeon's knife, whilst the edges of the eyelids retain their full sensibility.'[3]

In April 1857, in his 144th case under amylene anaesthesia, Snow had his first death from this agent. Another death followed in July, in his 238th case. ' I have no doubt ', wrote Snow, ' that in each of these accidents the patient must have taken into his lungs at one moment air containing upwards of thirty per cent. of vapour of amylene. And there is no doubt that the cause of this was the unsteady boiling-point of the agent.'[4]

Up till then, Snow had been using the apparatus which, ' for ten years, whilst exhibiting chloroform ' (see Fig. 41), had enabled him ' to give four per cent. of the vapour, probably without ever allowing the quantity to exceed six per cent '. ' In the future cases in which I employ amylene ', he wrote, ' it is my intention to administer it from a bag or balloon, putting in so

[1] Snow, J. 1858. *On chloroform and other anaesthetics.* London. 373, 374, 384, 386.
[2] *Ibid.* 384, 387.   [3] *Ibid.* 389, 398.   [4] *Ibid.* 408, 411, 415, 416.

much of the liquid as will make fifteen per cent. of vapour when
the bag is filled up with air.   In this manner the variability in the
boiling-point of the amylene can have no influence whatever
on the amount of vapour which the patient breathes ; and if
the vapour be breathed over again, within certain limits, in the
manner of nitrous oxide gas, there will be a great saving in the
amount of amylene consumed.' [1]

'Although amylene was largely used in Paris, Strasbourg,
Montpelier, and Lyons, soon after I published my first account
of it,' wrote Snow, 'and although I have lately heard that it is
still employed in Paris and Berlin, nearly eighteen months after
its first use in these places, I am happy that I have not heard
of any accident from its use except the two which happened in
my own hands.'   He recorded, however, that the Académie de
Médecine, in Paris, had 'recommended the disuse of amylene
on account of the accidents which had happened in my hands'. [2]

During 1857 two important discussions on amylene as an
anaesthetic had been held by members of the Académie de
Médecine.[3]   It was agreed among them that amylene was in no
way superior to chloroform and was in many respects greatly
inferior.   To the French, one of the most serious disadvantages
of amylene was the fact that it could not satisfactorily be administered like chloroform, from a *compresse* or a sponge, but
necessitated the use of an apparatus such as Charrière's (see
Fig. 40).   It was the surgeon, Velpeau, who, at the close of the
second discussion, expressed the opinion that since in Snow's own
hands the drug had proved fatal ' it must be absolutely banned '.[4]

In 1893, when a purified form of amylene, called pental, was
attracting a certain amount of attention, Hewitt wrote of Snow's
two fatalities, ' in discussing these by the light of our present
knowledge it is questionable whether they should be directly
attributed to the influence of the anaesthetic . . . it is quite
possible that other factors than the toxic action of the amylene
may have been at work.   These, however, are mere conjectures '.[5]

Amylene, the anaesthetic from which Snow had once hoped
so much, was finally relegated by him to second place ' between
chloroform and ether in respect to its comparative safety by the
ordinary methods of administration '.   To the end ether held, in

[1] Snow, J. 1858. *On chloroform and other anaesthetics.* London. 416, 417.
[2] *Ibid.* 417, 419.
[3] *Bull. Acad. Méd. Paris,* 1856–7, **22,** 751–68, 1118–32.   [4] *Ibid.* **22,** 1130–1.
[5] Hewitt, F. W. 1893. *Anaesthetics and their administration.* London. 266.

theory, the first place in Snow's esteem ; in practice he allowed chloroform to usurp it.[1]

At about the time when the surgeons of Paris tried and then rejected the use of amylene, Ozanam, in a series of papers addressed to the section of chemistry of the Académie des Sciences, was attempting to introduce the clinical use of carbon dioxide gas as a general anaesthetic.

In 1856 he asserted what Nunneley had suggested in 1849 (see p. 212), ' that the whole series of volatile and gaseous carbons is endowed with anaesthetic powers ', and later added that ' the higher the proportion of carbon the greater the power '. In 1857 he stated :

' I have confirmed this law through making a study of carbon monoxide gas. Following up these researches I have now demonstrated that the ethers act as anaesthetics only after breaking down into carbon dioxide gas and precisely because they are able so to break down. If one considers, indeed : (1) that ether is a body containing a high proportion of carbon ; (2) that in the etherized animal carbon dioxide is exhaled in double the quantity (Ville and Blandin's researches [cf. Snow's finding, p. 218]); (3) that the inspiration of a gas not containing carbon does not result in this increase of carbonic acid ; one is justified in drawing the legitimate conclusion that, in the case of etherization, production of a fresh quantity of carbonic acid occurs at the expense of the only new body which has been absorbed.

' In other words, when one breathes ether, it breaks down in the blood stream, and this decomposition, which is nothing more than a process of combustion, gives rise to the formation of abundant carbonic acid gas.

' We already know the anaesthetic properties of carbon dioxide gas : the arrest of bleeding, paralysis of the nervous system, all the phenomena of insensibility to the point of apparent and then actual death. It is evidently in this new form and as a result of its decomposition, therefore, that ether exercises its stupefying action upon the nervous system.

' What happens in the case of ether doubtless happens also with chloroform, amylene and other anaesthetic bodies ; each of them, according to its chemical affinities, breaks down either into carbon dioxide or into carbon monoxide.'

In a further paper on the subject, in 1858, Ozanam continued :

' I was thus led, by reasoned deduction, to use the inhalation of carbonic acid gas as a general anaesthetic. Ether was no more

[1] Snow, J. 1858. *On chloroform and other anaesthetics.* London. 418.

indeed, than a useless and sometimes dangerous intermediary, of which one could neither consistently calculate the dose, nor with certainty foresee the effects. I believe I can to-day present to the Académie a serious study of a body powerful enough to arrest sensibility, manageable enough to enable one to prolong its administration, yet so innocuous that one need no longer fear sudden death.'

Ozanam proceeded to support his fallacious argument with an account of twenty-seven experiments on rabbits. He claimed that carbon dioxide produced an anaesthetic effect very similar to that of ether but more fugitive.[1]

Neither Ozanam's theory of anaesthetic action nor his proposal that carbon dioxide should be used clinically as a general anaesthetic was adopted.

[1] *C.R. Acad. Sci., Paris*, 1856, **43,** 1187–3 ; *ibid.*, 1857, **45,** 348 ; *ibid.*, **46,** 417–20.

CHAPTER VIII

CHLOROFORM IN PRACTICE *c.* 1850-70

Chloroform in France—Nasal Inhalation—Dosimetric Inhalers—Open
Administration

Chloroform Anaesthesia in France

AT the time of Snow's death in 1858 the tide which had swept
chloroform into favour was already on the turn in England,
although as yet the ebb was scarcely perceptible. But on the
European Continent it was during the eighteen-fifties that
chloroform anaesthesia became firmly established and rules for
the guidance of administrators which were then formulated
continued to influence practice, so far as the average surgeon
was concerned, until the eighteen-nineties when a general
revival of the use of ether began to take place (see p. 410 *et seq.*).

In France Charrière's chloroform apparatus (see Fig. 40)
continued an existence which was now little more than nominal,
but about 1857 Duroy, a Parisian pharmaceutical chemist,
devised an ' ingenious but very complicated ' *anaesthesimeter* (see
Figs. 45 and 46) in which the quantity and rate of supply of the
liquid chloroform allowed to fall upon the evaporating surface
could be regulated and the area of the evaporating surface itself
correspondingly increased or decreased. Despite its ingenuity,
however, the apparatus appears to have had little to recommend
it to the clinician.[1]

Among other unfavourable comments made by Snow, he
wrote : ' M. Duroy . . . follows the rude and objectionable
plan of using a nose clasp, and thus compelling the patient to
breathe by the mouth alone '[2] and Duroy's fellow-countryman,
Robert, speaking of the *anaesthesimeter* at a meeting of the
Académie de Médecine in Paris, in June 1857, said that it took
from twenty-five to thirty minutes to establish anaesthesia with
it, in an adult male.[3]

[1] Gaujot, G., and Spillmann, E. 1867. *Arsenal de la chirurgie contemporaine.* Paris.
1, 16-21 ; *Pharm. J.*, 1856-7, **16**, 274.
[2] Snow, J. 1858. *On chloroform and other anaesthetics.* London. 86.
[3] *Bull. Acad. Méd. Paris*, 1856-7, **22**, 969.

225

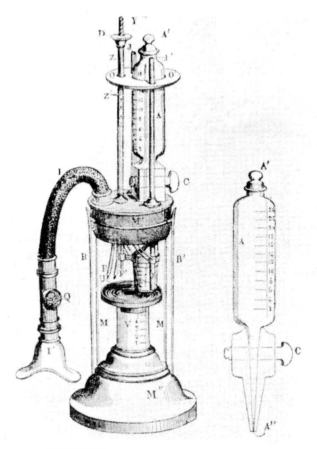

FIG. 45.—DUROY'S ' ANAESTHESIMETER ' (Paris, 1857)

MM. Glass cylinder enclosing evaporating mechanism.
M′. Cork-lined ebony stopper closing MM.
M″. Ebony base.   R, R′. Metal supports.
I, I′. Inhaling tube and mouthpiece, with expiratory valve Q, and inspiratory valve
 (also at Q, not shown).
 A. Graduated chloroform reservoir with stopper, A′, control tap, C, and dropper,
  A″.
 Z. Tube, with scale Z′, through which rod Y, with pointer Y′ (for scale Z′) was
  raised or lowered by the screw D (see Fig. 46 for detail).
J, J′. Tubes through which air entered MM.
 K. Graduated receptacle (see Fig. 46) kept filled with chloroform from A, by a
  constant level device.
F, F′. Curved tubes through which ran wicks. One end of each tube dipped into the
  chloroform in K (see Fig. 46) the other end hung over the concentrically
  grooved evaporating plate, U. In the centre of U was a hole communicating
  with the graduated receptacle, V, below (see Fig. 46).

226

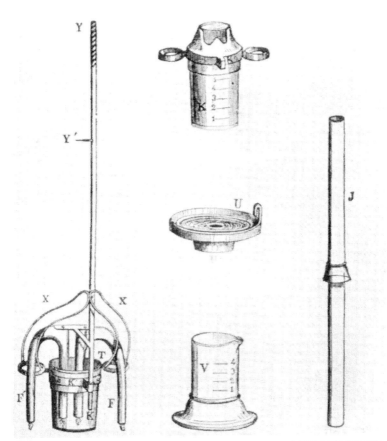

FIG. 46.—COMPONENTS OF DUROY'S 'ANAESTHESIMETER'

(*Left.*) Mechanism whereby chloroform was dropped by the wicks in F, F', from K on to U (see Fig. 45)—the movable rod Y, passed through a collar K', fixed round K. The T-shaped bar, projecting from Y, attached F and F' to itself by pivots, so that they were raised or lowered by the movement of Y. F and F' passed through X and X, guide rails fixed to K.

When Y was raised, by turning the screw D (see Fig. 45), F and F' penetrated less and less deeply into K, so that the path travelled by the chloroform along the wicks was lengthened and the distance between their free ends and the evaporating plate U was increased. Simultaneously X and X caused the free ends of F and F' to swing towards each other. Thus the field of evaporation was reduced in area and more of the liquid chloroform fell through the hole in U into V, beneath. This resulted in a smaller proportion of chloroform being vaporized and taken up by the stream of air entering the body of the apparatus MM, through the tubes J, J', and passing through I, I' to the patient.

In Fig. 45, the relative positions of F, F' and U, when Y was at its highest point, are shown ; Fig. 46 shows their relative positions when Y was at its lowest.

Robert, incidentally, seems to have been almost the only Frenchman to recommend and use Snow's chloroform inhaler ; but then the number of his countrymen who still used any kind of mechanical apparatus was relatively small.[1]

The two most usual methods of administering chloroform in France were : either to give it, after the Scottish manner, sprinkled in repeated doses on a pad (*la compresse*) of some kind of woven material (or occasionally on a sponge) held just sufficiently far above the patient's nose and mouth to allow the free admixture of atmospheric air with the vapour ; or to give it from a truncated cone made, as a rule, from pasteboard. The open base of the cone fitted over the patient's nose and mouth and through the opening in the top chloroform was sprinkled, as in the ' *compresse* ' method, on to a sponge or a wad of lint placed in the upper part of the cone.[2]

French faith in the administration of chloroform by the simplest, non-mechanical means was no doubt strengthened by the experience of military surgeons during the Crimean War (1854–5). At a meeting of the Académie des Sciences, in 1855, Baudens, who had been officially concerned in organising military hospitals for the reception of Crimean wounded, reported that he had been assured by the Surgeon-in-Chief of the French Army, that in more than 25,000 cases of chloroform administration not a single accident had occurred. Baudens stressed the usefulness of chloroform in enabling gunshot wounds to be investigated and in making possible the conservative surgery of limbs. ' It had only remained for chloroform to prove itself on the battlefield ; ' he said, ' its triumph has been complete.'

Mounier, who had served during the war, described his experiences :

' During six months spent as Surgeon-in-Chief of the Dolma-Bagtché Hospital at Constantinople, I had occasion to use chloroform several thousands of times . . . and I have the satisfaction of being able to tell the Académie that administrations have always been crowned with complete success.

' The apparatus I invariably used was extremely simple ; it consisted of a paper cone sufficiently open at its base to include both the nose and mouth of the patient, and truncated at the apex so as to allow the free entry of air during inspiration ; a pinch of lint introduced into the end of the cone took the place of a sponge. Twenty or thirty drops of chloroform were poured

---

[1] *Bull. Acad. Méd. Paris*, 1856–7, **22**, 831, 968.   [2] Cf. *Ibid.* **22**, 967.

into the cone and absorbed by the surface of the lint. The wounded man was laid flat on his back. Experience having taught us that bright light and noise appreciably retarded, if they did not preclude, the action of chloroform, a pad was laid over the patient's eyes and silence was observed by everyone assisting. An intelligent assistant timed pulse and respiration rates by the second hand of a watch. The cone was alternately lowered and raised for a few seconds from the patient's mouth ; and, according to the degree of anaesthesia manifest, the apparatus was held nearer to the face and for a longer time. The patient's sensibility was tested by pinching the skin, his mental reaction by repeated questions. The patient's silence was, for us, the indication for beginning to act and that moment has always been the start of the operation.

'If the operative procedure lasted for a long time, a second or third dose of chloroform, which was always inspired intermittently, was dropped into the cone.

'Such has been the method of chloroforming used for all the wounded of Alma and Inkerman brought to my hospital, and we have never had a death or even an accident. . . .

'The popularisation of the use of chloroform and the practising of operative procedure on the cadaver, which I taught the students of the Medical School at Constantinople, are two good works which, I hope, will leave permanent traces of French military medicine upon the Orient.'

Mounier, in view both of his own experience and of Flourens's theory that chloroform acted first upon the mental faculties, then upon sensibility and finally upon the power of movement (cf. p. 160), believed it unnecessary ever to 'push the absorption of chloroform to the point of abolishing the movements'. If excitement occurred Mounier claimed that he was able to control it not by increasing the dose of chloroform but by raising the cone from the patient's face for a few seconds until the stage which he considered the normal one for beginning the operation —the stage in which sensation was abolished—was re-established.[1]

That anaesthesia should not be allowed to progress beyond this stage had indeed been emphasized by Baudens, who cited Flourens as his authority, and he reported that during the Crimean campaign French surgeons generally, were careful to observe this precaution.[2]

The cone for administering chloroform was common also to French naval surgery and continued to be in general use

[1] *C.R. Acad. Sci., Paris,* 1855, **40,** 530–2.   [2] *Ibid.* 1855, **41,** 1076.

during the remainder of the nineteenth century. In the last quarter of the century the cones were still made from pasteboard, but the evaporating surface for the chloroform consisted of a diaphragm, placed across the upper third of the cone, composed of two or three layers of lint and having a hole in the centre to allow the patient to draw in sufficient fresh air (see Fig. 47).[1]

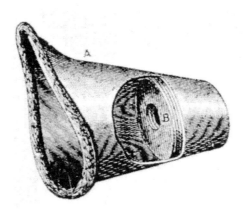

FIG. 47.—CONE, MADE FROM PASTEBOARD, FOR ADMINISTERING CHLOROFORM

A type of inhaler used in France, particularly in naval hospitals, from 1848 until 1900 and after.

A. End of cone, with padded rim, adapted to fit the patient's face, 14 cm. across at the widest point.
B. Diaphragm composed of two or three rounds of lint lightly stitched together, on to which the chloroform was poured. The diaphragm was placed across the cone about 9 cm. from the wide end ; it was about 4 cm. across, corresponding in diameter to that of the truncated end of the cone ; its central perforation had a diameter roughly double that of the trachea.

Although many French surgeons, in the early years of the use of chloroform, attempted to avoid the already obvious dangers of the agent by keeping the patient in an analgesic rather than a completely insensible state, this procedure was not approved by all. Sédillot, of Strasbourg, for instance, who always used a handkerchief for giving chloroform, said at a meeting of the Société de Chirurgie in Paris, in October 1851 :

' If I am to believe a certain medical journal and what I myself have seen, a large number of our colleagues employ

[1] Cf. *Bull. Soc. Chirurgie Paris*, 1861, N.S. **2,** 501, 502 ; Rottenstein, J. B. 1880. *Traité d'anesthésie chirurgicale.* Paris. 141–3 ; *Gaz. Hôp., Paris*, 1891, No. 129, 1191.

chloroform in such a way that it ceases to be of use either to patient
or surgeon, on the pretext that the dangers attributable to complete anaesthesia are averted. . . . I must deny this doctrine and
I have no hesitation in stating that this agent, properly administered, in a pure state, never kills, even if its action is prolonged
for a considerable time. . . .

'We generally avoid the period of excitement,' Sédillot
continued, 'which with us, occurred most frequently with
alcoholic men.

'I always wait to begin operating', he said, 'until muscular
relaxation is obtained, so that the patient remains quite motionless
under the application of the instruments.

'To proceed otherwise seems to me irrational, because one
is deprived of the greatest benefit of anaesthesia, the immobility
of the patient being operated upon, yet is not protected against
accidents, for death has been observed to follow immediately upon
the first breaths of chloroform.' [1]

In the discussion following Sédillot's remarks, Maisonneuve
maintained that an excitement stage was practically inevitable.
In Paris, at any rate, so he said, it was in order to avoid the
difficulties of this stage that surgeons hastened to operate before
it became established ; he himself believed, however, that the
operation should not be begun until the stage was passed and
the patient breathed tranquilly.

Sédillot replied that although an excitement stage was liable
to occur in alcoholic men, he could not agree that it occurred
in all or even the majority of patients.

Chassaignac stated that he never applied the knife to living
tissues until chloroform anaesthesia was completely established.
He added that he preferred to make his patient breathe
through the nose rather than the mouth, because he believed the
vapour acted more promptly by this route and the patient was
less liable to spasms.

'As I have just said,' remarked Sédillot, 'the excitement
stage is generally absent ; but if it does occur the action of the
chloroform should nevertheless be continued, but with great
prudence. One may, in some cases, bring about relaxation by
making the patient take deep inspirations, if respiration is not
obstructed ; otherwise it is wiser to wait a moment and continue
the administration as the agitation begins to subside.'

With reference to Sédillot's assertion that if a fatality occurred

[1] *Bull. Soc. Chirurgie Paris*, 1851-2, **2**, 336.

under chloroform anaesthesia it must be due either to impurity in the drug or to maladministration, Forget expressed the opinion that pure chloroform *could* kill.[1]

Nearly forty years later, in 1889, and on this occasion also during a meeting of the Société de Chirurgie, Sédillot's assertion was recalled by Reynier :

' Pure chloroform, well administered, cannot kill, Sédillot said, and this phrase has been often repeated and discussed by surgeons, almost all of whom have rebelled against its apparent dogmatism and the great measure of responsibility which, at the same time, it imposes upon them. Although my own observations have led me to accept his opinion in its entirety, I do not wish to begin a similar discussion to-day and I will deal only with part of Sédillot's phrase, to which he attached so great an importance —the purity of chloroform. . . .' [2]

Opening the discussion on Reynier's paper, Lucas-Championnière remarked : ' One may effectively establish in principle that with pure chloroform, properly administered, anaesthetic accidents are extremely rare. It must be added that, in fact, it is very rare to have pure chloroform '.[3]

The question of the great responsibility imposed upon the administrator, which Sédillot's statement implied, was raised at the meeting in 1851 by Hugier.

' From the medico-legal point of view ', he said, ' M. Sédillot's proposition may be a grave source of inconvenience to the surgeon, if one admits that chloroform never kills ; for, since fatal accidents have occurred and may occur again, it follows that the surgeon will be prosecuted [4] and often convicted. The chloroform question is by no means yet resolved ; surgeons are not yet in agreement as to the method of administration, dosage, and the duration of administration. Well, then, in the presence of these uncertainties *ought* one always to push the administration of anaesthetics to the final stage ? ' [5]

---

[1] *Bull. Soc. Chirurgie Paris*, 1851–2, **2**, 338–40.
[2] *Ibid.* 1889, **15**, 618.   [3] *Ibid.* **15**, 623–4.
[4] Snow recorded : ' A person named Breton, a dealer in porcelain, died in Paris, in the early part of 1853, immediately after a few inspirations of chloroform, which was administered with the intention of removing a tumour of the cheek. An action was brought against Dr. Triquet and M. Masson for causing death by imprudence in this case ; and at the trial which ensued, various interesting opinions were given, and the accused practitioners were ultimately exonerated (*Gaz. Médicale*, 1853, p. 304). I have not, however, met with any record of the symptoms which occurred in the case.' (Snow, J. 1858. *On chloroform* . . . London. 200.)
[5] *Bull. Soc. Chirurgie Paris*, 1851–2, **2**, 341.

Sédillot replied :

' I cannot allow that a question bearing upon legal judgment should be opposed to the truth. We all make mistakes and the wisest of us is he who makes the least mistakes. The magistrates' bench in France usually knows how to judge sensibly the cases brought before it, and it is perhaps not a bad thing that the professional man should not be absolutely free to do what he pleases without any responsibility. I must add in closing, that I have never seen a refractory patient under chloroform and that no accident has ever happened to me.

' This discussion, in which the majority of the members of this Society have boldly declared themselves in favour of complete anaesthesia, will have, I hope, a happy influence upon surgical practice, giving to it greater security and bringing back rational and efficient methods in the use of anaesthetics.' [1]

The discussion on amylene (cf. p. 222), which occupied much of the time of the Académie de Médecine, during the early summer of 1857, gave rise indirectly to an equally lengthy discussion upon the use of inhalers as opposed to the use of a *compresse* or cone for chloroform administration. Velpeau, with a very large majority of his colleagues behind him, set himself at the head of the winning side of *compresse* and sponge users. ' I discarded a long time ago the more or less complicated apparatus of Charrière and others ', he said. In support of similar views, another member of the Académie, H. Larrey, cited Porta, of Milan, Constantini, of Rome, and the Russians, who never gave chloroform by any other means than on a folded cloth or a sponge, and the Americans who used a sponge for ether inhalation.[2]

Nasal Inhalation

In 1859 Faure, of Paris, adopted the practice of administering chloroform through one nostril. This new method was, in fact, very similar to Malgaigne's original method of giving ether (see p. 135). Like Malgaigne's, Faure's apparatus was ' of the simplest : one end of a rubber tube is inserted in the nostril [later Faure fitted a conical nozzle to the tube] the other opens into a flask containing chloroform. The interior of the flask communicates freely with the air '. This it did by means of an unstoppered glass neck the aperture of which could be closed

[1] *Bull. Soc. Chirurgie Paris*, 1851–2, **2**, 341, 342.
[2] *Bull. Acad. Méd. Paris*, 1856–7, **22**, 764, 828, 953, 1084, 1087, 1097.

by the anaesthetist's finger. ' In order to decrease, abolish or restore sensibility it is only necessary to move the tube further into or out of the nostril or to shake the flask so as to cause increased evaporation at any given moment.' Faure appears to have ignored the possibility of the patient snuffing up liquid chloroform.

He claimed that the depth of anaesthesia was readily controllable by this method and that the patient was spared all unpleasant feelings of suffocation. It was in the course of making experiments upon animals with chloroform vapour given through one nostril that Faure decided to adopt nasal administration, for he observed that in this way ' an animal might be anaesthetised with chloroform while still receiving into the lungs a column of fresh air equal in quantity to half that breathed in a normal state '.[1]

Benjamin Ward Richardson, who had an eye for anything new and useful in anaesthesia, immediately saw the possibilities of applying Faure's technique in operations in and about the mouth ; the only method then in current use being to give the anaesthetic intermittently, a whiff at a time, so as not to obstruct the operative field. Richardson's first case using Faure's method of nasal administration was one in which Spencer Wells removed half the lower jaw. His enthusiasm for it disappeared, however, after one or two further cases in which ' great danger had arisen therefrom '.

In May 1861, A. E. Sansom also administered chloroform nasally, using an apparatus similar to Faure's. As Richardson had proposed, he reserved the method ' for prolonging anaesthesia in cases of operation in which the ordinary means for the exhibition of chloroform interferes with the manipulation of the operator, in operations on the mouth, etc.' [2]

Early in 1862 the dental surgeon, Alfred Coleman, who was responsible for a number of ingenious pieces of apparatus, including the forerunner of the Mason gag,[3] adapted a modified Snow's chloroform inhaler (see Fig. 50) for nasal administration (see Fig. 48). He took the chloroform chamber, attached a 10-inch length of tubing and to its free end added a brass cap with a ' valve opening outwards '. To this cap he

[1] *Arch. gén. Méd.*, 1859, **1**, 633 ; *Bull. Acad. Méd. Paris*, 1859–60, **25**, 115.
[2] *Med. Times, Lond.*, 1861, i, 550.
[3] See *Med. Times, Lond.*, 1861, i, 105 : ' An instrument for keeping the mouth open in operations under chloroform.'

' attached the nose-piece—a silver tube flattened on its upper surface, and having soldered into its end, at a right angle, two smaller tubes of an oval form, these converge[d] slightly towards each other at their extremities, and by means of a slide the distance between them [could] . . . be diminished or increased '. Coleman attached a rubber hand-bellows to the chloroform chamber ' to enable the administrator to force a stream of air through the instrument into the patient's nose ', because he had found that in some cases when the mouth was open the full effects of the chloroform could not be maintained.

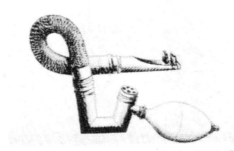

FIG. 48.—COLEMAN'S NASAL INHALER
FOR CHLOROFORM, 1862

The two small tubes were inserted into the nares and a stream of air was pumped through the chloroform chamber by the hand-bellows, the air-inlet holes of the chamber being closed by the administrator's thumb.

Incidentally Coleman seems here to have been the first to make use of the ' blow-over ' method in a piece of anaesthetic apparatus, as distinct from the ' draw-over ' method.

Coleman did not induce anaesthesia nasally but used an ordinary Snow's facepiece until the patient was ' sufficiently insensible ', then the facepiece was removed and the nose-piece substituted.[1]

J. T. Clover, about 1862, introduced a nasal cap shaped like a miniature facepiece, for maintaining anaesthesia. He explained : ' I merely exchange the face-piece of my inhaler [see p. 242] for a nose-cap provided with valves and apply it over the nose. It is retained *in situ* by a strap which goes round the back

[1] *Lancet*, 1862, i, 42.

of the head, and thus the chloroformist has his hands at liberty to watch the pulse or to afford assistance to the Dentist in managing the gag [cf. p. 298] or in sponging the gums in those cases where much difficulty is experienced in extracting roots '.[1]

The idea of using a miniature facepiece to fit over the nose

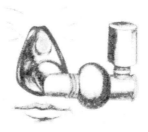

FIG. 49.—CHLOROFORM APPARATUS
WITH A MINIATURE SNOW'S TYPE
OF FACEPIECE, USED BY COLEMAN
FOR NASAL ADMINISTRATION

The graduated drop-bottle containing chloroform either hung down from the tube, into
which its mouth opened, or it could be
inverted (as shown) so that chloroform fell
on to a sponge within the tube. The end
of this tube was covered by a wire-mesh cap
through which air was drawn in by the
patient's inspiration. 'The expanded portion
[of the tube] has in front of it a piece of fine
wire gauze, which has the object of thoroughly
mixing the chloroform-vapour and air together, rendering the vapour less pungent.'
(Coleman, A., 1888. *Manual of dental surgery*.
London. 275, 276.)

was also adopted by Coleman, whose apparatus is shown in Fig. 49.

Dosimetric Inhalers

Many English anaesthetists during the early eighteen-sixties, continued to use Snow's chloroform inhaler (see Fig. 41) or modifications of it. Of these modifications a popular one was Arthur Ernest Sansom's.

[1] *Brit. J. dent. Sci.*, 1868, **11**, 128.

Sansom had been House Physician at King's College Hospital in Snow's day, and had often worked with him. In 1865 he wrote on the subject of the chloroform inhaler :

' Dr. Snow's instrument has certainly proved of immense value in regulating and methodising the administration of chloro-

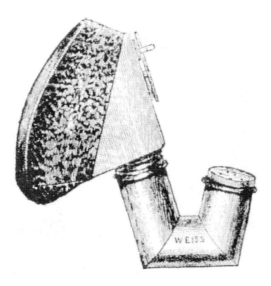

FIG. 50.—A SO-CALLED 'MODIFICATION OF SNOW'S CHLOROFORM INHALER' (cf. Fig. 41)

Made by Weiss, *c.* 1865. The original model was made by Matthews, of Portugal Street, London, during the eighteen-fifties.
The vaporizing chamber was simply a bent metal tube with a close-textured sponge filling the arm farthest from the facepiece. This arm was fitted with a screw cap perforated by seven holes, set in a rosette, each $\frac{1}{8}$ inch in diameter.

form. There are, however, in my opinion, certain objections to it. Its water-bath makes it heavy and cumbrous ; its long flexible tube is often in the way. It does not provide at the early stage a sufficiency of dilution to make the patient take kindly to the vapour and to prevent the occurrence of spasm or cough, and, lastly, the general proportion which it supplies (5–6 per cent.) is too high.' [1]

[1] Sansom, A. E. 1865. *Chloroform : its action and administration.* London. 125.

By greatly modifying Snow's inhaler Sansom considered that he had remedied these defects. His inhaler (see Fig. 51) consisted of a cylindrical metal vaporizing chamber, ' its height about three inches, its diameter about an inch and a half'. He

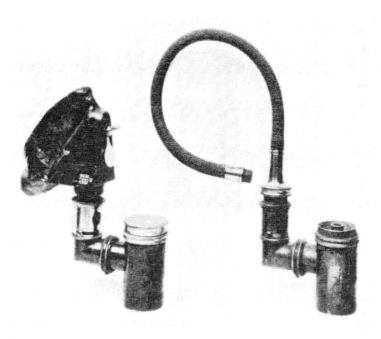

FIG. 51.—SANSOM'S CHLOROFORM INHALER (c. 1865)

(*Left.*) The air-inlet holes of the vaporizing chamber are covered by a cap, which was removed when the inhaler was in use. The air port in the tube beneath the facepiece can be seen.

(*Right.*) The tube for nasal administration, its nozzle missing, has been substituted for the facepiece. The cap of the vaporizing chamber has been removed, but the ring of holes, at the bottom of a saucer-shaped depression, can scarcely be seen.

(Original in the Wellcome Historical Medical Museum.)

retained Snow's perforated disc for the ingress of air, but in place of the wire frame within, supporting rolls of blotting-paper, Sansom filled his cylinder with loosely crumpled blotting-paper or ' what is better, a rolled piece of lint '. He discarded the water-jacket and instead insulated his cylinder with a layer of gutta-percha. This, he claimed, ' allowed even a greater percentage of vapour to be given off than the . . . [water] did.

' But ', Sansom added, ' . . . the difficulty is not so much in keeping up this high proportion as in preserving it sufficiently low. I fulfilled the indication of diminishing the proportion by reducing the cylinder in size and bulk, and I was led to consider that the value of the gutta percha was not so much to keep the chloroform warm, as it were, but rather to prevent the metallic surface getting too warm from being held in a hot hand.'

Sansom also discarded Snow's long, flexible tube linking the facepiece with the vaporizing chamber. Instead, ' an exit tube passes at right angles from this receptacle [the vaporizing chamber], it being attached a little above the centre, so that a cup may be kept for the retention of any liquid chloroform which may be more than sufficient to moisten the blotting-paper or lint '. To the free end of this exit tube, which ' was again bent at a right angle before ending at the mouth-piece ', Sansom attached a Snow's (he called it ' Sibson's ', cf. Figs. 28 and 41) facepiece. This could be pivoted to suit the position of a patient either sitting or lying down.

In order to ensure proper dilution of chloroform vapour with air just before the mixture reached the patient, Sansom had the tube immediately behind the facepiece made ' double, an external rotating upon an internal ; both are perforated, front and back. Thus, in one position air enters freely ; by slightly turning the outer tube the apertures are partially closed, and by turning it still more they are covered completely ; the unperforated portions of one tube cover the perforations of the other '.[1]

As an alternative to the facepiece, for anaesthesia in dentistry, Sansom provided a length of flexible tubing with a nozzle to fit into one nostril, such as he had used with Faure's type of apparatus in 1861 (see p. 234).[2]

By 1865 it was generally admitted that Snow's inhaler had considerable drawbacks of the kind recorded by Sansom. Nevertheless the principle on which the inhaler was based remained unshaken. Snow provided the water-jacket to supply heat to the evaporating chamber to compensate for heat lost through the evaporation of the volatile substance within, so that by keeping the temperature constant the amount of vapour taken up by the air passing through the chamber was also kept constant. In ' improving ' upon Snow's work by insulating the vaporizing

[1] Sansom, A. E. 1865. *Chloroform : its action and administration.* London. 127–9.
[2] *Ibid.* 186.

chamber with gutta-percha, Sansom in fact travestied that principle.

Another inhaler which became popular was that introduced by Weiss, the surgical instrument maker, in 1859. It was described in enthusiastic terms in an annotation in the *Lancet* for March 12, 1859 :

'Whenever we have had occasion of late to deplore the loss of life from the administration of chloroform, we have also to regret that more exact means were not adopted for regulating the quantity of chloroform and its proportion to the air inspired. In all those cases the chloroform had been administered loosely on a handkerchief, or, as the French have it, on a simple sponge. . . . We have not hesitated to declare it to be a failure of duty in any surgeon to administer, or to permit the administration of, this powerful agent by so irregular and imperfect a method when a more careful adjustment might be attained by the use of Snow's inhaler with Sibson's mask. . . .

'We are glad to find . . . that the ingenuity of Mr. Weiss has introduced a new chloroform inhaler, in which . . . the quantity of chloroform is registered, the proportion of air is controlled and indicated, while the considerations of convenience, cleanliness, and portability are amply consulted. . . . We think that this instrument is an important improvement . . . and it is now less than ever defensible to administer chloroform habitually on a handkerchief or sponge.' [1]

The apparatus (see Fig. 52) was illustrated, but inadequately described, on another page of the *Lancet* (p. 267). It consisted of a graduated glass container from which, by turning the stop-cock above it, liquid chloroform was allowed to drop into the vaporizing chamber beneath. This drum-shaped chamber was encased in a water-jacket. Between the chloroform reservoir and the vaporizing chamber was a 'valve-box', the effect (but not the mode of action) of which was described as follows :

'The valve-box is so constructed that when its index points to A (air) [letter not shown in Fig. 52], the patient inhales pure air only, and the vapour is gradually mixed with the latter to the degree required by turning the valve-box towards C (chloroform) [letter not shown in Fig. 52], at which point the full strength of the vapour is administered.'

Any of three different-sized facepieces could be fitted to this apparatus. The tube connecting the facepiece to the apparatus

[1] *Lancet*, 1859, i, 273.

was jointed and covered with flexible tubing so that the face-piece could be turned at various angles to accommodate the apparatus to the position of the patient. The *Lancet*, however, thought this a less manageable arrangement than Snow's length of tubing, particularly when the apparatus was being used for operations in the region of the mouth.

Of all Snow's contemporaries and immediate successors, by far the most important to the development of anaesthesia was Joseph Thomas Clover. His was an original genius but it was

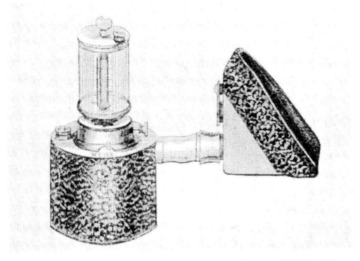

FIG. 52.—DOSIMETRIC CHLOROFORM INHALER
Made by Weiss, of London, 1859.

to a certain extent moulded in the likeness of Snow's. But whereas Snow's greatness lay primarily in his power to grasp and formulate the physiological processes of anaesthesia and after-wards to harness them to the service of practical anaesthetists, Clover's chief claim to eminence lay in his resourcefulness and his inventiveness in devising apparatus and methods of adminis-tration based on scientific principles.

Clover first began to play a dominant part in anaesthetics in 1862, when he produced a chloroform apparatus which was essentially Snow's balloon apparatus (see p. 194) redesigned and modified in certain respects. It was exhibited among the surgical instruments at the International Exhibition held in

London in 1862 and was favourably noticed in the medical journals. An account of it in the *Medical Times* ran as follows :

' This instrument has been contrived in order to regulate with precision the mixture of air and chloroform vapour, and to limit the proportion of the latter to four and a-half parts in a hundred. It consists of a bag made of air-proof cloth, which has a flexible tube leading from it and connected by means of a bayonet-joint with a mouth-piece. The latter is furnished with two valves made of thin plates of ivory supported by spiral springs, and contained in a sort of box, in order to prevent them from getting out of order, which render it impossible for the patient to breathe the expired air a second time. The bag is suspended from the collar of the administrator's coat . . . the tube passing over his shoulder.'

In thus slinging the bag (which was shaped like a large pillow-case) on his back (see Fig. 54) Clover overcame Snow's chief objection to the balloon, namely, that it got in the way. It soon became quite the fashion among anaesthetists to hang various bits of apparatus from the lapel of the professional frock-coat, just as it was the thing to carry a stethoscope wedged in the crown of the top-hat.

The account in the *Medical Times* continued :

' To prepare the apparatus [see Fig. 53], a bellows, in shape like a concertina, is fastened to the edge of the table. The nozzle of the bellows is fitted to a metallic box, and the latter to the inhaling tube, the mouth-piece having been removed. . . . The metallic box is arranged to secure the evaporation of all the chloroform supplied to it, every time a bellowsful of air passes through it. It contains a metallic bottle for hot water, which is covered with blotting paper, to distribute over a large surface the chloroform which falls upon it. The lid of the box is per-forated by a short tube lined with cork, into which a glass syringe fits. The syringe is graduated, and its capacity is limited to forty minims by means of a screw-nut on the piston-rod.

' The capacity of the bellows is 1000 cubic inches, and while this quantity is measured and forced through the evaporating vessel with the left hand, 40 minims of chloroform (the equivalent of 45 cubic inches of chloroform vapour) are supplied by means of the syringe with the right. This process is repeated three or four times ; all the chloroform is found to have been evaporated by the air passing over it and, consequently, the mixture of chloro-form vapour and air is in the proportion of four and a-half parts in a hundred. . . . The proportion . . . is sufficiently strong to render any person insensible in four minutes. . . .

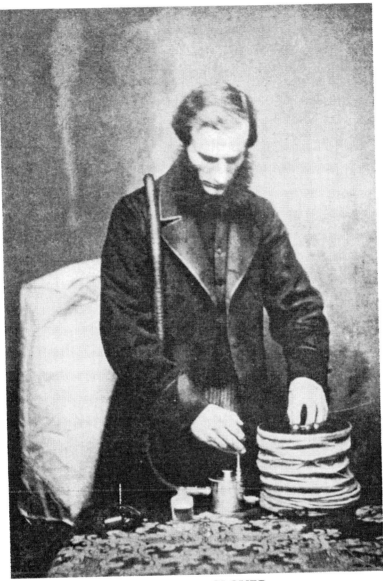

FIG. 53.—J. T. CLOVER

filling the reservoir bag (seen over his shoulder) of his chloroform
apparatus, 1862, with a mixture of $4\frac{1}{2}$ per cent. chloroform vapour
in air.

(From the original photograph, presented by his daughter, Miss Mary
Clover, to the Nuffield Department of Anaesthetics, Oxford.

243

' In order to dilute the vapour there is an aperture in the mouth-piece, large enough to admit as much air as is wanted in ordinary respiration. This aperture is left open at first, and when the patient has gained confidence and breathes freely, it is gradually closed by moving a sliding plate. Anaesthesia having been induced, the aperture is again opened to about half its full size, so that the patient then breathes an atmosphere containing about one and a-half per cent., which is sufficiently strong to keep up perfect insensibility.

' This ', the reporter concluded, ' is undoubtedly the safest instrument which has yet been devised for the administration of chloroform, and would surely be generally adopted if it could be rendered a little less cumbersome.[1] It is, however, admirably suited for Hospital use, and I believe its inventor has employed it in a very great number of instances without the occurrence of a single accident.' [2]

Among the hospitals which adopted Clover's chloroform apparatus were St. Mary's, Guy's and the Westminster Hospital. Clover himself used it constantly during the next six or seven years, for in addition to hospital practice his services as an anaesthetist were much in demand within a large circle of the leading London dentists.

Nevertheless the *Medical Times* was, in the main, right. Clover's chloroform apparatus was too clumsy to be generally adopted and the mere sight of it had been known to appal a nervous patient.[3]

Open Administration

A reaction from complicated to simplified apparatus was, indeed, just then making itself felt in England. ' You have twice too many instruments in London ', said Professor Simpson to Charles Kidd ; ' you do not give enough chloroform ; you are

[1] A far more effective apparatus, based on a principle similar to Clover's, was devised in 1898 by Robert Marston, a dental surgeon practising in Leicester. Marston made possible for the first time the administration not only of a quantitative anaesthetic mixture but one automatically diluted by measured quantities of air. His apparatus consisted of a pressure chamber in which a highly concentrated mixture of a volatile anaesthetic with compressed air or nitrous oxide was prepared. The flow of this mixture, when released from the pressure chamber, actuated an injector (Marston's most important contribution) which, according to the setting of a dial, drew in predetermined amounts of air to dilute the mixture to the required degree. The diluted mixture accumulated in a reservoir bag before passing to the patient. (British Patent Specification No. 17237, 1898.) This apparatus appears to have been completely ignored by Marston's contemporaries.

[2] *Med. Times, Lond.*, 1862, ii, 149.

[3] *Brit. J. dent. Sci.*, 1868 **11**, 129 et seq.

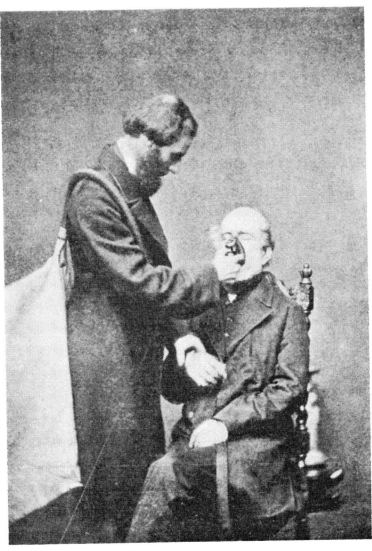

FIG. 54.—J. T. CLOVER

demonstrating how chloroform was administered with his apparatus.

(From the original photograph, presented by his daughter, Miss Mary
Clover, to the Nuffield Department of Anaesthetics, Oxford.

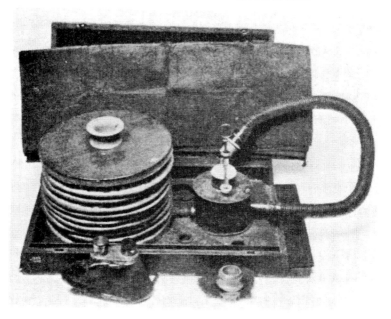

FIG. 55.—A CLOVER'S CHLOROFORM APPARATUS

Probably made about 1870, showing carrying case, folded reservoir bag made of impermeable material, hand-bellows, chloroform vaporizing chamber with graduated glass syringe for injecting liquid chloroform and connecting tube reinforced with a wire coil to prevent kinking. In the foreground, Clover's facepiece with an inflatable rubber rim—a feature which came into use with nitrous oxide anaesthesia (*c.* 1870), and the metal junction, which has become detached from the filling tube and reservoir bag.

(Original in the Wellcome Historical Medical Museum.)

too much afraid of it ', and Kidd readily agreed, adding that ' It frightened men in the country.' [1]

In 1861 Joseph Lister contributed the first of a periodical series of anaesthetic commentaries to Holmes's *System of surgery.* He wrote :

'. . . With the view of preventing fatal syncope, Dr. Snow contrived an inhaler for regulating the amount of chloroform vapour in the inspired air, and used it in upwards of four thousand cases, of which only one was fatal [cf. p. 202]. . . . Finding his ingenious efforts crowned with success . . . and assuming that when chloroform is given from a folded cloth it is apt to be in too

[1] *Brit. J., dent. Sci.* 1868, **11**, 133.

concentrated a form, he attributed most of the deaths that have occurred to paralysis of the heart from this cause.

' But the cloth being the means which has been used from the first in Edinburgh, with success even superior to Dr. Snow's, I have been long satisfied that his argument was fallacious ; yet . . . I have thought it worth while to subject a matter of such great practical importance to experimental inquiry. . . . I find that, so far from the amount of chloroform given off from the cloth being in dangerous proportion to the air inhaled, the whole quantity which evaporates from the under surface, even when the rate is most rapid, viz. just after the liquid has been poured upon it, is below Dr. Snow's limit of perfect security against primary failure of the heart.' [1]

Lister had been Syme's pupil and was his son-in-law, and for eight years he had been following both Syme's teaching that ' every case for operation is a case for chloroform ' and method of administration :

' A common towel being arranged so as to form a square cloth of six folds, enough chloroform is poured upon it to moisten a surface in the middle about as large as the palm of the hand, the precise quantity used being a matter of no consequence whatever. The patient having been directed to loosen any tight band round the neck, and to shut his eyes to protect them from the irritating vapour, the cloth is held as near the face as can comfortably be borne, more chloroform being added as may be necessary.' [2]

When Lister recommended this method in a standard textbook on surgery, Simpson had already abandoned it in favour of dropping chloroform on to a single layer of material (see pp. 192–3). It was not until some twenty years later, however, that Lister forsook Syme's method to follow Simpson's (see pp. 540–1).

In the autumn of 1862 Thomas Skinner, Obstetric Physician to the Dispensaries, Liverpool, published an account of a new way of giving chloroform. This was to drop it from a specially adapted bottle on to a small wire frame covered with domette (a wool and cotton fabric) and held over the patient's face (see Fig. 56). His instrument was the origin of a long line of descendants.

' For all that I know ', wrote Skinner, ' the means may be nothing new, but they suggested themselves to me on hearing of

[1] *The collected papers of Joseph, Baron Lister.* Oxford, 1909, **I**, 140.
[2] *Ibid.* **I**, 143.

the method lately introduced by Professor Simpson, of administering chloroform by drops on a muslin or cambric handkerchief, which method . . . is subject to two objections, namely : (1) The difficulty of dropping the chloroform and of seeing where you are dropping it ; and (2) The difficulty of protecting the patient's face . . . even by inunction with olive oil. . . .

'The apparatus is extremely simple, and is composed of a mask . . . for receiving and evaporating the drops of chloroform, and a bottle with a peculiar form of drop-tube attached.

' 1. The inhaler is a mask, the framework of which is of tinned iron or German silver wire. It somewhat resembles a fencing mask, excepting that it is covered with thin coarse domette instead of wire gauze, and that it covers only the lower half of the face.

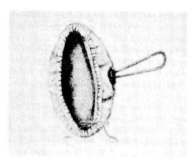

Fig. 56.—SKINNER'S MASK FOR CHLOROFORM
(1862)

The single wire forming an arc across the long axis of the oval, wire rim, can be seen raising the flannel cover into a dome.

For convenience, it has a movable handle, and is otherwise made to fold up so that it may be carried in the pocket, hat, or case.

' 2. The drop-tube is a tube of glass about two inches long, sealed at one extremity, so that a silver wire ligature only can pass ; it is then thrust through a perforated cork which is inserted into a three or four ounce phial, and it is ready for use. . . .

' On inverting the bottle and drop-tube with chloroform in it, at no single inversion can more than thirty nor less than ten minims escape until it is reinverted.' [1]

Although Skinner saw nothing unhygienic in carrying his chloroform mask, neatly folded, in his hat, he nevertheless indignantly wrote in 1873 :

' If there be one evil more crying, more disgusting than another, in the practice of inducing anaesthesia, it is the use of

[1] *Retrosp. practical Med.*, 1862, **46**, 185.

inhalers. . . . There is not one inhaler, my own excepted, where every patient is not made to breathe through the same mouth-piece, tube, and chamber. . . . Sweet seventeen is made to follow a bearded devotee to Bacchus, saturated with the smoke of cigars and the exhalations of cognac ; or another whose nasal and pulmonary mucous membrane, leave alone the cutaneous surroundings of the mouth and nares, may be exhalant of all odours but those of purity and innocence, and when looked into may be found sensible to sight as well as smell. . . . The mouth-piece in time becomes loaded with grease, and filthy enough to upset any one's digestion and sleep for a considerable time to come. . . .

'Speak of refinement! We turn up our noses if we have not a clean table-napkin every day, if our knife, fork, spoon and plate

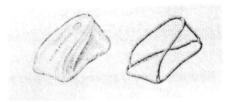

FIG. 57.—MURRAY'S MASK FOR CHLOROFORM
(1868)

(*Left.*) The frame covered with woven material, showing the circular hole to admit air.
(*Right.*) The frame uncovered.

be not cleaned or changed after every dish, or course at dinner ; . . . but when we come to inhalation . . . after twenty-five years' experience . . . we remain the merest barbarians, every-one breathing after his neighbour. . . . These remarks do not apply to such inhalers as those which are extemporised out of a bedroom towel, lint, flannel, sponge, and the like, all of which are readily renewable, or easily washed clean. . . .' [1]

In England Skinner's compact little mask proved popular and it was soon imitated ; John Murray's mask (Fig. 57), for example, described as fitting, with its 1½ ounce bottle, into a case to be carried in the breast-pocket, appeared in 1868. The announce-ment in the *British Medical Journal* stated :

'This inhaler consists of a folding up frame-work of strong wire, and a removable cover of flannel or fine and closely-made cotton cloth, which being several plaits thick in the centre, absorbs from half a drachm to a drachm of chloroform, and at

[1] *Brit. med. J.*, 1873, i, 353.

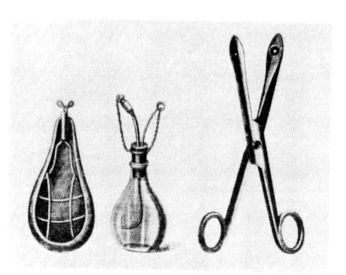

FIG. 58.—ESMARCH'S MODIFICATION OF SKINNER'S MASK

Interior view, showing the domed, wire frame and surgical gauze cover. The drop-bottle and tongue forceps, which were standard accompaniments of the mask, are shown also.

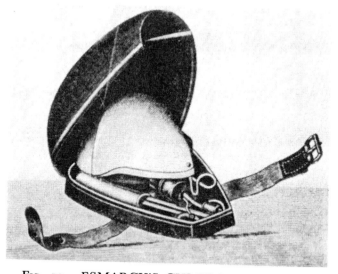

FIG. 59.—ESMARCH'S CHLOROFORM MASK,

drop-bottle and tongue forceps packed into the carrying case. The exterior of the mask is shown with the handle which could be hooked through a band passing round the patient's head to make the mask self-supporting over the face.

the same time allows of as equable and proper an evaporation of chloroform as possible under the circumstances.

' An aperture in the cover admits air, which, if necessary, may also be allowed to enter at the sides. The shape of the inhaler is made to suit any face, by applying the lower end above or below the chin, as may be found desirable.' [1]

On the Continent, particularly in Germany, Skinner's mask was frequently used. At the Bethanien Hospital in Berlin, for instance, it was the routine method of administering chloroform until 1882 (see pp. 267–8).

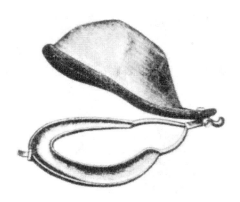

FIG. 60.—KIRCHHOFF'S CHLOROFORM MASK

with a hinged upper wire frame to support the cover and a shallow trough-shaped rim, to prevent liquid chloroform from dropping on to the patient's face, secured to the upper frame by a clip.

An important Continental modification of Skinner's mask was the ' simplified ' version of it devised by the German military surgeon, Friedrich von Esmarch (see Figs. 58 and 59). Whereas Skinner's frame was elliptical with the handle at right-angles to the long axis, Esmarch's was oval with a curved handle in line with the long axis. This handle could be hooked through a band passing round the patient's head so that the mask hung down over his face by itself.[2]

Writing in 1880 Kappeler stated that then the most usual

[1] *Brit. med. J.*, 1868, i, 535.
[2] Esmarch, F. 1879. *Chirurgie de Guerre.* Paris. 112, 113.

way of administering chloroform in Germany was to use either Esmarch's or Murray's modification of Skinner's mask.[1]

Towards the close of the nineteenth century chloroform masks were commonly furnished with a hinged trough-shaped rim to catch surplus chloroform and prevent it running on to the

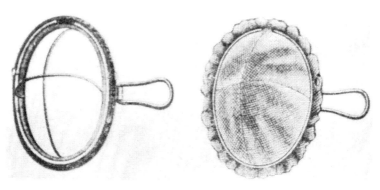

FIG. 61.—THE SCHIMMELBUSCH MASK (1890)

with a rim to prevent the anaesthetic liquid touching the patient's face. The mask, covered with permeable material, was used for chloroform; it could also be used for ether, in which case an impermeable outer cover of waxed cloth was drawn over the permeable material.

patient's face (see e.g. Fig. 60). Of this type of mask that designed in 1890 by Curt Schimmelbusch, of Berlin, is the best known (see Fig. 61).[2] This mask was intended for administering either chloroform or ether; when it was used for ether, however, a waxed-cloth outer cover, impermeable to air, was drawn over the mask in accordance with the method of etherization intro-duced by Julliard, of Geneva, in 1877 (see pp. 405–6).[3]

[1] Kappeler, O. 1880. *Anaesthetica : Deutsche Chirurgie*, **20**. Stuttgart. 144.
[2] *Ill. mschr. ärztl. Polyt.*, 1890, **12**, 203; ref. taken from *Index medicus*, 1890, **12**, 615.
[3] Dumont, F. L. 1903. *Handbuch der allgemeinen und lokalen Anaesthesie*. Berlin and Vienna. 71.

CHAPTER IX

THE CHLOROFORM COMMITTEE OF 1864

Royal Medical and Chirurgical Society's Chloroform Committee (1864)—
The Use of Anaesthetic Mixtures Suggested—Anaesthetic Sequences

The Royal Medical and Chirurgical Society's Chloroform Committee (1864)

BY 1863 the number of cases in which death ' could be positively assigned to the inhalation of chloroform ' had reached the formidable total of 123. ' Even this large number is probably far short of the aggregate mortality which must have been due to its use in various parts of the world. Many of these deaths, moreover, happened during trivial operations, which, without chloroform, are not attended with risk to life. Added to these, there are cases still in which life is placed in imminent jeopardy during the administration of chloroform, although it is not actually lost.'

' Facts so important ' led the Royal Medical and Chirurgical Society (now the Royal Society of Medicine) to appoint a Committee ' to give their anxious attention to devise means for· obviating such accidents '.[1] Among the distinguished members of the Committee were T. B. Curling, the Chairman, George Harley, William Marcet, Richard Quain and Francis Sibson. B. W. Richardson and Charles Kidd, both in the front rank of practising anaesthetists, were called in in an advisory capacity ; and J. T. Clover, ' although not a member of the committee, attended at their request nearly all the meetings for experiments, administered the chloroform, and contrived, from time to time, with remarkable ingenuity, special apparatus for carrying them out '.[2]

A long report was published in the *Medico-chirurgical Transactions* in 1864.[3]

' The committee ', it began, ' have chiefly confined their physiological report to observations which they have themselves

---

[1] *Med.-chir. Trans.*, 1864, **47**, 339.
[2] *Ibid.* **47**, 441, 442.   [3] *Ibid* **47**, 323–442.

253

made. Without overlooking or neglecting the labours of former
investigators, they have endeavoured rather to furnish an accurate
account of experiments which they have observed carefully and
together, and to compare the results thus obtained and agreed
upon, with the phenomena of cases in which death or peril of
life has arisen from the inhalation of chloroform in the human
subject.'

In fact a large number of the Committee's conclusions had
already been reached by John Snow.

Experimenting on dogs, the Committee observed the physiological effects of different percentages of chloroform vapour on
various organs and functions of the body, in particular, upon
the heart and upon respiration. They proceeded to make
similar tests with ether and compared the two sets of results.
Their final conclusions were almost identical with those of
Snow (cf. pp. 179, 200). 'Whilst . . . [a] general similarity
may be traced in the action of ether and of chloroform, there
is an important contrast in their influence on the heart. Chloroform depresses the action of that organ, and frequently kills by
inducing syncope. Ether, on the other hand, exerts but a very
slight depressing influence on the force of the heart's action.

'Hence death, when produced by ether, is almost invariably
due to the failure of the respiratory movement, and the heart is
generally found to continue its pulsations for some time after
the respiration has ceased.'[1]

In addition to investigating the effect of chloroform upon
the heart under normal conditions the Committee also carried
out experiments to test the action of chloroform on the heart
when the vagal nerves had been severed, either before or during
chloroform inhalation :

'It is well known that if, in a healthy animal, one of the
pneumogastric nerves be divided, very little immediate effect is
produced. If both nerves be severed the number of the respirations
is at once reduced by about one half, and the frequency of the
heart's action is increased in an inverse ratio. . . .

'If, now, an animal is placed under the influence of chloroform before the nerves are divided, these phenomena become
modified, and are even in some cases absent. The respiration
became only slightly less frequent than before the division of the
nerves, and sometimes there was no perceptible alteration of the
number of respirations. The pulse, however, became extremely

[1] *Med.-chir. Trans.*, 1864, **47**, 333.

rapid, though even thus it failed to reach the rate observed in cases in which the animals had not taken chloroform. In like manner, if chloroform was inhaled after division of the pneumogastrics, the discomfort of the animal was manifestly relieved, the breathing became more frequent and easier, and the chloroform appeared to bring about greater toleration of the loss of the function of these nerves.' [1]

In experimenting with dilute anaesthetic mixtures the Committee used 'Mr. Clover's apparatus [see p. 242], in consequence of the exactness with which the quantity of chloroform administered through it can be regulated. The effect of air impregnated with from 1 to 15 per cent. of the vapour was thus observed '.[2]

'If', said the Committee, 'a mixture composed of from 2 to 4 per cent. of chloroform vapour and 98 or 96 per cent. of atmospheric air be inhaled, there is little or no risk to life.

'In some cases it is indispensable to employ as much as $4\frac{1}{2}$ or even 5 per cent. of the vapour. But if a larger dose (one 10 per cent.) be inhaled, alarming symptoms are liable to supervene. At times, even with every care, and with the most exact dilution of the vapour, the state of insensibility may in a few moments pass into one of imminent death.

'It is therefore extremely desirable to obtain an anaesthetic agent which shall be capable of producing the requisite insensibility, and yet is not so dangerous in its operation as chloroform.

'Ether, to a certain extent, fulfils these conditions, but its odour is disagreeable, it is slow in its operation, and gives rise to greater excitement than chloroform. The committee therefore concur in the general opinion which in this country has led to the disuse of ether as an inconvenient anaesthetic.' [3]

The Use of Anaesthetic Mixtures Suggested

Instead, the Committee strongly advised the use of mixtures of chloroform and ether, with or without the addition of ethyl alcohol. Such mixtures were not new. John Gabb, of Bewdley, not long after the introduction of chloroform, in May 1848, suggested that it might 'be desirable to add a little of the stimulating effect of the ether to the directly sedative influence of the chloroform'. He asked, 'Could not this be done by mixing the

[1] *Med.-chir. Trans.*, 1864, **47**, 331.   [2] *Ibid.* **47**, 324.   [3] *Ibid.* **47**, 339–40.

two agents in properly ascertained proportions ? I should think
. . . about one part ether to two parts chloroform would be
the best proportion for the majority of cases '.[1] But Vaughan
Jones, of Westminster, replied to Gabb ' that the administration
. . . would not be found practicable, on account of the difference
in specific gravity of the two agents '.[2] A year later (1849)
John Snow also pointed out this essential impediment :

' As the most desirable strength of a volatile narcotic liquid,
not requiring great care in its use, is between that of chloroform
and that of sulphuric ether, it might be supposed that by mixing
the two medicines the desired end would be attained : but such
is not the case : they have been so mixed by some practitioners,
and I have tried them together, but the result is a combination
of the undesirable qualities of both, without any compensating
advantage. Ether is about six times as volatile as chloroform. . . .
When the two liquids are mixed, although they then evaporate
together, the ether is converted into vapour much more rapidly ;
and in whatever proportions they are combined, before the whole
is evaporated the last portion of the liquid is nearly all chloroform ; the consequence is that at the commencement of the
inhalation the vapour inspired is chiefly ether, and towards the
end nearly all chloroform : the patient experiencing the stronger
pungency of ether when it is most objectionable, and inhaling
the more powerful vapour at the conclusion, when there is the
most need to proceed cautiously.' [3]

Probably because of Snow's authoritative condemnation,
anaesthetic mixtures of chloroform and ether had not been
adopted in England and Charles Kidd was, apparently, the
only Englishman of note who, previous to 1864, habitually used
the two agents together (cf. p. 179).

About 1860 George Harley, a man of great versatility, who
was very familiar with contemporary Continental pharmacology,
suggested a mixture of ethyl alcohol, chloroform and ether
which became famous as the ' A.C.E. ' mixture—these being
the initial letters of its constituents in the order of least to greatest
proportion : Alcohol, 1 part ; Chloroform, 2 parts ; Ether,
3 parts.

When in 1864 the Committee of the Royal Medical and
Chirurgical Society advocated the trial of mixtures they mentioned three : Mixture A, which was their colleague Harley's

[1] *Lancet*, 1848, i, 521.   [2] *Ibid.* i, 610.
[3] *Lond. med. Gaz.*, 1849, **8**, 983.

A.C.E. mixture ; Mixture B : Chloroform 1 part, Ether 4 parts ; and Mixture C : Chloroform 1 part, Ether 2 parts. The Committee stated their belief that both B and C had ' been extensively used in America '.

After carrying out experiments the Committee discarded B because ' it was found that the physiological effects . . . were very similar to that of simple ether . . . the mixture, however, was open to the same objections as ether itself, the chief of which was the slowness of its operation '. In regard to A and C the Committee found that they ' were very similar to each other in their action ', which was ' intermediate between that of ether and that of chloroform. . . . Insensibility might be induced . . . with sufficient rapidity ; that is to say, in from four to eight minutes in animals, and in from ten to fifteen minutes in man '. Both mixtures ' exercised a much less depressing effect upon the action of the heart than chloroform alone '. Although suggesting that both mixtures ' should be more extensively tried than they have hitherto been in this country ', the Committee expressed a preference for mixture A, ' on account of the uniform blending of the ether and chloroform when combined with alcohol, and probably the more equable escape of the constituents in vapour '. It was noted, but without comment, that ' ether is a more volatile fluid than chloroform, and in a mixture of the two the ether evaporates more quickly than the chloroform '.

At the time when the report was published the Committee were able to say that at their request mixtures A and C had been tried in ' about seventy cases in the London hospitals, and the evidence of this limited experience tends to show that they may be given with safety and with complete effect, although they take a longer time than chloroform (ten to fifteen minutes) to procure anaesthesia '.[1]

Directions for administering anaesthetic mixtures were not explicitly given. ' The mixture of chloroform, ether, and alcohol should be given in the same way as chloroform alone, care being taken, when lint or handkerchief is used, to prevent the too free escape of vapour '.[2]

The dangers and the drawbacks of chloroform anaesthesia to which the Committee drew attention were already well-known, and for the generality of the medical profession the advantages

[1] *Med.-chir. Trans.*, 1864, **47**, 339–43.   [2] *Ibid.* **47**, 354.

9

of chloroform—speed of action and simplicity in use—still out-weighed the disadvantages. Nevertheless the publishing of the Committee's report on chloroform in 1864 marks the end of a clearly defined phase in the history of inhalation anaesthesia in England—the period of chloroform's supremacy in this country. While the prestige of chloroform as an anaesthetic was not seriously affected (indeed chloroform continued to be of the first importance in Great Britain, as on the Continent, until well into the present century), from 1864 onwards in England other anaesthetic agents came to be acknowledged as having equal and in many circumstances greater importance.

During the eighteen-fifties anaesthetic researches in England had been characterized by the endeavour to find the perfect substitute for chloroform. Reluctantly in 1864 the Chloroform Committee abandoned that search. Instead they turned the attention of anaesthetists back from the unknown to the known, in fact to ether. They suggested its use merely as an auxiliary to chloroform. Within a few years it was to be considered a rival.

Anaesthetic Sequences

The ' mechanical mixtures ' (Hewitt's term) recommended by the Committee in 1864 did not become immediately popular. Clover himself thought them unsatisfactory because they caused greater excitement than chloroform and in bringing the patient through this difficult state there was more danger of giving an overdose.[1] But as an indirect outcome, and an important one, of the Committee's recommendation a small number of men began to try anaesthetic sequences, usually establishing anaesthesia with chloroform and maintaining it with ether. A. E. Sansom, for instance, is reported as having said at a meeting of the Obstetrical Society of London during February 1866, ' that it was his constant practice to administer ether if in any case chloroform seemed to produce a depressing effect. Indeed usually, in pro-longed operations, he thus maintained the anaesthesia. . . . He always found that the plan answered admirably '.[2]

In 1866 the first piece of apparatus intended for giving an anaesthetic sequence was devised by Robert Ellis, Obstetric Surgeon at the Chelsea and Belgrave Dispensary.

[1] *Brit. J. dent. Sci.*, 1868, **11**, 128.
[2] *Lancet*, 1866, i, 288.

The mixing mechanism of the original apparatus (see Fig. 62A) was described by Ellis as follows :

' The part of my instrument which is peculiar is the receptacle for chloroform and the corresponding one for the alcohol and ether. This part consists of two separate pieces, an upper and a lower (Figs. 1 and 2 [see Fig. 62A]) ; the upper fitting as in a socket into the vertical part of the lower tube. The upper part consists of a tube (a) of a little more than two inches diameter,

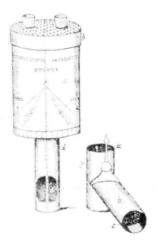

FIG. 62A.—ELLIS'S APPARATUS
(Feb. 1866)
For administering ether-alcohol and
chloroform vapours, either mixed or
in sequence.

and is three in height. It is fitted with a perforated lid (b), at each side of which is a small funnel (c). This tube is divided through its whole length by a metal diaphragm (e), which also runs down into the smaller tube fitted into it at the bottom. The whole forms one compact piece from top to bottom, and enclosing two entirely distinct spaces, one of which is reserved for the chloroform, and the other for the alcohol and ether. These have no communication with each other, but have a common opening of an elliptical figure at the bottom (e) of the smaller tube. This smaller tube (d) is accurately fitted, so as to work easily round in the vertical piece of the other part (Fig. 2) of the instrument. In so doing it necessarily exposes, according to the direction in which the larger tube is turned, first one side of the opening (say that leading to the chloroform). It is thus seen that we can perfectly control the nature of the vapour allowed to pass into the other part of the instrument, accordingly as we cause it to turn to the right or to the left.

'The second part (Fig. 2) of my instrument forms the receptacle for the socket (d) of the first, and carries the vapour up to the mouth-piece. But in order thoroughly to mix the separate vapours before they are breathed, a piece . . . of perforated gilt metal is fixed [at (c)] inside the horizontal arm (b) of this piece, and the diffusion thus caused effects a complete mixture before the vapours rise to the mouth. This same horizontal arm carries the index-finger, which points to the scale engraved at the upper part of the receptacle, and by this means (the scale having been carefully adjusted by experiment to the openings below) the quantity and the quality of the vapour are at once read off. What is told by this scale is represented below in the diagram. The rise of the lines exhibits the gradual increase of aperture. The graduated marks answer the double purpose of an index and a safeguard ; for the index-finger fits into them with a spring, and holds the apparatus at the required degree until it be desirable to shift it farther. The instrument may thus be consigned to a nurse for a time, and the operator feel secure that no excess of chloroform can be accidentally administered.'

With this apparatus Ellis administered an ether-chloroform sequence. In this he differed from most of his colleagues, who gave a chloroform-ether sequence, to avoid the difficulties of induction with ether. Ellis adopted his sequence because he believed that the action of ether was stimulant whereas that of chloroform was depressant.

'Reflecting on the commoner causes of fatal chloroform accidents', he wrote, 'the conviction is impressed on me that we commence our anaesthetic induction with the wrong agency. Chloroform, however diluted, is unsuitable for the *early stages* of inhalation, and it is in these especially that fatal results have been most frequent. At this period the emotional causes of danger are most active, the resistance greatest, and the danger also greatest. . . . What it seems to me to require, therefore, is to commence the anaesthetic operation with some of those substances which will give a gentle stimulus to the patient [1],

---

[1] Early attempts to establish ether anaesthesia were characterized by a prolonged excitement stage which resembled alcoholic intoxication. The popular fallacy that alcohol is a stimulant is old and very tenacious and it is easy to see how ether also came to be considered as a stimulant (cf. Gabb, p. 255). The fresh demonstration, by the Chloroform Committee in 1864, that chloroform is a depressant and kills by paralyzing the heart, whereas ether kills by paralyzing the respiratory mechanism, the heart remaining active for a time, revived and appeared to confirm the view that ether was a stimulant, particularly a cardiac stimulant. (Cf. *Med.-chir. Trans.*, 1864, **47**, 335.)

sustaining the heart-power, tranquillizing the emotional condition, and thus gradually introducing to the stage of first partial, and then complete insensibility. In the method I would now introduce, this is effected by a means so simple and secure, that I have good hope it may commend itself to the judgment of many of our profession. . . .

'. . . The patient begins to inhale, and receives into his lungs a mixed vapour of alcohol and ether. . . . *Then*, when the heart and the nervous system have fully experienced the power of this excitant, a little turn [of the cylinder upon the tube] . . . brings in the chloroform vapour, by such gentle gradations that the patient passes insensibly from the milder influence of the one agent into the anaesthetic power of the other ; and by still further rotating the instrument, he is made to breathe only chloroform vapour just at the time when he is ready for the further proceedings of the surgeon. . . .

' The question will be asked as to the value of using these anaesthetics in a separate form, when all can be had combined in the mixture so strongly recommended by the Chloroform Committee. The principal and most important advantages are these : that we thus isolate and have under our control a perfectly safe stimulant and mild anaesthetic, while in the same instrument we have at command a most valued and powerful agent for the abolition of pain. And these are capable of being so united and blended together in any desired quantities as to give us such control over the individual case operated on as that may seem to require. We are able to produce any degree of anaesthesia by this means, from the slight dreamy unconsciousness to the deepest coma ; and by aid of the index we can at any moment observe what is the precise amount .of either or both agents which is being employed.' [1]

In March 1866, Ellis published a small book, *On the safe abolition of pain in labour and surgical operations* (London), in which he described an improved version of his inhaler (see Figs. 62B, 62C and 62D).

' I must now draw attention ', he wrote, ' to a very peculiar feature in this apparatus, and one to which no small importance must be attached. It is the method by which the evaporation of the ether and chloroform are regulated. The alcohol representing chiefly the vehicle for the others, it appeared to me of the greatest consequence to contrive some simple plan by which only a certain portion of ether or chloroform could be liberated in a given time. . . .

[1] *Retrosp. practical Med.*, 1866, **53,** 386 *et seq.*

'After making trial of numerous plans, it occurred to me to imitate the lubricating arrangements adopted in steam-engines and other machines, namely, to pour a definite quantity of the fluid into a little cup, and then to cause it to liberate itself by inserting in it a few strands of cotton wick. The capillary attraction instantly makes itself felt, and the fluid leaves the cup in a beautifully gradual manner. . . . In proportion to the number of the strands of wick is the evaporation and the loss of fluid ;

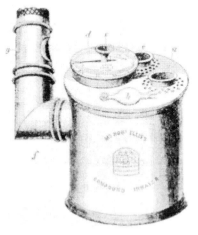

FIG. 62B.—ELLIS'S IMPROVED APPARATUS
(March 1866)

a. orifice for alcohol ; *b.* orifice for ether, with cover to reduce evaporation loss ; *c.* orifice for chloroform ; *d.* indicator, moved over scale by screw *e*, and showing the degree to which the outlets of the vaporizing chambers for ether-alcohol and chloroform were opened ; *f.* elbow tube leading vapours to facepiece ; *g.* air inlet valve, used to dilute the anaesthetic vapours during induction. The apparatus was 3 in. high by 2¾ in. diameter.

and this can be so timed that a definite percentage of either chloroform or ether is given off for every inspiration drawn through the apparatus. . . .

'Within the compartment for chloroform, and in that for ether, is fastened a little ring, and into this is dropped a small glass tube having from six (for ether) to eight (for chloroform) strands of cotton wick, hanging down on opposite sides, making twelve to sixteen strands for evaporation. The tube holds about sixty minims. At the bottom of the compartment is a little cambric frilling, placed so as to catch any drops which may fall from the wick. This is the whole arrangement. Immediately that the fluid is poured in, it begins to ascend the wick, becomes exposed to the inspiratory draught, evaporates, and is steadily replaced by fresh, until the whole is used up. The regularity with which this most simple contrivance does its duty is most satisfactory, and I commend it to any who, not caring to adopt the whole of my principles of anaesthesia, may be glad of an adjustment so perfect in action and so incapable of derangement.

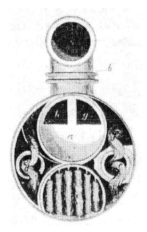

FIG. 62C.—ELLIS'S APPARATUS (see Fig. 62B)

With the lid removed, seen from above.

a. mixing chamber from which the vapours passed into the elbow tube *b.* At the bottom of this chamber is seen a diaphragm perforated by the openings *g,* into the chloroform compartment, and *h,* into the alcohol and ether compartments. A disc, removed with the lid, could be turned over the diaphragm (by *e,* in Fig. 62B) to occlude *g* and *h,* either more or less. *c.* test tube from which strands of cotton wick *f,* depended to the bottom of the compartment. *d.* tube for ether, with wick. *e.* alcohol compartment with frame laced with cambric hanging in parallel folds.

' The device by which I have effected the large evaporation of alcohol, according to my views, essential to the system of mixed vapours [is as follows]. With a few pieces of brass wire a little cage is made, in miniature representing the arrangement adopted in floor-cloth factories, but really designed from a consideration of the respiratory apparatus of fish. After much trial, the very best material for evaporating the alcohol was found to be the beautiful cambric frilling made at Coventry, and perfectly free from all " dress ". This fabric, an inch in width, was passed alternately over cross-wires at the top and bottom of this little frame, until 50 inches of it were contained in a space not more than 3 inches in depth, by one inch and a quarter in diameter. Thus hanging in vertical folds, the air inhaled passes over it without impediment ; and in its course robs it of the alcohol which is poured on from above.' [1]

Ellis's inhalers, remarkably ingenious though they were, do not appear to have been much used by other anaesthetists.

In 1867, however, two pieces of apparatus appeared, which subsequently became famous, one in connection with chloroform, the other with ether. These were Junker's inhaler (see Fig. 63)

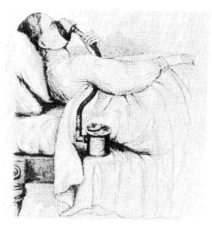

FIG. 62D.—ELLIS'S APPARATUS IN USE

and Rendle's inhaler (see Fig. 67). Both were originally intended for administering a new anaesthetic agent, bichloride of methylene.

This agent, which was given the formula CH_2Cl_2, in practice was generally found to consist of a mechanical mixture of chloroform and methyl alcohol. It was introduced in 1867 by Benjamin Ward Richardson who, in the old tradition of searching for a substitute for chloroform, had been making an intensive trial of the hydrocarbons, familiar and unfamiliar.[2] During the eighteen-seventies and eighties bichloride of methylene had a sporadic, but always transient, popularity on the Continent as well as in England. Spencer Wells, however, the man who first gave the

---

[1] Ellis, R. 1866. *On the safe abolition of pain in labour and surgical operations.* London. 66-70.
[2] *Lancet*, 1867, ii, 524.

vapour clinically, in 1867, continued to give it with success in abdominal surgery, using Junker's inhaler, for more than twenty years.[1]

Writing of the administration of bichloride of methylene Hewitt, in 1901, stated that 'Junker's apparatus has been found to be the best for the purpose. Rendle's mask is used by some, but with this apparatus the danger of an overdose, and of asphyxial troubles, is certainly greater than with Junker's inhaler. As the liquid is more volatile than chloroform, an open mask such as Skinner's is not so applicable. . . . Difficulty may be experienced in obtaining true surgical anaesthesia in many cases, especially when using Junker's inhaler [because it was not possible with that apparatus to administer a sufficient concentration of bichloride of methylene in the inhaled mixture]. . . . The anaesthesia produced by " methylene " is, in fact, comparatively superficial, and would hardly satisfy most surgeons of the present day '.[2]

F. E. Junker, who was a Doctor of Medicine of the University of Vienna and a Member of the Royal College of Surgeons of England, was physician to the Samaritan Free Hospital, but on the outbreak of the Franco-Prussian war, in 1870, he left England and, after serving at Bazeilles, became for a time Surgeon-in-Chief of the German Hospital at Saarbrucken. The Samaritan Hospital continued for many years to be a stronghold of ' methylene ' anaesthesia, until the drug was ' eventually replaced by its former rival, chloroform '.[3]

Junker's inhaler was designed on the ' blow-over ' principle. By means of a hand-bellows (a device much in the public eye in 1867, owing to Richardson's recent introduction in 1866 of the ether spray for local anaesthesia) a stream of air was driven through a length of narrow tubing into a graduated glass flask not more than two-thirds filled with the liquid anaesthetic. The flask was housed in a ' stand of non-conducting material lined with velvet ' to prevent the methylene from boiling, should the room be hot. The stand containing the flask was hooked into the administrator's lapel. From the flask another length of tubing led the anaesthetic-air mixture to a vulcanite facepiece which ' has the shape of one half of a hollow spheroid. . . .

[1] *Brit. med. J.*, 1888, i, 1211 ; *ibid.* ii, 72, 203 ; Hewitt, F. W., 1893, *Anaesthetics and their administration.* London. 249–52.
[2] Hewitt, F. W. 1901 (2nd ed.). *Anaesthetics and their administration.* London. 399.
[3] *Ibid.* 1893. 251.

9*

The rim has notches for the prominences of chin and nose '. There was an expiratory valve opening out of the wall of this facepiece.[1] The facepiece itself, however, was not intended to fit more than lightly over the face. This facepiece was the first important departure, in England, from the type of facepiece introduced by Snow and subsequently modified by Clover (cf. p. 242). The makers of the apparatus were Krohne & Sesemann, of London.

Junker, describing his original apparatus, wrote :

It ' differs in principle from the usual methods of producing narcosis . . . the anaesthetic fluid is not brought to evaporation immediately before the mouth and nostrils of the patient, as in other contrivances for narcotisation, Mr. Clover's bag excepted. With such the vapours are inhaled in an unequally varying proportion, depending upon the quantity of fluid allowed to evaporate, and upon such diffusion in air as the ordinary mouthpieces, the porous surface of Skinner's mask, or the more or less near proximity of a saturated sponge and napkin to the patient's mouth, admit. The vapours also soon become mixed with the expired moisture, and are thus frequently reinspired. Besides, it is often beyond the power of the narcotiser to regulate the exact quantity inhaled by each inspiration. Most of these drawbacks I believe to be obviated in my apparatus. Here continually fresh air is driven through the fluid itself, and, according to the fixed laws of diffusion, only a certain quantity of the anaesthetic can be taken up by the former. . . . The expired air passes off through the valve, and it is perfectly within the power of the narcotiser to regulate, by pressure of the bellows, the fresh supply of the diluted anaesthetic unvitiated by the expired air, with the strength and the rhythm of the inspirations. When the bellows are at rest . . . the supply of anaesthetic . . . [is] stopped . . . no loss or waste of the anaesthetic ensues from evaporation, which is often so unpleasant to those around the patient during the operation.' [2]

Clover disapproved of Junker's apparatus on the grounds that it occupied both the anaesthetist's hands, one in working the bellows, the other in applying the facepiece.[3] Nevertheless, the inhaler proved extremely well adapted to administering chloroform, and from 1867 until the end of the century and afterwards it was indisputably the most popular piece of mechanical apparatus for that purpose in England.

[1] *Med. Times, Lond.*, 1867, ii, 590.   [2] *Ibid.* 1868, i, 171.
[3] Cf. *Brit. J. dent. Sci.*, 1868, **11**, 127.

During the eighteen-seventies Junker's inhaler began to be used for administering chloroform by certain surgeons in Switzerland and Germany, in particular by Edmund Rose, of the Zurich Clinic, later Director of the Department of Surgery at the Bethanien Hospital in Berlin, and Kappeler of Münster-

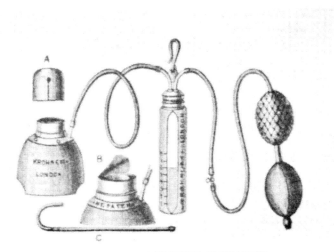

FIG. 63.—JUNKER'S INHALER

of the original pattern (1867), except for the expiratory valve which, in the first model had no feather indicator and was placed somewhat below the highest point of the domed, vulcanite face-piece. The case containing the chloroform (or bichloride of methylene) bottle was suspended by the hook from the lapel of the administrator's coat.

A. Cap for covering the valve when the instrument was not in use.
B. Valve with feather indicator.
C. Pharyngeal tube for injecting the anaesthetic mixture into the mouth when it was inconvenient to use the facepiece. (This was an addition to the apparatus made after 1867.)

lingen. This is noteworthy because the use of any kind of regulating inhaler was then unusual on the Continent.

Rose stated that at the suggestion of Junker himself he first tried the apparatus, using methylene bichloride of English manufacture, but almost immediately changed to the use of chloroform (also of English manufacture). When, in 1881, Rose assumed his directorship at the Bethanien Hospital, Skinner's mask (see Fig. 56) had for many years been in general use there.

Soon afterwards Rose substituted Junker's inhaler and the hospital records (covering an eight-year period) showed that during 1882, the first year of its exclusive use, although the number of major operations was greater the consumption of chloroform was actually less than in any previous year.[1]

Kappeler, like Clover, found the fact that Junker's inhaler occupied both the administrator's hands a disadvantage and he also complained of the kinking of the tubes but continued to use it because of the very small consumption of chloroform as compared with other methods of administration. In 1880 Kappeler was using Teuffel's modification of Junker's original apparatus.[2] Later he himself was responsible for a modification which allowed graduated chloroform-air mixtures of known percentage, and dilute mixtures especially, to be administered.

This apparatus consisted of a double hand-bellows, having a capacity of 110 c.c., a valved facepiece with an inflatable rubber rim and a chloroform bottle (see Fig. 64) bearing three scales, etched in distinguishing colours : red, white and blue. The capacity of the bottle was 50 c.c. and when it was filled the tip of the tube B (connecting with the hand-bellows) was only 1 mm. from the surface of the liquid. The tube C passed directly from the cap, A, of the bottle to the facepiece. The middle scale, D, indicated the amount of chloroform in the bottle.

Scale E was used when induction was begun with the bottle fully charged. When the hand-bellows pumped thirty times a minute the initial composition of the anaesthetic mixture was 14·8 grams of chloroform in 100 litres of air.

Scale F was used when induction was begun with the bottle charged with not more than 45 c.c. chloroform. The tip of tube B then being some distance from the surface of the liquid, the initial composition of the mixture was 7·5 grams of chloroform in 100 litres of air. When the level of the liquid fell below 30 c.c. (usually after 3 to 4 minutes' pumping) scale F went out of commission and the percentage of chloroform in the mixture was read from scale E. The lowest percentage obtainable, when the level of the liquid had been reduced to 25 c.c., was 2·8 grams of chloroform.

For anaesthetizing women induction was, as a rule, begun with 45 c.c. chloroform in the bottle, and for children 40 to 35 c.c.[1]

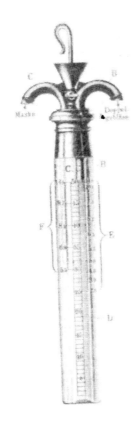

FIG. 64.—THE CHLOROFORM BOTTLE
OF KAPPELER'S MODIFICATION OF
JUNKER'S INHALER

Numerous modifications of Junker's inhaler were made in England, notably by the original manufacturers Krohne & Sesemann, by D. W. Buxton (see Figs. 118, 120) and by F. W. Hewitt.   A primary aim of almost all modifications of the apparatus was to prevent the afferent length of tubing being

---

[1] Dumont, F. L.   1903.   *Handbuch der allgemeinen und lokalen Anaesthesie.*   Berlin and Vienna.   77–8.

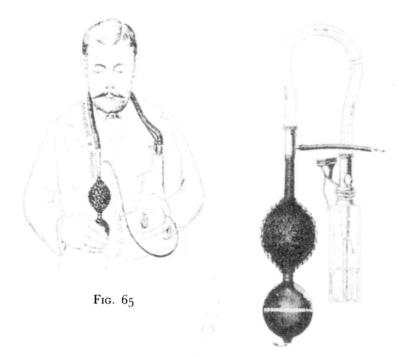

FIG. 65

FIG. 66

HEWITT'S MODIFICATION OF JUNKER'S INHALER

Fig. 65 shows the chloroform bottle stowed in the administrator's pocket and the flannel-covered face mask.

Fig. 66 shows how the tube carrying the anaesthetic mixture to the face mask ran through the afferent air tube connected with the hand-bellows.

coupled up with the efferent metal tube of the chloroform bottle and *vice versa*, which could result in a jet of liquid chloroform being pumped into the facepiece.

' A somewhat similar accident has also been known to occur by the chloroform bottle becoming tilted during the administration ', wrote Hewitt. ' As one or two fatalities have arisen from these accidents I thought it worth while to modify the inhaler with the object, not only of preventing the possibility of the tubes being wrongly adjusted, but of rendering the bottle less likely to become tilted during use. . . . [Figs. 65 and 66 show this modification.]   Air enters as usual through the hand-bellows. The afferent india-rubber tube is made much larger than that ordinarily used, and the same may be said of the long metal tube of the bottle with which it becomes continuous.   The efferent system commences in the wall of this long metal tube at the little orifice shown.   From this orifice the efferent tube passes through the larger afferent one, and emerges at the hand-bellows. . . .   The air entering the bellows passes along the afferent tube system and bubbles up as shown, through the chloroform.   It then escapes by the efferent system. . . .

' Other modifications have been made in this inhaler.   In addition to the replacement of the vulcanite facepiece by the flannel mask [' a kind of Skinner's mask, shaped to the face '] Messrs. Krohne and Sesemann have interposed in the afferent rubber tube a little stopcock ; and when this is nearly closed it offers such obstruction to the bellows that a more or less equable chloroform vapour is continuously transmitted.   These makers have also added a feather to the vulcanite facepiece, so that the respiration of the patient may be observed. . . .' [1]

To return to Richard Rendle's inhaler (cf. p. 264), which was introduced for the administration of bichloride of methylene in 1867, soon after the original Junker's inhaler, Rendle's own description of it ran as follows :

' It was suggested by Mr. Bader, who had seen [bichloride of methylene] so used by a dentist in Brighton, that, if I could succeed in making the patient inhale a large quantity of the bichloride in a short space of time, anaesthesia would be rapidly induced. For this object, I constructed a cylinder of cardboard, seven inches long, and about three in diameter, perforated at the sides, and covered inside and out, and at one end, with some absorbent yet porous material.   The other end was left open, and shaped to fit closely over the nose and mouth.

' I have had several modifications made, in size, shape, and material. . . . They are made in various sizes, of leather sufficiently thick to retain the shape, yet thin enough to yield a little in fitting on the face.   The top is dome-shaped, and per-forated to admit just sufficient air to enable one to breathe with-out effort.   The sides are not perforated, and the open end is shaped to fit nose and chin.   In the interior is a flannel bag, the mouth of which is turned over the edge of the leather, and secured by an elastic band.   Thus the edge is made soft to the face ;   and the flannel lining is kept in position, and, when soiled, can be readily changed.   Into this inhaler, for an adult, one fluid-drachm of the bichloride of methylene is sprinkled, and

[1] Hewitt, F. W.   1893.   *Anaesthetics and their administration*.   London.   195-7.

the inhaler applied closely over the nose and mouth. . . . In some cases, the respiration proceeds naturally ; in others, chiefly from fear, there are convulsive efforts at inspiration for a few seconds. This generally ceases, and respiration becomes natural.

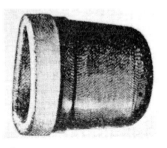

FIG. 67.—RENDLE'S INHALER

Showing the perforations in the dome of the leather cup to allow air to be drawn in, and the removable flannel lining turned back over the edge of the inhaler to give a comfortable fit on the face.

If not, it is advisable to remove the inhaler, and allow one inspiration only ; and then reapply it ; and all goes well. But all unnecessary admission of air must be avoided, as the rapid effects are dependent on the rapid inhalation of the bichloride with a minimum of air.' [1]

[1] *Brit. med. J.*, 1869, ii, 413.

PART FOUR

REVIVED USE OF NITROUS OXIDE
AND OF ETHER

CHAPTER X

NITROUS OXIDE

Reintroduction into American Dental Practice—Introduction into Continental
and English Practice—The Use of Nitrous Oxide Established.

Reintroduction into American Dental Practice

IN 1862, by an odd turn of circumstance, nitrous oxide anaesthesia was again introduced into American dental practice
indirectly by Gardner Quincy Colton (cf. pp. 94–5). He still
toured the States giving his popular lectures and he described
how the revival came about, as follows :

' Not being a dentist or a surgeon, I had no use for the gas
as an anaesthetic. But I remembered the experiment with Wells,
and often recounted the . . . facts in my introductory lectures.
On one occasion, at New Britain, Conn., during the summer of
1862, after stating the above facts respecting Wells, a lady asked
me if I would administer to her the gas, and have a dentist—
whose office was in the building—extract some teeth. I consented, and the dentist, whose name escapes me at this moment
[it was Dunham], extracted teeth not only for this lady, but for
two others. This dentist was so delighted with the operation,
that he insisted upon my instructing him how to make the gas.
A year passed, when I returned to New Britain again, in 1863,
to give another series of lectures and exhibitions. I learned that
this dentist had used the gas during the past year with entire
success, giving it, as he stated, to over six hundred patients. I
told him that he was the first dentist whom I had been able to
persuade to try the gas. As I was going to New Haven to lecture,
I asked him if he would come there, and we would extract teeth
for one week with the gas, as I wished to establish its anaesthetic
power. He came, and we commenced in the office of Dr. J. H.
Smith, where, with the aid of Dr. Smith, we continued the
business for three weeks and two days, in which time we extracted

something over three thousand teeth and stumps. This I thought was a little better business than lecturing, often to " a miserable account of empty boxes ", and determined me to come to New York, and establish an institution devoted exclusively to extracting teeth with the gas. As my name has been for so many years identified with laughing gas, I called it the " Colton Dental Association ".

' It will be seen by the above that I claim no honour in the discovery of anaesthesia, that honour belongs to Dr. Wells ; but I confess to some pride in being the occasion of the discovery, and of having given the gas to Dr. Wells for the first operation ever performed with an anaesthetic.[1] If any honour is due to me, it is in reviving and establishing the use of the gas after it had lain dead and forgotten for twenty years.' [2]

In reintroducing the anaesthetic use of nitrous oxide Colton at first followed the traditional methods of the ' frolics ' for administering the gas—methods which had failed Wells at the crucial moment in 1845. Later he adopted a more scientific and satisfactory technique both for administration and for generating the gas itself from heated ammonium nitrate (see Fig. 68).

' Now, in regard to the best apparatus for making the gas ', Colton wrote. ' For twenty years I used a very primitive apparatus which I invented ; but soon after I commenced using the gas as an anaesthetic, Mr. A. W. Sprague, of Boston, Mass., invented an apparatus, which I now use in my office, and find it altogether the best I have ever seen. It is the best in several important particulars. First. The *beginner* can hardly fail to make pure gas with it, provided he has pure nitrate of ammonia. Second. After being started, and the ammonia melted, it requires no watching, or even attendance. . . . Third. The passage of the gas through the four washing glass jars (there never should be less than four) controls a " regulator ", through which the common coal-gas passes to the burner under the retort, so that *one uniform degree of heat is applied to the retort*, thus preventing the possibility of too great heat. Fourth. The glass tubes in each jar are so made as to break up the nitrous oxide into very minute bubbles in its passage, and thus thoroughly wash it before it reaches the gasometer. It can be breathed from the gasometer while being generated ! ' [3]

[1] The general recognition of Long's prior discovery was largely due to the efforts of J. M. Sims a few years later. (Sims, J. M. 1877. *The discovery of anaesthesia.* Reprinted from *Virginia med. (Semi-) Mon.*) (cf. pp. 90–3).
[2] *Mon. Rev. dent. Surg.*, 1873–4, **2**, 28–9.
[3] *Brit. J. dent. Sci.*, 1868, **11**, 256.

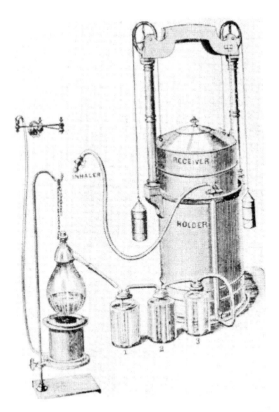

FIG. 68.—TYPE OF APPARATUS DESIGNED BY SPRAGUE
(c. 1863) FOR GENERATING, PURIFYING AND COLLECTING
NITROUS OXIDE GAS

The retort contained granulated ammonium nitrate, which was
heated by a coal-gas burner controlled by a ' regulator ' to maintain
a uniform degree of heat. The nitrous oxide liberated in the retort
passed through (in this instance three, but often four) wash-bottles ;
1 and 2 contained a solution of ferrous sulphate, 3 (and 4) fresh water.
A stick of caustic potash was sometimes placed in 3, to remove traces
of chlorine. The purified gas was stored in the counter-poised holder.
From the holder ran a length of tubing terminating in a mouth-tube
(in this case controlled by a stopcock, but sometimes by a valve)
through which the patient breathed the nitrous oxide directly from
the gas holder.

The gas was led off from the gasometer to the patient through a length of tubing terminating in a valved mouth-tube ' having an aperture of a full half inch diameter to breathe through. . . . Instruct the patient ', Colton advised, ' to take full, deep, and *slow* inspirations of the gas, and hold the lips and nose so as to allow *no particle of common air to enter and dilute the gas.* By this means, anaesthesia will be reached in from forty-five to sixty seconds '.[1] Colton's alternative method of bringing the gas to the patient was to draw off a quantity from the gasometer into a large rubber bag fitted with the same kind of mouth-tube as that just described.

In evolving these new methods Colton probably owed something to H. J. Bigelow, who had successfully used nitrous oxide anaesthesia on a single occasion in 1848, for the removal of a breast tumour. In Bigelow's case :

' The patient, having been placed on the operating table, was made to respire nitrous oxide gas through a valved mouthpiece and a flexible tube leading through a bladder to two large copper reservoirs filled with the gas. After several inspirations, the patient's lips and the most vascular part of the tumor began to assume a purple color. She remained quiet, however, and in a short time was evidently insensible, though the muscles were not perfectly relaxed. The tumor was then encircled by a double incision. . . .

' The patient made no outcry or other sign of suffering until some time during the ligation of the arteries, when she expressed a little uneasiness. . . .

' During the above operation, the patient inhaled about sixty quarts of the gas, which was delivered under a moderate pressure from two large gasometers. By means of the double valvular mouthpiece, the inspired gas was exhaled into the apartment, and a constant supply of fresh gas insured.' [2]

Despite his success Bigelow considered nitrous oxide inferior in every way to ether and after this one trial in 1848 he completely ignored the gas until Colton revived its use in 1863.

By 1864 news of the American revival of the use of nitrous oxide in dentistry reached England, mainly, it appears, through J. S. Latimer's brief account of Colton's methods published in 1863 in the *Dental Cosmos*.

[1] *Brit. J. dent. Sci.*, 1868, **11**, 256.
[2] Bigelow, H. J. 1900. *Surgical anaesthesia—addresses and other papers.* Boston. 97–8.

Latimer stated that he had witnessed several dental operations in which ' Dr. Colton administered the gas as for ordinary entertainment save, that . . . *the inhalation was continued much longer.* Two minutes were required to induce complete anaesthesia. . . . There was no indication of excitement, and the anaesthesia was perfect '.

It was upon the lines indicated in this rather misleading account of Colton's work that Samuel Lee Rymer, in London, decided to investigate the matter. Accordingly he and an assistant, Mr. Tribe, a chemist on the staff of St. Thomas's Hospital, carried out a short series of clinical experiments at the National Dental Hospital. Rymer published his results in the *Dental Review* for January 1864. After describing the production of nitrous oxide, Rymer proceeded to describe the manner of the inhalation (cf. Fig. 69) :

' The usual method of inhaling nitrous oxide is from a bladder filled with the gas, and to which is attached a tube of wood. The mouth-piece is held by the right hand of the person inhaling the gas, the nostrils being closed with the left. The tube is placed in the mouth, and the gas breathed from and into the bladder.

' For a practical purpose, such as the extraction of a tooth, the orifice of the tube must be much larger than for common experiments—in other respects, the inhalation is conducted after the same manner, except that it ought to be under the direction of a professional man, and it is desirable that two persons should be in attendance on the patient—one to administer the gas, and the other to extract the tooth. . . .

' In the experiments, a vulcanized india-rubber bag and a bladder were alternately used to hold the gas. The tube or mouth-piece was of *large aperture* to admit of *quick* inhalation—an all-important point where excitement is not wanted.

' These experiments ', Rymer stated, ' were not further extended as the means of producing the gas at the Hospital were limited, and consequently a sufficient supply could not, at the time, be obtained. . . .

' I have been asked ', Rymer ended, ' whether I think nitrous oxide will produce all the satisfactory results claimed by Dr. Colton. To this question . . . I would not venture to hazard a decided opinion. Nevertheless, I may say, I have not much doubt that transient anaesthesia may, in almost all cases, be produced safely by the *proper* inhalation of the gas : by which I mean not only the exhibition of pure nitrous oxide, quickly, but the exercise of some discrimination in allowing its exhibition at all—thus excluding persons suffering from disease of the vital organs. . .

'Granted that this gas shall be proved generally reliable, what advantages has it . . . in Dental Surgery, over chloroform ?

'The reply will be that it has not been found unsafe.' [1]

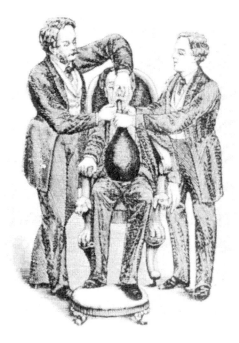

FIG. 69.—THE METHOD OF ADMINISTERING
NITROUS OXIDE

used by Samuel Lee Rymer, in London, during a few trial administrations in 1863. This method is similar to that used by Horace Wells during the winter of 1844–5. The patient is seen inhaling from a rubber bag containing the gas while an assistant pinches his nostrils shut.

Referring to a letter [2] on the subject of nitrous oxide anaesthesia by Alfred Coleman, which appeared in December 1863 in the *British Journal of Dental Science*, Rymer stated :

'Reference is made to the difficulty and expense of preparing the gas pure, as a drawback to its use. It is so, undoubtedly ; but if it be once found to combine the advantages already spoken

[1] *Dent. Rev.*, 1864, N.S. **1**, 1, 6, 8.   [2] *Brit. J. dent. Sci.*, 1863, **6**, 552–3.

of, we may be tolerably sure that suitable apparatus and means for readily producing it will be contrived. Even now there is an advertisement in the December number of the *Dental Cosmos* of an improved apparatus designed by an American firm. . . .

' In conclusion, I have to add that the *uniform* success claimed by Dr. Colton is to me a matter of perplexity ; for . . . I . . . am led to conclude that the action of nitrous oxide varies very considerably in different individuals. . . .' [1]

After Rymer's trial of nitrous oxide the gas was again forgotten in England.

Introduction into Continental and English Practice

In 1867 Colton demonstrated his apparatus for making and administering nitrous oxide in Paris, where the fourth of the many great international exhibitions arranged in the capital cities of Europe during the nineteenth century was in progress, and where also the First International Congress of Medicine was that year held.

While in Paris Colton made contact with Dr. T. W. Evans, an American dentist whose practice in that city was one of the most fashionable. At Evans's request Colton taught him the art of making and administering nitrous oxide. Evans immediately became enthusiastic and to Colton's 24,000 cases he was soon able to add another 1000.

Evans was not only a successful man, he was also a philanthropist. In March 1868 he came to England, bringing with him a Sprague's apparatus, such as Colton used for making nitrous oxide, and several ' Colton's bags ' for administering it. On arriving in London he booked a room at the Langham Hotel and there proceeded to fix up the Sprague's generator, drawing off the gas into the bags. These he took round with him to the house of one of the leading London dentists, David Hepburn, where he gave his first demonstrations of nitrous oxide anaesthesia. Through Hepburn and another well-known dentist, Underwood, both of whom were members of the Odontological Society, Evans arranged to give a series of demonstrations of nitrous oxide anaesthesia at the Dental Hospital of London, Moorfields Hospital and elsewhere.[2]

---

[1] *Dent. Rev.*, 1864, N.S. **1**, 9.
[2] *Brit. J. dent. Sci.*, 1868, **11**, 196–215, 385–6.

Evans's demonstrations were attended by the leading metropolitan anaesthetists and dentists and were soon afterwards described by Clover as follows :

' The results of his cases were on the whole in favour of the gas but the appearance of the patients, their lividity and convulsive movements, were regarded as alarming, and a few of his patients were evidently insufficiently narcotized. . . .

' Dr. Evans brought the gas in a large india rubber bag which was placed on the floor, a tube of several feet led from this to the mouth-piece—a flat piece of ebonite which was placed between the patient's teeth.' [1]

Evans's visit to London was brief, but he had every reason to congratulate himself on the results, and on his return to France he wrote, on April 5, 1868, to James Parkinson, President of the Odontological Society :

' Sir,—Upon my return to Paris I hasten to address to you, as the chief officer of the Society, my thanks for the sympathetic and generous reception which was given by my confreres of London, and beg you to transmit to them the expression of my gratitude.

' The experiments which I had the honour to make in their presence in the hospitals of London seeming to excite their interest, I think it right and proper to call again your attention to this anaesthetic. Constantly occupying myself with the means of mitigating human sufferings, and being much impressed both with the advantages and inconveniences which attend the employment of ether and chloroform, I interested myself with anaesthetical researches made in Europe and America, and more recently especially with those experiments made in the United States in view of rendering practicable the employment of nitrous oxide gas for surgical operations.

' After having been convinced . . . of the real utility of this agent, I made arrangements with Dr. Colton, in order that, utilising his large experience and adding my own observations and my conscientious investigations, I might surely and effectually introduce the employment of this anaesthetic in Europe.

' The results that I had in Paris were so satisfactory that I felt it my duty to make them known to my fellow-practitioners of England, and the generous and unanimous approbation they have given to my demonstrations have proved to me that I was right to rely upon their collaboration.

---

[1] Clover, J. T. MS notes, now in the possession of the Nuffield Department of Anaesthetics, Oxford.

' Convinced of the utility of nitrous oxide gas as an anaesthetic agent when kept from the hands of quacks and unprincipled persons, and desirous that the largest possible number, and especially the poor of London, should benefit by the advantages . . . of this agent when administered by skilful hands and competent men, I beg to offer to the Dental Hospital of London " one hundred pounds ", to be used for the purchase of apparatus and materials to manufacture the nitrous oxide gas.

' However, if, after more experience, our common hope should not be entirely realised, and the officers of the Hospital should decide to discontinue its use, they would be authorized to employ the remaining sum for the employment of any other anaesthetic that in their judgment would better fulfil the object we have in view. At all events I shall have pleasure in feeling that this contribution may be the beginning of a permanent fund destined to render operations upon the teeth less painful to the poorer classes of London.' [1]

Evans had no need to fear apostasy among his converts. ' The value of an agent evidently so safe, and so well suited for dental purposes, was only too apparent,' wrote Alfred Coleman, ' and within a week of witnessing Evans's administration we had arranged an apparatus, prepared the gas, and given it successfully to four patients.' [2]

Nevertheless there were several people whom Evans failed to convince, most notably B. W. Richardson, then President of the Medical Society of London. During a discussion on nitrous oxide, at a meeting of the Society held soon after Evans's visit, ' a question on the subject addressed to . . . Dr. Richardson . . . drew from him a clear and careful summary of its action. It was painful, he remarked, to see the childish excitement with which nitrous oxide and its effects had recently been dwelt on. The gas had been treated as an unknown, wonderful, and perfectly harmless agent ; whereas, in simple fact, it was one of the best known, least wonderful, and most dangerous of all substances that had been applied for the production of general anaesthesia. No substance had been physiologically studied with greater scientific zeal or more rigid accuracy ; and no substance had been more deservedly given up as unfit and unsafe for use. . . .

[1] *Brit. J. dent. Sci.*, 1868, **11**, 196–7.
[2] Coleman, A. 1881. *Manual of dental surgery and pathology.* London. 255.

'Respecting the mode of action of the nitrous oxide, Dr. Richardson explained that it was not, in the true sense, the agent that caused the insensibility. It acted indirectly, and the immediate stupefier was really carbonic acid. In fact, nitrous oxide is an asphyxiating agent. There are two explanations of this. It may be that the nitrous oxide quickens the oxidation of the blood, and so causes accumulation of carbonic acid in the blood ; or it may be—and this is most probable—that it acts by checking the outward diffusion of carbonic acid.' [1]

'Dr. Sansom greatly agreed with the President. . . . Nitrous oxide is greatly inferior to chloroform, both as to its manageability, and its prospects of safety.' [2] But Charles Kidd,[3] who had written to the *Medical Times* in 1864 at the time of Rymer's experiments, protesting against the use of the gas in dentistry and reporting the death of ' a fine young woman, in perfect health, who was induced to have this anaesthetic rather than chloroform ',[4] now wrote to the *British Journal of Dental Science* :

' . . . In this gas (why termed " laughing " does not well appear) the Dentist has certainly a most extraordinary and ready mode of rendering the Dental patient insensible to the agony of extraction. Its quickness of action and the fugitive character of the insensibility mark it out from all other anaesthetics. Some say, no doubt, it is not an anaesthetic at all, tied down as they are to certain chemical theories of cardiac syncope, deficient oxidation, synthesis of disease, etc. That it takes away consciousness of pain is very certain, and, in strict etymology, is an anaesthetic, there cannot be two opinions.' [5]

Events soon led Richardson to modify his opinion that nitrous oxide was the ' most dangerous of all ' anaesthetics ; but his assertion that the gas was not a true anaesthetic but an asphyxial agent gained many adherents—partly because it provided a ready explanation of the alarming appearance of cyanosis observed in patients during the inhalation, partly because, as the *Lancet* commented, Richardson's ' authority on such a point cannot be questioned '.[6]

Soon after the publication of Richardson's carbonic acid accumulation theory, an alternative hypothesis to account for the

[1] *Lancet*, 1868, i, 507–8.   [2] *Med. Times, Lond.*, 1868, i, 459.
[3] Kidd favoured empirical methods in anaesthesia and was scornful of the theorizing of ' Snow, Sansom, Richardson, etc.' (Cf. *Brit. J. dent. Sci.*, 1868, **11**, 318–20.)
[4] *Med. Times, Lond.*, 1864, i, 301.
[5] *Brit. J. dent. Sci.*, 1868, **11**, 318–20.   [6] *Lancet*, 1868, i, 507.

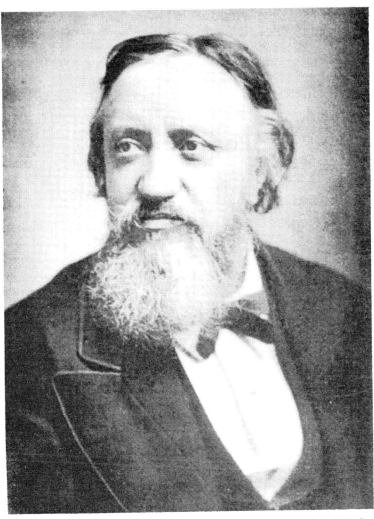

FIG. 70.—BENJAMIN WARD RICHARDSON M.D., F.R.S.
(1828–96)

Knighted in 1893. Physician. He carried out numerous experiments on the action of anaesthetics and introduced into practice the use of bichloride of methylene and of the ether spray for producing local anaesthesia by refrigeration. He was the friend and biographer of John Snow and the editor of Snow's textbook on anaesthetics published posthumously.

283

physiological action of nitrous oxide was put forward by W. H. Broadbent, George Johnson (Professor of Medicine at King's College, London), and others. It was ' that the anaesthetic effect of nitrous oxide is simply due to apnoea, that is, to the privation of oxygen '. This hypothesis that nitrous oxide was merely an oxygen replacer was discussed in the *British Medical Journal* for June 13, 1868 :

' If this explanation were true, it would have an important practical bearing ; for if the exclusion of oxygen be all that is requisite, it can be effected without interfering with the mechanism of respiration by causing a patient to inhale nitrogen, a gas which has no physiological action of its own, and produces effects which are exclusively negative.' [1]

In order to test this latter supposition J. Burdon Sanderson and John Murray carried out two short series of experiments on dental patients at the Middlesex Hospital, using nitrous oxide in one series and the inert gas nitrogen in the other and comparing the results. Sanderson also carried out a few experiments on animals.[2]

' From his observations, which were about six in number, it came out perfectly clearly that, as regarded the action of nitrous oxide on the circulation and respiration, there was no material difference between it and apnoea [' privation of oxygen ']. The action of nitrogen as a neutral gas, compared with nitrous oxide, upon the respiratory movements, was nearly identical, and he had at first felt inclined to come to the conclusion that no difference existed between them. In man, as in animals, the action of the two gases was similar, so far as related to their effect on the heart and breathing. Both also produced anaesthesia. When nitrogen was used, this did not occur until the patient was already asphyxiated, *i.e.* after three minutes or so of inhalation ; whereas nitrous oxide rendered the patient insensible in less than a minute, *i.e.* before the apnoeal state had come on. In other words, nitrogen produced anaesthesia by means of apnoea ; nitrous oxide independently of apnoea, by its direct action on the nervous system.' [3]

To return to the spring of 1868 and the events which more immediately followed the receipt of Evans's letter to Parkinson ;

[1] *Brit. med. J.*, 1868, i, 593.   [2] *Trans. odont. Soc.*, 1869, N.S. **1,** 53–4.
[3] Nitrogen anaesthesia was also demonstrated at the Radcliffe Infirmary, Oxford, during the meeting of the British Medical Association held in Oxford in August 1868, by John Murray, while Charles James Fox, the London dentist, extracted teeth (see also p. 296). (*Brit. J. dent. Sci.*, 1868, **11,** 413–14.)

the letter itself was read by Parkinson to a meeting of the Odontological Society on April 6. At the end of the meeting a member moved that ' a committee should be appointed, consisting of gentlemen practising as Dentists and Surgeons, and of the chloroformists Mr. Potter and Mr. Clover, who had specially given their attention to anaesthesia ; that that committee should operate upon animals, should make the most full and perfect experiments, and should report to the Society the results of their labours '. The motion was adopted and it was unanimously agreed that Clover and Potter should be among the investigators. Tomes, Coleman, Hepburn, and Underwood, with the President of the Odontological Society and certain members of the staff of the National Dental Hospital, were later elected to form a joint committee.

The Use of Nitrous Oxide Established

While Clover was attending Evans's demonstrations it struck him that his own chloroform apparatus (see Fig. 54) was well suited to administering nitrous oxide. Like Evans's apparatus it had a large reservoir bag (which could, moreover, be stowed at the anaesthetist's back instead of cumbering the floor) and a length of wide-bored tubing (with the additional advantage that a spiral wire round it prevented kinking—a salient fault of Evans's tubing).[1] Best of all Clover's own apparatus had a delicately valved, accurately fitting facepiece [2] instead of the clumsy and often inefficient mouth-tube.

---

[1] Cf. *Brit. J. dent. Sci.*, 1868, **11**, 213–485.

[2] Clover's apparatus was also provided with a nosepiece (cf. p. 295) which, with chloroform, had proved useful in dentistry. For a time Clover tried this cap for nitrous oxide.

' In dental operations it is often desirable to carry the inhalation to the extent of stertor and diminished rate of breathing,' he wrote in August 1868, ' for the mouth being wide open recovery is quicker than it could otherwise be and although the anaesthesia may be prolonged by giving the gas by means of a nose cap it will not always last long enough. I have lately found this form useful, the bag allowing a supply to be ready to pass into the nostril readily. In such cases I have sometimes commenced with the gas and then kept up the insensibility with chloroform.' (MS notes in the Nuffield Department of Anaesthetics, Oxford.)

Coleman also tried giving nitrous oxide nasally. To ensure that the patient breathed through the nose when unconscious he thought it necessary to cover the mouth during induction ; but Clover merely encouraged his patients ' to try to " snore " ', for he found that in this way nasal respiration continued throughout administration. (See *Brit. J. dent. Sci.*, 1868, **11**, 128 ; *Trans. odont. Soc.*, 1871, N.S. **3**, 236–7.)

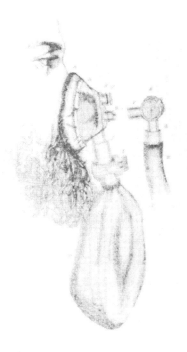

FIG. 71.—CLOVER'S REBREATHING BAG
called by him the Supplemental Bag, for nitrous
oxide administration (1868). The type of facepiece and the stopcock also devised by Clover
are shown.

'The woodcut represents the face-piece applied, with the
supplemental bag, M attached. A. Soft pad of India rubber.
C. The valve opening during expiration. D. The mount upon
which the stopcock, F, G, fits; the spindle part of the inspiring-
valve is seen projecting. E. Opening in the stopcock of
inhaling tube, which permits air to be breathed whilst the
face-piece is adjusted. When the little knob is turned down
to G, the opening, E, is closed, and the supply tube, H, leading
from the bag of gas, is opened. M. The supplemental bag
to be used or not by turning the stopcock, L.'

'As my chloroform apparatus was well fitted to serve for
giving Nitrous Oxide', wrote Clover, 'I lost no time in commencing to use it. In a few cases it answered very well, in
others—such as those who had thin cheeks which were drawn in
during inspiration, and those who had much hair on the face—
the results were often unsatisfactory. The facepiece was made
larger and very carefully fitted [with a padded rubber rim] but

yet the patient would sometimes draw air under it. As this appeared to me to arise from the gas not being able to travel quickly enough along the tube during the forced movements of respiration I added a supplemental bag holding about 200 inches, connecting it with the face-piece by means of a tube in which was a stopcock [see Fig. 71].

' This bag should be empty at first and remain so till by 6 or 7 full inspirations the residual air of the lungs has been replaced by N[itrous] O[xide]. The stopcock is then opened and it receives a portion of the *ex*pired gas—at the next *in*spiration the patient has not only the fresh gas from the supply bag as at first, but also that which is contained in the supplemental bag, and thus it is so rapidly supplied that no vacuum is formed under the face-piece and consequently unless the face-piece is carelessly applied no air at all is drawn in. This is an economical method also,' Clover continued, ' but it may appear objectionable because some gas is breathed twice. Practically it is of no importance, and we see why when we remember that we are always breathing air over and over again since the lungs do not entirely empty their contents.' [1]

Besides Clover, the other prime mover in developing nitrous oxide anaesthesia in England was the dentist, Alfred Coleman.

' Mr. Coleman ', wrote Clover, ' has contrived a very in-genious apparatus for both economizing the gas and also obviat-ing this supposed objection [the objection to rebreathing]. He takes a gallon of gas into a bag and makes the expired gas pass over slaked lime contained in a glass tube before it reaches the bag again [cf. Fig. 72]. I do not think enough gas is saved to pay for the trouble of its purification and as yet I do not think his results are better than my own.' [2]

Coleman's was the first clinical use of a carbon dioxide absorber in anaesthesia, although Snow had used a similar device while experimenting on himself with chloroform and ether (see p. 218), and Lavoisier and Seguin had used carbon dioxide absorbers to keep animals alive in closed vessels during experiments on respiration (see p. 60.)

Coleman's suggestion was not adopted by his contempor-aries, but he himself used a carbon dioxide absorber at the

---

[1] Clover, J. T. MS notes now in the possession of the Nuffield Department of Anaesthetics, Oxford.
[2] *Ibid.*

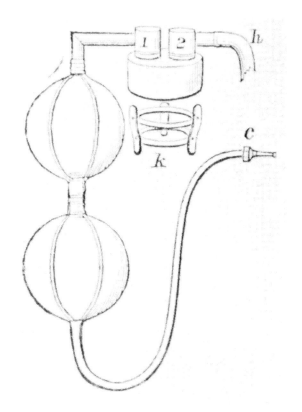

FIG. 72.—COLEMAN'S 'ECONOMISING APPARATUS'

for absorbing carbon dioxide from the patient's exhalations during
to-and-fro breathing in nitrous oxide anaesthesia.

k. frame which supported the ' economiser ' on the top of the gas cylinder.
c. point of junction between apparatus and gas cylinder.
h. wide-bored tubing leading to the facepiece.

Narrow-bored tubing led the gas into the lower reservoir bag. The only inspiratory valve in the apparatus was situated in the tubing between the two bags so that
gas passed from the lower to the upper bag but could not return.

The ' economiser' itself consisted of a round tin box divided internally by a vertical
diaphragm half the height of the box and attached to its lid. The box was filled
with small pieces of lime, dropped into it through two holes in the lid closed by :
cap 1, into which opened one end of the angle tube connecting with the upper
reservoir bag ; cap 2, from which wide-bored tubing led to the facepiece.

The reservoir bags were first filled with nitrous oxide, then the facepiece was
applied and the patient was allowed two or three breaths which he exhaled through
an expiratory valve in the facepiece. Then the valve was held down by the administrator and the patient breathed to and fro, from and into the upper reservoir bag,
the diaphragm compelling the mixture to pass through the lime. As gas was lost
from the circuit the pressure in the lower bag raised the inspiratory valve and allowed
fresh gas to flow into the upper bag until the pressure was again equalized.

Dental Hospital of London,[1] and for many years he hoped that the principle of conserving anaesthetics exhaled from the lungs would eventually be generally adopted, particularly in hospital practice, where the expense of anaesthetic drugs was such an important factor governing their use.[2]

That Clover's apparatus for administering nitrous oxide was superior to Evans's was quickly apparent to the Londoners; but for the first three months after the introduction of nitrous oxide into English dental practice the bulkiness of the gas itself and the difficulty of making it, or obtaining it ready made, and of storing it, constituted formidable obstacles to its general adoption. Only the most enterprising or the most prosperous dentists felt able to fit up Sprague's generating apparatus, for this entailed appropriating a room adjoining the surgery or at least partitioning off part of the surgery in order to set up the retort, the wash-bottles, and the counter-poised gas receiver. Once made the gas was either drawn off into rubber bags from the receiver or inhaled directly from the generating apparatus by means of a pipe line running through the partitioning wall into the surgery ' where issuing from the wainscot in front of the chair there is nothing more alarming to be seen by the patient than a few feet of india-rubber tubing, with Mr. Clover's face-piece attached'.[3] The alternative to this procedure was to obtain the gas in large rubber bags from the various manufacturing chemists and surgical instrument makers.

Ernest Hart, editor of the British Medical Journal, took the initiative in attempting to simplify this state of affairs. On April 11, 1868, the following announcement was made in that journal:

' It is understood that there will be no difficulty in obtaining the gas in a pure, and probably even in a portable form, if desired. Mr. Ernest Hart, availing himself of the known properties of the gas, proposes to obtain it in the liquefied form, by which means twenty gallons of the gas may be compressed into a small-sized vessel, and readily carried about. In this way, it may, if necessary, be made pure and on a large scale, and carried about in steel cylinders for all surgical purposes.' [4]

In the following July nitrous oxide compressed into metal cylinders, although not sufficiently to liquefy the gas, was for

---

[1] Brit. J. dent. Sci., 1869, **12**, 443.   [2] Brit. med. J., 1881, ii, 1056.
[3] Brit. J. dent. Sci., 1868, **11**, 528-9.   [4] Brit. med. J., 1868, i, 355.

10

the first time produced on a commercial scale by the firm of Barth.

' Into an iron bottle with a capacity of two quarts, fifteen gallons of gas are compressed by force-pumps. This gas could not be retained under the pressure by any ordinary stop-cock . . . nor could it be delivered properly from the bottle ; . . . but the bottle is fitted with a screw and india-rubber valve, which allows the gas to pass out in a full stream, or as gently as desired, by merely turning the valve screw. Where the Surgeon or Dentist has not leisure to make his own gas, this is a very convenient form in which to obtain it, and, if in the country, almost the only one in which it can be supplied to him. It retains its properties unimpaired when confined in the iron bottle, for any length of time, the inventor assures us, which is a very great advantage, as it cannot be kept long in an india-rubber bag. The bottle is of wrought iron, about the size of a Winchester quart, and weighs about fifteen or sixteen pounds. The gas can be used either with a bag or gasometer, or other suitable apparatus. Those who use it must buy their own gas bottles, which can be recharged with gas when empty. . . . As the demand increases (and there need be little doubt as to increase) Mr. Barth expects he will be able to reduce the price of the gas. We hope he may accomplish this for few will give the time, take the trouble, and risk broken retorts, etc., if they can be supplied with pure gas already prepared, and in such a handy and manageable form as this is presented in. The little gasometers for use with the compressed gas are got up in the neatest and most elegant manner, and would be an ornament in any operating-room.' [1]

Not long afterwards Coxeter & Son similarly succeeded in compressing nitrous oxide gas and they also provided gasometers into which the gas could be decanted. The vogue for these gasometers, which were usually surmounted by a statuette— a baroque angel sounding a trumpet, Mercury, a nymph, or a stag couchant (cf. Fig. 73)—persisted until well into the eighteen-eighties when, perhaps no longer considered an ornament to the dental surgery, they were one by one discarded.

For hospital use and for those who preferred the utilitarian to the decorative in the dental surgery, Coxeter, in August 1868, produced an apparatus which enabled the compressed gas to be inhaled directly from the cylinder. This apparatus is important in that it was the basic model for similar apparatuses during the rest of the nineteenth century. It was a composite

[1] *Brit. J. dent. Sci.*, 1868, **11**, 394–5.

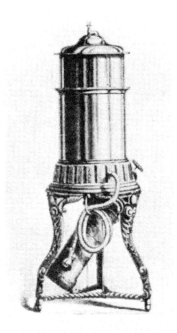

FIG. 73—ORNAMENTAL RESERVOIR FOR
NITROUS OXIDE GAS

to stand in the dental surgery. Underneath the reservoir
is the cylinder from which the compressed gas is emptied
into the reservoir. Looped up at the side is the inhaling
tube and, in this particular instance, a mouth-tube, fitted
with an expiratory valve.

affair, embodying the ideas of several of the leading men engaged
on nitrous oxide anaesthesia (see Fig. 74) ; the following account
of it was given in the *British Journal of Dental Science* :

' Mr. Clover's facepiece, with inspiratory and expiratory
valves of ivory is too well known for it to be necessary for us to
describe it minutely here [1] ; but in order to allow of the

[1] Clover himself described this facepiece as being ' made of sheet lead, so as to be
easily moulded to the face, and edged with india-rubber tubing, so that nose and mouth
may be covered with an air-tight cap. Two valves prevent the gas being breathed a
second time '. (*Brit. J. dent. Sci.*, 1868, **11**, 486). Later the facepiece was made with an
expiratory valve only and although Clover continued to use ' sheet lead or composition
metal, capable of being bent to the form of the face and covered with leather ', Coleman
found the metal apt to break away and preferred to use a thin but unyielding metal
edged with ' an air or water-pad where it meets the patient's face, which makes it fit
airtight '. (Coleman, A. 1881. *Manual of dental surgery and pathology*. London. 262.)

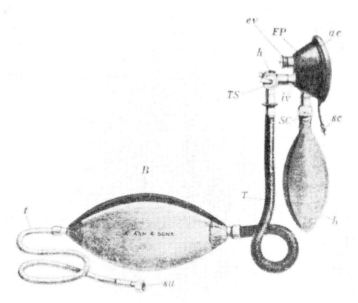

FIG. 74.—LATER MODEL, *c.* 1890, OF THE TYPE OF NITROUS OXIDE APPARATUS

first put on the market by the firm of Coxeter & Son in August 1868.

su. single union to cylinder of compressed gas.
t. narrow-bored rubber tubing leading the gas into
B. Cattlin's reservoir bag ; the gas then passed through wide-bored tubing to the inhaling apparatus the three main parts of which were :
TS. two-way stopcock (Clover's),
FP. facepiece (Clover's), and
b. Clover's ' supplemental bag '.
h. air-hole in two-way stopcock, so that air or nitrous oxide might be breathed by the patient as the administrator wished.
ac. air cushion (in the 1868 model) the facepiece was rimmed with rubber, covering padding (cf. Fig. 71).
sc. stopcock for inflating rubber rim.
iv and *ev.* inspiratory and expiratory valves, ' two circular horn valves working upon delicate spiral springs '.
SC. stopcock opening or closing the mouth of the rebreathing bag, *b.*

occasional holding down of the expiratory valve, so as to econ-omize the gas, Messrs. Coxeter and Son have prolonged the central pivot of the expiratory valve, so that it can be readily kept down with the forefinger. . . . We would take this opportunity of directing attention to Mr. Clover's two-wayd stopcock . . . by which, whilst the instrument is being adjusted to the patient's face, he is enabled to respire air freely . . . until ready to receive the gas. . . . Where it is desired to make use of a supple-mental bag as used by Mr. Clover for economizing the gas by

partial reinhalation . . . Messrs. Coxeter prefer to use a material called Indianette, as being more durable than the ordinary India rubber, the bag being removable at pleasure. . . .
'For the inhalation of Barth's compressed gas direct from his bottles, Messrs. Coxeter have arranged (from Mr. Cattlin's [1] suggestion) a bag connected by an india-rubber tube and stopcock to Barth's bottle at the one end, and by another tube to the ordinary mouthpiece [*i.e.* Clover's]. The object of this arrangement is both portability and economy of gas, inasmuch as, if the contents of a Barth's bottle are discharged into a large bag, there will, in many cases, be a larger quantity left which cannot be returned into the bottle, and must, therefore, be wasted (as it does not keep in the bag). . . . We are informed by Mr. Fox that he has found this an exceedingly convenient form of using the gas when administering it in the wards of the Great Northern Hospital.' [2]

Meanwhile T. W. Evans, in Paris, during the early summer of 1868 was attempting to solve the problem of liquefying (as distinct from merely compressing) nitrous oxide [3] on a commercial scale and to popularize its use among dentists. [4]

In July 1868 Evans brought over to England ' a single bottle of liquid gas '. Charles James Fox stated :

' I had the pleasure of operating with it at the Dental Hospital of London, Mr. Clover administering the gas ; but there the matter ended. Although I have applied to the maker in Paris of this single bottle, I have never been able to get more than an assurance that it would be ready when certain great difficulties were overcome. . . .
' At last, one night at the Medical Society of London, I saw the large bottles of compressed oxygen and hydrogen, which were employed by Dr. Thudichum [cf. p. 308] in his illustrations of spectral analysis. In them I saw—at least, for a time—the solution of the difficulty, and happily succeeded in convincing

---

[1] W. A. N. Cattlin was a prominent member of the Odontological Society. Clover wrote in 1868 : ' Mr. Catlin of Brighton connects the bottle [cylinder] of gas with a bag holding about 400 inches and allows this small bag to receive a supply during the inhalation. He placed this bag about a foot from the mouthpiece with which it was joined by a large tube '. (MS notes now in the Nuffield Department of Anaesthetics, Oxford.) The standard type of reservoir bag fitted to nitrous oxide apparatus during the remainder of the nineteenth century was commonly known as a *Cattlin's bag*.

[2] *Brit. J. dent. Sci.*, 1868, **11**, 444–6.

[3] That nitrous oxide liquefied under a pressure of 50 atmospheres at a temperature of 45° F. had been observed by Michael Faraday in 1823. *The liquefaction of gases. Papers by Michael Faraday, F.R.S. (1823–1845)*. Alembic Club Reprint, No. 12. Edinburgh and London, 1896. 16.)

[4] *Brit. J. dent. Sci.*, 1868, **11**, 382.

Messrs. Coxeter & Son that if these bottles could be filled in a similar manner with compressed nitrous oxide a great want would be partially met.

' They at once set to work energetically in response to my appeal . . . to supply us with the vessels containing respectively forty-five and ninety gallons of gas, which are now [April, 1870] so well known. Still, although a great improvement, this was not yet sufficiently portable to win the support of the surgeon. . . . I never dropped the hope that liquid gas might be produced at a moderate cost, and never ceased to persecute Messrs. Coxeter on the subject.'

Finally, during February 1870, Coxeter & Son succeeded ' in producing a supply of liquid gas, from the first hundred gallon vessel of which', wrote Fox, ' I administered the gas with uniform success to several patients at the Dental Hospital of London on Monday, Feb. 21st, 1870 '.[1]

By May 1870 the firm of Barth, as well as Coxeter, was manufacturing and supplying liquid nitrous oxide to the medical profession on a large scale.[2] Coxeters' charge for exchanging filled for empty cylinders was ' 3d. per gallon '.[3] This firm's apparatus for administering liquid nitrous oxide was copied by Johnston Bros., of New York, and by 1873 was on the American market.[4]

Already by the end of 1868 nitrous oxide was firmly established in place of chloroform for dental work among the London dentists and nearly 2000 successful administrations were reported from the provinces. In Paris it was ' used daily by at least twenty gentlemen ' and its popularity was growing in Liège, in Brussels, and in Sweden and Germany. Colton, who had personally given demonstrations of nitrous oxide anaesthesia in London during June 1868, was able, by December, to report from New York that he and his assistants had ' now given it in 40,000 cases without a fatal result '. The Colton Dental Association then had branches in all the principal cities of the United States.

The year 1868 closed with the reading of the eagerly awaited report of the Nitrous Oxide Committee appointed by the Odontological Society. The report was announced as being a preliminary one only, as the ' Committee, owing to the short time

[1] Lancet, 1870, i, 516.
[2] Brit. J. dent. Sci., 1870, 13, 145 ; Brit. med. J., 1870, i, 496.
[3] Coxeter, J., & Son. 1870. Catalogue of surgical instruments and apparatus. London. 120.
[4] Brit. J. dent. Sci., 1873, 16, 195.   [5] Ibid. 1868, 11, 626.

placed at its disposal had prepared a somewhat hurried report'
in order to satisfy at least in part, the ' anxiety of the profession '
to receive early information.[1] A digest of the report appeared in
the *British Medical Journal* on December 12, 1868 :

' The Committee . . . proceeded, in the first place, to consider in detail how far nitrous oxide gas is an efficient anaesthetic.
To ascertain this, experiments upon various lower animals were
instituted. From these, they arrived at the conclusion that it
was [,] free from atmospheric air, a powerful anaesthetic, more
rapid in its action, although more evanescent, than chloroform
and other anaesthetics ; and that although, if pushed, it produced death, still the animals were often speedily brought round,
when apparently dead, by the admission of air.

' They next proceeded to arrive, if possible, at the conclusion
whether, as an anaesthetic in man, it was as safe as, or safer than,
those in general use. To this they give a guarded answer for the
present ; stating, however, that it is at least as safe, for short
operations, as any other anaesthetic.

' They next enumerate the conclusions arrived at, founded
on 1380 cases watched and carefully reported on by the various
members of the Committee, and on 1051 reported to them on
trustworthy authority, as to the advantages and disadvantages of
the gas. The advantages are shortly, these : the rapidity of its
effects in producing anaesthesia, the shortest time being twenty-
five seconds ; rapidity in recovery ; its agreeable nature ; its
being tasteless and less irritating ; almost entire freedom from
nausea and vomiting, occurring in less than 1 per cent. ; absence
of headache and vertigo, as a general rule, after complete recovery
from the anaesthesia. The disadvantages are noted as consisting
in its unsuitableness for long operations, on account of the
rapidity of recovery ; in the difficulty of making and transporting
the gas, and also in the expense of the agent ; in its being troublesome to make, and requiring unusually complicated apparatus
in its administration ; in the undesirability of quick recovery in
operations followed by much pain ; in the administration being
occasionally accompanied by twitchings which render it unsuitable for delicate operations.

' The Committee next took up the physiology of its action,
with the view to obviate, if possible, any serious results which
might follow in its administration. They confess they are as yet
unable to explain the *rationale* of its action ; but recommend,
from experience with lower animals, that, when dangerous
symptoms appear, the exhibition be at once suspended, and,
should respiration not take place, artificial respiration be resorted
to. . . .

[1] *Trans. odont. Soc.*, 1869, N.S. **1**, 31.

'. . . In its administration, they observe that, whatever instrument is employed, [1] it ought to be as air-tight as possible ; but they offer nothing fresh, of importance, in this respect, or in the mode of administration. . . .

' As regards the question, whether there are any special conditions of the system contraindicating its use . . . they . . . advise caution, especially in those affected by diseases of the heart, vessels, or lungs. . . . They propose to prosecute further experiments.' [2]

Although this report was not in itself very important, merely recapitulating findings which had already been made public in the journals, either by individual committee members or by others working independently along similar lines, that the Committee, composed as it was of members of the Odontological Society and the National Dental Hospital, should have been set up was of the first importance. It concentrated the attention of some of the most able anaesthetists and dentists in London upon investigating the use of nitrous oxide and they, individually and collectively, were largely responsible for guaranteeing the worth of this agent to the cautious British medical profession as a whole. They also gave to the technique of nitrous oxide administration a number of characteristic features which persisted during the remainder of the century and after.

Another important factor in establishing the use of nitrous oxide in England was the meeting of the British Medical Association held in Oxford at the beginning of August 1868. The attractions of Oxford made the meeting one of the best attended and most successful which had up to that time been held ; and among outstanding papers was J. T. Clover's on ' Nitrous oxide gas '. During the course of the meeting Clover also gave a demonstration of nitrous oxide anaesthesia for dental extractions at the Radcliffe Infirmary ' in the presence of many members of the Association '.[3]

In 1872 the Joint Committee made a second and final report on nitrous oxide, which was as disappointing as the first had been (a fact admitted by the President at the conclusion of the

---

[1] ' The Committee, after having seen several tried, would recommend that introduced by Mr. Clover, which is a slight modification of his well-known apparatus for administering chloroform.' It was admitted, however, that there was and probably always would be ' a difference of opinion on this point '. (*Trans. odont. Soc.*, 1869, N.S. **1**, 40.)

[2] *Brit. med. J.*, 1868, ii, 622.   [3] *Ibid.* ii, 201.

report). The report served, nevertheless, to indicate the trend of development in nitrous oxide anaesthesia.

The chief point with which the Committee dealt was ' the manner in which the agent acted as an anaesthetic ', and as it was found impracticable ' to undertake *en masse* special experiments in regard to [this] . . . point, . . . this duty was delegated to Dr. Frankland, Mr. Coleman and Mr. Braine '. Frankland's investigations were concerned only with animals, Coleman's were clinical ; Braine failed to make a report in time for publication. Both Frankland and Coleman concluded ' that nitrous oxide gas when inhaled underwent very little if any change '. ' The general conclusion to be drawn from the experiments was that nitrous oxide induced anaesthesia by preventing oxidation.'

The only other point of interest, the third of six on the original agenda, was that dealing with ' the possibility and best mode of prolonging the anaesthetic effect of the gas '. The Committee advocated that in operations ' on the mouth ' the administration should be continued by means of a ' nosepiece, or by jetting the gas into the mouth at each inspiration, the nose being closed by a spring clip '. In operations not involving the mouth the Committee advised keeping up anaesthesia by the intermittent application of the facepiece, a method which, indeed, had been in general use for prolonging the effects of volatile anaesthetics since the inception of the use of anaesthesia.

The Committee regretted ' that inasmuch as anaesthesia can be kept up for several minutes, the gas was not used in place of chloroform more frequently in the many minor operations of surgery, and they wished to direct the attention of surgeons to this point '.[1]

At the time of this second report apparatus for administering nitrous oxide fell roughly into three groups. Those dentists who in the early days had gone to the trouble and expense of fitting up the American type of combined apparatus for generating and delivering the gas to the patient (see Fig. 68) naturally continued to use it. A larger section of the dental profession obtained the gas in cylinders from Barth's or Coxeters' and emptied it into a receiver standing in the surgery from which the patient inhaled directly (cf. Fig. 73). Finally there was the type of apparatus used by the specialist anaesthetist. Of this

[1] *Lancet*, 1872, ii, 687.

type Coxeters', for compressed gas (see Fig. 75), put on the market in 1869, and Barth's 'liquid nitrous oxide bag' (1871) were popular examples. Barth's apparatus was described as ' a conveniently fitted little [leather] bag, with every appliance for the administration of nitrous oxide '. The bag contained two 25-gallon copper cylinders of liquid gas, two or more facepieces, a Cattlin's bag of 4 gallons' capacity, ' and a pair of vulcanite gags '.[1]

From the point of view of dental surgery an important outcome of the adoption of an anaesthetic agent so transient in its action as nitrous oxide was the development of a type of mouth-gag which could be easily and, above all, speedily inserted. Mouth-props, made most commonly from a cork, from boxwood, or from vulcanite, either with or without a string tied round them in case they should be swallowed, were familiar to the leisurely chloroformist, and Clover and Snow each referred to two steel plates (covered in Snow's instance by leather, in Clover's by bone), controlled by a screw, which rested on the teeth and kept the jaws apart during chloroform anaesthesia.[2]

In 1868, as it happened, Thomas Smith had just invented a new gag for use during cleft palate operations.and in the same connection Francis Mason was already working on the original of his now famous gag (cf. p. 234). But the form of gag which was first introduced in connection with nitrous oxide anaesthesia was the telescopic, spring gag and from this the swivel gag soon developed.

As usual, Clover was early in the field with a gag shaped like an ordinary mouth-prop but having a spring in the shaft so that the gag could be compressed, secured by a small bolt on a handle, and inserted between the teeth. The bolt was then withdrawn and the spring coming into play forced the tooth plates apart—with a loud and startling click, so one of his colleagues said. The gag was made of vulcanite and was soon ' improved ' almost beyond recognition by various makers of surgical instruments and by individual dentists.[3]

The first of the swivel gags was sponsored by Coleman in 1871. This rather dangerous-looking instrument was devised

[1] Brit. J. dent. Sci., 1871, **14,** 589.
[2] Cf. Snow, J. 1858. *On chloroform and other anaesthetics.* London. 299, 316.
[3] Brit. J. dent. Sci., 1869, **12,** 41–2.

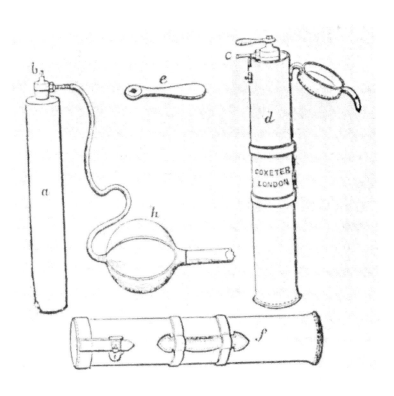

FIG. 75.—COXETERS' PORTABLE APPARATUS FOR COMPRESSED NITROUS OXIDE (1869)

(Left.)

a. iron vessel holding 36 gallons of compressed gas ; length 28½ inches, diameter 4½ inches, weight 23 lb. The outflow of gas at *b* was controlled by the handle, *e*. Narrow tubing led the gas into

h. Cattlin's reservoir bag. Wide tubing joined the bag to ' the usual stopcock and facepiece ' (not shown).

(Right.)

c. screw union where narrow tubing joined cylinder.

d. leather case with firm base which allowed the cylinder to stand upright during administration.

(Below.)

f. the cylinder packed in its carrying case.

by S. J. Hutchinson, then a student at the Dental Hospital of London.

' It consisted of a horse-shoe form of spring, to the extremities of which were attached pieces of metal guarded with gutta-percha, which, when the instrument was used, were adapted to the incisors of the upper and lower jaws. The tooth plates were attached to the arms of the spring by swivels, so that the spring portion of the instrument could be moved to either side of the mouth, and quite out of the way of the operator : a stop regulated the distance ; the mouth when acting upon the spring, could be closed to.'

This gag had, Coleman thought, ' the great merit of simplicity, and appeared to him to fulfil everything the designer of the instrument intended '.[1] Certainly this type of gag proved popular both in England and on the Continent.

Another advance in the administration of nitrous oxide came about, although slowly, by the evolution of the reducing valve. Warwick Hele, of Carlisle, was the first to devote attention to this particular aspect of gas anaesthesia. He noticed the resistance which the long lengths of tubing linking the gas receiver with the facepiece offered to the passage of the gas and stated, in a paper read at a meeting of the Odontological Society in November 1873 :

' After many efforts at providing some intermediate apparatus between the gasometer and patient, whereby such a supply of nitrous oxide should be yielded as to make the respiration of it no more difficult than air, I adopted [a regulator]. . . .
' I was led to the adoption of this regulator by a consideration of the fact that a law governs the flow of fluids, by which they invariably take the shortest road of escape from confinement. . . .
' The apparatus consists of a two-gallon bag and a three-wayed tube, by which it is attached to, and dependent from, the inhaling tube, and should be brought as near the patient as possible. . . .
' When the gas is turned on from the gasometer . . . the flow of nitrous oxide, governed by the above law, causes its escape first into the bag, when, having accumulated within to such an extent that the pressure of the bag's elastic walls overcomes the friction against the onward flow of the gas along the straight tube to the face-piece, the administration should be commenced. . . .
' The patient obtains, in consequence of the easily contractible walls of the bag, a free supply of gas, also supplemented by the amount flowing direct to the facepiece.'

[1] Trans. odont. Soc., 1871, N.S. **3**, 236.

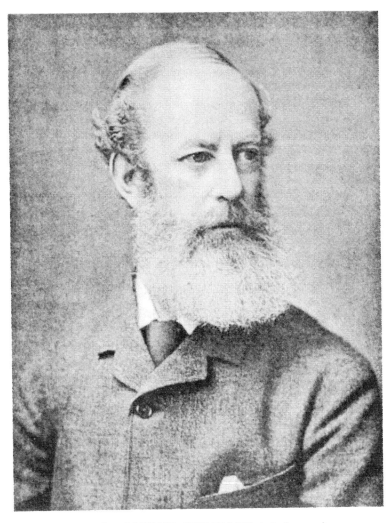

FIG. 76.—ALFRED COLEMAN (1828–1902)

Dental surgeon, who made a number of important contributions to anaesthesia, particularly nitrous oxide anaesthesia.

(From the original photograph lent by his son, Dr. Frank Coleman).

This device was only partly successful. Hele's next regulator was a more ambitious affair called a ' governor ' (see Fig. 77).

In this apparatus the outlet tube (A) from the main gas receiver led into a second, miniature, receiver—the ' governor '. The bell and counterpoise of this miniature receiver were supported by the outlet tube (A) ' by means of a double sextant, which revolves at its centre a stop-cock within the inlet tube (A). The Governor is provided with an outlet tube which permits the passage of gas to the patient. . . .

' When the amount of gas driven over from the large gasometer exceeds the quantity inhaled by the patient, it raises the bell of the Governor, and in so doing gradually closes, and finally shuts the inlet tube by means of the sextant levers and the stop-cock thereby revolved. . . . But the quantity of gas within the bell of the Governor being exhausted by the next inspiration, the way is again opened by the depression of the bell reversing the stop-cock.'

Hele next adapted his ' governor ' for use with a cylinder of compressed gas. This he did by adding a regulator (between the cylinder and the ' governor ') which consisted of a valve chest, with inlet and outlet tubes, topped by a flexible diaphragm with two fixed diaphragms below to act as baffle plates. To the centre of the flexible diaphragm was fixed a rod, the other end of which, terminating in a ball, dropped down into the inlet tube. As the pressure of gas entering the valve chest rose, so the diaphragm rose, carrying the rod with it, until the ball finally engaged with the orifice of the inlet tube and so cut off supply until the pressure was once more reduced by the escape of gas through the outlet tube. Hele called this regulator the ' elastic valve trap ' (see Fig. 78).[1]

A little time before this development of Hele's, about 1870, various ingenious but laborious devices had been introduced for use in connection with nitrous oxide gasometers for ' ascertaining at a glance how much gas has been inhaled by the patient and with what degree of rapidity '. A typical example described in the *British Journal of Dental Science* [2] was that of J. B. George, of the Rue de Rivoli, Paris, but in all of them the principle was similar. A scale graduated in quarts and based on the capacity of the gasometer was set up and a pointer directly linked by a cord to the bell of the gasometer, ran up and down it accordingly

[1] *Trans. odont. Soc.*, 1873, **5**, 95–116.   [2] *Brit. J. dent. Sci.*, 1870, **13**, 42–4.

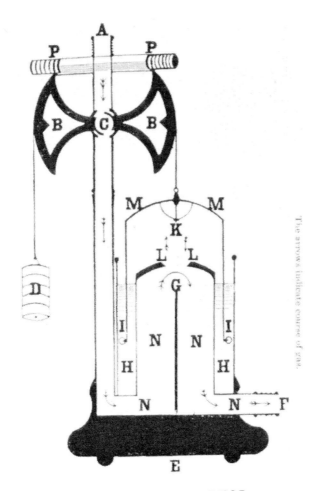

The arrows indicate course of gas

FIG. 77.—HELE'S GOVERNOR

to control the flow of nitrous oxide from the gas reservoir
to the patient (1873).

'NITROUS OXIDE GOVERNOR—*Sectional View.*

'*Drawn to scale, ¼ real size.*

'A. Inlet to Governor.
B. Double Sextant.
C. Stopcock revolved by B.
D. Counterpoise.
E. Stand.
F. Outlet from Governor.
G. Central Diaphragm.

H. Water Chamber.
I. Friction Wheels.
K. Cover for Core.
L. Circular depression for K.
M. The Bell.
N. Position of Pipes—interior.
P. Shifting Counterpoise.'

303

as the volume of gas within the receiver caused the counterpoised bell to rise or fall. 'A black-headed pin is each time stuck into the board at the point where the needle has stopped. After 30 quarts inhaled by a lady,' wrote George, 'or 90 by a gentleman, I invariably perform the operation, even though the insensibility obtained be not complete, which, however, is a very rare case.'

In England a popular device for marking the duration of nitrous oxide anaesthesia, though it did not gauge the quantity

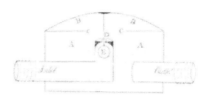

FIG. 78.—HELE'S REGULATOR

for controlling the flow of nitrous oxide from a cylinder of compressed gas to the patient (1873). This regulator was situated between the cylinder and the ' governor ' (see Fig. 77).

'A. Valve Chest.   C. Fixed Diaphragm.
B. Elastic Diaphragm.   D. Socket for reception of E.
E. Ball which, rising into D, shuts Inlet.'

of gas inhaled, was Dennant's ' Seconds Indicator ' (1869). It consisted simply of a clock mechanism, dial, and pointer enclosed in a box. The dial was divided into seconds and ' a clear sonorous little bell . . . strikes every time the hand points to the 30 or the 60 (thus marking every half minute) '. True, it was necessary to have an assistant present to count and note down the half minutes ; nevertheless Charles James Fox, among others, found this instrument ' a most useful companion when giving nitrous oxide ' in his dental practice.[1]

In both Paris and London, in the early days of nitrous oxide anaesthesia, Colton's edict that the gas must be given not only pure but entirely free from atmospheric air was faithfully observed.

Clover, still essentially the chloroformist, in adapting his chloroform apparatus to gas at the time of Evans's demonstrations in April 1868, tentatively suggested, however, that an

---

[1] *Brit. J. dent. Sci.*, 1870, **13**, 38-40.

important advantage of his apparatus over Evans's was 'the means of *regulating* the percentage of air when it is found necessary to diminish the strength of the vapour '. With reference to his first seventeen gas administrations he noted :

' To-day I gave the gas at University College Hospital to three patients. . . . One of them (excision of two enlarged bursae patellae) was unconscious for seven minutes, except for a few seconds when I had ceased giving the gas. I found it much better to continue giving the gas with not more than an equal quantity of air than to take away the face-piece, on account of the brief period which suffices to restore the patient to semi-consciousness when breathing pure air.' [1]

In December 1868 Fox, the dentist, who was an enthusiastic user of nitrous oxide, wrote to the *Lancet* :

' My present theory is, that although the admixture of atmo-spheric air with the gas when first administered tends to induce excitement, yet when once the patient is fully anaesthetized, the anaesthesia may be kept up for an indefinite period by continued administration of the gas, diluted with certain pro-portions of atmospheric air without any excitement supervening. I have had some instruments constructed by Mr. Coxeter to effect this measured admixture, so as to pursue my experiments with greater exactness.'

What was the nature of these instruments Fox did not state.

'. . . Meanwhile ', he added, ' I throw out these hints in order to secure the early co-operation of my medical friends in this path of investigation, and I have no doubt, with their aid, some means will be found of prolonging the anaesthesia induced by nitrous oxide, either by the admixture of atmospheric air or some other chemical agent.' [2]

Fox's plans did not mature, but the idea of using a mixture of nitrous oxide and oxygen had already been conceived and put into practice in America by E. Andrews, Professor of Principles and Practice of Surgery in the Chicago Medical College. An account of his work by Andrews, reprinted from the *Chicago Medical Examiner*, appeared in the *British Journal of Dental Science* for January 1869 :

' Every surgeon who has seen the prompt and pleasant anaesthetic action of the nitrous oxide gas, so much used by Dentists, has wished that in some way it might be made available

[1] *Brit. J. dent. Sci.*, 1868, **11**, 274-5.   [2] *Lancet*, 1869, i, 32.

in general surgery. . . . There have been, however, great obstacles to the use of the gas, owing to its evanescent action. The oxygen contained in it is in a state of chemical combination, so that it is not available for oxygenation of the blood ; hence, if any attempt is made to continue its action, the patient becomes purple in the face, showing all the signs of asphyxia . . . and, if allowed nothing but pure nitrous oxide, would doubtless die in a few minutes.

' I have for some time been experimenting, to see whether by the addition of free oxygen to the nitrous oxide, a mixture would not be obtained, by which a patient might be anaesthetized for an indefinite period without danger of asphyxia, and thus render the gas available for the most prolonged operations of surgery. These experiments are not yet finished, but they have advanced far enough to show that the preparation, which I have named the Oxygen Mixture, is certainly available for a large part of our operations, and that for pleasantness, and probable safety, it is infinitely superior to chloroform, ether, or unmixed nitrous oxide.'

Andrews briefly described five experiments on animals by which he had tested this theory. He then gave the results of four clinical cases in which patients had inhaled the Oxygen Mixture, two for the manipulation of ankylosed joints, a third for a dental extraction, and the fourth for the removal of toe-nails. All four cases were very satisfactory. Andrews also stated that one or two dentists in Chicago had tested the Oxygen Mixture in practice and had found it act ' more agreeably than unmixed nitrous oxide '.

' The above experiments ', Andrews concluded, ' are by no means sufficient to settle the value of the Oxygen Mixture, but they give strong reason to think that it will prove the safest, and by far the pleasantest, anaesthetic known. . . .
' It is my impression that the best proportion of oxygen will be found to be one-fifth by volume, which is the same as in the atmospheric air.'

No new apparatus was devised in connection with the Oxygen Mixture. The nitrous oxide was generated and passed into the receiver in the usual way and the oxygen was then generated and passed into the same receiver.

' As the nitrous oxide is fifty per cent. heavier than oxygen . . . the oxygen coming afterward, passes through it, and hastens the mixing. It is better to let them stand a day or two, if possible, before using, to complete the mixture, but this is not essential.'

The prepared mixture was led off through a length of tubing and a mouth-tube to the patient.

'As the oxygen dilutes the nitrous oxide, it is necessary to be very careful to exclude all atmospheric air, or else the anaesthetic will be imperfect', wrote Andrews. 'The inhaler must be taken into the mouth, the lips very carefully closed around it, and the nares compressed by the person administering the anaesthetic.'

The only serious drawback to his Oxygen Mixture which Andrews could find was 'its great bulk. For office use, and also in hospitals, this is no objection, as it can be kept in a gasometer ; but for outside patients it can only be carried in a large rubber bag '.[1]

Andrews's report on the use of the Oxygen Mixture made little impression outside Chicago. In England mixtures of oxygen and nitrous oxide were tried during 1870, independently of American suggestion, by E. Frankland in the laboratory while carrying out physiological researches for the Second Report of the Nitrous Oxide Committee, and in the same connection by Coleman clinically (cf. p. 297). When the question of the use of such mixtures was raised during a discussion on the Report at the Odontological Society in December 1872, Coleman confined himself to the statement ' that mixtures of nitrous oxide and oxygen in various proportions had been employed, but that they had not been attended with success ; they produced much struggling and excitement, with but imperfect anaesthesia '.[2]

In America after Colton's introduction in 1863 of Sprague's generating and inhaling apparatus (see Fig. 68) and of the use of large rubber bags into which the gas could be drawn off for inhaling—methods which proved adequate to the needs of the average dental surgeon—further development tended to be slow. During the eighteen-seventies the use of compressed nitrous oxide was adopted and some features of English apparatus, notably Cattlin's type of reservoir bag, were copied (cf. p. 294) ; but as late as the eighteen-eighties and nineties the mouth-tube and compression of the nostrils remained the most usual method of introducing the gas into the patient's lungs. Laurence Turnbull, of the Jefferson Medical College

[1] *Brit. J. dent. Sci.*, 1869, **12**, 22–6.   [2] *Trans. odont. Soc.*, 1873, **5**, 50.

Hospital, Philadelphia, stated indeed in 1880 that 'inhalers which cover the face or any part of it are objectionable '.[1]

In France and Germany the development of nitrous oxide anaesthesia was seriously retarded by the intensive preparations which preceded the outbreak of the Franco-Prussian War in the summer of 1870.

'We understand ', wrote the editor of the British Journal of Dental Science, 'that the practice of several eminent German Dentists has been interrupted by the outbreak of war, in a way they could scarcely have contemplated when adopting the speciality of Dental Surgery. The greater number of German Dentists, being qualified medical men, are now called upon to serve in the military hospitals as surgeons, while their unqualified assistants are enrolled in the army. . . .

'In the earlier days of the war, Dr. Thudichum [J. L. W. Thudichum, a German settled in England and at the time in question Lecturer on Pathological Chemistry at St. Thomas's Hospital and Director of a newly founded chemico-pathological laboratory there [2]] made an earnest appeal in the papers in favour of the use of nitrous oxide in military surgery. His letters were somewhat snubbed by the medical papers, which we think was a pity. There could never be a better opportunity for testing the great question as to whether nitrous oxide can be used with success in general surgery. If it is valueless it will soon fall of itself. Meanwhile we are happy to learn from the Times of September 26, that £184 10s. [has been] contributed to the Nitrous Oxide Fund. . . .

'Messrs. Coxeter & Son, to meet the great demand upon them for nitrous oxide, have fitted up extensive machinery by which they can make and liquefy immense quantities of gas at the shortest notice. To Dr. Thudichum, who is at the seat of war, they have forwarded 3000 gallons, and to Paris about three weeks ago 2000 gallons. . . . We shall look with much interest to the report of those who may use the gas in the military hospitals. Meanwhile our earnest sympathies are with the wounded and suffering of both the great nations now engaged in this sad warfare, which will, we trust, terminate in a solid and lasting peace.' [3]

Despite the efforts of Thudichum and Coxeters', however, chloroform was the anaesthetic almost exclusively used by both sides during the war, and it continued to be so when peace came. Even in Paris Evans's example in the use of nitrous

[1] Turnbull, L. 1880 (2nd ed.). *The advantages and accidents of artificial anaesthesia.* London. 164.

[2] *Brit. med. J.*, 1901, ii, 726.   [3] *Brit. J. dent. Sci.*, 1870, **13**, 498–9.

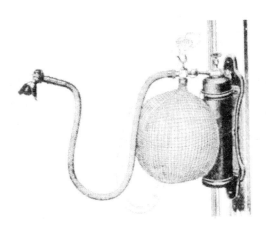

FIG. 79

Wall-bracket for nitrous oxide cylinder. The control handle on top of the cylinder regulated the flow of gas. Behind the mouth-tube, with a flange to cup the outside of the mouth, is the expiratory valve.

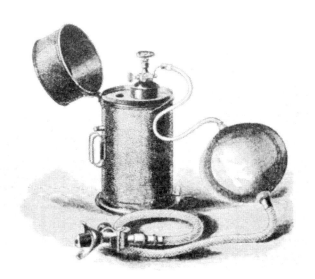

FIG. 80.—' SURGEON'S UPRIGHT CASE '

For nitrous oxide anaesthesia. The reservoir bag could be filled and detached from the 100-gallon cylinder if the administrator so desired. Both this apparatus and that shown in Fig. 79 were in use in America at the close of the nineteenth century.

oxide no longer carried weight. His influence before the war had no doubt been heightened by his close connection with the Court of Napoleon III, and at the downfall of the Empire he is said personally to have escorted the Empress to the coast, ' whence she sailed to England in a private yacht '.[1]

During 1873 F. Jolyet and T. Blanche published the results of researches on animals carried out in the Physiological Laboratory of the Faculté des Sciences in Paris. These researches, they believed, demonstrated that

' the anaesthesia which is manifest at a certain stage, in animals breathing pure nitrous oxide, ought not to be attributed to the presence of that gas in their arterial blood, but to the privation of oxygen in the blood. Experiment has shown, in fact, that anaesthesia, in animals breathing pure nitrous oxide, supervenes when they begin to have only from 2 to 3 per cent. of oxygen in the arterial blood.'[2]

This view (cf. pp. 282–4) appears to have been endorsed by Claude Bernard[3] and, chiefly on that account, to have been widely accepted in France.

For example during a discussion on anaesthetics held by the Société de Chirurgie in Paris in 1875 Trélat said :

' It is established by M. Claude Bernard's experiments that the action of laughing gas constitutes a true asphyxia, of which anaesthesia is one of the symptoms and lasts only as long as the inhalation of the asphyxial gas. . . .'

On that occasion this opinion was expressed in very similar words by several other members present.[4]

It was not until late in 1878 that Paul Bert pointed out that the anaesthetic effects of the gas were being obscured by asphyxial symptoms which were inevitable only so long as patients were made to inhale 100 per cent. nitrous oxide (see pp. 356–7).

[1] *Brit. med. J.*, 1897, ii, 1538.
[2] *C.R. Soc. Biol.*, Paris, 1873, **5**, 223, 224.
[3] In his book *Leçons sur les anesthésiques et sur l'asphyxie* (Paris, 1875, pp. 44–5) Bernard wrote, however, as follows :

' Ether . . . and chloroform are not the only substances which possess anaesthetic properties ; the researches occasioned by the discovery of etherization have led to the finding of many others which possess the same properties in various degrees. One may cite, besides these two bodies, the majority of ethers, . . . benzine, aldehyde . . . amylene . . . nitrous oxide, etc.

' Chloroform and ether are the only anaesthetics used in surgical practice or in physiology and consequently we will speak only of these two substances. . . .'

[4] *Bull. Soc. Chirurgie Paris*, 1875, N.S. **1**, 213, 216.

CHAPTER XI

ETHER IN ENGLAND

Revived Use of Ether in England and its Subsequent Development

ON October 24, 1871, J. Warrington Haward, Surgical Registrar and chloroformist at St. George's Hospital, at a meeting of the Royal Medical and Chirurgical Society, read a paper on ' Ether and chloroform as anaesthetics '. ' The statements of Dr. Bigelow and other American Surgeons ', he is reported to have said, ' showed that ether as an anaesthetic had been to our detriment neglected.' He himself ' had, during the past year, practically investigated the subject, and had arrived at the conclusion that ether was, for several reasons, to be preferred to chloroform.' Briefly these reasons were that ether was not so marked a cardiac depressant as chloroform, that it was ' antagonistic to the effects of the shock of an operation ', and that it was less likely to produce post-operative sickness.

His fellow members, remembering the conclusion reached in 1864 by the Society's Chloroform Committee, that the use of ether as the sole anaesthetic was inexpedient despite its greater safety as compared to chloroform (see p. 255), received Haward's paper with little enthusiasm.

The President, Mr. Curling, F.R.S., in opening the discussion merely regretted that no notice had been taken of the recommendation of the Society's Chloroform Committee ' to use the mixed vapours of alcohol, ether, and chloroform '. Spencer Wells pointed out that in Vienna, where mixed vapours had long been used, it was found that ether evaporated first, and after it had gone the patient was drenched with chloroform. He added that ' he had tried ether . . . but it was so troublesome that he was glad to take to bichloride of methylene ' (see p. 264). Charles Kidd also said that he had tried ether and found its use tedious. Nevertheless he advocated putting the patient under the influence of chloroform and then keeping up the anaesthesia with ether. This method, Sansom claimed, had been devised by himself ' some time ago ' (cf.

p. 258). A certain Mr. Holmes said that he too had made a trial of the use of ether. ' He tried to favour the escape of the vapour by using a hot sponge, and it blistered the face of the patient. Violent convulsive movements were also induced by it in certain patients.' J. T. Clover then stated that he ' had been in the habit of giving nitrous oxide first, and then ether, as the great difficulty was to get patients to inhale it freely '.[1]

Clover, in using this new sequence, had once more adapted his chloroform inhaler (see Figs. 53 and 54) to his needs and simply by reducing the size of the reservoir bag had provided himself with an ether inhaler. His method was to induce anaesthesia with the ordinary type of nitrous oxide apparatus (cf. Fig. 74) and then quickly substitute his ether inhaler for maintaining anaesthesia.

Haward, in administering ether alone, followed the American method, using ' a cone of felt, into which a small sponge was introduced, and which was so constructed that the ether could not drain down on to the patient's face '. Unlike the Americans, however, he lowered the cone gradually over the patient's face until anaesthesia was established.

Commenting upon Haward's work at St. George's during 1871[2] the *Lancet* expressed the opinion that ' the only outward difference between the administration of ether and that of chloroform appeared to be the more frequent replenishment of the inhaler, and the very appreciable extent to which the theatre became pervaded with the vapour of the anaesthetic '.[3] This latter drawback Haward attempted to overcome soon afterwards by enveloping his felt cone in a mackintosh cover.

Despite Haward's not unsuccessful application of American methods of etherization in his own practice, it needed an apostle from America to bring about the general revival of the use of

---

[1] *Med. Times, Lond.,* 1871, ii, 603–4.

[2] This was not the first revival of the use of ether at St. George's since Snow had so successfully administered it there during 1847 (cf. p. 18). In 1861 Thomas Jones, R.M.O. and administrator of anaesthetics to the hospital, gave ether in a number of cases from ' a large conical sponge '—' a very objectionable method ', Jones afterwards came to think. But although his cases were on the whole successful he discarded ether in the following year, except in cases ' which were considered unsafe for chloroform ', because of the inconvenience to those present which the smell of ether caused ' and from the time it took in some cases to get the patient under its influence '. (*Brit. med. J.,* 1872, ii, 603.)

[3] *Lancet,* 1871, ii, 778.

ether in England. This man was B. Joy Jeffries, an ophthalmic surgeon of Boston, Massachusetts.

' My student life in Europe in 1858–59 ', Jeffries stated, ' taught me that English and Continental surgeons were generally unacquainted with ether and its administration as an anaesthetic, to such an extent as to readily explain their adoption and continued use of chloroform, notwithstanding its frequent fatal effects. Hence, I have from that time thought it would be doing good service to show our medical brethren, the other side of the water, our method of giving ether, and thus, perhaps, give them the confidence in it which we have in Boston, where it was first used and has never been superseded.' [1]

Jeffries came to London in August 1872, primarily to attend an international congress of ophthalmologists, but with the further intention of spreading information about American methods of etherization among the British and Continental chloroformists also attending the congress. He opened his campaign by delivering a provocative paper on ' Ether in ophthalmic surgery '.

'. . . I do not advocate the use of ether because I come from the city where its employment in surgery was discovered and promulgated,' he said, ' but because I believe that there are others like myself who do not desire to run the risk of killing a patient with chloroform, and who, perhaps, would gladly avail themselves of ether were they rendered as familiar with its administration and harmlessness as we are in America. Let me be clearly understood. I use and advocate ether because it is as effectual as chloroform, and not dangerous to life. . . . Ether, at the worst, is but a profound intoxicant, and not unlike a drunken fit. On the other hand, thousands inhale it without trouble. . . .
' A towel rolled into a cone, with a napkin or sponge pushed to the top of the inside, is all we need to pour our ether on, whilst our fingers can mould it over any mouth and nose. Some years ago I often heard in Europe medical gentlemen say, " But there are so many people who cannot take ether ". I have yet to see one. The truth is, I believe, that surgeons who use chloroform are afraid of ether, and do not dare to give enough of it at once in the commencement. Now if the patient is warned that the ether will choke him, and told when this occurs to take long breaths to relieve it, and not to struggle and endeavour to push away the sponge, many will go to sleep quietly and without trouble to themselves or the surgeon. I have but one other

[1] *Boston med. surg. J.*, 1872-3, N.S. **10**, 225.

point to speak of in reference to giving ether. When the patient, whether old or young, struggles, and asks for a respite and fresh air, do not yield. Hold them down by main force, if necessary, and at any rate, keep the sponge tight over the mouth and nose till they finally take long breaths and then soon go off into ether-sleep. Doing this prevents their remembering anything about their struggles. It is absurd to stop the ether and try to reason with adults excited by the anaesthetic, and cruel not to push on quickly with children. This may sound almost puerile to my American brethren, but my personal experience tells me that those who use chloroform have somehow a sort of dread of ether, as if it was to be suddenly fatal, and hence fail to give a patient enough to intoxicate him quickly. This arises from lack of familiarity with its use and administration.' [1]

At the conclusion of Jeffries's paper Brudenell Carter said, ' I much regret . . . the absence from among us of a gentleman who, more than any other in London, is in the habit of adminis-tering ether,—Mr. Warrington Hayward [sic]. . . . He has advocated very strongly the use of ether in general surgery, but his experience is, and I must say that mine entirely coincides with it, that ether as an anaesthetic agent does not produce sufficient muscular relaxation to fulfil all the requirements of the ophthalmic operator . . . and after some experience both Mr. Hayward and myself have determined to lay it aside, and return to our old and trusted friend chloroform. . . . I shall be grateful ', he added, ' if Dr. Jeffries will come to St. George's Hospital and administer ether for us, that we may see whether our past dissatisfaction with it may be in any way due to our faults of administration '.[2]

Jeffries readily complied with this request, and during his brief stay in London gave seventeen demonstrations at various hospitals.[3]

His forceful, slap-dash American technique was indubitably successful. Though it startled the cautious London chloro-formists, at the same time it left them convinced at last that ether was not only safe but, when suitably administered, effectual.

On his return to America Jeffries had some droll stories to tell.

' When I asked the object of measuring the chloroform used,' he said, ' I was told, with a smile, " for the benefit of the coroner's

[1] Lancet, 1872, ii, 241–2.   [2] Ibid. ii, 242.   [3] Brit. med. J., 1872, ii, 499.

jury ". This explained to me the looks and expressions of astonishment when I lavishly poured out ether on my towel cone, which I purposely did to prove there need be no fear of the anaesthetic, the important point being how much the patient got, not how much was in the sponge or other apparatus.

'As may be well imagined, I had to answer many questions. . . . To the very frequent one as to relative expense, I replied by showing them that if ether was manufactured and sold only as cheaply as in the United States, and not wasted in administration, its cost was little, if any above that of chloroform. Politeness, of course, prevented my adding what was naturally in my mind, namely, that probably any gentleman who had had one fatal case from chloroform would gladly deduct from his fee any difference in price of the anaesthetic to avoid another. . . .

'As to the relative disagreeabilities of ether and chloroform, I frankly told them I was not in a position to judge, for I had never administered the latter and was not an etherist ; in fact, we had and needed none among us, since surgeons in America gave ether themselves when operating, or it was exhibited by a surgeon assisting, or by a medical student. . . . There was evident surprise on finding . . . that I was simply an ophthalmic surgeon, and not in any way an etherist, as they have chloroformists. It was a good argument in favor of ether.' [1]

After Jeffries's demonstrations ether was applied in general surgery by certain of the specialist anaesthetists, particularly those who had actually been present, with as much alacrity as, four years earlier, nitrous oxide had been applied in dentistry after Evans's demonstrations (see p. 279 *et seq.*).

For example Charles Bell Taylor, Surgeon to the Nottingham and Midland Eye Hospital, wrote to the *Lancet* in December 1872 :

'It was not until I had the pleasure of meeting Dr. Joy Jeffries, of Boston, at the College of Physicians . . . that my difficulties respecting ether were overcome.'

He added, however :

'I don't think that ether will ever take the place of chloroform ; but it is unquestionably a valuable anaesthetic in cases where chloroform is inadmissible.' [2]

As a body chloroformists were not easily to be transformed into etherists, despite the obvious success of American methods

[1] *Boston med. surg J.*, 1872-3, N.S. **10**, 226.   [2] *Lancet*, 1872, ii, 879-80.

of administration and well-authenticated evidence that these methods were safe. On November 16, 1872, however, the British Medical Association, through its *Journal*, stated that, ' In the face of the great mortality from chloroform, and of the almost deathless record of ether, it has become our duty to interpose, to call the urgent attention of professional men throughout the country to the claims which ether has upon their confidence, and to urge that the anaesthetic which was thrust out of repute by the ready and convenient fluid introduced by Simpson, shall have an extended and a fair trial. We are glad to find ourselves supported in this view by many experienced manipulators. . . . We shall be glad to hear further on the subject from all whose experience can contribute to the speedy decision of a question of capital importance. . . . We shall be glad to receive for publication short notes of the results, of course, whether favourable or unfavourable '.[1]

The result of this appeal was encouraging. ' Three weeks ago ', wrote the editor of the *British Medical Journal*, on November 23, 1872, ' the administration of ether was a rare exception ; we have reason to believe that it is already becoming the rule. . . . Thus far only the most favourable verdicts reach us '.[2]

On December 21, the editor was able to note ' that at the London Hospital, where Mr. Couper has for some time used it . . . the whole surgical staff have resolved to give it an exclusive trial in the operating-theatre. Circumstances have prevented us from recording the successful results of the administration of ether at the Royal Infirmary at Edinburgh, the early cradle of chloroform, and at the Leeds Infirmary. We shall shortly do so. . . .'[3]

For some months, after the beginning of January 1873, the *Journal* contained weekly reports illustrating the growing use of ether anaesthesia in the London and provincial hospitals. Among the first of these reports were the following:[4]

From G. Everitt Norton, Chloroformist to the Middlesex Hospital :

' For the past three months, ether has been generally administered at this hospital with satisfactory results. The longest time during which its inhalation has been continued was an hour. . . . It is administered at this hospital mixed with air, passed

[1] *Brit. med. J.*, 1872, ii, 556.   [2] *Ibid.* ii, 583.
[3] *Ibid* ii, 689.   [4] *Ibid.* 1873, i, 35–6.

over a vapour of ether at a temperature of 70 deg. Patients find its inhalation by this method far more pleasant than by the ordinary methods. . . . The average time required for an adult is from three to four minutes. . . .'

From Lewis Mackenzie, House Surgeon at the London Hospital :

' Our four surgeons almost universally use ether now. Mr. Hutchinson makes the exception in the case of old people, for whom he prefers chloroform. . . . We generally use a towel, in form of a cone, with a sponge.'

From Walter Rigden, Resident Medical Officer at University College Hospital :

' I have as yet only administered ether twelve times. . . . The plan of administration has been that recommended by Dr. Joy Jeffries—i.e. a towel folded into a cone and a piece of lint eight inches square screwed up and put into the inside. I then pour on to the lint as much ether as I can get it to absorb without soaking through to the towel—generally about an ounce and a half—and tell the patient to breathe deeply. . . .'

From J. W. Plaxton, House Surgeon at the Hull Infirmary :

' Ether, so far as I can ascertain, has never been used as an anaesthetic in this infirmary. It will be so used, for the first time, on Wednesday next, January 1st, 1873.'

A report from the Charing Cross Hospital stated that ' Ether . . . is to be tried shortly '.

Frank H. Hodges, House Surgeon at the York County Hospital, wrote :

' Ether as yet has only been employed in the operations performed by Mr. Husband (our other two surgeons being perfectly satisfied with chloroform) in four cases. . . . Mr. Husband is very favourably impressed with the action of ether, and is resolved to give it a fair trial. I employ a large hollow sponge, four thicknesses of towel being stitched round it ; over this I place gutta-percha tissue, and carefully exclude all air till the induction of anaesthesia. I then keep up the action of the agent as it may be required.'

On January 18, Carey of Guy's Hospital reported twelve

cases of ether anaesthesia. On January 25, a report from the Hospital for Sick Children [1] stated :

'For some time past ether has been given here by Mr. Fletcher Beach, the registrar, as an anaesthetic. The apparatus used is simply a cone of felt covered with oil silk or Lister's protective ; and in the cone is inserted, after having been wrung out in hot water, a sponge, which can be changed from time to time, if necessary. Sufficient ether is poured on the sponge to saturate it, and the cone is applied as closely as possible to the face of the child. By pushing the ether from the first, struggling is considerably reduced. Two or three minutes suffice for the production of anaesthesia. Air is excluded as much as possible at the commencement, but is admitted afterwards, according to the state of the patient and the length of the operation. Ether is added, from time to time, as it is required.' [2]

On February 1, the House Surgeon wrote from the Birmingham and Midland Eye Hospital :

'During the last three months ether has almost entirely taken the place of chloroform in this hospital. It has been administered in several different ways, and it has been found that, the nearer the approach to a total exclusion of atmospheric air, the more satisfactory are the results obtained. . . . The apparatus which I at present always use is a simple leather cup, five inches in depth, and shaped so as to fit pretty accurately to the face, covering the mouth and nose. In the bottom of the cup, out of reach of the patient's face, is placed a sponge. An ounce of ether, to begin with, is poured upon the sponge and the patient is allowed to take two or three inspirations freely diluted with air . . . and the inhaler is then held firmly over the face, and surrounded with a fold of towel.' [3]

On the first occasion on which ether was used at the Stamford Infirmary, a large sponge was covered with a towel for the administration ; on the second occasion, however, in order to avoid the diffusion of ether in the operating theatre, ' a cone of pasteboard, eight inches deep, was cut so that the wide end would fit the face fairly well, and a sponge was fixed close to the small upper opening. Two ounces of ether were sufficient to produce complete anaesthesia, and an ounce was afterwards needed to keep up the effect ' during the excision of an epithelial growth from a man's hand.

[1] Warrington Haward was Assistant Surgeon at this Hospital, and the method of etherization here described shows his influence (cf. p. 312).
[2] Brit. med. J., 1873, i, 88.　　　　　[3] Ibid. i, 116.

W. E. C. Nourse, of Brighton, also advocated 'cheap and simple inhalers made of card or paper. . . . They consist of short open cones, fitting the face, and containing a piece of sponge '.[1]

These various accounts show that during the first six months of the revived use of ether in England our anaesthetists were strongly influenced by American methods of administration— methods which included the use not only of cones made from a folded towel, but from felt, cardboard,[2] and leather. This was to be expected, for American methods succeeded whereas English methods, on the whole, had failed.

It was soon discovered, however, that the leather cone devised by Rendle in 1867 for bichloride of methylene (see Fig. 67), and a somewhat similar leather cone first used by B. W. Richardson in November 1872 for his then newly introduced mixture, methylene ether (dichloromethane and diethyl ether), could equally well be used to administer sulphuric ether. (Cf. Appendix D, p. 591.)

In 1873 C. S. Tomes, an English dentist of some standing, while on a visit to the United States, wrote an account of the anaesthetic procedure at Boston :

' It was at the Massachusetts General Hospital, Boston, that ether was first administered . . . and I cannot do better than describe the course of the procedure at this institution which . . . unquestionably takes the first place among the hospitals of this country.

' The patients are etherized in small ante-rooms adjoining the operating theatre, the ether being administered by one of the junior house officers, who is, in nine cases out of ten, not yet qualified. Two or three ounces of pure anhydrous ether are poured upon a conical sponge which has been previously moistened with water ; this is at once placed over the patient's mouth and nose. If he struggles, which he generally does, as he experiences the suffocating sensation produced by the pungent vapour, he is held down by main force till he succumbs to its influence. Ether is lavishly poured upon the sponge, so that it often runs down the patient's face and neck, and half a pound is not rarely used for a single administration.

[1] *Brit. med. J.*, 1873, i, 142, 154.
[2] Horatio C. Wood, of Philadelphia, in the seventh edition of his text-book *Therapeutics : its principles and practice* (London, 1888 (7th ed.), p. 142) stated that a stiff paper cone enclosing a sponge or napkin, on to which about an ounce and a half of ether was poured, was the ' ordinary method of the administration of ether in Philadelphia '.

'Not uncommonly there is a good deal of spasm of the expiratory muscles, stridulous breathing, and laryngeal spasm, and I have several times seen a degree of asphyxial lividity transcending that which I have ever observed during the administration of nitrous oxide. Though these asphyxial symptoms are strongly pronounced, not the smallest anxiety is felt ; the sponge is merely removed for half-a-minute, or a minute, the blood at once recovers its colour, and the administration is proceeded with. . . . I do not remember to have ever seen the administrator feel the patient's pulse. When anaesthesia is complete, the patient is picked up and carried in the arms of a stout attendant into the theatre, and when there, no special attention is given to his position. Should it happen to be more convenient, he is placed upright, in a sitting position, in Dr. H. J. Bigelow's admirable operating chair. . . .

'To one familiar with the dangers of chloroform . . . the whole procedure, from first to last, looks perfectly reckless, and yet it is fully justified by experience, for at the hospital, which almost monopolises the operative surgery of New England, and presents a very large weekly list of operations, there has never been any misadventure attendant on the use of ether.' [1]

Although the rank and file of English anaesthetists seemed prepared to accept, with modifications, the 'reckless' American way of etherization, which made use of carbon dioxide accumulation within the inhaler as a means of intensifying the anaesthetic effect, many specialist anaesthetists, almost immediately after Jeffries's demonstrations, turned their attention to devising methods more in keeping with English anaesthetic tradition.

G. Everitt Norton was among the first, in the autumn of 1872, to produce what can be described as a typically English ether inhaler.

'The apparatus consists of an application of one of the principles employed in Dr. Smith's carbonic acid apparatus (*Philosophical Transactions*, 1859–61) by which a current of air is made to travel over the largest amount of surface in the smallest compass.'

The inhaler was made by Hawksley, of Oxford Street, and consisted of a metal box measuring 7 by 4 by 3 inches and divided into six compartments horizontally by five flannel-covered shelves. Each shelf had a hole in the middle and a row of holes at one end. The shelves were so arranged that the row of holes

[1] *Brit. med. J.*, 1873, i, 297.

on alternate shelves came at opposite ends of the box, but all the holes in the middle coincided. About two ounces of ether were poured into the box through a funnel in the top, the flow being controlled by stopcocks. The ether fell on to a metal plate which scattered the liquid in drops and these showered through the hole in the middle of each shelf and were soaked up by the flannel. A length of tubing passed from the bottom compartment of the box to a Snow's facepiece. The patient drew in air through an inspiratory valve in the top of the box. The small size of the holes at the ends of the shelves compelled each inspiration to pass over the surface of the shelf before reaching the tube and facepiece.[1] Norton claimed that this inhaler worked well, but had the drawback that it was not easy to perceive when all the ether in the box had evaporated. He discarded it, about March 1873, for another inhaler also made by Hawksley.

' The apparatus consists of an ordinary Wolf's bottle, capable of containing a pint of ether, having on its upper surface three openings, through the left-hand one of which a tube, graduated so as to indicate the amount of anaesthetic the patient has taken, passes down into the ether. The upper end of this is guarded by a valve, through which the patient inhales the air. The centre one is only used when it is wished to give the ether in the form of a spray, on Richardson's principle, in mouth and similar operations [2]. In the right-hand opening a long elastic tube is fixed, with a face-piece like Snow's. The tube is furnished with an expiratory valve, to which is attached a second tube, through which the expired air is passed on to the ground. Much unpleasantness to those around is thus avoided. In front of the face-piece is a revolving shutter, which allows the patient to inhale pure air when desirable. The bottle stands in a bath surrounded with warm water, at a temperature of 70 deg. Fahr. ; and by that means the patient inhales an uniform mixture of ether and air, of probably about 60 per cent. of the former. The bottle is half filled with ether, and the inspiratory tube is pushed down to the surface of the anaesthetic ; but if it be wished to give the

---

[1] *Brit. med. J.*, 1872, ii, 629.
[2] Describing Norton's inhaler, in 1874, Clover stated that in such circumstances a nose-cap was commonly substituted for the facepiece after anaesthesia was well established. He added that ' In such cases, it is well to be provided with a tin tube an inch in diameter and a foot long, lined with blotting-paper ; and, if required, to pour ether into it, and hold it near the mouth, so that the weight of the vapour will cause it to flow into the mouth during inspiration. Ether is well suited to these operations ', Clover added, ' because, if the administration have been continued long enough to get the tissues well soaked with ether, the anaesthesia is kept up longer than is usual after the withdrawal of other anaesthetics.' (*Brit. med. J.*, 1874, i, 202.)

II

patient a stronger dose, the tube is pushed into the fluid. Suspended in the bottle is a flannel bag, intended to promote the surface of evaporation of the ether.'

Norton stated that the average time for induction with the apparatus was four minutes in an adult. In two cases of ovariotomy, one lasting 45 minutes, the other 1 hour and 40 minutes, the consumption of ether was, in the first-mentioned

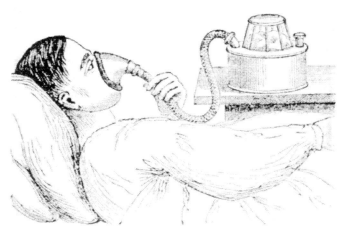

FIG. 81.—MORGAN'S ETHER INHALER (November 1872)

Showing the round metal box with the filling port for ether, covered by a screw cap, the rubber diaphragm which rose and fell with the patient's exhalations and inhalations, the flexible tubing, and the valveless facepiece.

case, $3\frac{1}{2}$ ounces, and in the second, 5 ounces. In a haemorrhoidectomy in a strong, alcoholic man, however, the consumption was $2\frac{1}{2}$ ounces for a 12-minute anaesthesia.[1] This inhaler was popular for several years and Hawksley brought out an improved model in 1876.

An inhaler which aimed at putting fully into practice the American dictum that ether anaesthesia should be induced as rapidly as possible, and with a minimum of air, was invented, during the autumn of 1872, by J. Morgan, of Dublin.[2] This inhaler (see Fig. 81) was described by Clover as ' a metallic

[1] Brit. med. J., 1873, i, 353.   [2] Ibid. 1872, ii, 575.

vessel with a diaphragm of india-rubber membrane, which rises and falls with the breathing. This arrangement effects the same result with ether which I produced by the supplemental bag of my nitrous oxide apparatus [see Fig. 71]. The patient inhales almost the same atmosphere over and over again, the ether and the carbonic acid increasing and the oxygen diminishing. I have tried it ', added Clover, ' and found it economical and effective, but I think those patients who used it complained more than others of headache afterwards '.[1]

It was some time before Clover, whose conception of the correct way of administering volatile anaesthetics was still essentially that of Snow, could fully reconcile himself to the American conception of etherization. He continued to disapprove of American practical methods. ' I should be afraid of giving *pure* ether by means of a large warmed sponge to a patient already well narcotized ', he wrote in February 1874.[2]

The first inhaler which Clover himself designed exclusively for administering ether, he called the ' double-current inhaler ' (see Fig. 82).

' I do not now use . . . [the modified chloroform apparatus, cf. p. 312] for ether ', he wrote in March 1873, ' except in operations about the mouth, as I have succeeded in supplying the ether-vapour with sufficiently uniform dilution by the inhaler which I am about to describe. It consists of a facepiece without any valves ; a metal box measuring six inches by four, and five deep ; and an elastic tube five-eighths of an inch in diameter, to connect them. The box is either suspended by a ribbon from the administrator's neck, or placed upon the patient's bed. Inside the box is a tube of very thin copper, which conveys the expired air through it, and is then provided with a valve which opens only during expiration. The tube is broad enough to extend across the box, and undulating, in order to present a large surface, which is covered with cloth to absorb the ether. Plates of metal are so disposed as to direct the current of air, which enters through a valve during inspiration, over the surface of the tube. . . .

' The flexible tube leading to the face-piece joins it at B. The part of the vessel containing ether-vapour is marked E. When the patient *in*hales, air enters at A and follows the course marked by the arrows ; when he *ex*hales, the current in the flexible tube

---

[1] *Brit. med. J.*, 1874, i, 201 ; Clover, J. T. MS. notes in the possession of the Nuffield Department of Anaesthetics, Oxford.

[2] *Brit. med. J.*, 1874, i, 201.

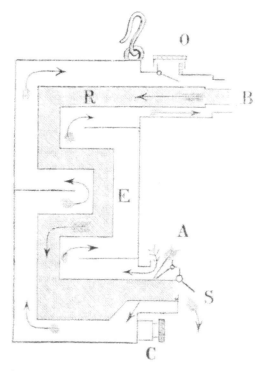

FIG. 82.—CLOVER'S ' DOUBLE-CURRENT INHALER '
FOR ETHER (March 1873)

A. Inspiratory valve.
B. Junction between inhaler and flexible tubing leading to the facepiece
    (the last two items not shown).
C. Filling and emptying port for ether.
E. Vaporizing chamber.
O. Sliding shutter and valve admitting fresh air to dilute the ether-air
    mixture before it entered the flexible tubing. The valve prevented
    the air from flowing back into the body of the inhaler.
R. Metallic tube, covered with absorbent cloth, through which the patient's
    exhalations passed back to the expiratory valve, S, thus warming
    the vaporizing chamber.

is reversed, and enters the metallic tube marked R, and escapes
at the valve S. The opening for supplying and removing the ether
is at C.

' It will be observed that the part where the greatest cold is
produced, by the current of fresh air passing over the ether,
corresponds with the termination of the *exhaling* tube, and will
condense much of the ether-vapour breathed back by the patient ;
also, that the current of air towards the patient goes over a surface
which has been warmed by the patient's breath as it passes

outwards through the tube. A sliding shutter at O regulates the admission of air, without passing through the ether-chamber ; but the egress of the patient's breath at the same opening, in expiration, is prevented by a valve. A similar valve and shutter are placed at the end of the flexible tube, near the facepiece. Both should be open at first and closed gradually, that coughing and struggling against the pungency of the ether may be avoided.

' After supplying about 6 or 8 ounces of ether, the inhaler should be shaken, to diffuse the liquid over the cloth which covers the exhaling tube. At the conclusion of the operation, a considerable quantity of ether and some water will be found condensed inside this tube, and may be poured out at S by inclining the inhaler. The ether thus saved can be rectified and used again. . . .

' The chief advantage of this apparatus is, however, in the comparative uniformity of mixture with air which it effects, and which, whilst securing complete quietude of the patient, prevents the unpleasant results of an over-strong dose. Although this double-current inhaler could be modified so as to make it useful for other anaesthetics, it is for ether that I have now introduced it.' [1]

Clover showed this inhaler at the London meeting of the British Medical Association in 1873, but although he himself used it apparently with success for more than a year it was never generally adopted.

During 1874 and the two years following Clover spent most of his spare moments in the workshop attached to his house, devising new apparatuses for his gas-ether sequence (cf. p. 312).

He referred in 1874 to two methods of administering it which he had previously used. ' By means of a bag of gas,' he wrote, ' I make the patient unconscious, and then give ether as usual.' Alternatively he induced anaesthesia ' by using a small bag which is supplied with gas during the inhalation ', and maintained it ' by diverting the current of gas and making the supply of gas pass over ether, as soon as the patient loses consciousness '.[2] It was the latter method which Clover developed from the spring of 1874 onwards.

He first publicly described his new apparatus at the meeting of the British Medical Association which that year (1874) was held in Norwich, the city in which he had been educated and where his grandfather had practised as a farrier and maker of veterinary instruments, winning more than local fame by his skill and learning.[3]

[1] *Brit. med. J.*, 1873, i, 283.   [2] *Ibid.* 1874, i, 203.
[3] Cf. *Dictionary of national biography.* London, 1908, **4,** 587.

The new gas-ether apparatus was noticed briefly in the *British Medical Journal* and Sir J. Rose Cormack's opinion was quoted : ' It was unquestionably a most admirable invention, but its cost and complexity must prove fatal to its introduction into general use '.[1]

Sir J. Rose Cormack was wrong. Despite this not entirely favourable review and despite the complexity of the apparatus the anaesthesia obtained by its use was found to be so easily induced and so satisfactorily maintained that a number of London hospitals, during 1875 and 1876, thought it worth while to install Clover's apparatus.

Clover continued to improve upon it and by July 1876 it had taken its final form.[2]

' The apparatus about to be described [see Figs. 83, 84, and 85] ', wrote Clover in July 1876, ' is, in principle, like the one shown at the Norwich Meeting in 1874, with some improvements. It has been used at St. Bartholomew's, University College, St. Mary's and the Dental Hospitals ; and I have myself placed under the influence of ether with it two thousand, three hundred cases. . . . The apparatus is made by Mayer and Meltzer of Great Portland Street, and consists of a thin bag, oval in shape and fifteen inches long ; at one end connected with the ether vessel, at the other with the facepiece. Inside the bag, there is a flexible tube, also connected with the facepiece and ether vessel. By turning the regulator . . . the patient is made to breathe, either directly into the bag, or indirectly through the tube and ether vessel. When the letter G is visible [on the dial], the way to the gas-bag is open ; when the letter E is visible, the only way to the bag is through the tube and ether vessel, so that the more the regulator is turned towards E, the more ether is given, and *vice versâ*. The ether vessel contains a reservoir of water, to prevent the temperature of the ether becoming too low. This is to be kept full. The ether vessel is to be rather more than half filled, the precise point being marked against the glass gauge. A thermometer inside this gauge tells the temperature of the ether. Before using it, the vessel should be dipped into a basin of warm water, and rotated until the thermometer stands at about 68 deg. If the room be cold, and if the patient have thin cheeks and large whiskers, the temperature may be 73 deg. It is important that the face-piece should fit closely against the face. Those made by

[1] *Brit. med. J.*, 1874, ii, 382.
[2] It is frequently and, in fact, usually stated in textbooks on anaesthesia, written after 1876, that Clover first introduced his gas-ether sequence in 1876. This error is probably due to the fact that far wider publicity was given to the apparatus and to the method in that year than in previous years.

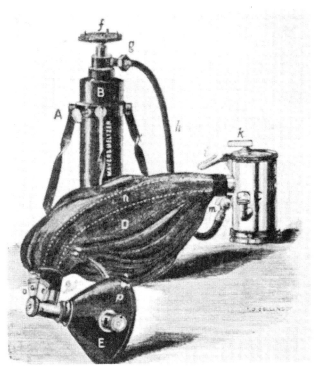

FIG. 83.—CLOVER'S ' COMBINED GAS-AND-ETHER
APPARATUS ' (1876)

A. Stand for nitrous oxide cylinder.
B. Cylinder, actuated by foot-key, *f*.
g. Union between cylinder and tubing, *h*.
m. Stopcock.

When the administrator wished to administer nitrous oxide alone,
he set the regulating stopcock, O, behind the facepiece, E, for ' gas '.
The stream of gas then passed into the inhaling bag, D, and so to the
facepiece. The exhaled gas escaped through the expiratory valve, *p*.

When he wished to administer a mixture of nitrous oxide and ether,
he set O accordingly and turned the tap, *k*, on top of the ether reservoir, C.
The stream of gas then circulated through C before passing down the
flexible tube, *n* (within the bag, D), to the facepiece.

By turning the stopcock, *m*, the supply of gas was shut off and the
patient could then breathe ether alone, to and fro through the inhaling bag, D.

(For details of the ether reservoir and the regulating stopcock
see Figs. 84 and 85.)

The ether level gauge and thermometer, mentioned on p. 326.
are not shown in Figs. 83 and 84.

327

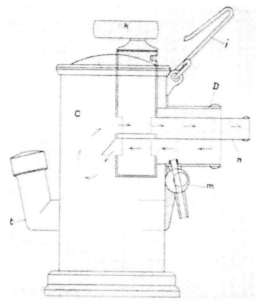

FIG. 84.—DIAGRAM OF THE ETHER VESSEL
OF CLOVER'S 'COMBINED GAS-AND-ETHER
APPARATUS', IN SECTION

i. Hook for suspending the vessel from a strap round the administrator's neck.
t. Filling tube for ether.
The flexible tube joined the ether vessel at *n*.
The bag joined the ether vessel at D.

When the control tap, *k*, was opened the interior of the ether vessel, C, was in direct communication with the bag, D and the tube, *n*.

The flow of nitrous oxide from the cylinder into the ether vessel was controlled by the stopcock, *m*. Arrows indicate the direction of the stream of gas passing through the ether vessel.

Mayer, of solid leather framework supporting a collar of inflated India-rubber, are the best, but sometimes they require to be warmed before using.

' *For giving nitrous oxide only.*—The regulator is turned to G. The stopcock of the ether vessel is closed. This vessel is hooked upon the strap round the [administrator's] neck. The strap is adjusted so that the ether vessel stands at a higher level than the facepiece. The gas being turned on, by rotating the foot-key with the foot, the gas-bag is kept filled as fast as it is emptied

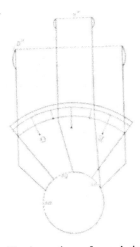
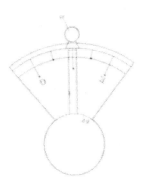

Fixed portion of regulating stopcock, O, with three slots, *sa*, *sg*, and *se*, for air, gas, and ether. Slots shown in dotted line.

Rotating portion of regulating stopcock, O, with one slot, *eg*, shown in dotted line. Handle, *w*, now half-way (=half gas and half ether). The fixed dial-plate on which *w* moves is also shown.

FIG. 85.—DIAGRAM OF THE REGULATING STOPCOCK OF CLOVER'S 'COMBINED GAS-AND-ETHER APPARATUS'

n″. Junction between stopcock and tube, *n*.
D″. Junction between stopcock and bag, D.

The diagram shows how the slots in the rotating part of the stopcock could be made partially or wholly to coincide with the orifices of the bag, D, and the tube, *n*; and how these orifices could be occluded and the air slot made patent.

by the patient. When the latter breathes out, the supply of gas is stopped; and after the bag is fully distended, the escape-valve opens, and allows the expired gas to escape. . . .

' *If Ether is to be used without Gas.*—The gas-tube should be taken off the ether vessel; the regulator should be turned to G, and the face-piece should be first applied to the face during an expiration. . . . The regulator is gradually turned towards E, and thus the way is opened to the inner tube. The air breathed through it carries vapour from the vessel into the distal end of the bag. As soon as one-half of the air passes through the ether vessel, the vapour becomes strong enough to cause insensibility in about two minutes, usually without any coughing. . . .

' By far the easiest and least unpleasant way of getting a patient ready for a surgical operation is to use gas and ether combined; the gas being given pure during 4 or 5 respirations,

11*

and the ether gradually added as above described. The supply of gas should cease when the ether is turned on.' [1]

Some models of the gas-and-ether apparatus had a cylindrical expansion chamber fitted to the outlet of the cylinder (at (g), Fig. 83). This Clover called the ' gas-rarefier ' and wrote of it :

' Sudden distension and bursting of the gas-bag can scarcely happen when the gas-rarefier is used ; but if this be not used, or if the gas-bottle have become frozen [owing to the presence of water vapour as an impurity in the nitrous oxide] it is desirable to warm the bottle, and in doing so the tap end should be more warmed than the other.' [2]

Towards the close of 1875 the *British Medical Journal* undertook a census among the London hospitals to discover which anaesthetics were in general use, in what circumstances and by what means they were administered, and the reasons for their adoption in the first place. In particular the *Journal* sought to assess the relative popularity of chloroform and ether. The principal hospitals of London were accordingly sent a questionnaire arranged to cover four main lines of inquiry :

' 1. What anaesthetics are now in use ; and for what cases is either [*i.e.* chloroform or ether] anaesthetic preferred ? 2. What methods of administration are employed? 3. Has any change been made within the last four or five years in the anaesthetic used, or its mode of administration ? and, if so, what were the reasons for the change ? 4. Can any suggestions be made by the adoption of which the safety of the anaesthetised patient might be more completely secured, or any improvement in the production of anaesthesia for surgical operations be effected ? ' [3]

The answers received to these questions were published in the *Journal* periodically between late December 1875 and the end of February 1876, under the heading ' Reports of medical and surgical practice in the hospitals and asylums of Great Britain '. They furnish an interesting survey of anaesthetic practice during the early eighteen-seventies.

Among the first to reply was the chloroformist to St. Bartholomew's Hospital :

'. . . The anaesthetics now in use [December 1875] . . . are ether, chloroform, and nitrous oxide gas ; ether preceded

[1] *Brit. med. J.*, 1876, ii, 74.   [2] *Ibid.* ii, 75.   [3] *Ibid.* 1875, ii, 781.

by nitrous oxide gas is used in by far the greater number of cases. Chloroform is used for very young children, and in operations about the mouth and nose which are likely to last some time. Nitrous oxide gas is employed for short operations, such as extraction of a tooth or opening an abscess. Nitrous oxide gas and ether are administered by means of Mr. Clover's apparatus, which is admirably adapted for the purpose. Chloroform is given on lint, from a drop-bottle. Until January 1875, chloroform was used for nearly all cases. . . . Chloroform is used in long operations about the mouth and nose, because : 1. The narcosis of chloroform lasts longer than that of ether ; 2. In many operations, as for cleft palate . . . it is necessary to keep a gag in the mouth, which comes very much in the way of a facepiece, such as is necessary for the administration of ether ; while chloroform can very conveniently be given on a piece of lint ; 3. In operations for cleft palate, too, there is another objection to the use of ether, in the fact that it excites a flow of viscid saliva, and is apt to induce coughing. . . . In cases of fracture which require an anaesthetic whilst the parts are being placed in apposition during the time the muscles are relaxed, chloroform is preferable, because patients recover from its effects quietly, the inhalation of ether being generally followed by a state of noisy delirium and struggling which would be likely to displace the fractured ends and necessitate their readjustment.'

The Surgical Registrar of Guy's Hospital replied :

' 1. In the surgical wards and surgery of Guy's Hospital, chloroform is the anaesthetic which is almost invariably administered ; occasionally only, the mixture of alcohol, ether, and chloroform, as recommended by the Committee of the Royal Medical Chirurgical Society [see pp. 356-7], and, more rarely still, ether alone. In some cases, anaesthesia first produced by chloroform, is continued by " the mixture " or by ether alone ; this especially in cases in which chloroform does not appear to be well borne. 2. Chloroform is given from a piece of lint, fitted into a metal nose-piece for convenience sake alone, a few drops being poured from a stoppered bottle as often as required. The mixture is generally given on flannel, adapted as the loose lining of a cylindrical paste-board or leather inhaler ; and ether on a sponge at the bottom of a deep cylindrical leather inhaler fitting closely round the mouth. 3. During the last four or five years, all the anaesthetics, old and new, ether, chloroform, nitrous oxide, bichloride of methylene, the mixture of alcohol, chloroform, and ether, etc., have been used to a very considerable extent at Guy's ; but, chloroform being found much the most convenient in administration, and, as a rule, well borne in surgical operations, and much less frequently followed by the disagreeable after effects—headache, vomiting, etc.—which were observed to be especially severe and prolonged in the case of ether, it has again become the anaesthetic in common use. In the eye wards, however, " the mixture ", is still generally administered. . . .'

The late resident medical officer of the London Hospital wrote :

' 1. The anaesthetic chiefly employed . . . is ether ; it was introduced . . . in the early [*sic*] part of the year 1872. . . . Mr. Jonathan Hutchinson prefers the use of chloroform in old people with rigid or brittle arteries, as he considers the arterial tension produced by ether a condition very likely to give rise to cerebral haemorrhage. . . . Chloroform is more used in the maternity department than any other of this hospital ; but, in obstetric operations, ether has been chiefly given. . . . In the dental department . . . nitrous oxide gas [is used]. . . . Bichloride of methylene was used for a short time in our ophthalmic department, but was abandoned in consequence of its acquiring a bad reputation in other hospitals. [Chloroform was preferred to ether in this department because it was thought to produce less congestion of the " eyeball and orbit ".] 2. It has been the invariable rule at the London Hospital to have as little apparatus in the administration of anaesthetics as possible. . . . Ether is administered in cones, made with new stiff towels, with sponges in them. Chloroform is always given with a simple Skinner's inhaler [see Fig. 56]. . . . Several leathern inhalers have been tried with ether, but the towel, in form of a cone, seems still most popular. 3. A great revolution in the administration of anaesthetics took place in this hospital in 1872 ; at that time, ether became almost universally substituted for chloroform. Since the introduction of ether, the hospital has not contained any case in which death has resulted from its use nor during its administration. . . .' [1]

Despite the alleged dislike of the London Hospital authorities for apparatus, during 1876 J. E. Adams succeeded in installing in the operating theatre a non-portable apparatus for ether administration. It consisted of a large water-bath screwed to the wall, the water being kept at a temperature of 100° F. ' so as to secure the boiling of the ether ', and fixed to it with a clamp, the ether-bottle of Hawksley's inhaler (see p. 321). A length of tubing, carried above the heads of the assistants and sufficient ' to extend over the whole area of the theatre ', joined the vaporizer to a facepiece. ' By having this arrangement,' wrote

[1] *Brit, med. J.*, 1875, ii, 781–2.

Adams, ' the apparatus is always at hand and not in the way.' [1]

The reply to the questionnaire which came from the Charing Cross Hospital, was made by Woodhouse Braine, ' chloroformist ' to that hospital and to the Dental Hospital :

' 1. Nitrous oxide is given to render the patient insensible and the anaesthesia is kept up by means of ether.' (Clover's combined gas-ether apparatus was not used. Nitrous oxide was first administered from an ordinary type of apparatus and ether was then given from a felt cone.)

The ' chloroformist ' to St. Mary's Hospital stated that ' chloroform has been almost exclusively given here during the last five years ', by Clover's apparatus (see Figs. 53 and 54), ' and the ether ', given from a felt cone containing sponge, ' has only been adopted as an experiment, in deference to its reputation for safety '. But Sydenham J. Knott, late anaesthetist to the hospital, wrote independently : ' I am now in the habit of using ether, nitrous oxide, or both combined. . . . And I never give chloroform except when requested to do so by the operator, and that is now very seldom '.

G. E. Norton replied from the Middlesex Hospital :

' I am in the habit of administering chloroform, ether, and nitrous oxide gas. . . . Chloroform I prefer for children and elderly people . . . [and] in operations about the mouth . . . [and] eye operations. . . . Chloroform I administer on a small frame covered with flannel, with a piece of sponge inside, on which the chloroform is poured. . . . Ether I administer with one of Hawksley's inhalers. . . .'

The Surgical Registrar at St. Thomas's Hospital made the orthodox statement that chloroform was given to children and old people, ether to adults for general surgery and nitrous oxide to dental patients. Where speed was especially important, in general surgery, a chloroform-ether sequence was used. He gave the impression, however, that despite new-fangled ideas, chloroform was still the anaesthetic of choice at St. Thomas's.

' Chloroform ', he wrote, ' is always administered by an instrument known as Millikin's modification of Snow's inhaler. When employed in the wards, it is merely given on a fold of lint. The instrument used for administering ether is Golding

[1] *Brit. med. J.*, 1876, ii, 113, 168.

Bird's [¹]. Millikin's modification of Snow's instrument has been in use since 1856. All changes have been tried within the last three years. For a time, a mixture of ether, chloroform, and rectified spirits in equal parts was tried, but was discontinued on account of its being very slow in taking effect, whilst the after-effects were unsatisfactory. Clover's [chloroform] bag was tried for a few months, but was discontinued on account of the house-surgeons (there being no special chloroformist) preferring the instrument which had been so long in use, and finding the bag cumbrous. . . . Also, on students leaving the hospital, they preferred to be acquainted with an instrument which, when in the country, would be more portable and more easy of application.' 'Chloroform', he added, 'should always be administered, as it is at this hospital, in a small room adjoining the theatre, previously to the patient being brought in for operation, as he does not then become excited, and is more quickly brought under the influence. Great objection should be made to the administration of chloro-form in the wards.' ²

The Resident Medical Officer and chloroformist at University College Hospital replied that a nitrous oxide-ether sequence, administered from Clover's apparatus, was in use for all cases except short operations (for which nitrous oxide alone was used), operations on young children, and operations in or about the mouth (for which chloroform was preferred). Ether had been in use only since the beginning of 1875, ' chloroform having been previously employed, given either on lint or by means of Mr. Clover's chloroform apparatus. The change to ether was made in deference to the generally expressed opinion of the profession that ether was much safer than chloroform. Before the introduction of Mr. Clover's [" combined "] apparatus, the inconveniences of ether, especially in unpractised hands, were much felt, and some of the surgeons always preferred chloroform ; but the efficiency of the present method, and the time saved, have produced an universal revolution of opinion in its favour '.

At the Westminster Hospital chloroform was preferred for children ; Clover's apparatus was used. In other operations

¹ Golding Bird's inhaler was a leather cylinder with an inspiratory valve at one end, the other being open and adapted to fit tightly over mouth and nose. As in Rendle's inhaler (see Fig. 67), a flannel bag and sponge could be inserted. Just behind the nick in the rim, accommodating the inhaler to the bridge of the nose, was an expiratory valve. Bird claimed this valve as an advantage but in fact it prevented the volume of the mask from being used as an addition to the ' physiological ' dead space. (*Med. Times, Lond.*, 1875, ii, 281.)

² *Brit. med. J.*, 1876, i, 12–13.

ether was reluctantly given by Mr. Beer in a cone of felt containing sponge. 'After using chloroform in three thousand cases without accident', protested Mr. Beer, ' the outcry raised by the journals has compelled me to substitute ether. I believe one cannot abolish sensation and motion by any known means without a certain amount of risk. It appears to me that one thing most essential to the safe administration of any anaesthetic is, that the person administering it should attend to the patient only, and not to the operation. With this precaution, and, if the administration be prolonged, with the use of Clover's apparatus, I believe that chloroform is practically as safe as it is certainly convenient.' [1]

The House Surgeon and chloroformist at the Royal London Ophthalmic Hospital wrote :

' We used bichloride of methylene almost exclusively . . . until about a year ago [the early part of 1875] but it is now entirely abandoned in favour of ether and chloroform. The methylene bichloride was in use at the Ophthalmic Hospital for about five years and was administered at least five thousand times without a fatal case occurring. . . . At length a fatal case occurred [about December 1874] and the feeling in favour of ether, already strong, gained the upper hand, and led to the disuse of methylene.'

He further stated that ether was given on a towel cone or conical sponge. In very delicate eye operations, however, to avoid both irritation of the larynx, provoking coughing, and post-operative excitement a preliminary dose of chloroform was customary. In such cases Hawksley's ether inhaler was used, which ' answers very well for the purpose. A small cup is adapted near the mouth-piece for containing chloroform, which may be used to begin the inhalation, and may then be shut off. . . .' [2]

Alfred Coleman, who was dental surgeon to both St. Bartholomew's Hospital and to the Dental Hospital of London, wrote :

' 1. The anaesthetics I employ are nitrous oxide alone, or in combination with ether, both in dental cases. 2. I use a method of my own, an apparatus [see Fig. 86] which has an arrangement for passing nitrous oxide through ether when desired ; it is upon the plan adopted by Mr. Clover, only much simpler. . . . 3. I have quite given up chloroform. . . . 4. I can only state

[1] Brit. med. J., 1876, i, 13.   [2] Ibid. i, 73.

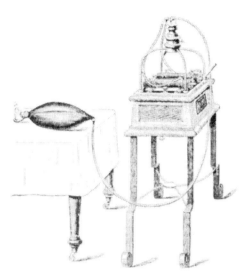

FIG. 86.—COLEMAN'S APPARATUS FOR NITROUS
OXIDE AND ETHER

Coleman in 1881 described it as follows :

'It consists of an iron stand with drawer to hold necessary
appliances. The stand supports two bottles of gas so
arranged that in case of one failing the other can be
employed (Barth's plan, we believe). The gas passes from
either bottle to a sausage-shaped bag, and directly from this
to the face-piece, a two-way stopcock only intervening.
This arrangement (Clover's) possesses great advantages, as
the gas comes to the patient more readily than when its
progress is impeded by the friction of a tube. Above the
gas bottles is shown an arrangement for administering ether
with the gas. It consists of a vessel to receive the ether,
under the surface of which a tube dips ; by turning a two-
way stopcock the current of gas is made to pass through
the ether. An outer vessel for holding hot water is also
shown, but we have not found it necessary even in the
coldest weather.'

that I think the method pursued by Mr. Clover of administering
nitrous oxide, then nitrous oxide and ether, and finally air and
ether, the safest and most perfect method of administering
anaesthetics yet introduced, the only drawback being the cost
and complicated nature of the apparatus in its present form.' [1]

[1] *Brit. med. J.*, 1876, i, 74.

John H. Morgan, lately house surgeon at St. George's Hospital, wrote that he was in the habit of using ether for adults in all cases and also for children, except very young ones. At that time, January 1876, Morgan used a sponge enclosed in a felt cone for giving ether. In May of the same year the *British Medical Journal* published a short description of an inhaler invented by Morgan, who was then Surgical Registrar at St. George's. It consisted of a double-walled metal case into which fitted a felt cone with a sponge in the apex. Air was drawn in by the patient, through an inspiratory valve in the lower wall of the inhaler, just behind its apex, and passed through the ether-soaked sponge. The exhaled mixture found its way, through a valve set at a little distance behind the inflatable rubber rim of the inhaler, into the space between the double walls of the metal case. Having circulated round the inhaler, to restore heat lost through the evaporation of the ether (cf. Fig. 82), the exhaled mixture passed out through a third valve and was led away from the immediate neighbourhood of the patient, through a long length of tubing (cf. Hawksley's inhaler, p. 321).[1]

A. E. Sansom (cf. pp. 236–9), who in 1876 was Assistant Physician at the London Hospital, stated in his reply to the *British Medical Journal's* questionnaire, that he now used nitrous oxide, chloroform, chloroform mixed with absolute alcohol, and ether.

For children under seven he gave ' pure chloroform . . . drop by drop upon a cambric handkerchief. . . . There should never be more than 5 drops at one time upon its surface. When chloroform and alcohol are used ', he added, ' the quantity applied is almost (or even quite) immaterial '.

Sansom advocated the use of an ether inhaler extemporized from a newspaper folded in three and covered ' while flat with an ordinary cambric pocket-handkerchief, leaving a small portion of the latter below the edge, and then rolling the whole so as to form a hollow cylinder about four inches in diameter. The free portion of the handkerchief closes one extremity, the ether is poured into the interior of the cylinder, and the other extremity is closely adapted over the nose and mouth of the patient. . . . I have always looked upon chloroform as a dangerous agent,' he wrote, ' though I believe its dangers early

[1] *Brit. med. J.*, 1876, i, 567.

in the administration to be solely due to the *brusque* administration of a too strong atmosphere ' (cf. p. 200, Snow's opinion).[1]

Moss, of King's College Hospital, wrote :

' When the choice of anaesthetic is in my hands, I usually prefer chloroform, provided, after examination of the patient, there are no reasons to contraindicate its use.'

When the choice did not rest with Moss, however, he compromised. ' When I give ether to adults,' he explained, ' I commence with a short inhalation of chloroform well diluted with atmospheric air, and keep up the state of insensibility with ether.'

A chloroformist who was quickly becoming converted to the use of a gas-ether sequence was G. Eastes of the Great Northern Hospital.

' 1. I have administered chloroform extensively for the last twelve years in all kinds of surgical cases ', he wrote, ' and, upon the whole, have had much cause to be satisfied with it. A few years ago, I used bichloride of methylene ; I have also within the last year given ether alone in many cases, and am now beginning to use nitrous oxide gas and ether . . . for operations in adults lasting more than a minute. . . . I have given chloroform by Clover's apparatus since 1865, always with most satisfactory results. Ether I have given upon a sponge, gas and ether I am now administering by means of Clover's newly introduced apparatus [Fig. 83]. The bichloride of methylene was always given in a leathern cone lined with flannel.' [2]

G. C. Coles, formerly chloroformist at the Great Northern Hospital, also replied :

' 1. The anaesthetics I have mostly employed have been chloroform and bichloride of methylene, although, at the suggestion of my friend Dr. B. W. Richardson, I have frequently experimented with others, such as hydramyl [pentane, C_5H_{12}], methylic ether, etc. I have also used a mixture of equal parts of chloroform and ether successfully . . . which was the anaesthetic constantly resorted to at the London Surgical Home. Ether alone and nitrous oxide I have not tried, being satisfied with chloroform.

' 2. The apparatus I have and still do employ is the one known as Snow's Modified Inhaler, with this modification of my own in the valves, viz., that, instead of india-rubber valves, which from moisture and mucous expectoration are frequently rendered

[1] *Brit. med. J.*, 1876, i, 74.　　　　[2] *Ibid.* i, 162.

incompetent, I have had valves made of brass foil, and lined with chamois leather. In the case of infants, I use simply a piece of lint quadrupled, and pressed over the nose, the lower part remaining open, so that the carbonic acid exhaled may find a ready exit. . . .

'I trust you will be able to obtain the opinions also of Dr. Richardson, Messrs. Clover, Woodhouse Braine, Dr. Jones (late of St. George's), Mr. Warrington Haward, Dr. Potter and Mr. Peter Marshall. It will be interesting to compare these various opinions, as in medicine there is always, apparently to me a popular, or rather, perhaps, a fashionable method of proceeding, which lasts only temporarily, and frequent recourse is again had to remedies long since sunk into oblivion.' [1]

Dr. J. M. Crombie, late Resident Medical Officer at the Cancer Hospital, wrote :

'I invariably use chloroform, except when expressly requested to employ ether or nitrous oxide.'

Dr. E. Holland, Assistant Physician to the Hospital for Women, wrote :

'For eighteen years, my attention has been much occupied by the subject of anaesthesia. . . . Of the three standard anaesthetics now in vogue, chloroform, ether and bichloride of methylene, recent experience leads me to feel pretty sure that ether is the safest of the three, and not inferior . . . to either of the others. In midwifery practice, I invariably give chloroform, and desire no better anaesthetic. . . . I usually administer it by my modification of Junker's inhaler ; or on a square (five inches) of amadou [porous tissue derived from fungi], or on a pad of lint, made of five thicknesses, five inches square, and tacked together. . . .'

From these answers it appears that about three-quarters of the important London hospitals had abandoned the general use of chloroform anaesthesia—half in favour of ether, a quarter in favour of Clover's gas-ether sequence. The majority of anaesthetists changed willingly, from a genuine belief that ether or gas-ether anaesthesia was safer than chloroform ; a few changed reluctantly in obedience to the dictates of public opinion. At the rest of the London hospitals administrators showed the courage of conviction and continued to use chloroform as the anaesthetic of choice in general surgery.

[1] *Brit. med. J.*, 1876, i, 163.

The majority of anaesthetists, even the most enthusiastic users of ether or gas and ether, continued, however, to use chloroform in certain types of operation and of patient : (i) in operations in or about the mouth, nose, and throat ; (ii) in operations on the eye ; (iii) in setting fractures ; (iv) in midwifery (although not in gynaecological operations) ; (v) in young children (under 5 years old) ; and (vi) as a general rule, in the elderly (over 60 years old).

Considering each of these six classes in turn, one may find the following reasons why the use of chloroform was retained :

(i) At this date (1876) when endotracheal anaesthesia was in its extreme infancy (cf. Appendix E) and when methods of anaesthesia other than by inhalation were the exception and never the rule, in operations anywhere in the region of the face and neck the difficulties of maintaining anaesthesia and at the same time leaving the operative field clear for the surgeon were very great. Existing methods of administering ether necessitated the close and often prolonged applications of either a cone or a Clover's type of facepiece.[1] The powerful action of chloroform, on the other hand, made the patient deeply insensible very quickly and by intermittent readministration, using the open-drop method with a Skinner's mask or folded lint held above the patient's face, anaesthesia could be maintained, with a reasonable degree of effectiveness, over long periods without seriously hindering the surgeon or necessitating the removal of instruments from the region of the nose and mouth.

The greatly increased mucous secretion caused by ether (and not checked at this time by premedicating the patient with atropine) was another disadvantage of its use in this type of operation ; and as it had not yet become practicable to pack off the throat, the danger of the patient aspirating operative debris into the lungs during coughing provoked by the irritant qualities of ether was formidable.

(ii) The application of a cone or facepiece was a hindrance in ophthalmic operations. In addition to the simplicity of its administration chloroform was thought by many to cause less turgescence in the eye, and despite a greater tendency to vomiting the patient was likely to be more tranquil both during anaesthesia and in the post-operative period under chloroform than under ether. Nevertheless Butler, of the Royal London

---

[1] Similar drawbacks were entailed in the use of gas or gas and ether anaesthesia.

Ophthalmic Hospital, stated that ether was extensively used there (cf. p. 335).

(iii) It was feared that the newly reunited ends of fractured bones might become deranged during the turbulent recovery period which frequently followed ether anaesthesia.

(iv) The custom of maintaining an analgesic rather than an anaesthetic state during normal labour was firmly established (cf. p. 193), and for this chloroform was found to be admirably suited. It was administered in small intermittent doses so that the danger of an overdose causing cardiac syncope (unless through gross carelessness) was held to be negligible. The occurrence of ventricular fibrillations (see pp. 452–4) was not yet envisaged nor was the danger of serious damage to the liver generally appreciated.

(v) Very young children were found to take chloroform more readily than ether. Nineteenth century beliefs in this connection were summarized in 1901 by F. W. Hewitt as follows :

' The upper air-passages of *infants and very young children* are so sensitive that ether often causes some irritation and respiratory difficulty. This has led many to prefer chloroform which is certainly inhaled with comparative ease by children. It is a mistake, however, to suppose that children are not so susceptible as adults to the toxic effects of this agent, and that with them fatalities are practically unknown. It is true that children inhale chloroform freely, and that they are not as prone as adults to certain forms of respiratory embarrassment. It is certain also that children may be rescued from conditions of respiratory and circulatory depression which in adults would be attended by more immediate risk to life.' [1]

More than thirty years earlier, in 1867, Giraldès, a member of the Société de Chirurgie, in Paris, had said during a discussion on chloroform :

'. . . I wish to protest against the immunity [from accidents due to chloroform] which people are disposed to attribute to childhood. That immunity does not exist.' [2]

(vi) Before it became customary to premedicate patients with atropine before ether anaesthesia the increase in mucous

---

[1] Hewitt, F. W. 1901 (2nd ed.). *Anaesthetics and their administration.* London. 116.

[2] *Bull. Soc. Chirurgie Paris*, 1867, **6,** 314.

secretion very frequently led to post-operative chest complications. This proved a serious deterrent from the use of ether for old people (cf. pp. 420–2, 588). Nevertheless, in cases where vascular or cardiac disease was known or strongly suspected to exist, even the most diehard chloroformist was apt to remember that the Chloroform Committee of 1864 had found chloroform to be a cardiac depressant, and in spite of the risk of bronchitis it was customary to administer ether to such patients.

In 1876 administration of ether by some form of cone was still the most prevalent method. But in the following year two inhalers were produced, one by Clover the other by Lambert H. Ormsby, Surgeon to the Meath Hospital, Dublin. Both these inhalers quickly captured the popular fancy.

Clover briefly described his new apparatus (see Figs. 88 92), which he called the 'Portable Regulating Ether-Inhaler', on January 20, 1877, in the *British Medical Journal* : [1]

'. . . 1. It has no valves ; 2. It supplies the vapour so gradually that patients breathe quietly ; 3. It produces sleep in two minutes ; 4. It does not require fresh ether during the continuance of an operation ; 5. The recovery from a short operation is more speedy than with most other inhalers ; 6. It does not need to be warmed before it is used ; 7. No sponge or felt is required ; 8. Ether left in the inhaler can be saved for another time.

'The face-piece is edged with an air-cushion. The ether-vessel and water-chamber rotate upon the mount of the face-piece. When the instrument is first applied, the stopper should be towards the patient's forehead, and now he breathes in and out of the bag directly. As the ether-vessel is turned round, the air is obliged to enter the ether-chamber and pass through it before it reaches the bag ; and, when the vessel is turned half-round, so that the stopper is opposite the patient's chin, all the air going in and out of the bag must pass through the ether-vessel. Two ounces of ether (specific gravity 735) are enough for a long operation. Usually, an ounce and a half is the proper charge. The opening for supplying the ether is arranged to prevent an excessive quantity being supplied, but, to guard against the possibility of a few drops escaping through the inner openings, there are two recesses made to catch them, and prevent the liquid ether from reaching the patient's lips.

'The ether-vessel is spherical in shape, and one half is surrounded by a closed water-compartment, to prevent the ether

[1] *Brit. med. J.*, 1877, i, 69.

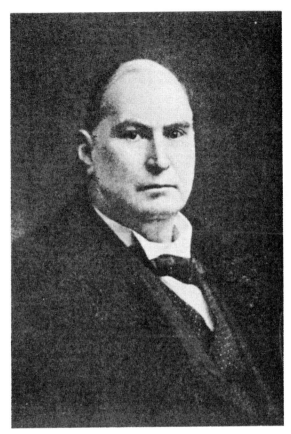

FIG. 87.—LAMBERT HEPENSTAL ORMSBY
(1850–1923)

Born in New Zealand, but removed to Ireland at
an early age ; surgeon, knighted in 1903. Inventor
of the ether inhaler which bears his name.

from becoming too cold. The bag . . . can be kept on one side so as not to obstruct the light in operations on the eye. The instrument is intended for giving ether without gas, but, by connecting the bag with a supply of nitrous oxide, it forms a tolerably efficient substitute for the gas- and ether-inhaler.'

This is the inhaler by which Clover is chiefly remembered. Ironically enough, Clover himself never cared for its use. ' My experience with this Portable Inhaler is limited ', he wrote, ' simply because I prefer my original Gas and Ether Inhaler '.[1]

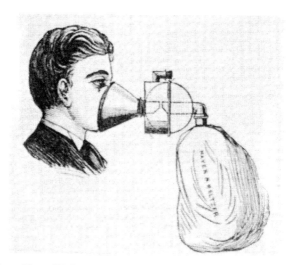

FIG. 88.—CLOVER'S ' PORTABLE REGULATING ETHER INHALER ' (1877)

The original portable inhaler certainly had several awkward features which Clover himself would probably have corrected had he used the instrument more. A serious objection to it was its inflexibility. This shortcoming was not successfully remedied until 1891 when, only a few weeks before his death, Charles E. Sheppard (cf. p. 474), a young anaesthetist of great promise, devised an angle-piece so that the inhaler could be used for a patient in the lateral or in the prone position (see Fig. 91).[2]

[1] Clover, J. T. MS. note now in the possession of the Nuffield Department of Anaesthetics, Oxford.
[2] *Brit. med. J.*, 1891, ii, 68.

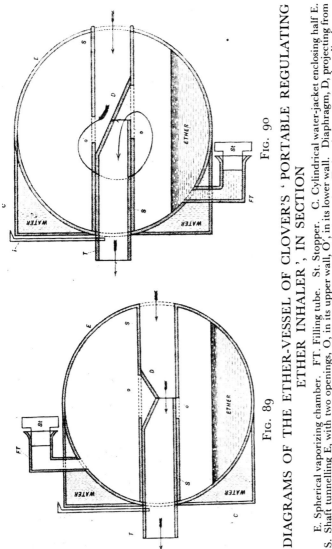

Fig. 89

Fig. 90

DIAGRAMS OF THE ETHER-VESSEL OF CLOVER'S 'PORTABLE REGULATING
ETHER INHALER', IN SECTION

E. Spherical vaporizing chamber. FT. Filling tube. St. Stopper. C. Cylindrical water-jacket enclosing half E.
S. Shaft tunnelling E, with two openings, O, in its upper wall, O', in its lower wall. Diaphragm, D, projecting from
the upper wall of S, closed half the shaft diagonally. Into S fitted a tube, T, bearing at one end a diaphragm
similar to D, its other end attached to the facepiece.

S, carrying the sphere and water-jacket with it, turned through a half circle upon T. When FT was at the top
(Fig. 89) the diaphragms and walls of S and T were in such relation to each other that O and O' were closed. The
patient then breathed air directly from and into the bag. As S was turned O and O' became increasingly opened and
the diaphragms deflected an increasing amount of air into E. The proportion of air passing into E was indicated
by a scale engraved on C and the index-finger, i, fixed in the wall of T.

345

It was left, however, for Frederic Hewitt to make the most important amendments (see Fig. 93). Hewitt described his own version of Clover's ' portable regulating ether inhaler ' in the second edition of his textbook on anaesthetics, in 1901 :

' It differs from Clover's original pattern in the following particulars : (1) Its internal calibre or air-way is very much larger ; (2) Instead of the ether rescrvoir rotating upon the central tube, the central tube rotates within the fixed reservoir ; (3) The face-piece is screwed into the ether reservoir so that the latter cannot be unexpectedly detached from the former ; (4) The ether reservoir can be adjusted, whatever the position of the patient may be, so that ether may be poured into it through its wide-mouthed filling-tube without removing the inhaler from the face. In order to secure these improvements, I found it necessary to materially modify the internal mechanism of Clover's original apparatus, and to have two separate inner tubes which are made to revolve as one tube by the indicating handle which fits into each. The large bore of the apparatus is distinctly of advantage, not only in lessening the initial unpleasant sensations of re-breathing, but in reducing asphyxial phenomena (stertor, cyanosis, and laboured breathing) of well-established ethcr anaesthesia. . . . In cold weather, and particularly when about to anaesthetize powerfully-built or alcoholic subjects, partly immerse the ether reservoir in warm water for a few moments.' [1]

Hewitt had previously modified the original type of ' Clover ' for giving a nitrous oxide-ether sequence (cf. p. 344) :

' In addition to a Clover's portable regulating ether inhaler ', wrote Hewitt, '. . . and a cylinder or pair of cylinders for thc supply of nitrous oxide . . . all that is needed is a gas-bag capable of holding about, but not more than, two gallons of gas, and furnished with the special form of stopcock . . . which I find to give the best results in ordinarily administering nitrous oxide [see Fig. 125, pp. 476-80]. The ether chamber, which should be slightly warmed in cold weather . . . should be charged with an ounce and a half of ether, and its indicator turned to " O ". The gas-bag should be filled or nearly filled with gas, according to the age and strength of the patient. . . . The bag should be disconnected from the gas supply tube and placed near at hand. A face-piece of appropriate size should be fitted to the ether chamber. . . . The face-piece with the charged ether chamber is then applied during an expiration. . . . When the respiration [of air] is seen to be proceeding freely . . . the charged gas-

[1] Hewitt, F. W. 1901 (2nd ed.). *Anaesthetics and their administration*. London. 277-8.

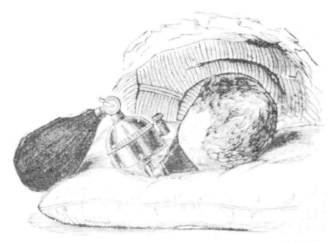

FIG. 91.—SHEPPARD'S 'ANGULAR ADJUSTER' (1891)

Attached between the facepiece and ether vessel of Clover's
'Portable Regulating Ether Inhaler'.

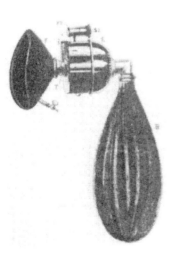 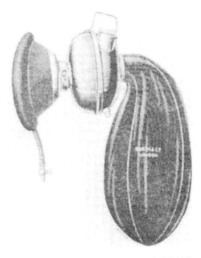

FIG. 92.—THE ORIGINAL
TYPE OF CLOVER'S
'PORTABLE REGULAT-
ING ETHER INHALER'
For comparison with Fig. 93.

FIG. 93.—HEWITT'S MODI-
FICATION OF CLOVER'S
'PORTABLE REGULATING
ETHER INHALER' (c. 1901)

347

bag is attached to the ether chamber. Air will still be breathed, but now through the valves of the special stopcock. When the valves are heard to be working properly gas is turned on, and likewise breathed through the valves. Three or four respirations (or about one-half of the contents of the bag) are allowed to escape. The valve action is now stopped by turning the tap at the upper part of the stopcock. At the same moment at which

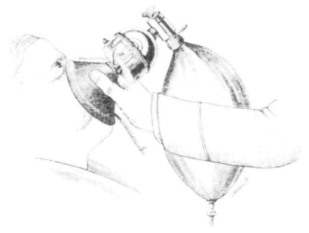

FIG. 94.—HEWITT'S ADAPTATION OF CLOVER'S
' PORTABLE REGULATING ETHER INHALER '

for administering a nitrous oxide-ether sequence—showing the detachable bag of gas and between it and the ether reservoir Hewitt's stopcock (for diagram of which see Fig. 125).

In this inhaler, as in all but the earliest ' Clovers ', the inter-relation of the tubes and diaphragms (cf. Figs. 89 and 90) was controlled not by rotating the ether reservoir but simply by moving the indicator handle, here seen with its pointer between the figures ' 1 ' and ' 2 ' engraved on the outside of the water-jacket. In this position nearly half the stream of nitrous oxide was deflected through the ether reservoir.

the patient begins to breathe gas backwards and forwards, the rotation of the ether chamber, for the addition of ether vapour, should be commenced. . . . The administrator will . . . find that he can, in a few seconds from the commencement of the administration, rotate the ether chamber as far as " 1 " or " 1½ ". . . . Should swallowing or coughing arise, he must rotate more slowly. Respiration soon becomes deep and regular, and more and more ether may be admitted.' [1]

[1] Hewitt, F. W. 1893. *Anaesthetics and their administration.* London. 183.

Ormsby had tested his inhaler over a period of nine months before he described it in the medical journals, a week or two after the first account of Clover's portable regulating ether inhaler had appeared. The inhaler consisted of :

' (*a*) An india-rubber flexible bag, covered over with a network, to prevent undue expansion during expiration. (*b*) A soft metallic mouthpiece which allows of adaptation to any face ; . . .

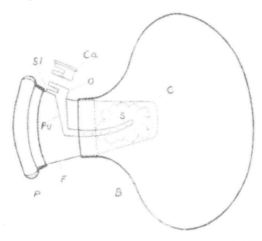

FIG. 95.—DIAGRAM OF ORMSBY'S ETHER INHALER
(1877)

P. Indiarubber pad. F. Zinc facepiece. B. Breathing bag. C. Wire cage fixed in the mouth of B, containing S : sponge. Fu. Funnel-shaped tube passing downwards into the inhaler from the outside of the facepiece. Where it turned inwards, it divided into two arms (one shown) pierced with holes. These arms penetrated the sponge. In the widened part, O, of the tube, Fu, which rose above the facepiece, was a slot, Sl. O was covered by a cap, Ca, similarly slotted. By turning Ca upon O, so that the two slots coincided, air could enter the interior of the inhaler.

along the border applied to the face it is lined with india-rubber tubing, in order to fit more closely, and thus prevent the ingress or exit of air.'

In the facepiece was a simple sliding valve, ' so as to admit air if required and allow its escape if necessary. In the body of the inhaler there is a cone-shaped wire cage, into which fits a similarly shaped hollow sponge, into which the ether is poured, and the inhaler is then ready for administration. If it is necessary to give more ether, in a prolonged operation, there is a tube passing down to the centre of the sponge, into which the ether can be poured without raising the mouthpiece from the face '.[1]

Ormsby's inhaler achieved a more immediate popularity than Clover's ' portable ', possibly because Clover himself was

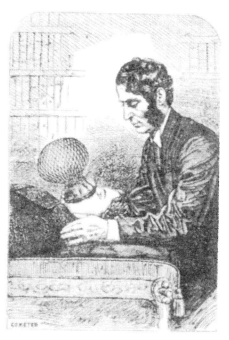

FIG. 96.—ORMSBY'S INHALER

in use, showing the soft metallic facepiece moulded to the patient's face and the bag enclosed in a net to prevent over-distension.

not enthusiastic about his own inhaler and gave only a brief description of it in a single journal. Writing in June 1877, Ormsby was able to say, ' I have been informed by Messrs. Coxeter & Son . . . that many of the leading hospitals in London, Dublin, and the provincial towns of England, including those of Manchester, Birmingham, Leeds, and Liverpool, are using the ether inhaler suggested by me '.[2]

[1] *Lancet*, 1877, i, 218.   [2] *Ibid.* i, 863.

Sixteen years later Hewitt compared the two inhalers :

' For *inducing* anaesthesia by means of ether there is no apparatus which can be compared to that invented by Clover, for the anaesthetic vapour may be admitted so gradually that

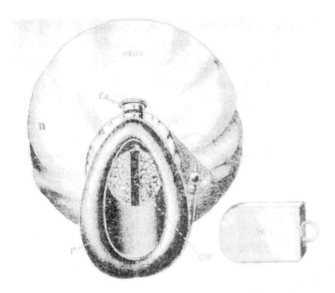

FIG. 97.—ORMSBY'S INHALER

(Woodhouse Braine's pattern) with Hewitt's modification— the addition of a compartment, CW, dividing the sponge cage longitudinally. Into CW was inserted ' a small metal water chamber ', W, which prevented the sponge freezing during administration (a fault of the original ' Ormsby ').

    P. Inflatable rubber rim to facepiece.
    CW. Compartment to receive W.
    W. Water container.
    Ca. Cap controlling the entry of air into the inhaler.
    B. Bag.

the initial discomforts are reduced to a minimum. But for *maintaining* ether anaesthesia Ormsby's inhaler is equal, and in many cases superior to Clover's. I have on several occasions changed from a Clover's to an Ormsby's inhaler with marked improvement in the symptoms of the patient. For example, I have often known cyanosis to quickly vanish and the breathing to become less hampered by effecting this change of inhalers during deep ether anaesthesia.'

'The Ormsby's inhaler which I myself employ . . .' Hewitt stated, 'is identical in its general construction with Mr. Woodhouse Braine's pattern; [*i.e.* "an inhaler possessing no filling tube and having a very capacious bag of red rubber without a network covering"] but it possesses a simple internal arrangement . . . for preventing the temperature of the sponge becoming too low during administration. There has always been this objection to Ormsby's inhaler. It may, of course, be overcome by simply wringing out the sponge in hot water before commencing, by warming the body of the inhaler, by replacing the frozen sponge during the administration, or by other devices. But the best plan that I know is to have the cage of the inhaler so made that it will allow of a small portable metal water-chamber being introduced. By having the sponge cage longitudinally divided into three compartments, and using the central compartment . . . for the water-chamber, the two side partitions are left for the sponge or sponges. By placing the little chamber in warm water for a few minutes it takes up heat, and will thus either prevent the tendency of the sponge to freeze, or, should it have become frozen, will quickly thaw it. . . . If one has a hand basin of hot water it is very easy to keep the water-chamber warm by immersing it and replacing it from time to time.'[1]

While anaesthetists in England and Ireland were thus busily developing what Hewitt termed the 'close' methods of administration, and which he defined as the use of a 'bag inhaler . . . so that to-and-fro breathing is permitted, and the supply of air during the inhalation of ether-vapour is intentionally restricted', in America the first signs of a tendency towards 'open' methods of etherization (see Appendix D) with free access of air were just beginning to be noticeable.

The inhaler which marked the inception of this new phase in American anaesthesia was O. H. Allis's, although in fact the large 'dead space' in the inhaler allowed carbon dioxide from the patient's exhalations to accumulate. 'The instrument', wrote Laurence Turnbull, 'was first exhibited before the Philadelphia County Medical Society on October 14, 1874, and described in a paper . . . published in the *Philadelphia Medical Times*, No. 162'. It consisted of a stout metal cage-work, oval in section and 'sufficiently large to cover the lower part of the face. A bandage was laced between the bars (which were $\frac{1}{4}$ inch broad and $\frac{1}{4}$ inch apart) across and across 'dividing the instrument into parallel sections' lengthwise. When the lacing

[1] Hewitt, F. W. 1893. *Anaesthetics and their administration*. London. 150, 151.

ALLIS'S ETHER INHALER

in use in the United States from 1874 onwards.

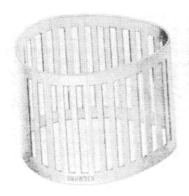
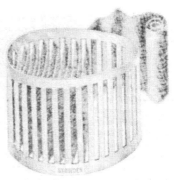

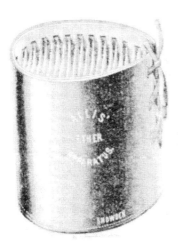
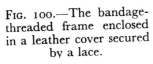
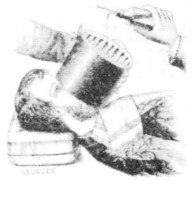

Fig. 100.—The bandage-threaded frame enclosed in a leather cover secured by a lace.

Fig. 101.—Administration with Allis's inhaler—ether is being dropped on to the bandage from a drop-bottle.

was completed a leather cover, shaped rather like a detachable shirt-cuff, was fastened round the inhaler, but leaving both ends free.[1]

The inhaler was ' placed upon the face of the patient dry ' and the ether gradually poured on from a drop bottle. ' When the effect of the anaesthetic is apparent, a single layer of a coarse towel may be laid over the nose and mouth, and the instrument replaced. This is a wise precaution against vomiting or spitting.' It was claimed that ' the average time required for the production of complete unconsciousness was eight minutes and that the average amount of ether used during half an hour of anaesthesia was one to two ounces '.[2]

The advantages claimed for Allis's inhaler over the towel cone method of etherization were as follows :

' 1st. It presents a large surface for the liberation of ether vapor. The partitions are made of thin bandage, and the air coming to both sides of each layer, sets the ether vapor free more rapidly than is possible in the use of a towel or sponge.

' 2d. It is open at the top, and ether can be added constantly if desired, and in small quantities, without removing from the face. The sponge and towel require removal, and the ether is usually poured on them in quantities.

' 3d. The ether vapor falls by its weight, as it is heavier than the air ; and as the instrument fits the face the patient gets the full advantage of it.

' 4th. It does not cover the patient's eyes, does not terrify him, and he often passes under its influence without a struggle.

' 5th. By its proper use the laryngeal irritation may be wholly avoided, the anaesthetic effect as easily gained as is possible with the use of ether, a great economy of ether and great comfort to the patient.'

In the opposite scale were set these disadvantages :

' 1st. That the exhaled vapor is . . . diffused in the air, to be breathed by the operator and his assistants. For a single operation, this is not of much importance, but where there are a number of cases the arrangement is not conducive to the comfort of the operator.

' 2d. The bandage of muslin across the bottom becomes clogged with moisture and saliva, and at times by discharges from the stomach, and cannot be so readily removed.

---

[1] Turnbull, L. 1880 (2nd ed.). *The advantages and accidents of artificial anaesthesia.* London. 237.
[2] *Trans. int. Congr. Med.,* 1890, **1,** 143.

' 3d. Owing to the peculiar arrangement of the muslin strips, it is tedious when it is required for a number of patients to remove or replace them.' [1]

These disadvantages weighed lightly, however, and the inhaler became popular in the United States. Nevertheless by the end of the century some anaesthetists had lost sight of Allis's original intention that the access of air should be quite free. There was a marked tendency to elongate the outer cover (made during the eighteen-nineties of rubber, not leather) into a truncated cone and to pinch together or fold over the apex ' in order to increase the air space above, and the nose space below ' and to ' prevent the escape of ether, and administer it in more concentrated form '. The frame itself was no longer closely approximated to the face but was supported just above the tip of the nose by the walls of the cover. Nor was it threaded with bandage but was loosely packed with gauze, a gauze diaphragm closing the end of the frame nearest the face, to prevent liquid ether splashing through.[2]

Although Allis's inhaler was described in some of the English medical journals in the year following its introduction into American practice, and although it was ' confidently recommended ' by Martin Oxley, Physician to the Liverpool Infirmary for Children, who had seen it used in New York, it never became popular in this country.[3]

[1] Turnbull, L.   1880 (2nd ed.).   *The advantages and accidents of artificial anaesthesia.* London.   239–41.
[2] *Med. Rec., N.Y.*, 1899, **56,** 953–6.
[3] *Lancet,* 1875, ii, 874 ; cf. Hewitt, F. W.   1893.   *Anaesthetics and their administration.* London.   136.

PART FIVE

CONTINENTAL DEVELOPMENTS

CHAPTER XII

PAUL BERT'S CONTRIBUTION

The Revival of Interest in Anaesthetic Problems in France.

BETWEEN 1878 and 1885, a time when English anaesthetists were settling down to consolidate the gains of some thirty years of varied anaesthetic experience, Paul Bert made a serious attempt to persuade French surgeons to adopt new methods of inhalation anaesthesia based, as he believed, upon sounder principles than were those in general use among them. He succeeded in interesting only a very small number of his immediate contemporaries, although eventually his work on anaesthesia had a wider influence.

He began, in November 1878, by reading before a meeting of the section of physiology of the Académie des Sciences a paper ' On the possibility of obtaining prolonged anaesthesia with nitrous oxide and upon the harmlessness of that anaesthetic '.

Bert's own interest in this particular subject was directly due to his researches into the physiological effects of atmospheric pressure. His monograph, ' La pression barométrique ' had appeared earlier in 1878.

In this first paper on nitrous oxide anaesthesia Bert, referring to the current methods of administration, pointed out that ' this form of insensibility cannot be prolonged because at the very moment at which it becomes adequate, asphyxial symptoms appear and these soon become formidable. . . . This is because anaesthesia can only be achieved by making the patient breathe pure nitrous oxide without any admixture of air ; as a result asphyxia goes hand in hand with anaesthesia. I proposed ', he said, ' to remedy this serious inconvenience and I am now able to obtain an indefinitely prolonged anaesthesia without the least danger of asphyxia.

' The fact that nitrous oxide must be administered pure indicates that in order to be absorbed by the organism in sufficient quantity, the tension of the gas must be equal to one atmosphere. In order to achieve this at normal pressure, the gas must be in the proportion of 100 per cent. But let us suppose that the patient is placed in an apparatus where the pressure can be increased to two atmospheres ; then one could submit him to the desired tension by making him inhale a mixture of 50 per cent. nitrous oxide with 50 per cent. air. Thus one could achieve anaesthesia while maintaining the normal quantity of oxygen in the blood, and it follows that the normal conditions of respiration would be preserved.

' This is what, in fact, has been done ; but I must add that up to the present I have experimented only upon animals.'

After giving details of these experiments Bert concluded :

' I now feel justified by the results of my experiments on animals, in most strongly recommending to surgeons the use of nitrous oxide under pressure in order to obtain an anaesthesia of long duration. . . .

' I see only one difficulty—the apparatus necessary for administering nitrous oxide under pressure. I realize that this is an insuperable obstacle for military surgeons and for country practitioners. But most large towns, and it is there that almost all major operations are performed, have [therapeutic] establishments which specialize in compressed air bathing. The installation of a chamber to accommodate, besides the patient and the operator, some dozen assistants, would not cost more than 10,000 francs, a trifling expenditure in hospital administration.

' There are, also, minor difficulties the solution of which rests with the surgeons ; it is up to them to solve all the many questions of detail which the application of a new therapeutic agent always raises. For my part it must suffice that I, as a physiologist, have drawn attention to this agent, have shown the immense advantages of its use and have stressed, among other things, its remarkable, yet easily explicable, safety.' [1]

If existing compressed air chambers were to be used it was unavoidable that not only the patient but also the surgeon and his assistants must equally be submitted to increased atmospheric pressure. Nevertheless by July 1879 Bert was able to state at a meeting of the Académie des Sciences :

' Two surgeons from Parisian hospitals, MM. Labbé and Péan, have responded to the appeal I made to practitioners. . . . As a

[1] *C.R. Acad. Sci., Paris*, 1878, **87**, 728–30.

typical example [of the new method] I will describe M. Labbé's first operation :

'The operation was the removal of an ingrowing nail and nail-bed, the patient an extremely nervous girl of twenty. We entered the large sheet iron chamber of Dr. Daupley's [aero-therapeutic] establishment and the atmospheric pressure was, in the course of a few minutes, gradually increased by 17 cm. (total pressure 92 cm.). The patient lay down on a mattress and M. Préterre applied the valved facepiece, which he was in the habit of using for the inhalation of pure nitrous oxide, the bag of the apparatus being filled with a mixture containing 85 per cent. nitrous oxide and 15 per cent. oxygen. I was holding the patient's wrist, the pulse being rapid, when suddenly, without any warning change in the pulse rate, in the respiration or the colour of the skin or the expression of the face and without any stiffening, struggling or excitement, about ten to fifteen seconds after the first inspiration of the anaesthetic gas, I felt the arm become completely limp. Both insensibility and muscular relaxation were established and the cornea itself could be freely touched. The operation began and the bandaging followed without a single movement on the part of the patient, who slept calmly. The pulse rate had returned to normal. At the end of four minutes, just as M. Labbé finished the bandaging, a slight contracture occurred in one arm, then in one leg. Everything being over, the facepiece was removed, whereupon the contractures ceased. For thirty seconds the girl continued to sleep ; then, someone having tapped her on the shoulder, she woke and looked at us with a surprised air. . . .

'On the way back to hospital ', Bert added, ' she complained so bitterly of being hungry that we had to stop and get her something to eat.'

Bert also referred to sixteen operations performed by Péan, at Dr. Fontaine's therapeutic establishment. These included three excisions of the breast, four operations on the bones, six extirpations of tumours, a nerve resection, and two reductions of three- and four-day-old dislocations of the shoulder. The duration of anaesthesia varied from four to twenty-six minutes.

In Bert's opinion the most frequent complication—and one which might appear quite serious—arising during this type of anaesthesia was contracture of the limbs. This, he thought, was due to insufficient tension of the gas and in order to remedy it, all that was necessary was to increase the pressure by two or three centimetres. As a general rule the total increase in pressure varied between 15 and 22 centimetres.

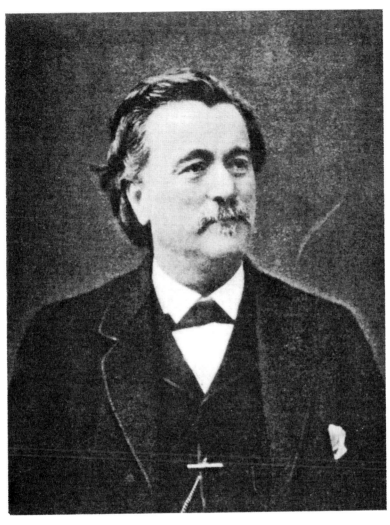

FIG. 102.—PAUL BERT (1833–86)

Physiologist and politician. Appointed Professor of Physiology at the Sorbonne in 1869. Bert made important contributions to the theory and practice of anaesthesia, particularly in connection with nitrous oxide and chloroform.

' The employment of compressed air ', wrote Bert, ' makes modifications in the dosage of gaseous agents easily possible. Nothing would be more difficult than to alter the proportions in a gaseous mixture, nothing is simpler than to vary the tension and thus the physiological dose. . . . I must thank Doctors Labbé and Péan, whose bold initiative, justified by the results of my previous experiments, has allowed me to pass on the use of nitrous oxide from the physiological laboratory to the operating theatre.' [1]

Meanwhile Fontaine, at whose establishment Péan's earlier operations were done, had been improving the facilities for nitrous oxide anaesthesia under pressure. In addition to a cast-iron chamber which could be installed in hospitals Fontaine succeeded, by 1879, in devising a mobile chamber (see Fig. 103), so that sometimes Labbé was able to operate in it at the Hôpital Larboisière and at other times Péan used it at the Hôpital Saint-Louis.

' This apparatus, mounted on a chassis . . . is painted white inside. It is lighted by ten portholes, the four above directly lighting the operating table. It is 2 metres wide, 3·50 metres long and 2·65 metres high. Ten or twelve people can be comfortably accommodated. . . . Pressure can be regulated and read on a manometer, either in or outside the car.' [2]   On a small trailer were mounted : (1) a two-handled pump, capable of delivering from 400 to 600 litres of air per minute ; (2) a refrigerator through which the compressed air passed, in summer, in order to keep the temperature inside the car no more than one or two degrees above that of the air outside—in winter the refrigerator was replaced by a hot-water heater ; (3) an iron cylinder containing 350 litres of nitrous oxide and oxygen under a pressure of ten atmospheres.

The anaesthetic mixture passed through tubing from the cylinder into a large reservoir bag placed under the operating table. To this bag the facepiece was attached by more tubing. The flow of the anaesthetic mixture was controlled by a stop-cock. Whenever it became necessary to have more air pumped into the car the pumping squad outside was warned of the fact by a blast from a whistle mounted on the wall inside the car.[3]

[1] C.R. Acad. Sci., Paris, 1879, **89**, 132–5.
[2] Rottenstein, J. B. 1880. Traité d'anesthésie chirurgicale. Paris. 324.
[3] Ibid. 323–4.

An account of this mobile chamber was given to the *British Medical Journal* by a Londoner, T. R. Allinson, in the autumn of 1881 :

' Last summer I was in Paris, and had an opportunity of seeing Paul Bert's anaesthetic car at work. . . . We—the patient, doctor [this was Péan, at the Hôpital Saint-Louis], and his students— went into the car ; the door, air-tight, was closed, and air forced

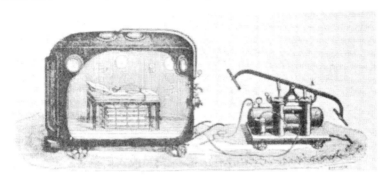

FIG. 103.—THE ' ANAESTHETIC CAR '

designed by Fontaine—a mobile, compressed air chamber serving as an operating theatre in which a mixture of nitrous oxide and oxygen could be administered to the patient under positive pressure, in accordance with Paul Bert's suggestion. The surgeon and his assistants were also subjected to the increased atmospheric pressure. This ' car ' travelled round among various of the Paris hospitals, during 1880.

A. Double-barrelled air pump.
B. Refrigerator for cooling the air.
C. Iron cylinder containing 350 litres of gas and oxygen under a pressure
    of ten atmospheres.
D. Reservoir bag for the anaesthetic mixture.
E. Facepiece.

into the car, in a few minutes my ears began to feel strange, and I was told to swallow, yawn, and blow my nose, which I did every few minutes, and so made the pressure equal on both sides of the drums of my ears. The patient laid himself down on the operating-table, and the anaesthetic agent was given him. He took it very quietly, did not struggle, and was soon insensible. Whilst he was unconscious, an epithelioma was removed from his lower lip ; after the wound was sewn up, the compressed air was allowed to escape ; the patient got up from the table, walked out of the car and lay down on the grass ; he complained of no headache nor nausea, but said he felt just as usual. We also were glad to escape from the car, on account of the heat which was

12*

very intense. During the operation, all the assistants and the surgeon pulled off their coats and waistcoats, and yet they perspired very freely. The car is on wheels, and is carried about from hospital to hospital ; the hospitals being under Government, the car is a public one, and is taken all over Paris.' [1]

The vogue for giving nitrous oxide and oxygen under pressure was short-lived. Bert wrote in 1883 :

' I have no hesitation in saying that this method of anaesthesia as nearly as possible approaches perfection. . . . Unfortunately, the necessity for employing complicated and costly mechanical apparatus—cast iron chambers to withstand the pressure, pumps, steam engines—makes it possible for large hospitals only, to use this valuable method. In Paris a very fine installation has been made at the Hôpital Saint-Louis ; and I know of others, at Lyons [Claude Martin's apparatus, cf. Hewitt, F. W. 1893. *Anaesthetics and their administrations*. London. 117.] at Geneva, in Brussels and in some German cities. . . .

' In view of these material difficulties, I have been trying to discover whether it would not be possible to solve the problem another way ', Bert continued, ' and to use the gas at normal pressure during prolonged operations. . . .

' For a long time past in America, some major operations have been performed under nitrous oxide anaesthesia. The patient has been anaesthetized in the ordinary way and the operation begun ; when asphyxia became imminent the mask was raised, while the operation proceeded and during the next few succeeding seconds of anaesthesia the patient breathed air. Sensibility having returned, the operation was suspended while nitrous oxide was readministered, then begun again as the second anaesthesia was established, and so on.

' I have never seen this intermittent method applied in man ', Bert stated. ' But I must say that in dogs it produces the most deplorable spectacle. . . .

' The idea occurred to me, however, that a mixture of nitrous oxide and oxygen in proportions similar to those in which nitrogen and oxygen are found naturally together might be used.

' By first anaesthetizing the animal with pure nitrous oxide and then making it breathe the above-mentioned mixture, I was able to obtain and prolong insensibility for several minutes—a period quite sufficient to allow the blood to reabsorb the necessary oxygen. Since the high proportion of nitrous oxide in the mixture prevents the rapid elimination of the gas from the blood, its anaesthetic effect is consequently maintained. Upon then reapplying pure nitrous oxide I had no need to push anaesthesia to the dangerous verge of asphyxia; for I had, if I may thus express it, only a little gap to fill, and the first inspirations of pure gas brought about the required concentration of it in the blood.

'Neither asphyxia nor a return to consciousness is to be feared and thus the problem is solved. . . .

'I confidently suggest that surgeons try this very simple method on man. It needs only the ordinary facepiece and two rubber bags. But', Bert added, 'I wish first to determine, by a sufficient number of experiments, the exact proportions of oxygen and nitrous oxide which will give the most satisfactory mixture.' [1]

At this point Bert appears to have discontinued his investigation of nitrous oxide-oxygen mixtures. At all events he did not complete his series of articles on the subject in the *Comptes Rendus* of the Académie, by publishing the promised results of experiments to determine the most satisfactory mixture. He now turned his attention to chloroform and the problem of controlling the proportion of that drug in anaesthetic mixtures.

Bert's interest in chloroform anaesthesia was not new, for he made special reference to the subject in 1881 in a paper, published in the *Comptes Rendus* of the Académie des Sciences, entitled 'On the *zone maniable* of anaesthetic agents and on a new method of chloroforming.' [2]

'When', said Bert, in that paper, 'a volatile or gaseous anaesthetic is added in increasing proportions to air and the successive mixtures are administered to an animal, the moment arrives when anaesthesia is established. If one continues to increase the proportion of the drug the animal finally dies. The interval comprised between the anaesthetic dose and the lethal dose I call the *zone maniable*.

'In carefully determining the extent of this *zone maniable* for different anaesthetic agents (chloroform, ether, amylene, ethyl bromide, methyl chloride) and for different animals (dogs, mice, sparrows)', Bert continued, 'I arrived at this singular result, that in every case the lethal dose is exactly double the anaesthetic dose.'

Bert briefly described his experimental method which was to place the animal in a closed vessel already filled with the prepared mixture and sufficiently large to obviate asphyxial complications.

[1] *C.R. Acad. Sci., Paris*, 1883, **96**, 1271-4.　　[2] *Ibid.* 1881, **93**, 768.

'The use of potash to absorb carbon dioxide must be absolutely rejected,' he stated, ' at least in experiments with chloroform, which it rapidly breaks down. It was through failing to take this fact into account that certain investigators have been altogether misled as to the lethal proportion of chloroform in air.'

Bert contrasted the swift and tranquil anaesthesia obtained by administering ' a mixture corresponding to about the middle of the *zone maniable* ' with ' the results of ordinary methods of anaesthesia, using a compress, sponge, etc.' By these latter methods, he pointed out, according to the saturation of the compress and its proximity to the nose and mouth, the patient might breathe an anaesthetic-air mixture which was less than the anaesthetic dose, within the *zone maniable* or equal to and even greater than the lethal dose.

' The *zone maniable* ', Bert continued, ' is, in fact, singularly narrow, and a few additional drops of liquid may change the inspired mixture from an active to a lethal dose. This is particularly true of chloroform : 8 grams vaporized in 100 litres of air will not put a dog to sleep, 20 grams kills him. The margin is 12 grams. Ether, which has the same proportionate strength (the lethal dose being double the anaesthetic dose), nevertheless offers far less danger because there is a margin of almost 40 grams between the active and the lethal dose. Herein, incontestably, lies the reason for the relative harmlessness of which ether has given proof in surgical practice.

' When one reads accounts of longish operations, one notices that the surgeons do not omit to draw attention to the quantity of chloroform which they used, that is to say, poured on to the compress, but they do not mention the chloroform lost from the outside [of the compress] nor consider it otherwise than as having entered the patient's lungs. Such information is value-less. I can make a dog breathe an extraordinary quantity of chloroform without producing any anaesthesia, so long as I take care that its proportion in the mixture does not exceed 5 or 6 parts. Inversely, by using a mixture containing 30 parts of chloroform, a very trifling amount is sufficient to kill the animal stone dead. In other words, chloroform does not act according to the quantity inhaled but according to the pro-portion in which it is present in the inspired air. . . . For in both volatile and gaseous anaesthetics, particularly nitrous oxide, the action depends upon the tension [of the drug] in the inspired air, which regulates the proportion existing in the blood and tissues' (cf Snow's conclusions, pp. 188–91, 217).

In order to put this principle into practice and so bring ' to the use of every anaesthetic the same security as nitrous oxide under pressure gives', Bert advised abandoning the use of compresses and ' all the complicated apparatuses, based on the erroneous principle of quantitative administration, upon which surgeons and instrument makers have exercised their imagination'. He suggested instead, the use ' simply of a tube, a small facepiece and a suitably proportioned mixture of air and anaesthetic agent. There is no need', he added, ' to bother about the pulse or the respiration, and the temperature scarcely varies. The only things which are not thus avoided are the intrinsic inconveniences of the agent itself, the excitement of the induction period and subsequent nausea and vomiting.

' Measured mixtures have already been used, a few years ago, in my laboratory by two of my pupils', Bert said, ' and M. Gréhant, indeed, preceded them in this course. Snow in England and Lallemand, Perrin and Duroy [1] in France, have also made some reference to this subject. I think that the new researches on the *zone maniable* ought to determine surgeons to try the application of this method to man.'[2]

When in 1883 Bert returned to the subject of measured anaesthetic mixtures he read a paper (before the section of physiology of the Académie des Sciences) dealing with the reactions of dogs to variously proportioned mixtures of chloroform and air. These mixtures were delivered from a double gasometer, designed by Saint-Martin in the previous year, to which an inhaling mask was attached. At the close of the paper Bert strongly recommended the clinical use of such mixtures ' which would have the advantage of regulating administration—the success of which now depends entirely upon the skill of the surgeon—according to precise rules '.[3]

Early in 1884 Bert read a second paper on the subject of measured mixtures and was able to refer to twenty-two cases, from Péan's department at the Hôpital Saint-Louis, in which patients had been successfully anaesthetized from Saint-Martin's apparatus

---

[1] Lallemand, L., Perrin, M., and Duroy, J. L. P. 1860. *Du rôle de l'alcool et des anesthésiques dans l'organisme.* Paris. 354–8.
[2] *C.R. Acad. Sci.*, Paris, 1881, **93**, 768–71.   [3] *Ibid.* 1883, **96**, 1831–3.

with a mixture containing eight grams of chloroform vaporized in 100 litres of air.

' When the proportion [of chloroform] was reduced to 7, the sleep was less profound ', Bert stated. ' It seemed to me pointless to try a higher dose [than 8 grams].' [1]

Bert's method was adversely criticized by Gosselin and by Richet.

Gosselin chiefly condemned Saint-Martin's gasometer as being ' cumbersome, very heavy and difficult, if not impossible, to transport '. He contrasted its use with the method, ' so simple and so safe for those who thoroughly understand how to use it, which almost all of us employ—a compress or a hand-kerchief on to which one pours, little by little, the necessary doses of the anaesthetic agent.

' Moreover, in my opinion ', said Gosselin, ' M. Bert's meas-ured mixture might, on occasions, very well have detrimental effects on certain patients. The danger of chloroform lies in the susceptibility of the individual. Some go to sleep very quickly and may be deeply anaesthetized by doses which in others induce anaesthesia more slowly and gently. To avoid accidents arising from the exceptional cases of idiosyncrasy, chloroform must be given intermittently, in increasing doses, so as to accustom the body to it gradually. . . .

' What, in my eyes, makes the new procedure inferior to the usual practice, is that it delivers from the outset a uniform dose, which I find too strong for the initial inspirations ; with it one cannot (by beginning with a small dose and gradually increasing it) establish that tolerance which should be sought above all and which is found very quickly in sensitive subjects, more slowly in resistant subjects. M. P. Bert may, it is true, have met with surgeons who administer too great a quantity of chloroform, but they are very rare to-day.

' On the other hand, for those who persistently give too much chloroform at a time and for all those who, in the future, will have to familiarise themselves with the subject, M. P. Bert's procedure will have the advantage of demonstrating far better than we have been able to do up to the present, and in a thoroughly scientific way, how small a quantity of chloroform is necessary for anaesthesia. So far, in this respect, we have approximations only. But while we advocate progressive doses and while we think that, according to the patient, either more or less chloroform must be introduced into the circulation to induce and maintain

[1] *C.R. Acad. Sci., Paris*, 1884, **98**, 63-9.

anaesthesia, we think, also, that it is necessary to know far more about the matter than M. P. Bert has yet taught us. . . .

' M. P. Bert's new suggestion, by providing those who advise moderate but at the same time progressive doses, with a fresh argument, will have contributed towards making increasingly safe the simple process to which the majority of surgeons will always be obliged to give preference.' [1]

Richet, after agreeing with Gosselin's criticisms and describing three cases in which he himself had seen Bert's measured mixture administered by Dubois for Péan, at the Hôpital Saint-Louis, stated :

' Theoretically it seems to me, if not impossible at least very difficult, to admit that one could ever demonstrate the harmlessness of any anaesthetic method without first having discovered the cause of death from the inhalation of chloroform. But, up to the present, all is mystery and, in spite of the extremely numerous and painstaking researches of the physiologists, we must still fall back upon hypotheses. It is, indeed, a hypothesis which our learned colleague puts forward when he speaks of his *limited dose* and until we have a more complete demonstration I refuse to accept it. . . .

' I must say ', Richet added, ' that the dangers of death from anaesthesia have been remarkably exaggerated ; among more than a million individuals who have submitted to anaesthesia, one can only with difficulty muster 290 to 300 cases of death *attributed* to these inhalations. . . .'

Referring specifically to Bert's proposal that only measured mixtures should be used for anaesthesia, Richet said :

' About twenty-four years ago, the Chloroform Committee of the *Royal Medical and Chirurgical Society of London* recommended mixtures and that, above all, if one wished to proceed in relative safety, 3·50 per cent. of chloroform vapour in the air must not be exceeded. I will merely call to mind the apparatuses of Snow, Demarquay, Duroy, Sansom, Junker, Skinner, Esmarch and Billroth, and will single out Clover's alone, because it offers the strongest analogy to that of M. Bert [2]. The principles are the same ; only the form of the apparatuses differs. . . .

[1] *C.R. Acad. Sci.*, Paris, 1884, **98**, 121–4.

[2] During February, March, and April 1882, a discussion on chloroform anaesthesia was held among the members of the Académie de Médecine. In the course of this discussion Gosselin, among others, had had occasion to refer to Bert's researches of 1881 on measured mixtures of chloroform and air, and a fellow-member, Léon le Fort, then drew attention to the above-mentioned inhalers, and to the previous use of measured chloroform-air mixtures, particularly Clover's. (*Bull. Acad. Méd. Paris*, 1882, N.S. **11**, 180, 187, 258, 259.)

' Administration with Clover's apparatus succeeded, without any untoward happenings, not only in England but in France, where I remember having seen it used at the Charité by an Englishman in Velpeau's department, and, according to the authoritative statement of Professor Erichsen (*System of Surgery*, latest edition), 3000 administrations of chloroform have been completed without accident. [1]

' In 1867, however, a man needing the reduction of a dislocated thumb, submitted to the inhalation of chloroform from Clover's apparatus ; he had inhaled for scarcely three minutes when he abruptly died ; only 1·7 grams of chloroform (37 drops) had been used (*British Medical Journal*, 2 March 1867). . . .'

Richet, at this point, gave details of three further fatalities attributed to the use of Clover's chloroform apparatus. He continued :

' Finally, in 1874, a fifth death occurred, this time in the hands of Clover himself, fifteen minutes after the beginning of induction (*British Medical Journal*, 20 June 1874).

' What is instructive about this last happening is that, no doubt in order to exonerate his method from all blame, Clover decided that he himself must have made a mistake and added a little more chloroform than usual to the air. [2]

' These five fatal cases, which occurred within a short period, with an apparatus delivering a mixture containing a measured proportion of chloroform vapour, for which also relative safety had been claimed, appear remarkably to have cooled the enthusiasm of our neighbours for Clover's method, for one no longer hears any mention of it.' [3]

[1] Erichsen, J. E. 1884 (8th ed.). *The science and art of surgery*. London. **1**, 22. Here Erichsen, in fact, wrote as follows :

' Mr. Clover, to whom we are indebted for the most accurate and scientific of these instruments [for chloroform anaesthesia], used it himself many thousands of times without an accident of any kind.'

[2] In fact, in this particular case (the removal of adenoids from an adult male), Clover, after inducing chloroform anaesthesia with his usual apparatus (see Figs. 53-4), in order to allow the surgeon free access to the mouth, substituted what he termed ' the blowing apparatus '. This ' consists of a bellows moved by the foot, which drives air through a vessel containing chloroform, and forwards by means of a tube held in, or near the patient's mouth. A stop-cock regulates the current.' It was to the use of this latter instrument and not at all to his ordinary chloroform apparatus that Clover attributed the giving of an overdose which resulted in the patient's death. (*Brit. med. J.*, 1874, i, 817). William McCardie, however, in a note pencilled in the margin of his copy of Hewitt's textbook on anaesthetics (now in the Nuffield Department of Anaesthetics) recorded that Clover had two deaths when using his chloroform apparatus (one patient being an alcoholic man, the other a woman) and he repeated a malicious little anecdote : ' Dr. Milner Moore of Coventry told me, one he saw was never published, a reporter being paid two guineas to be silent.'

[3] *C.R. Acad. Sci., Paris*, 1884, **98**, 192-200.

Bert, in replying to his critics, and more especially to Richet, said :

' Many people . . . oppressed by their responsibility, have tried to regulate the amount of chloroform with the aid of various pieces of apparatus ; but these apparatuses have been abandoned for the good reason that they were all founded upon the erroneous principle of measuring the amount of chloroform used instead of the true principle—the measuring of the tension of the vapour. . .

' I have the temerity to say that it is not an apparatus but a new method which I am putting forward. My aim is to regulate and maintain constant in the system the quantity of chloroform necessary for anaesthesia and I am able to do so by causing the chloroform to be breathed at the necessary tension. . . .

' Thus the use of measured mixtures has the precision which gives security and the adaptability which will lend itself to all eventualities. One . . . can change the proportions and one can, obviously, administer intermittently if one wishes. What the method will not do is to allow danger to arise through the use of too strong doses. At one sure stroke, and mechanically, it achieves what the ablest practitioners search after and obtain only at the price of long and often painful experience. . . .

' Our learned colleague, M. Richet, must let me thank him for having drawn my attention to Clover's apparatus. I admit it was unknown to me. . . .

' The examination which I have made showed me at once that its inventor was not directed by the theoretical ideas which led me to propose my methods of anaesthesia by nitrous oxide, chloroform and ether.

' But since the measured mixtures used by Clover are analogous to mine, but a little weaker (30 to 40 minims in 1000 cubic inches is from 5 to 7 grams in 100 litres of air) I must try the method which has given such excellent results in thousands of cases.' [1]

Bert was criticized also in the *British Medical Journal* in an editorial note headed ' A rediscovery in anaesthetics ' :

' M. Paul Bert has been making experiments in anaesthesia with a mixture of chloroform-vapour and air. . . . He used an anaesthetic vapour composed of eight grammes of chloroform volatilized in 100 litres of air, and claims several advantages for this new method. . . . It will be at once evident that M. Gambetta's ex-minister [2] has been travelling over exactly the same ground as that which was completely explored fully five-and-twenty

[1] *C.R. Acad. Sci., Paris*, 1884, **98**, 265-72.
[2] Bert was a professional politician as well as a physiologist.

years ago by the late Mr. J. T. Clover [¹]. . . The proportion of chloroform-vapour to air was slightly less in the older English than in the new French apparatus ; but chloroform has, for some nine or ten years past, been practically superseded here by other still safer anaesthetising agents, such as nitrous oxide gas, ether, or the mixture of alcohol, chloroform, and ether. Of the advantages possessed by these anaesthetic agents in many cases over chloroform, however skilfully and exactly it may be administered, our French neighbours may (if they travel at M. Bert's rate of progress) possibly become aware at the dawn of the twentieth century.' ²

During 1884 and 1885 the physiologist Raphaël Dubois and an engineer named Tatin worked under Bert's supervision on an apparatus for delivering measured mixtures of chloroform and air, the clinical tests being made by Dubois during operations performed in Péan's department at the Hôpital Saint-Louis. In all, about 200 administrations were made, for a variety of operative procedures, and the patients' ages ranged from six months to sixty years.³

In laboratory experiments and in the first twenty-two or so clinical tests Saint-Martin's gasometer had proved reliable in delivering a single, constant mixture composed of 8 grams of chloroform vaporized in 100 litres of air. Bert soon aimed, however, at being able to vary the mixture easily during the course of the administration so as to have 10 grams of chloroform vaporized in 100 litres of air for induction and from 8 to 6 grams of chloroform vaporized in 100 litres of air for maintaining anaesthesia. ' In order to be able to dispense with the need for assistants and avoid the possibility of error ', it was necessary to design an apparatus to deliver these mixtures automatically.

The ' anaesthetizing machine ' which Raphaël Dubois designed for this purpose was worked by a handle. A measured volume of air was drawn into the apparatus by a pump and passed through a warmed evaporating chamber into which, simultaneously, a measured quantity of liquid chloroform was injected from a reservoir, by the stroke of a piston. The resulting chloroform-air mixture, after accumulating in the pump body, was blown through a long rubber tube to a valveless facepiece. So long as the handle was steadily turned this process was continuously repeated and the anaesthetic mixture was delivered at

---

¹ Clover died in 1882.   ² *Brit. med. J.*, 1884, i, 281.
³ *Rev. gén. Sci. pur. appl.*, 1891, **2**, 360.

the facepiece in an unbroken stream. If, for any reason, the anaesthetic stream became unduly slowed or interrupted, the patient breathed fresh air, presumably through some kind of open port in the facepiece which served also for the escape of

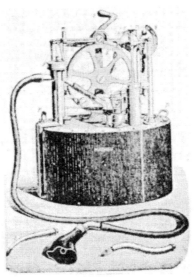

FIG. 104.—DUBOIS'S 'ANAESTHETIZING MACHINE'
(c. 1891)

designed on the principles of safe chloroform administration laid down by Paul Bert.

The handle actuated the mechanism which injected a predetermined quantity of liquid chloroform into a warmed evaporating chamber and simultaneously pumped through it a fixed volume of air. The resulting mixture accumulated in the drum-shaped body of the pump, on which the mechanism was mounted. Thence the mixture passed to the facepiece or, in operations in the region of the face and neck, to either the oral or the nasal tube (shown in the foreground).

the expired mixture. The pump body, which was described as being like ' a child's drum ', or alternatively, like ' a hat box ', gave to the apparatus its characteristic shape. On it were mounted the other component parts ; these, in later models, included a spirit lamp which warmed a metal plate in contact with the vaporizing chamber, and a setting dial for the mechanism regulating the amount of chloroform injected. In the

original model the change from one mixture to another necessitated substituting by hand small measuring cups of different
capacity one for another which, once in place in the apparatus,
automatically drew the requisite amount of chloroform from the
reservoir and emptied it into the evaporating chamber.[1]

Induction, the maximum duration of which with the
' anaesthetizing machine ' was said to be 7 to 10 minutes, was
effected with what Bert called the ' 10 per cent. mixture ', that is
to say 10 grams of chloroform vaporized for every 100 litres of
air blown to the facepiece. The regulator was then set for the
' 8 per cent. ' mixture and in a further 5 minutes, if the operation was to be of long duration, for the ' 6 per cent. ' mixture
(cf. p. 374).

Once anaesthesia was established, if the operation involved
the facial region or the air passages, a nasal or a buccal tube,
as the case demanded, was substituted for the facepiece. The
nasal tube could also be used for artificial respiration ; the
buccal tube very conveniently acted as a mouth-prop and
tongue depressor.[2]

Bert's interest in the practical application of his measured
mixtures of chloroform and air lasted until 1886, when he left
France to take up a political post in Annam. He died from
dysentery at Tonkin a few months after his arrival.

On the Continent the use of Dubois's ' anaesthetizing
machine ' was limited to a few hospitals where Dubois himself
had some personal link with the surgical staff—in Paris, at
Lyons, where he was Professor of Physiology, and at Ghent.

In England D. W. Buxton, in 1924, expressed the opinion
that Dubois's machine ' remains one of the best dosimetric
apparatus available '. He added : ' However, it has not received
much attention in this country, probably because of its size and
possibly because mechanical contrivances do not appeal to busy
practitioners '.[3]

Bert's theoretical work on chloroform-air mixtures, on the
other hand, exerted a considerable influence on the work of
British anaesthetists during the last decade of the nineteenth
and the first decade of the present century. Augustus D. Waller,
for example, one of the few British physiologists—among many

[1] *Rev. gén. Sci. pur. appl.*, 1891, **2**, 360–2.
[2] Dubois, R. 1894. *Anesthésie physiologique.* Paris. 111–12.
[3] *Brit. J. Anaesth.*, 1924, **2**, 9.

then investigating the problem of the correct dosage of anaesthetics—whose researches have proved of lasting importance, drew the attention of the Society of Anaesthetists [1] to Bert's work, in February 1896.

He pointed out that the conclusion reached by Bert that the lethal dose of chloroform was double the minimum anaesthetic

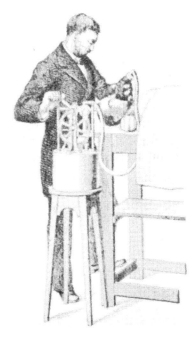

FIG. 105.—ADMINISTRATION WITH DUBOIS'S 'ANAESTHETIZING MACHINE'

dose had already been reached many years earlier by John Snow (see p. 190). He further pointed out that the amount of chloroform which each had determined by experiment as being necessary fully to saturate the body tissues was identical, namely 2 per cent. by volume of chloroform vapour in the body fluids (cf. p. 189). 'The coincidence', Waller is reported in the *Transactions* to have said, ' was veiled by the fact that different units [of measurement] had been used '. Waller explained that according to Snow the greatest amount of chloroform which the

[1] See footnote, p. 461.

fluids of the organism would hold ' lay between 18 and 36 minims, or between 1 and 2 c.c. of chloroform, or between 300 and 600 c.c. of chloroform *vapour*. . . . Taking 30,000 c.c. as the volume of fluid in the body, and taking Snow's figure of 300 and 600 c.c. as the anaesthetic and the lethal dose respectively, the percentages between which the patient should be kept, come out as being between 1 per cent. and 2 per cent. . . .

' Bert considered as fatal to his dogs 10 per cent., by which he meant 10 grammes per hundred litres ; 10 grammes = 2000 c.c. per hundred litres, namely 2 per cent. . So that Bert's 10 per cent. was in reality Snow's 2 per cent.'

Waller concurred in believing that ' the proportion of chloroform was not to exceed 2 per cent. ', but he believed that recent researches showed that ' in order to maintain within the fluids of that reservoir called the human body, a percentage of between one and two per cent. very much less chloroform was necessary than was stated by the earlier observers, even less than was stated by Snow, much less than was stated by Paul Bert '.[1]

---

[1] *Trans. Soc. Anaesth.*, 1898, **1,** 72, 74–5, 82–4

CHAPTER XIII

'MIXED ANAESTHESIA' AND PREMEDICATION

Bernard's 'Mixed Anaesthesia'—The Development of Pre-Anaesthetic
Medication and of Basal Anaesthesia

Bernard's 'Mixed Anaesthesia'

PRE-ANAESTHETIC medication, the administration of a
sedative drug or combination of drugs an appreciable time
before the administration of the principal anaesthetic in order,
by calming the patient mentally and physically, to lower his
resistance to anaesthesia and obviate as far as possible post-
operative shock, is to-day a generally accepted routine procedure, even for the ambulatory patient. During the first
half-century of anaesthetic practice this was by no means the
case although before that period, sedation with wine [1] or opiates
commonly played an important part in the preparation of the
patient for the operative ordeal and sedatives were also given
post-operatively.

An important early reference to pre-operative sedation occurs
in Georg Wolfgang Wedel's monograph on opium, *Opiologia*
(Jena, 1682).[2] Wedel stated that 'opium in a moderate draught'
might be given 'to the patient on the night preceding the
operation [amputation], for thus he bears the burning and
cutting of the limb with a readier spirit, and various [unpleasant]
symptoms will be averted '.[3]

---

[1] As late as 1874, J. T. Clover stated : ' I like to give a teaspoonful of brandy,
without water, a few minutes beforehand [*i.e.* before chloroform], but not so much
as a tablespoonful. If wine be given or if the patient must have some water in the
brandy, then they should be given half-an-hour before inhaling, to allow time for
absorption.' (*Brit. med. J.*, 1874, i, 202.) In England, at this particular time, some
such procedure as Clover described was the only kind of premedication attempted.

[2] Although pre- and post-operative sedation with opium was frequently employed, the giving of opium to procure surgical anaesthesia, although recognized
as a possible procedure, was condemned as unsafe by reputable surgeons. Wedel
himself stressed this point and quoted various authorities upholding it ; *e.g.* Fal-
lopius : ' " If soporifics are weak ", he said, " they will not help ; if they are strong
they are exceedingly dangerous " '. (Wedel, G. W., 1682. *Opiologia*. Jena. 130.)

[3] Wedel, G. W. 1682. *Opiologia, ad mentem academiae naturae curiosorum.* Jena.
129-30.

Cheselden, about 1731, recommended that a 'quieting draught' should be given where violent pain was present after lithotomy.[1] In 1820, John Hennen, Deputy Inspector of Military Hospitals, wrote :

'About his person each medical man, of course, carries a pocket case of instruments ; and I would strenuously recommend that he never omits a canteen of good wine, or spirits diluted. Many men sink beyond recovery for want of a timely cordial before, during, and after operations ; and many of the primary operations would be rendered much more favourable in their results, by the administration of a single glass of wine.' [2]

On page 116 of the same treatise Hennen wrote :

'The after management of compound fractures is a most serious duty, requiring industry, judgment, and humanity, as well as great discrimination in both the medical and surgical treatment. . . . Anodynes [i.e. opium in some form or other, cf. ibid. p. 199] are urgently called for in these cases, and are best combined with antimonials, to obviate their heating and constipating effects.'

When the use of ether anaesthesia was generally adopted, late in 1846, the idea that it might be desirable or even necessary to put the patient to some degree under the influence of a sedative drug (itself capable of producing full anaesthesia if given in sufficient quantity) as a preparation for inhalation anaesthesia, did not occur to medical men. Had it done so it would undoubtedly have been rejected as being dangerous. Among anaesthetic concepts that of premedication was extremely slow in growth and slower still in becoming widely accepted, even after a few anaesthetists had stressed its advantages.

By 1846 post-operative medication had fallen into disuse. It was again mentioned early in 1863, in the *Lancet*, as a new procedure in amputation used by Paget, of St. Bartholomew's Hospital. The annotation was headed 'Subcutaneous injection of morphia[3]

---

[1] Douglas, J. 1731. *Cheselden's method of performing the lateral operation for stone.* London. 35.

[2] Hennen, J. 1820. *Principles of military surgery.* Edinburgh. 27.

[3] Morphine, isolated by Sertürner about 1806 (*Journal der Pharmacie für Aerzte und Apotheker (und Chimisten).* Leipzig. 1806, **14,** 47), was substituted for opium as an anodyne, by Magendie about 1820. Magendie prescribed it by mouth, but the 'inoculation of morphine' by dipping the point of a lancet in an aqueous solution and inserting it for a few seconds 'horizontally about one line in depth beneath the epidermis' was proposed by Lafargue, of Saint-Émilion, in 1836. (*Bull. Acad. Méd., Paris,* 1836, **1,** 13.)

The prototype of the modern hypodermic syringe seems to have been an instru-

after operation before restoration of consciousness after chloroform '. It read as follows :

'   . . . After the stump was dressed a subcutaneous injection of a solution of a third of a grain of morphia was practised, with a view of inducing freedom from pain, and some refreshing sleep after a return to consciousness.   This practice, as Mr. Paget remarked, has been in use for some time at the Middlesex Hospital, and has afforded much comfort and ease, especially after many of the more important and painful operations.   From a quarter to one third of a grain, or if necessary even half a grain of morphia may be employed according to circumstances.' [1]

One of the first events which seems to have had an indirect influence in turning attention towards the subject of premedication was a case occurring in the practice of the Viennese surgeon Pitha, which was reported in the medical journals in England and on the Continent.   In 1861, Pitha, after experiencing the utmost difficulty in anaesthetizing with chloroform and ether (presumably the Vienna mixture, 1 part chloroform, 3 parts ether) a patient about to be operated on for incarcerated hernia, proceeded to give an enema containing ' a scruple of the extract of belladonna.[2]   . . . Some time after that, the patient appeared to be in a state of deep intoxication ;   and herniotomy was then performed.   The sopor resembled throughout a deep and tranquil sleep . . . and it was not until twelve hours after the operation that the patient awoke. . . . Professor Pitha thought that the anaesthesia was due to the combined action of chloroform, ether and belladonna ;   and he recommended a mixture of atropine and chloroform to be administered for inducing anaesthesia in cases of chloroform réfractaires '.[3]

In spite of the publicity given to Pitha's suggestion it appears that no one else at the time adopted it in practice.   Nevertheless

ment devised by C. G. Pravaz, of Lyons, about 1853, for injecting iron perchloride into an artery for the cure of an aneurysm.   It consisted of a very fine gold or platinum trocar which was to be introduced obliquely through the artery wall ' with a kind of screwing movement'.   The trocar was attached to a syringe, the piston of which turned on a spiral thread, so that the liquid in the syringe was expelled in a steady, controllable stream.   (*C.R. Acad. Sci., Paris*, 1853, **36**, 88.)

    [1] *Lancet*, 1863, i, 148.

    [2] Atropine was first prepared from the plant *Atropa belladonna, Linn.*, by Mein, and by Grieger and Hesse, in 1833.   The use of various parts of the plant itself as soporofics was traced back with certainty to 1450, by Flückiger and Hanbury and was probably much older.   (Flückiger, F. A., and Hanbury, D.   1879.   *Pharmacographia.* London.)

    [3] *Med. Times Lond.*, 1861, ii, 121.

the case was subsequently widely quoted as being the first known instance of anaesthesia produced by the association of an alkaloid with an inhalation anaesthetic.

In 1855 Alexander Wood, lecturer on the Practice of Medicine, at Edinburgh, proposed a 'new method of treating neuralgia by the direct application of opiates to the painful points'. It had in the past been Wood's practice to treat neuralgia by applying 'a succession of small blisters *over the points* in the course of the nerve which are painful on pressure'. The next step in the treatment was to apply ' an ointment containing morphia to dress the blistered surface '. It was to this part of the treatment that Wood ascribed most of the benefit. ' It has frequently occurred to me, however ', wrote Wood, ' that a more direct application of the narcotic to the affected nerve, or to its immediate neighbourhood, would be attended with corresponding advantage. . . . In pursuit of this object, I have made several attempts to introduce morphia directly by means of acupuncture needles and otherwise, but without success.

' Having occasion, however, about the end of 1853, to endeavour to remove a naevus by injection with the acid solution of perchloride of iron, I procured one of the elegant little syringes, constructed for this purpose by Mr. Ferguson of Giltspur Street, London [cf. footnote, p. 376]. While using this instrument for the naevus, it occurred to me that it might supply the means of bringing some narcotic to bear more directly . . . on the affected nerve in neuralgia.'

Soon afterwards a case presented itself to Wood—that of an old lady suffering from cervico-brachial neuralgia.

'. . . At 10 p.m. . . . I inserted the syringe within the angle formed by the clavicle and acromion, and injected twenty drops of a solution of muriate of morphia [morphine hydrochloride]. . . .

' In about ten minutes after the withdrawal of the syringe the patient began to complain of giddiness and confusion of ideas ; in half an hour the pain had subsided, and I left her in the anticipation of a refreshing sleep.

' I visited her again about 11 a.m. . . . [and] was a little annoyed to find that she had never wakened ; the breathing also was somewhat deep, and she was roused with difficulty. Under the use of somewhat energetic stimuli, however, these symptoms disappeared, and from that time to this the neuralgia has not returned.' [1]

[1] *Edinb. med. J.*, 1855, **82**, 265.

Wood's method of injecting morphine for the relief of neuralgia rapidly came into general use.

In 1864 Nussbaum, of Munich, during an operation on a patient, and Claude Bernard, experimenting on an animal, accidentally discovered that an injection of morphine appeared to intensify and prolong chloroform anaesthesia. The discovery was made independently by Nussbaum and by Bernard, curiously enough at almost the same time.

In Nussbaum's case he had already given chloroform for about an hour, during the extirpation of a malignant tumour, when, fearing to prolong the inhalation, he decided to substitute the use of morphine. The subcutaneous injection of 1 grain in solution, not only provided satisfactory anaesthesia for the completion of the operation, as Nussbaum expected, but it also produced a long period of post-operative tranquillity.[1] Nussbaum was much struck by this latter phenomenon and decided to turn it to account in future operations. The technique which he developed was first to establish chloroform anaesthesia and then to inject hypodermically, half a grain of acetate of morphine. This, he claimed, gave 'five or six hours' tranquil sleep' post-operatively, during which time the patient was spared both pain and restlessness. A report on Nussbaum's work was made by a special committee appointed by the Versailles Medical Society. After experimenting on dogs the committee pronounced itself satisfied 'that the prolongation of chloroform anaesthesia by means of hypodermic injections of the salts of morphia may be regarded as an established fact'.[2]

Bernard, at the time in question, was engaged in research on the physiological action of opium alkaloids. A chloroformed dog on which he was experimenting recovered consciousness, whereupon Bernard injected what he knew to be an anaesthetic dose of 5 cg. morphine hydrochloride (*chlorhydrate de morphine*). Not only did the animal become unconscious but, to Bernard's surprise, it also showed symptoms of renewed chloroform anaesthesia. Having several times repeated this experiment with similar results Bernard reversed the process, first injecting morphine and then inducing chloroform anaesthesia. 'When one begins with chloroform', he stated, 'the unconsciousness

---

[1] Bernard, C. 1875. *Leçons sur les anesthésiques et sur l'asphyxie*. Paris. 226 ; *Dent. Rev.*, 1864, N.S. **1**, 203.

[2] *Med. Times, Lond.*, 1864, i, 259.

produced is long drawn out as a result of the influence of the morphine, but by giving the morphine first . . . scarcely is the inhalation of chloroform interrupted before sensibility returns. Thus one has a rapid means alternately to suspend and re-establish sensibility and this is important in certain cases. . . . In giving an injection of morphine first and then administering chloroform a much smaller quantity of the latter is needed. In this way one obtains anaesthesia without so pronounced a stage of excitement and above all without running so great a risk of accident as one does with large and repeated doses of chloroform '—advantages which, Bernard suggested, ought to recommend the method to surgeons.

These researches on the combined use of morphine and chloroform formed part of a series of lectures on anaesthetics and asphyxia which Bernard delivered to students at the Collège de France during 1869 and 1870 ; they were published, as two lectures, during 1869 in the *Revue des cours scientifiques*.[1]

From 1869 onwards a few French surgeons, most of whom, as students, had witnessed Bernard's demonstrations of what he termed ' mixed anaesthesia ', applied the method ' both in operating and during childbirth '. In 1875 Bernard stated that such practical applications were still infrequent ; nevertheless his recommendation of mixed anaesthesia exerted an increasing influence, although for more than a decade this was noticeable only on the European Continent and especially in France.

Guibert, of Saint-Brieuc (who had attended Bernard's lectures at the Collège de France), about 1870, was among the first to test the combined action of morphine and chloroform clinically. ' I obtained ', he wrote, ' two distinct states . . . 1. analgesia, 2. anaesthesia '. It was with the analgesic state that Guibert chiefly concerned himself.

' 1. *Analgesia.*—In the patient who has had a hypodermic injection of from 1 to 2 centigrams [1/6–1/2 grain] of hydrochloride of morphine, the initial effect of an ordinary chloroform inhalation is to produce an analgesic state. Consciousness and voluntary movement are retained but this state is sufficient very noticeably to blunt sensibility to pain during parturition and in minor surgery.

' 2. *Anaesthesia.*—When sufficient chloroform is uninterruptedly inhaled a state of anaesthetic sleep is achieved, with the muscular relaxation which is essential for major surgery. . . .

---

[1] Bernard, C. 1875. *Leçons sur les anesthésiques et sur l'asphyxie.* Paris. 234.

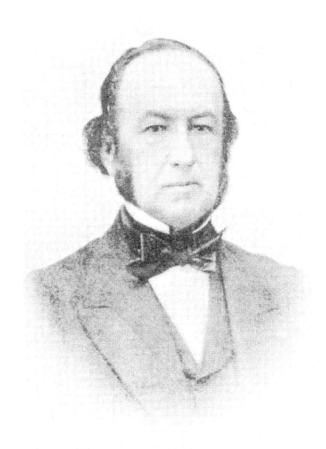

FIG. 106.—CLAUDE BERNARD (1813-78)

Professor of Physiology at the Sorbonne and in 1868 appointed to the newly created Chair of Physiology at the Jardin des Plantes. He carried out many experiments upon the physiology of anaesthesia and recommended the clinical use of a preparatory dose of morphine before chloroform inhalation—this he termed 'mixed anaesthesia'.

'Most of my cases', wrote Guibert, 'belong to the first of these states, analgesia—a state which has not yet been described and of which advantage is never deliberately taken in therapeutics.[1] My observations, some thirty in number, of which fifteen relate to childbirth, seem to me to show that this analgesic state will be of great service in cases of difficult labour, in operations where there is no lesion of the nerve trunks, and in very painful ailments such as lead colic and colic of the liver and kidneys. The dose of morphine varies from 1 to 2 centigrams. It is more difficult to give the exact dosage of chloroform, because of evaporation. The case of a patient suffering from a violent attack of lead colic goes to prove that the amount is small, for the analgesic state was satisfactorily maintained during several hours simply by intermittently breathing chloroform vapour rising from an uncorked bottle.

'In parturition', Guibert explained, 'I proceed as follows : I give a subcutaneous injection of about 1 centigram of hydrochloride of morphine into the forearm, at the moment when uterine contractions begin to become unbearable. . . . A quarter of an hour after the injection I begin chloroform inhalation . . . at a time when the woman announces the beginning of another contraction. After ten or so inspirations the woman ceases to feel acute pain although the contraction continues. I suspend the inhalation before the end of the contraction and continue in this manner throughout labour, allowing chloroform to be inhaled only during contraction. If when the head enters the perineum an increase in pain is seen to be imminent and if the analgesia is becoming less pronounced, one need not fear to give a fresh injection of half a centigram of morphine, which, added to the original dose, will make the pain of the passage of the head bearable.'

During a mastectomy performed under mixed anaesthesia Guibert noticed a fall in pulse rate from 100 to 54. 'No doubt the life of the patient was in no serious danger', Guibert commented. 'Nevertheless, this observation discloses a very remarkable effect on the circulation against which one should be on guard. Half an hour after the end of the inhalation the pulse rate slowly rose to 80'.[2]

The Development of Pre-anaesthetic Medication and of Basal Anaesthesia

The best-known exponents of Bernard's method were L. Labbé, of the Pitié, and his collaborator E. Guyon (also spelt Gujon). Labbé first used mixed anaesthesia at the Pitié

[1] In Great Britain obstetricians had long been in the habit of utilizing the analgesic state, cf. p. 193, footnote.   [2] *C.R. Acad. Sci., Paris*, 1872, **74,** 815.

on January 27, 1872. The patient was a youngish man, the operation a malleolar excision. Twenty minutes before the operation 0·02 g. morphine was injected into the inner side of the thigh. The subsequent chloroform inhalation caused a slight degree of excitement. Anaesthesia was complete at the end of 7 minutes and persisted some time after the operation which lasted 27 minutes. Twenty-eight grams of chloroform were used.

On the same day Labbé and Guyon repeated this anaesthetic experiment on another patient for an operation on the great trochanter. Chloroform was administered 20 minutes after the injection of morphine and complete anaesthesia was established in 6 minutes. The operation lasted 32 minutes and 25 grams of chloroform were used. The patient passed through a comparatively long period of excitement before becoming completely anaesthetized. In a third case (anal fistula) chloroform inhalation was induced a quarter of an hour after the injection of 0·02 g. morphine. Anaesthesia was complete in 5 minutes and 18 grams of chloroform were used. In a fourth case (ovariotomy in a girl twenty years old) 0·02 g. of morphine were given 20 minutes before chloroform inhalation. Anaesthesia was complete in 6 minutes and the operation lasted 1 hour 45 minutes, during which time 48 grams of chloroform were used. Anaesthesia and recovery were uneventful.

Summing up the results of these four cases Labbé and Guyon stated :

' 1. That, as M. Cl. Bernard demonstrated in animals, in man anaesthesia can be achieved far more rapidly by combining the action of chloroform with that of morphine.

' 2. That this anaesthesia is of longer duration and can be maintained for extended periods with smaller doses of chloroform, and that by this method the risk of fatal accidents is considerably diminished.'

' We also believe ', they wrote, ' that the dosage of morphine in the preliminary injection might without drawback be slightly increased ; furthermore, there might be an advantage in giving the injection a little longer before the operation than we have done. We have noticed, we think, that the whole amount has not been absorbed between the time of the injection and the beginning of the operation.' [1]

[1] C.R. Acad. Sci., Paris, 1872, **74,** 627.

Labbé and Guyon do not appear to have followed up this latter observation. Had they done so they would have found that the absorption of morphine by the body and the accompanying depressant action of the drug on the respiratory centre may continue for a very much longer period than they suspected. The practice to-day is never to inject morphine less than from $1\frac{1}{2}$ to 2 hours before an inhalation anaesthetic—'sufficiently early for . . . maximum respiratory depression to be manifest before the anaesthetic is begun '.[1]

In 1869 considerable interest was aroused by Oscar Liebreich's use, in Berlin, of chloral hydrate [2] as a hypnotic. It was known that when treated *in vitro* with an alkali, chloral decomposed, forming chloroform. Liebreich postulated that similarly when chloral is introduced into a living body the action of the blood alkali upon it must cause a gradual liberation of chloroform. He proceeded to test his hypothesis on animals.

He found that the effects of chloral could be divided into three stages : ' first the period of sleep, then follows the period of anaesthesia ; lethal doses produce paralysis of the heart. Here then is an effect completely analogous to the effect of chloroform. . . . Each of these phases ', he added, ' lasts for a considerable time. . . . The complete success of the experiments on animals encouraged me to repeat them in man.

' Chloral is soluble in water ; in solution it is without irritant effect and lends itself well to absorption by the system. This property led me to make use of subcutaneous injection.' [3]

Liebreich's first clinical case, reported in the *comptes rendus* of the Académie des Sciences, was that of an insane epileptic to whom ' an injection of 157 centigrams [of chloral hydrate in solution] was given. Five minutes later he fell into a profound sleep which lasted for four and a half hours. On waking the patient ate a meal in his normal manner '. In the same report two cases in which chloral was given by mouth to induce sleep were also described. In one case a man suffering from pleurisy supervening on a crushed foot was given ' 210 centigrams of chloral hydrate ' by mouth. He slept for nine hours. In the other case a woman suffering from an acute arthritic pain in her

[1] Macintosh, R. R., and Bannister, F. B. 1943. *Essentials of general anaesthesia.* Oxford. 95.
[2] Chloral, which is formed by the action of dry chlorine upon alcohol, was discovered by Liebig in 1832 and subsequently investigated by Dumas.
[3] *C.R. Acad. Sci., Paris*, 1869, **69,** 486.

hand, which was immobilized in plaster, was given 2 grams of chloral in a glass of water. During the sleep which followed the plaster was changed. Hitherto this had proved a painful procedure, but now, although she once or twice opened her eyes, the woman was unaware of what was being done, so she afterwards affirmed.[1]

In France a number of physiologists tested the effects of chloral on animals. The most important outcome of these investigations was the conclusion drawn by J. Personne, that although chloral is in fact at one stage split up into chloroform and formic acid in the blood it is ultimately converted into sodium chloride and sodium formate.[2]

From 1869 to 1874 chloral was widely used on the Continent as a sedative and soporific in such ailments as neuralgia, tetanus, delirium tremens, eclampsia, and for patients who were restless from pain.[3]

In England Benjamin Ward Richardson, at the Exeter meeting of the British Association in 1869, was asked by the President of the Physiological Section if he would undertake an investigation of Liebreich's findings in regard to chloral hydrate.

' An important series of experiments upon animals and birds was accordingly carried out in the laboratory of the Devon and Exeter Hospital, by Dr. Richardson. . . . The results of his researches were, that chloral is decomposed in the living body, as Liebreich affirms. It gives off chloroform, and it forms a formiate of soda with the blood. The chloroform, thus liberated produces sleep, which is in every sense the same as the sleep from chloroform itself. Two parts of hydrate of chloral are equivalent in physiological value to seven of chloroform ; the sleep it produces may be made to extend over four or even five hours ; but vomiting is frequently produced previously to sleep, and there is only a brief period of actual insensibility, the body being, if anything, hypersensitive to touch and pain, even during stupor. . . . Death is very liable to be induced by slight excess of the quantity administered. . . . He did not think that the hydrate of chloral would practically supersede opium, chloroform, and similar narcotising agents now in medical use. On the contrary, he believed that the decomposition of blood which it induces by the formation of formiate of soda is detrimental.' [4]

<hr />

[1] *C.R. Acad. Sci.*, Paris, 1869, **69**, 486.   [2] *Ibid.* **69**, 979.
[3] Chloral hydrate was first used as the sole anaesthetic in 1874 by Oré, of Bordeaux, who gave it intravenously in minor surgery. (*C.R. Acad. Sci.*, Paris, 1874 **78**, 515, 651.) A few among Oré's contemporaries adopted the method, but after a series of fatalities had occurred it was abandoned.
[4] *Brit. med. J.*, 1869, ii, 243.

13

About two months after the publication of this report, in a lecture on the subject of chloral, Richardson referred to his most recent experiments on animals which showed that chloral caused a ' great decrease of animal temperature ' and that the inhalation of an ethereal solution of chloral produced a deep and prolonged narcotic state. ' During a portion of the period of narcotism,' said Richardson, ' there may be complete anaesthesia with absence of reflex actions ; a condition, in short, in which every kind of operation fails to call forth con-sciousness. Therapeutically, the agent is to be accepted as the rival of opium. It promises to be useful in cases where there are increment of animal heat, muscular spasm, and pain. It will be worthy of extensive trial, in tetanus especially. The dose of hydrate of chloral for a child is seven grains ; for an adult, the dose may be twenty grains.' Richardson is not reported as having specified whether this dose was to be injected or given by mouth.[1]

During March 1870 an interesting discussion which showed, incidentally, the influence that Bernard's recommendation of mixed anaesthesia was already exerting in France, was held on the subject of chloral in association with inhalation anaesthetics, at a meeting of the Société de Chirurgie in Paris. The discussion was opened by Liégeois :

' In the course of the last few days ', he said, ' I have had occasion to operate in a case of phagedenic ulcers, and chloral having produced sleep, as is usual, but not anaesthesia, I chloro-formed the patient. Great was my astonishment to find that this association, far from producing an intensified effect, produced only a state of excitement which persisted so long as I continued the inhalation. I should like very much to be able to explain this result, which is contrary to the identity of action which Liebreich thought he had found between chloral and chloroform, a finding with which others have since agreed.'

The next speaker was Giraldès. He said :

' My procedure has been somewhat different. In several cases where children proved obstreperous after chloroform I administered a dose of chloral by mouth. The effect of this association was to induce tranquil sleep for the following five to eleven hours. Since that time I have frequently used a dose of chloral by mouth or in a rectal douche when excitement persists after children have been chloroformed, and always with success.'

[1] *Brit. med. J.*, 1869, ii, 400.

Liégeois replied that the results of his own case and those of Giraldès's were analogous to Claude Bernard's finding that the effects of morphine following chloroform and *vice versa* were exactly contrary.

Demarquay stated :

' I have got into the habit of giving all my patients post-operatively from 2 to 5 grams of chloral in syrup. This has the effect of calming them during the rest of the day and of relieving severe post-operative pain.'

The discussion was closed by Giraud-Teulon, who said :

' In the case of children I use ether for preference. On one occasion having given chloral to a little boy I tried to anaesthetise him with ether but only succeeded in strongly exciting him. This confirms what M. Liégeois said just now about the association of chloral and chloroform and shows that things turn out similarly with ether. It would be interesting to follow up this line of research to discover if it is the same with other anaesthetics.' [1]

No such investigation as Giraud-Teulon suggested appears to have been made, but four years later the attention of the Société de Chirurgie was once more directed to the association of chloral with chloroform when, in November 1874, a member named Lannelongue gave a verbal account of a new method of anaesthesia originated by Forné, a naval surgeon.

' The method ', said Lannelongue, ' is based on Claude Bernard's principle of the association of a narcotic agent with an anaesthetic agent. . . . [In Bernard's case] the narcotic agent was opium. . . . For opium M. Forné substitutes chloral and instead of the subcutaneous injection he recommends one or other of the natural routes by which drugs can be introduced —the mouth or the rectum. This is how he proceeds :

' At the first suitable opportunity he gives his patient a single dose of chloral, which varies from 2 to 5 grams, according to the patient's age, and waits until sleep has been established. . . . This generally takes about an hour. He then proceeds to administer chloroform, using a cone similar to those used in naval hospitals [see Fig. 47] . . . except that it has no partition across it and is lined with felt—an apparatus, in short, which allows the free access of air.'

Lannelongue explained that Forné's object in thus putting his patient to sleep before beginning to administer the anaesthetic

[1] *Bull. Soc. Chirurgie Paris*, 1870, **11**, 102.

was to overcome, as far as possible, the resistance of the patient to the inhalation—both resistance due to emotional disturbance, particularly fear, and the involuntary resistance of the body itself. These, Lannelongue said, were considered by Forné to be of paramount importance among the dangers of chloroform anaesthesia :

' It is for this reason that the patient is placed in a preliminary state of sleep. . . . In effect one annihilates the patient's resistance, removes the influence of fear and relieves the system by inducing sleep, which may be considered as being the first stage in the progress of anaesthesia towards complete insensibility.'

Unfortunately, when Lannelongue made his report to the Société de Chirurgie, Forné had used his new technique in only two operations and these were very minor ones. The first case was an exploration of the urethra in a girl four years old.

' The child was given 2 grams of chloral at 7 a.m. By eight o'clock she was sleeping peacefully. Anaesthesia was induced with 2 grams of chloroform and a further 4 grams sufficed for the operation. She did not wake until one o'clock in the afternoon.'

Forné's second patient was a robust young man of twenty and the operation was the lancing of an abscess in the anal region. Five grams of chloral were administered at 4 p.m. An hour later he was sleeping soundly and 5 grams of chloroform were administered from a cone and the operation was performed. ' While sufficient to establish the merit of the procedure ', said Lannelongue, ' these two cases are in themselves insufficient authority for making any comparison between this procedure and ordinary methods. Furthermore I can only accept with the greatest reserve M. Forné's conclusion that " chloroform inhalation ceases to be dangerous when it is administered during sleep induced by chloral, from an open apparatus which allows of the dosimetric administration of the anaesthetic agent ".'

The general trend of the discussion which followed Lannelongue's account of Forné's work indicated that minor operations upon patients chloroformed while already more or less under the influence of chloral were by no means uncommon ; chloral, in these cases, having been given as a sedative and not deliberately as an adjuvant to chloroform anaesthesia. Almost

all those members who spoke agreed, however, that they had
been seriously alarmed by the unusually protracted period of
post-operative unconsciousness.   More than one admitted,
indeed, that it was only while seeking an explanation of the
occurrence of such a state that the fact emerged of the patient
having previously taken chloral.   In the opinion of the meeting
more evidence was needed to prove whether or not the method
was safe—evidence relating not only to more numerous but also
to more important cases—before Forné's suggestion could be
seriously considered.[1]

In spite of these criticisms Forné had made a positive contribution to anaesthesia.   He was the first to propose what
to-day is known as basal anaesthesia—the induction of sleep
peacefully and pleasantly by a sedative drug and the super-
imposition of an inhalation anaesthetic given by an easily-
controllable method.[2]

In May 1858 Benjamin Bell had read a paper before the
Medico-Chirurgical Society of Edinburgh on ' The therapeutic
relations of opium and belladonna to each other '.   This paper
had drawn attention to the then recently proposed theory—
soon afterwards to become widely accepted—that morphine and
atropine are mutually antagonistic in their action on the human
body.

' I have often thought ', said Bell, ' that less attention has been
given than its importance deserves, to a doctrine which seems
to be undergoing gradual development, namely that opium and

---

[1] *Bull. Soc. Chirurgie Paris*, 1874, **3**, 619.

[2] The present-day attitude towards basal anaesthesia is summarized by Macintosh
and Bannister :

' For some reason for which no adequate explanation can be offered drugs given
by mouth, rectum, or subcutaneous or intravenous injection produce a more pleasant
transition from consciousness than do drugs which must be inhaled.   With basal
anaesthetics the onset of narcosis is almost imperceptible and so much resembles
normal sleep that resistance to anaesthesia is not mobilised as often as by inhalation
anaesthetics. . . .

' Some writers have stated that the preliminary use of a basal anaesthetic increases
the risk of post-operative morbidity which accompanies the administration of an
inhalation anaesthetic.   This view is erroneous, although it is true that return to
consciousness is usually delayed by a basal anaesthetic, so that the patient needs
longer post-operative care.

' The one tenable argument against most basal anaesthetics is that the prolonged
period of unconsciousness which they produce increases the period, pre- and post-
operative, during which the patient must not be left without skilled supervision.   For
this reason a shortage of nursing staff prevents a fuller use of basal premedication.'
(Macintosh, R. R., and Bannister, F. B.   1943.   *Essentials of general anaesthesia*.
Oxford.   100.)

belladonna are mutually remedial, when either of the two has entered the circulation in a poisonous dose. The earliest step towards this opinion appears to have been a suggestion thrown out about twenty years ago, by Dr. Corrigan of Dublin, while attending along with the late Dr. Graves, a case of typhus fever. . . . During the course of the illness . . . [the patient's] head became greatly implicated, with a remarkable contraction of the pupil. Tartar emetic with opium . . . was prescribed, but without good effect, and the patient died. Dr. Corrigan suggested, during . . . subsequent conversation, that, under similar circumstances, *narcotics which produce dilatation of the pupil might be beneficial.* The observation struck Dr. Graves as being curious and important, and . . . he determined to put it to the test of experiment on the first favourable opportunity.

' The result of his various observations and experiments seemed to be this—that the internal use of belladonna is a valuable remedy in cases of cerebral excitement coming in the course of fever, when there is a marked tendency to that very unfavourable symptom contraction of the pupil ; and that, under such circumstances, opium in every shape, is injurious. . . . [See *Dublin J. Med. Sci.*, 1838, **13**, 351.]

' In the winter of 1853, Dr. Thomas Anderson . . . was engaged in a series of experiments on the therapeutic action of belladonna, and having satisfied himself, by repeated clinical observation, of the soundness of the opinions entertained by Dr. Graves, he went a step further, and conceived the idea, that belladonna might perhaps be found beneficial in relieving the coma with contracted pupils caused by poisoning with opium, and a favourable opportunity having soon occurred, he submitted his hypothesis to the test of experiment . . . [and succeeded in reviving a patient]. Another step in advance is taken by Dr. Garrod, who, in . . . October 1854, hazarded the suggestion, that . . . probably in poisoning by belladonna, opium may be found advantageous.'

From the experience gained in two cases of atropine poisoning occurring in his own practice Bell declared, ' I am quite satisfied . . . that the injection of morphia had a powerful effect in modifying and controlling the poisonous influence of the atropia. I have had no opportunity, in the human subject, of putting the converse doctrine regarding morphia, to the test of experiment ', he added, ' but [on] the evidence of facts already brought together in support of it . . . I should confidently have recourse to the injection of atropia in a suitable case of poisoning with opium or any of its preparations '.[1]

[1] *Edinb. med. J.*, 1858–9, N.S. **4**, 1.

At this time atropine was commonly used in ophthalmic practice as a mydriatic and in general therapeutics as an anti-spasmodic, in asthma, tic, and epilepsy for example ; at this time also Wood's method of injecting morphine for the relief of neuralgia was extremely popular, so that it is not remarkable that cases of both atropine and morphine poisoning quite frequently occurred.

Three years after the publication of Bell's paper the theory of the antagonistic action of atropine and morphine was well-established. Albrecht von Graefe, the most important ophthal-mologist of the period, speaking at a meeting of the Berlin Medical Society in 1861 said :

' When a solution of atropine has been injected hypodermic-ally, three or four minutes afterwards the pupil becomes dilated, the pulse rises to 140–160, and other symptoms of narcosis by atropine are observed. If morphia is then injected all these phenomena, which would otherwise last for hours, disappear in a very short time.' [1]

In the previous year, 1860, Brown-Séquard, according to his own statement made many years later,[2] guided by the know-ledge of the antagonistic effects of morphine and atropine was led to employ these two alkaloids in combination in all cases in which the use of either one of them was indicated. In cases where pain or spasm had to be combated (e.g. in tetanus, cata-lepsy, hysteria, or chorea so pronounced as to interfere with sleep) Brown-Séquard was struck by the following points in favour of the simultaneous employment of morphine and atropine : (1) that greater therapeutic power was manifest than when either drug was used singly ; (2) that the combined usage allowed a con-siderably larger dose of each drug to be administered with perfect safety. In 1883 Brown-Séquard made the further statement :

' For fifteen years I have recognized the importance of the addition of atropine to morphine from a motive distinct from those described above : this is the question of vomiting, so frequently produced by morphine alone, particularly when injected sub-cutaneously. In the very great majority of cases, the addition of a certain amount of atropine to the morphine prevents the vomiting and also the nausea occasioned by morphine alone. That the ill effects of a strong dose of morphine or of atropine can be noticeably

[1] *Med. Times, Lond.*, 1861, i, 533.   [2] *C.R. Soc. Biol. Paris*, 1883, **5**, 289.

diminished or may not even appear when the two drugs are combined is so certain that I can subcutaneously inject a solution containing 1 to 2 milligrams of atropine sulphate and 3 to 4 centigrams of morphine sulphate without producing a marked degree of gastric, cardiac or cerebral symptoms.'[1]

The three Goulstonian Lectures for the year 1868 were delivered at the Royal College of Physicians in London by John Harley, Assistant Physician at King's College Hospital. His subject was ' The physiological actions and therapeutical uses of conium, belladonna and hyoscyamus alone and in combination with opium '. His second lecture dealt specifically with ' The physiological action and therapeutical uses of belladonna ' :

' Observations were made upon man, the dog and the horse. The effects following the subcutaneous injection of increasing doses of the sulphate of atropia in man were first considered. The fiftieth of a grain of this salt is usually sufficient to produce the full effects of the plant ; and, briefly summed up, the following are the effects of a full medicinal dose : an acceleration of the pulse from twenty to seventy beats, with a slight increase in its volume, and a considerable increase in the force of the cardiac and arterial contractions ; a general diffusion of warmth throughout the cutaneous surface ; a slight throbbing or heaving sensation in the carotids ; a slight feeling of pressure under the parietal bones ; giddiness, heaviness, and drowsiness, or actual somnolency, accompanied by a tendency to quiet dreamy delirium and nervous startings ; complete dryness of the tongue, roof of the mouth and soft palate [2], extending more or less down the pharynx and larynx, rendering the voice husky, and often inducing dry cough and difficulty of deglutination ; a parched condition of the lips ; occasional dryness of the Schneiderian and conjunctival mucous membranes ; and increasing dilatation of the pupils.

' If ', said Harley, ' we take the simplest view of the action of belladonna, it is that of direct and powerful stimulation of the sympathetic nervous system. . . . During the operation of medicinal doses of belladonna the heart contracts with increased vigour, the arteries increase in tone and volume, and the capillary system fully participates in the general excitation of the circulation. . . . In all conditions and diseases, therefore, in which there is a depression of the sympathetic nervous influence, such as syncope from asthenia, or shock ; in the collapse of cholera ;

---

[1] *C.R. Soc. Biol. Paris*, 1883, **5,** 289.

[2] Alex. Fleming in 1862 seems to have been the first to record of atropine that painted on the mucous membrane of the mouth and throat, it dries the part, and—chiefly as secondary effects—impairs both feeling and movement '. (*Edinb. med. J.*, 1862–3, N.S. **8,** 777.)

in the failure of the heart's action from chloroform or other cardiac
paralysers—the subcutaneous use of sulphate of atropia, in doses
varying from the hundredth to the fortieth of a grain, is the
appropriate and most hopeful means of resuscitation.'

Harley also stated that after a dose of atropine ' no difference
will be observed in the state of the respiration . . . the breathing
will be as tranquil as before the injection '.

In his third lecture Harley dealt with the combined effects
of opium and belladonna :

' There are ', he said, ' a number of persons who accept the
general statement . . . that belladonna is antagonistic to opium
and *vice versa*, and they would not hesitate in a case of poisoning
by either of these drugs to give at once an equally poisonous dose
of the other as an antidote. . . . Feeling that the whole question
required more patient and careful examination I have devoted
much time during the past year to its elucidation. My observations have been made upon the horse and dog, and upon man.

' In turning to the consideration of the combined operation
of opium and belladonna in man, I must first concede that belladonna possesses an antagonistic influence to some of the earlier
effects of the operation of opium. The first effect of opium, in
many animals as well [as] in many of humankind, is a derangement of the vagus nerve, resulting in nausea and retching, faintness, and depression of the heart's action. . . . In my own
practice, I have had four or five patients in whom the subcutaneous use of seven drops of laudanum or of one-twelfth of a grain
of acetate of morphia, has produced faintness, nausea, ending in
vomiting and retching, with intervals of delirious somnolency
for eight or nine hours. By repeated experiments upon these
individuals I have found that the previous or simultaneous use of
a small dose (one-ninety-sixth of a grain) of sulphate of atropia
entirely prevents these distressing and often alarming symptoms.
. . . It is by virtue of its powerful stimulant effect upon the
sympathetic nervous system, that the derangement of the vagus
nerve, causing the above mentioned symptoms, is overpowered.
This is a most important fact ; for by the help of atropia, we may,
I believe, bring *all* individuals alike under the beneficial influence
of opium. The only question of antagonism that now remains,
is that which might be supposed to result from this same stimulant
effect of belladonna upon the heart ; and it may be asked, would
not this action alone be sufficient to arouse a patient in whom the
pulse and respiration were well nigh obliterated by the effect of
opium ?

' I answer, inasmuch as belladonna has no stimulant action
upon the vagus nerve, and therefore no influence upon respiration,

13*

394 CONTINENTAL DEVELOPMENTS

no other result can be expected from the operation of belladonna, in a case of poisoning by opium, than that which would
follow its administration in any other similar case of depression of
the cardiac and respiratory functions. It will doubtless arouse
the heart but there is little hope of increasing the breathing ;
while, on the other hand, the atropia, if given in a large dose, will
only deepen the stupor.' [1]

Harley's researches on the antagonism between atropine and
morphine had a considerable influence in concentrating the
attention of physiologists upon the question of ' the antagonism
of medicines ' in general. The British Medical Association
appointed a committee to investigate this subject and in 1874 a
report was made.

In the course of the committee's experiments .on ' the
physiological action of sulphate of atropia on the rabbit and
dog ', its effects upon the motor and vagus nerves were
demonstrated :

' *Experiment 314.*—The following experiment was made to
determine the action of sulphate of atropia on the nerves and
on the heart. A small terrier . . . weighing 11 lbs., had three-
fourths of a grain of sulphate of atropia in twenty minims of water
injected under the skin of the back. After the usual phenomena,
it was apparently unconscious thirty-eight minutes after the
exhibition of the dose. . . .

' (a) *As to Effect on the Motor Nerves.*—The sciatic nerve in the
right hind leg was exposed, and was stimulated by currents from
Du-Bois Reymond's electro-motor. . . . The strength of the
current employed was so weak as scarcely to be perceived by the
tip of the tongue. . . . The muscles of the hind limb at once
contracted, indicating that the motor nerve-tubes were not
paralysed. . . .

' (b) *As to the Effect on the Pneumogastric Nerve.*—The vagi on
both sides were exposed as quickly as possible. A pair of
electrodes was placed beneath each, and, by means of Pohl's
commutator, the electrical arrangements were so made, that
either the right or the left vagus could be stimulated alternately
or both at once. The result was, that stimulation of the vagus or
vagi produced no appreciable effect on the number of cardiac
pulsations. This . . . indicates that atropia, as is now recognised by all physiologists, paralyses either the trunk of the cardiac
branches of the pneumogastric nerves, or the intrinsic nerve-
centres in the heart with which the cardiac branches are connected. . . .' [2]

[1] *Brit. med. J.*, 1868, i, 319, 343.   [2] *Ibid.* 1874, ii, 518.

During the two years following, 1875 and 1876, W. Munro of Manchester was carrying out, also for the British Medical Association, a fresh series of experiments on the effects of chloroform on laboratory animals.

'In these experiments', wrote Munro, 'I found that in cats, when chloroform was rapidly administered (the best way in my opinion as avoiding that saturation of the blood with chloroform which is apt to be produced by slow administration, and which renders stoppage of the heart's action, if it do occur, almost surely fatal) the systolic action of the heart *invariably* ceased before respiration. . . .

'Wishing to protect the heart's action against the chloroform I, after several preliminary experiments, used a large, but not lethal, dose of atropine, injected about an hour previously to the administration of the chloroform. I now found that the respiration invariably stopped before the heart's action, stoppage of the latter being exceedingly difficult to produce in one case . . . and recovery after stoppage of respiration was generally spontaneous, respiration recommencing of itself; but where I pushed the chloroform till all signs of heart movement were stopped, the effects were the same as if no atropine had been given.'

Four years after making these experiments Munro stated that although he submitted his results to the Association 'the Committee, for reasons best known to themselves, have not published those results'.[1]

During the last four or five years of the eighteen-seventies, at about the time that Munro was experimenting with atropine used as a preventive of the cardio-inhibitory effects of chloroform, E. A. Schäfer and T. R. Fraser were also working independently upon similar lines.

Schäfer, writing to the *British Medical Journal* in October 1880 with reference to a recently published case in which atropine had been injected in an attempt to resuscitate a patient who had died during chloroform anaesthesia, said :

'It is well known that atropin paralyses the cardiac inhibitory apparatus, and since it is probable that death in these . . . cases results from a stimulation of this apparatus, either directly by the drug, or may be in some instances, in a reflex manner, by the stimulation of abnormally excitable afferent nerves during the actual performance of the operation, there undoubtedly seems good reason for the employment of atropin. But clearly, it should be given immediately before the administration of the chloroform,

[1] *Brit. med. J.*, 1880, ii, 240, 761.

as a preventive. . . . My attention has for some time past been directed to the probable value of a prior dose of atropin, as an antidote to the cardio-inhibitory effects of chloroform ; and I have made a number of experiments, as yet unpublished, on the subject. . . . The precaution would only be of value in those cases in which, with the greatest care in administration, death is liable to ensue from the sudden arrest of the heart's action ; but, since the idiosyncracy cannot be detected beforehand, the atropin should never be omitted.' [1]

After the appearance of Schäfer's letter a correspondent wrote to the *Journal* drawing attention to certain points. These points were incorporated by the editor in an annotation :

' Professor T. R. Fraser, of Edinburgh, . . . has shown atropia to be a cardiac stimulant, advisable when chloroform is to be given. It stimulates the heart, not only indirectly, by lowering the conductivity of the cardiac terminations of the vagi, and thus, of course, diminishing their inhibitory power [2], but also directly by stimulating the intramural motor ganglia of the heart ; and possibly, also, by raising the excitability of the accelerator nerve to the heart from the cervical sympathetic ganglia ; and perhaps it may even stimulate the cardio-motor centres in the medulla oblongata.'

Fraser, it was stated, ' considers it advisable to combine with the atropia a little morphia, say 1/120th to 1/60th of a grain of sulphate of atropia . . . and one-twelfth to one-eighth of a grain of acetate or hydrochlorate of morphia. These are injected about fifteen or twenty minutes before the administration of chloroform is begun ; and by this means, (1) not only is the patient in a less nervous state when the inhalation is commenced, but (2) less chloroform is required, and, (3) moreover, a very objectionable evil is got rid of, or, at all events, ameliorated, viz., the emesis which is apt to occur with chloroform. In the cases in which our correspondent has seen this method followed, there has been no vomiting whatever, although in some the inhalation was considerably prolonged '.[3]

Although, as this annotation implies, combined atropine and morphine injection before chloroform anaesthesia had, at Fraser's

---

[1] *Brit. med. J.*, 1880, ii, 620.
[2] The discovery that stimulation of the peripheral ends of the vagus nerves will inhibit the heart's action was made by the brothers Ernst and Eduard Weber in 1846. (Bayliss, W. M. 1918. *Principles of general physiology.* London. 683.)
[3] *Brit. med. J.*, 1880, ii, 715.

suggestion, been used with success in clinical practice before the close of 1880, the method was very far from being in general use either in Scotland or England.   For this two good reasons can be found : Fraser's fellow Scots, as a body, had such faith in chloroform that they considered it needed neither atropine nor morphine as an adjuvant, while the English, at this particular time, held chloroform to be so dangerous that they preferred to discard it almost entirely in favour of ether.

In France, J. A. F. Dastre, in collaboration with another physiologist, Morat, had also been working since about 1878 on the blocking of the vagus nerves by atropine before chloroform anaesthesia.   The steps leading up to the clinical method which he proposed were described by Dastre in 1883 :

' Vulpian ', he wrote, ' has shown [1] . . . that excitation of the vagus nerves arrests the heart more easily in the anaesthetized animal. . . . It is also known that atropine diminishes the excitability of the vagi.

' From the first of these facts one may conclude that cardiac syncope—of such frequent occurrence in chloroform anaesthesia —will be averted if one removes the influence of the vagus nerves upon the heart.   Experiments confirm this conclusion. We have in fact observed that dogs anaesthetized after section of the vagi do not present these fatal syncopes. . . . The second of these facts shows that the injection of atropine is a procedure equivalent to section of the vagi.   Hence the idea of preparing an animal for chloroform anaesthesia by an injection of atropine. We have succeeded by this method in carrying out prolonged operations on dogs without accident and without the constraint of a tiring and often ineffectual vigilance. . . . The primary arrest of respiration is not an accident in the true sense of the word ; because it occurs only when the anaesthetic has been suddenly pushed or unduly prolonged.   It is in fact a toxic effect. . . .

' After the preliminary experiments we proposed our present method to other investigators.   The method consists in preparing the subject to be anaesthetized with an injection of 6 to 10 centigrams of morphine combined with 3 to 5 milligrams of atropine. The morphine, we reasoned, will prevent the period of excitement and prolong anaesthesia (advantages pointed out by Claude Bernard).   The atropine, in addition to its safeguarding effect, will remove the drawbacks of morphine—particularly that of nausea.   It is up to the surgeons, we added, to test this method and judge the results.   What seems to us to be established, in physiological experiments, is that the method removes the

[1] *C.R. Acad. Sci., Paris*, 1878, **86**, 1303.

danger of accident to the heart leaving only (through abuse of the anaesthetic) the grave danger of overdosage.

'This appeal to surgeons was answered by M. Aubert (of Lyons), who has used the method in his hospital practice.' [1]

Aubert himself, during 1883, gave an account of the first sixty cases in which the method was used clinically over a period of five months. His formula was :

Morphine hydrochloride	.	.	.	10 cg.
Atropine sulphate	.	.	.	5 mg.
Distilled water	.	.	.	10 g.

For an adult 1½ grams of this solution were injected with a Pravaz's syringe (see p. 376, footnote) twenty to thirty minutes pre-operatively. For children Aubert never exceeded 1 gram of the solution.

In his earliest cases Aubert used ether (still the anaesthetic of choice at Lyons) for the inhalation ; but he soon became wholly converted to Dastre's proposal and in his later cases ' used nothing but chloroform ' administered on a compress. The advantages which Aubert claimed for Dastre's method were :

' 1. Safety ; 2, greater rapidity in establishing anaesthesia ; 3, absolute tranquillity in the patient ; 4, the facility with which consciousness returned ; 5, absence of after-effects, such as nausea and vomiting.' [2]

Notwithstanding the recommendations of Dastre and Aubert, French surgeons showed themselves reluctant to accept pre-medication as a routine procedure. In a discussion on the subject, held at a meeting of the Société de Chirurgie in Paris in 1890, this reluctance was clearly apparent.[3] In Geneva, however, Julliard, the pioneer of the revived use of ether on the Continent (see pp. 405–6), during the eighteen-nineties adopted the practice of preparing all his patients for ether anaesthesia with a preliminary injection of atropine and morphine.

Previously Julliard had been in the habit, ' in all operations of long duration ', of giving a subcutaneous injection of one-sixth to

[1] *C.R. Soc. Biol. Paris*, 1883, **5,** 242.   [2] *Ibid.* **5,** 626.
[3] *Bull. Soc. Chirurgie Paris*, 1890, **16,** 546.

one-third of a grain of morphine alone before ether anaesthesia,[1] in order to overcome the patient's initial resistance to ether and, by reducing the total amount of anaesthetic inhaled, to obviate as far as possible the occurrence of post-operative chest complications.[2]

Julliard further believed that the injection of morphine (and later atropine-morphine) prior to the inhalation anaesthetic was important because the patient thereby came to the operating theatre in a state of greater mental and physical tranquillity than he would otherwise have done. This latter consideration weighed far more heavily with Julliard than it did with others on the Continent who practised Bernard's or Dastre's methods of mixed anaesthesia ; in England this particular aspect of mixed anaesthesia was unfamiliar. Special reference was made to it, however, in an account of Julliard's use of morphine before ether which appeared in the *British Medical Journal* in 1891 :

'The injection is given to the patient in a quiet room, and he is encouraged to close his eyes to sleep. In about twenty minutes he is carried to the operating table where in quietness and without excitement he is etherised.' [3]

The findings of the Hyderabad Chloroform Commissions of 1888 and 1889 (see pp. 429, 433–5) gave fresh impetus to the revival of interest in that drug which had begun to be manifest in England about 1880. The thirteenth finding of the Second Commission was that 'a small dose of morphia may be injected subcutaneously before chloroform inhalation, as it helps to

---

[1] Although Julliard claimed that morphine given twenty minutes before ether was a satisfactory adjuvant to anaesthesia, O. Kappeler, who observed the effects of such a combination in a series of twenty-five cases, came to the conclusion that it was unsatisfactory. In particular he found that the excitement stage was intensified. (Kappeler, O. 1880. *Anaesthetica : Deutsche Chirurgie*, **20**. Stuttgart. 210.)

An explanation of this phenomenon was given by Macintosh and Bannister in *Essentials of general anaesthesia* (p. 96) :

'Before the beginning of induction the respiratory depressant effect of the morphia may not be obvious, but it becomes so immediately ether is used. The sensitivity of the respiratory tract is scarcely diminished by morphia, so that the irritant effect of ether on the larynx raises the threshold of the respiratory centre to CO_2 above the level to which it has already been raised by the morphia. Shallow and slow breathing results, and if the anaesthetist attempts to shorten the induction period by increasing the concentration of ether vapour frank laryngeal spasm raises the threshold of the centre still further. During this period the blood-ether will be absorbed by the body tissues and anaesthesia may even lighten instead of deepen.'

[2] Dumont, F. L. 1903. *Handbuch der allgemeinen und lokalen Anaesthesie*. Berlin and Vienna. 36.

[3] *Brit. med. J.*, 1891, i, 920.

keep the patient in a state of anaesthesia in prolonged operations.
There is nothing to show that atropine does any good in connexion with the administration of chloroform, and it may do a
very great deal of harm '. Nevertheless in 1891 G. Cockburn
Smith was ' surprised to find that no one made any remarks
at the Bournemouth meeting of the B.M.A. about the use of
atropine, with a view to annul the dangers attending upon the
administration of chloroform '.[1]

In a letter to the *Lancet* he wrote :

' For a long time, especially in France, atropine has been
employed more particularly as an adjunct to morphia, when the
latter is needed to relieve pain, etc., and Dr. Brown-Séquard
[see pp. 391-2] pointed out that the nausea and vomiting that
sometimes attend the hypodermic use of morphia may be done
away with by the addition of atropine to the solution. So we
have for years had a fair indication of the applicability of atropine
and morphia as a means of lessening risk attending upon the
administration of chloroform. Wishing to satisfy myself of the
action of hyoscine on the pneumogastric, I came to the Continent
to avoid the anti-vivisection laws and since being here the extreme
kindness of the surgeons has enabled me to satisfy myself that the
dangers of ether and chloroform can be greatly, if not entirely,
removed by the injection of one centigramme of hydrochlorate of
morphia and one milligramme of sulphate of atropia some twenty-
five minutes previously to their administration in adults. Much
less of the anaesthetic is needed to produce anaesthesia, and the
danger from its toxic effects is avoided. There is often no stage
of excitement perceptible, salivary secretion is checked [2], an
important point in ether inhalation, as swallowing and vomiting
do not occur, but above all, the temporary suppression of the
inhibitory action of the vagus over the heart removes the risk of
its reflex arrest. Dr. Aubert, to whom is greatly due the credit
of having practically introduced the mixed method of inducing
anaesthesia, says that the atropine as it is given beneath the skin,
does not affect the pupil. In several of my cases, however, I
have noticed a marked dilatation. . . . For my part, I have
found that by administering nitrous oxide gas immediately before
the ether, either after Clover's method or that of Brain, the patient
having been previously prepared as above described (the atropine
and morphia injection), the most rapid surgical anaesthesia can

[1] *Lancet*, 1891, ii, 843.
[2] Ebstein, of Berlin, used atropine clinically in 1873 to arrest salivation in a case
of hemiplegia. Subsequently he carried out experiments on the subcutaneous
injection of atropine to check salivation (*Practitioner*, 1873, **11,** 461). In the following
year, 1874, Rossbach, of Würzburg, wrote a paper on the subject. (*Verh. phys.-med.
Ges. Würzburg*, 1874, **7,** 20 ; cf. p. 392, footnote.)

be satisfactorily obtained. . . . So far as I can discover, only one doubtful accident has occurred under the mixed method, and as many thousands of operations must now have been performed during its use, I think that we may consider its success as established.' [1]

Cockburn Smith's letter on premedication with atropine and morphine seems to have had some influence in turning the attention of English anaesthetists to the subject. Hewitt, one of the most influential figures in British anaesthetic circles during the last decade of the nineteenth century, referred to it in 1893, in his book, *Anaesthetics and their administration* (p. 273). He implied that he himself had not used this combination but had used the injection of morphine alone before chloroform, although with misgiving :

' Whilst there can be no doubt that the use of morphine in conjunction with general anaesthetics is of distinct advantage in many cases ', he wrote, ' we must not lose sight of the fact that weighty objections to the routine employment of this mixed narcosis undoubtedly exist.'

Although little was written on the subject of atropine-morphine injection in England until 1912, when Bellamy Gardner drew attention to it as being indispensable before the open administration of ether, atropine alone, as an adjunct to ether anaesthesia, seems to have gained supporters between 1891 and 1906.

In the latter year, at a meeting of the Liverpool Medical Institution, W. Blair Bell read a paper on the general management of cases of abdominal section. He particularly stressed the ' value of atropine before the administration of the anaesthetic ' which, for choice, should be ether.

In the discussion which followed it transpired that ' Mr. Thelwall Thomas was a warm advocate of the administration of atropine before ether ' and ' Mr. W. Fingland referred to the administration of atropine before ether as a most valuable procedure which he had adopted as a routine practice for many years. It had the effect of abolishing salivation, diminishing after-sickness, and facilitating the administration of ether. In dental surgery it was equally valuable, as the operator had only the haemorrhage from the extractions to deal with '.[2]

---

[1] *Lancet*, 1891, ii, 843.   [2] *Ibid.* 1906, ii, 1514.

The injection of morphine combined with scopolamine (hyoscine) was introduced into anaesthetic practice in 1900 by Schneiderlin, of Emmendingen, who had previously used this combination as a sedative in treating mental patients. The preparatory pharmacological work on scopolamine had been carried out chiefly by E. Merck, of Darmstadt, during the years between 1893 and 1899.[1]

Schneiderlin intended morphine-scopolamine to be used as the sole anaesthetic in general surgery, not as an auxiliary to chloroform or ether anaesthesia. He advised making a trial injection of about 0·0003 g. scopolamine and 0·01 g. morphine and repeating the dose after an interval of from one to two hours ; alternatively the initial injection could be given on the evening before operation and followed, on the actual day of operation, by a bigger dose. Schneiderlin stated that it might be necessary in some cases to give from two to four preparatory doses before anaesthesia estimated to be adequate for the contemplated operation was achieved.

This lack of precision seemed to his colleagues to be the weak point in Schneiderlin's method and Berthold Korff, of Freiburg, in 1901, suggested standardizing both the dosage and the intervals at which the dose was injected. He further suggested that if anaesthesia proved to be inadequate during the operation it should be supplemented by small inhalations of either chloroform or ether.[2]

After testing various combinations of morphine and scopolamine during 1901 and 1902 Korff, in 1903, proposed a total dosage of 0·001 g. scopolamine hydrobromide and 0·025 g. morphine hydrochloride in 10·0 g. distilled water. This was to be given in three equal injections, the first two and a half hours, the second one and a half hours, and the third half an hour before operation. If an exceptionally painful operative stimulus made it necessary anaesthesia was to be supplemented by the inhalation of ' a few drops ' of ether or chloroform.[3]

In the same year, 1903, Carl Hartog, of Landau's Clinic in Berlin, recommended the injection of 0·0005 g. scopolamine and 0·01 g. morphine half to three-quarters of an hour before operation, as a routine preliminary to ether anaesthesia administered from a Wanscher's mask (see Fig. 113).[4]

[1] *Merck's A.R.*, 1893–99.   [2] *Münch. med. Wschr.*, 1901, **48** (ii), 1169.
[3] *Ibid.* 1903, **50** (ii), 2005.   [4] *Ibid.* 1903, **50** (ii), 2003.

The injection of morphine and scopolamine to act either as the sole anaesthetic (supplemented if necessary by ether or chloroform) or as a preliminary to inhalation anaesthesia, was widely used on the Continent from 1903 onwards. Both uses were regarded simply as being variations of the mixed anaesthesia originally suggested by Claude Bernard as a means of reducing the amount of inhalation anaesthetic necessary and furthermore of reducing or obviating vomiting and post-operative complications such as chest symptoms and damage to the liver and kidneys.

In America, however, and also in England G. W. Crile's pronouncements, during the first decade of the present century, on the importance of the psychological factor in the production of surgical shock and the desirability of bringing the patient to the operating table calm and reassured, had a considerable influence in establishing premedication as the best means to this end. The drugs originally favoured for this purpose were morphine and scopolamine combined.

Crile himself did not especially recommend premedication, although in 1908 he mentioned that giving ' a hypodermic of morphia half an hour before the patient leaves his room ' was often a good plan to follow.[1]

D. W. Buxton was among the first in England to recognize the psychological importance of premedication. Writing in 1909 he expressed the opinion that ' a terrified patient after a sleepless night is in the worst condition for an anaesthetic and an operation. In such patients ', he said, ' I am convinced that the use of scopolamine and morphine injections before a general anaesthetic is valuable '.[2]

In the following year, 1910, Clifford U. Collins of the St. Francis Hospital, Peoria, Illinois, wrote :

' With all the improvements in the choice of anesthetics and the method of their administration, there still remains with the patient a strong disinclination towards being put to sleep and passing through unknown dangers while utterly powerless to help himself in any way. This decided antipathy to being made unconscious amounts at times to a positive terror, and has been advanced as a cause of some of the sudden deaths reported under anesthesia. It was a desire to overcome this unpleasant feature

[1] *Boston med. surg. J.*, 1908, **158**, 961.
[2] *Proc. R. Soc. Med.*, 1908–9, **2** (i) (Sect. Anaesth.), 60.

that led me to use the combination of scopolamin and morphin
as a preliminary to general anesthesia on myself. . . . The
action of the preliminary was so satisfactory that I adopted its
use in my work. . . .'

Reporting his first series of cases, which numbered well over
a thousand, Collins stated that :

' Tablets are obtained containing a combination of scopolamin,
1/100 grain, morphin, 1/6 grain, and the solution is made just
before it is administered hypodermically, which is done one and
one-half hours before the operation is begun. . . . All necessary
manipulations and handling of the patient in the preparation
are completed before the hypodermic is administered. The room
is darkened and everything kept quiet, and he falls into a tranquil
slumber. About twenty minutes before the operation a layer of
damp cotton is placed over the eyes and the patient is taken to
the operating room and placed on the operating table. . . .' [1]

[1] *J. Amer. med. Ass.*, 1910, **54,** 1051.

CHAPTER XIV

ETHER ON TRIAL : SWITZERLAND—DENMARK—GERMANY—FRANCE

Switzerland

THE English revival (in 1872) of the use of ether in place of chloroform for inhalation anaesthesia, although directly due to American influence, was purely insular in effect. If European affairs had been as settled and as prosperous as British affairs at that particular time this might have been otherwise ; but the Continent continued to be shaken by the repercussions of the Franco-Prussian War, and in Germany it was almost twenty years and in France twenty-five before that most controversial of nineteenth-century anaesthetic questions—chloroform or ether ?—claimed the full attention of medical men.

In Geneva in 1877, however, the surgeon Gustave Julliard, after experiencing in his own practice a death under chloroform anaesthesia, was led to make a trial of ether. He was immediately convinced that ether was superior to chloroform as an anaesthetic and he proceeded to evolve a method of his own for administering it.

He made use of a wire-framed face-mask 15 cm. long, 12 cm. wide, and 15 cm. deep with an evaporating surface of some 750 sq. cm. (see Fig. 107). This mask, except that it was about double the size, was of the same type as Esmarch's (cf. Figs. 58–9) for chloroform ; but Julliard's new technique for ether bore no resemblance to the open drop method of chloroform anaesthesia.

Julliard's frame was enveloped in a waxed cloth cover over an inner layer of absorbent gauze, and in the dome of the mask was a rosette of flannel. On to this rosette 20 to 25 c.c. of ether were poured just before induction was begun. The business of lowering the mask so that its entire rim finally rested on the patient's face, although not closely, was carried out very gradually until resistance to the pungency of the vapour lessened. After the mask had rested lightly on the face for from one to two minutes it was raised and a second dose of ether, about equal in quantity to the first, was poured on to the rosette. A folded towel was then held round the mask to cover the junction between rim and face.

Once tranquil anaesthesia was established the mask was raised by turning it aside from the face at intervals of from one to two minutes throughout administration. This manœuvre, by allowing fresh air to replace the expired mixture collected within the mask, Julliard considered sufficient to prevent undesirable asphyxial complications.[1]

Within a few years of 1877 other surgeons in Geneva followed Julliard's example in changing from chloroform to ether

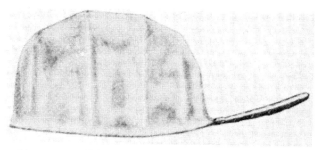

FIG. 107.—JULLIARD'S MASK FOR ETHER
(Geneva, 1877)
Exterior view showing the handle of the wire frame
and the impermeable, waxed fabric outer cover.

anaesthesia. They also copied his mask and technique of administration. By 1885 the method had spread to Lausanne, where C. Roux was its chief exponent ; he modified Julliard's technique, however, by first sprinkling only from 3 to 4 c.c. of ether into the mask and then, after a minute or two, adding a further 15 to 20 c.c., this latter dose being repeated.[2]

In the following year, 1886, the method spread farther northwards, to Berne. There it was again modified by F. L. Dumont and his colleague Fritz Fueter, the latter using a strong initial dose of about 50 c.c. ether.[3]

[1] Dumont, F. L. 1888. *Ueber die Aethernarkose.* Reprinted from *KorrespBl. schweiz. Ärz.*, 1888, **18,** 713.

[2] Dumont, F. L. 1903. *Handbuch der allgemeinen und lokalen Anaesthesie.* Berlin and Vienna. 40–1.

[3] Fueter, F. 1888. *Klinische und experimentelle Beobachtungen über die Aethernarkose.* Leipzig. 9.

Dumont added to Julliard's mask an inner wire frame (see Fig. 108), following the contour of the outer one and opening and shutting on a hinge. Between these two frames was sandwiched the gauze lining of the mask with the flannel rosette attached (see Fig. 112) ; by this means after each administration the soiled lining could readily be replaced by a clean one.[1]

During the late eighteen-eighties Julliard's method of etherization gradually found its way up from German-speaking Switzerland into South Germany, to Tübingen in Würtemberg.

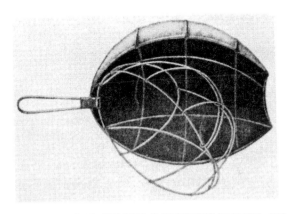

FIG. 108.—DUMONT'S MODIFICATION OF
JULLIARD'S MASK (c. 1885)

Showing the hinged frame which Dumont added to the original single frame, to hold in place the surgical-gauze inner cover with its rosette of flannel.

After Professor P. Bruns, of the Tübingen Surgical Clinic, and his colleague C. Garré (also written Garrè) had made a series of observations upon the physiological effects of ether in man, particularly its effect upon the blood pressure compared with that of chloroform, ether was for a time exclusively used in the Clinic. It was found, however, that chloroform anaesthesia was preferable for children under four years old and for all patients liable to develop chest complications ; but any suspicion of disease of the heart was invariably taken as an indication for the use of ether anaesthesia.[2]

[1] Dumont, F. L. 1903. *Handbuch der allgemeinen und lokalen Anaesthesie*. Berlin and Vienna. 33–41.
[2] *Münch. med. Wschr.*, 1891, **38**, 119 ; *Dtsch. med. Wschr.*, 1893, **9**, 958–9.

METHOD OF ADMINISTERING ETHER WITH DUMONT'S MASK

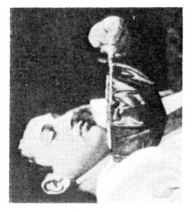 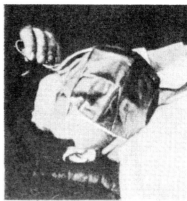

FIG. 109. FIG. 110.

FIG. 109.—The start of administration. The wire frame, with its impermeable outer cover and surgical-gauze inner cover with flannel rosette to receive the ether, has been charged with the anaesthetic dose and is gradually lowered over the patient's face.

FIG. 110.—The mask fully applied to the patient's face. Air filtered into the mask under its rim.

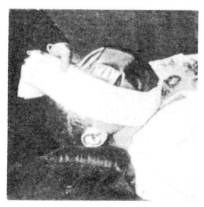 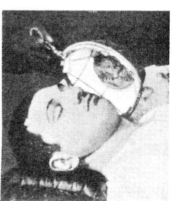

FIG. 111. FIG. 112.

FIG. 111.—The supply of air temporarily restricted, by a folded towel laid over the junction between the mask and the patient's face, in order to increase the proportion of ether vapour inhaled and so rapidly deepen anaesthesia.

FIG. 112.—The mask turned aside from the patient's face—this was done at intervals throughout administration to admit fresh air and allow the exhaled mixture to escape. The surgical-gauze inner cover with its flannel rosette to receive the liquid ether can be seen held in place by the hinged inner frame of the mask.

Denmark

The Continental revival of interest in ether anaesthesia was not entirely confined to Switzerland and South Germany. It appeared independently in Copenhagen about 1882.[1] Although no direct evidence upon the point has been brought to light it is possible that English anaesthetic practice had some influence on Danish in this connexion. After the publication of preliminary reports on anaesthesia by a committee of investigation (afterwards known as the Glasgow Committee) appointed by the British Medical Association during the autumn and winter of 1880 (see pp. 426–8), a long correspondence upon the question ' Ether or chloroform? ' appeared in the *British Medical Journal*.[2] The weight of opinion was heavily in favour of the use of ether. It so happened also that in the following year, 1881, the International Congress of Medicine was held in London. Several medical men from Copenhagen attended and as arrangements were made for members to visit various of the London hospitals daily the Danes almost undoubtedly saw ether anaesthesia used.[3]

In 1883 Oscar Wanscher, Professor of Surgery at Copenhagen, published a booklet on the use of ether as an inhalant for surgical anaesthesia which was entitled *Om Brugen af Aether som Indaandingsmiddel ved Chirurgisk Anaesthesi* (Copenhagen, 1883) ; and in 1884, in which year the Eighth International Congress of Medicine took place in Copenhagen, Wanscher read during the Congress a paper on the rectal administration of ether,[4] a method in which, he explained, he had become interested two years previously.[5]

Wanscher made no reference in this paper to the use of ethei as an inhalation anaesthetic, but during the next few years much of his interest appears to have been directed to the inhalation method of administering the drug.

[1] See, for example, an article by R. Paulli entitled ' Aether eller Kloroform? ', in *Ugeskr. Laeg.*, 1882, **6**, 156, 171, listed in the *Index medicus*, 1883, **5**, 262.

[2] *Brit. med. J.*, 1880, ii, 573, 760, 831, 866, 1000.

[3] Cf. *Trans. int. Congr. Med.*, 1881, **1**, xxxi ; *Brit. med. J.*, 1881, ii, 60.

[4] Axel Yversen, a fellow citizen of Wanscher's, visiting Lyons (the French stronghold of ether inhalation anaesthesia, cf. p. 423) at about this time, asked the surgeon Mollière by which route, rectal or respiratory tract, ether was administered at Lyons. This question prompted Mollière to try rectal ether and it was through his use of it that the method spread, in 1884, to the United States of America. (*Boston med. surg. J.*, 1884, **110**, 442, 451.)

[5] *Trans. int. Congr. Med.*, 1884, **2** (v), 186.

The inhaler which he devised (see Fig. 113) was not very different in outward appearance from Ormsby's (cf. Fig. 95). It consisted of a rubber bag attached to a Junker's type of face-piece. But instead of pouring the ether on to a sponge supported in a wire cage just behind the facepiece, as was Ormsby's method, Wanscher poured a measured quantity (up to 150 c.c.) directly into the bag. During administration he gently shook the bag from time to time to assist vaporization, which was still further facilitated by the warmth of the hand supporting the bag.[1]

In October 1890, during a visit to Dr. Landau's gynaeco-logical Clinic in Berlin, Wanscher stated the case for ether as

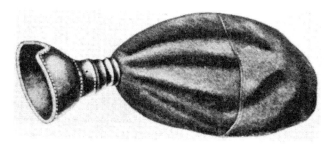

FIG. 113.—WANSCHER'S ETHER INHALER
First used in Copenhagen during the late eighteen-eighties, but adopted by Landau, of Berlin, in 1890. The liquid ether was poured straight into the bag. The vulcanite facepiece was valveless.

an inhalation anaesthetic so convincingly that Landau, although there had never been a fatality from chloroform at his Clinic, was persuaded that for the sake of his patients, many of whom were in an anaemic and debilitated state, he ought to abandon the use of chloroform in favour of the less generally-toxic anaesthetic, ether. So in 1890 ether, given from Wanscher's inhaler, became the routine anaesthetic at Landau's Clinic.[2]

At that date (1890) ether anaesthesia appears to have been in regular use at one other Berlin hospital,[3] the Berlin Eye Hospital, where Schweigger and his colleague Silex had for

[1] Dumont, F. L. 1903. *Handbuch der allgemeinen und lokalen Anaesthesie.* Berlin and Vienna. 41.
[2] *Dtsch. med. Wschr.*, 1894, **20**, 81 ; *Berl. klin. Wschr.*, 1894, **31**, 406.
[3] Ether was in use in Dresden in 1890, however, where Butter and Stelzner administered it from Dumont's modification of Julliard's mask and used Fueter's strong initial dose. (*Arch. klin. Chir.*, 1890, **40**, 66–71 ; cf. *Dtsch. med. Wschr.*, 1894, **20**, 56.)

many years been in the habit of administering it from a towel cone enveloped in an impermeable cover. Schweigger's adoption of ether apparently dated from about 1873, for in that year he read a paper on the subject before the Berlin Medical Society.[1] The facts that he was an ophthalmologist and that he was using the towel-cone method of administration in 1873 strongly suggest that he had been present at, or at least had carefully followed, the proceedings of the International Congress of Ophthalmologists in London in 1872, at which the American B. Joy Jeffries so effectively launched the revival of the use of ether in England (see pp. 313-4).

Germany

In 1890 the Tenth International Congress of Medicine was held in Berlin. To the English observer the evident lack of development in anaesthesia in Germany was no less remarkable than the advanced state of aseptic surgery everywhere prevailing. The *British Medical Journal* commented :

' It was evident on all sides at the Berlin congress, that antiseptic or rather aseptic surgery is held in the very highest repute in that city. A glance at the operating theatre of any hospital . . . was further sufficient to show the extreme care taken and the lavish expenditure that had been incurred so as to render all wounds perfectly aseptic. The surgical instruments are all kept in cupboards constructed solely of glass and iron, and consequently perfectly washable throughout ; the scalpels are all entirely composed of one piece of metal, a method that renders it impossible for dust or dirt to collect between the blade and handle ; the operation table is constructed of one slab of light green glass about an inch thick placed upon an iron frame, and running upon wheels with india-rubber tyres ; and in offices adjoining the theatre are ovens for the sterilization by means of dry or moist heat of everything (bandages, cotton wool, and dressings of all kinds) to be applied to wounds, or for use during surgical operations, which included even goloshes. . . . But in spite of the efforts to excel by this extreme attention to the details of antiseptic surgery that were everywhere observable, it was somewhat disappointing to learn that chloroform is still constantly employed for the production of general anaesthesia during surgical procedures, not only in Berlin, but throughout Germany.'[2]

[1] Cf. *Med. Times, Lond.*, 1873, ii, 556-7 ; *Berl. klin. Wschr.*, 1894, **31**, 415.
[2] *Brit. med. J.*, 1890, ii, 469.

This International Congress of Medicine held in Berlin in 1890 forms, in the history of anaesthesia, a parallel to the International Ophthalmological Congress held in London in 1872 ; for the Congress in 1890 helped to bring about a general revival of the use of ether in Germany as the Congress in 1872 had done in England. Again it was an American, this time Professor Horatio Wood, of Philadelphia, who by reading a paper on anaesthesia set the train of events in motion.

'The most brilliant modern achievements in the direct saving of life by the science of medicine are connected ', he said, ' with surgery. These great achievements have been rendered possible by two epoch-making discoveries, Antisepsis and Anaesthesia. . . . Antisepsis has outgrown the dangers of its youth, and to-day the measures that are meant to save, very rarely kill. On the other hand, the death-roll of anaesthesia is daily added to ; added to, according to my belief, at a rate that has not changed in forty years. . . .'

After referring at some length to the results of his own and other current researches upon the physiological effects of nitrous oxide, chloroform, and ether, with particular reference to the circulatory system, Wood proceeded to stress the superiority of ether over chloroform from the point of view of the safety of the patient.

Apart from mentioning O. H. Allis's inhaler (see Figs. 98–101) as being preferable to the folded towel and sponge, Wood did not concern himself greatly with methods of administration although the use of ether was unfamiliar to a number of his audience. In support of his argument that ether was comparatively safer than chloroform, he quoted statistics :

' It seems to me impossible ', said Wood, ' to get at the exact number of anaesthetic deaths, or the proportionate fatality of ether and chloroform. Lyman [American] considers that in regard to chloroform the ratio of deaths to inhalations is 1 in 5860 ; Richardson [English], that it is 1 in 2500 to 3000. Andrews [American] puts it for ether, at 1 in 23,204 ; and Lyman at 1 in 16,543.
' Without claiming strict accuracy for any of these figures, I think that it can be asserted that the probable ratio of deaths from chloroform is four or five times that of deaths from ether.' [1]

Earlier in the same year (April 1890), during the Nineteenth Congress of the German Surgical Society in Berlin, Oscar

[1] *Trans. int. Congr. Med.*, 1890, **1**, 133, 141.

Kappeler had expressed the opinion that the Americans were over-partial to ether and exaggerated the dangers of chloroform ; furthermore he stated his opinion that ' the use of ether is not without danger, as its partisans would have us believe '.[1]

In order to be able to draw its own conclusions as to the relative dangers of the two anaesthetics the German Surgical Society, in 1890, appointed Gurlt, of Berlin, to compile independent statistics relating to death or threatened death during anaesthesia. His first report to the Society was made a year later.

Gurlt stated that most of his data was of German origin, but records of a few cases came from abroad—three each from Austria and Russia, for example, two from Sweden, and one apiece from Holland and Belgium.

' In 22,656 chloroform anaesthesias 71 cases had been complicated by asphyxial symptoms and 6 cases had proved fatal ; in 470 ether anaesthesias there were no asphyxial complications and no deaths; in 1055 chloroform-ether anaesthesias, 5 cases had asphyxial complications but there were no deaths; in 417 ether - chloroform - alcohol anaesthesias, 4 cases had asphyxial complications ; in 27 ethyl bromide anaesthesias, no asphyxial complications and no deaths. This gives a total of 24,625 anaesthesias, 80 with asphyxial complications and 6 fatalities. Of these 6 chloroform anaesthesia had to its account one death in every 3776 cases and one case of asphyxial difficulty in about every 319 cases ; the figure for chloroform-ether anaesthesia is much smaller and the figure for ether-chloroform-alcohol anaesthesia is smaller still.'

Gurlt stated that only 470 cases of ether anaesthesia had come to hand

' and of these 304 came from Herr Stelzner of Dresden [cf. p. 410 footnote]. . . . The mixed chloroform-ether-alcohol anaesthesias (417 cases) came from Billroth and von Hacker [Billroth, in Vienna, used a mixture of three parts chloroform and one each of alcohol and ether]. On the question of morphine injection combined with inhalation anaesthesia there is a great deal of information ; some reporters stated that they made use of it in almost every case, others in a very large proportion of cases, still others, it seems, scarcely at all. 14 reporters with a total of 6806 cases between them, state that they used an injection of morphine in 2194 cases.' [2]

[1] *Sem. méd.*, Paris, 1890, **10**, 129.   [2] *Dtsch. med. Wschr.*, 1891, **17**, 599.

Again a year later Gurlt made a second report to the German Surgical Society. This time 62 returns had been submitted to him ; 52 came from Germany, the remainder from Austria, Switzerland, Denmark, and Russia. Out of a total of 84,605 cases 33 terminated fatally, so that taking the two years together out of 109,230 cases of anaesthesia, for which various agents had been used, 39 had ended fatally, giving a ratio of 1 death in 2800 administrations. For chloroform the return showed 1 death in 2614 administrations, for ether 1 in 8431. ' In Germany ', Gurlt said, ' ether has not yet received proper recognition of its worth. . . . Only Stelzner (Dresden) and Bruns (Tübingen) have made extensive use of it. Iversen, in Copenhagen,' he added, ' has recorded 2000 ether anaesthesias in three years without a death.' [1]

As Gurlt said, only a few Germans were using ether anaesthesia in 1892, but by the following year a considerable number were using it tentatively and these trial administrations were largely the effect of Gurlt's statistical assessment of the greater safety of ether as compared with chloroform. By 1894 the revival of the use of ether was well-established in Germany.

Soon the Germans were divided into two rival camps over ether anaesthesia. There were those who followed Garré, of Tübingen, in using Julliard's, or as it was also called, the Geneva method, and those who followed Landau, of Berlin, in using Wanscher's method.

The Geneva method soon came to be classed by Wanscher's followers with the American towel cone method, which Wanscher himself referred to as the ' asphyxiating method ' (*asphyxirende* or *Erstickungsmethode*). His own method he called the ' intoxicating ' (*berauschende*) method.[2]

O. Grossmann, of Giessen, in an article in the *Deutsche medizinische Wochenschrift* in January 1894,[3] forcefully contrasted anaesthesia by Garré's method and by Landau's, both of which he knew at first hand. He stated that by Garré's method about 10 to 20 c.c. were poured into the mask and the patient was allowed to become a little accustomed to the ether vapour before the mask was completely lowered. Almost immediately, after as little as half a minute, the mask was held

---

[1] *Dtsch. med. Wschr.*, 1892, **18**, 735.

[2] Cf. *Dtsch. med. Wschr.*, 1894, **20**, 79–81 ; *ibid.* **20**, 81–5 ; *Berl. klin. Wschr.*, 1894, **31**, 405–9.

[3] *Dtsch. med. Wschr.*, 1894, **20**, 55–8.

tightly to the face and again very soon (within two minutes) a further 30 c.c. of ether was shaken into the mask. The rim of the mask was then overlaid with a towel to prevent, as far as possible, the dilution of the vapour with air. For the events which followed, Grossmann quoted Garré's own words, taken from his book *Die Aethernarkose* (Tübingen, 1893) :

' " With the first inspirations of ether the respiratory rhythm becomes accelerated and shallow. This is apparently a reflex action caused by the irritant effect of the vapour on the nose. Only a few patients are able to tolerate the vapour without opposition and breathe regularly and deeply. Often the inhalation of ether vapour provokes coughing but this is soon over. In the excitement stage the breathing is very much disturbed, now quick and regular, then suddenly interrupted through powerful spasm of the respiratory muscles. The patient becomes cyanotic and struggles violently and there is tonic spasm in the muscles of the extremities. This state of affairs can seem very alarming, but it will pass without our interference. . . . In other cases respiratory movements are so shallow that they can only be followed with difficulty. With the onset of muscular relaxation breathing becomes deep and, often, stertorous. If, as is frequently the case in protracted anaesthesia, there is now a large quantity of mucus collected in the pharynx, this may be churned up by the inspired mixture itself, into fine snow-white froth. When this happens the breathing takes on an extremely unpleasant rattling tone. This indicates no danger to the patient, however. But were this chloroform narcosis such wheezing and apparently distressed breathing would create the most painful impression." '

' The " painful ", " distressing " and indeed " alarming " impressions which the first case of ether anaesthesia with Julliard's mask that I saw at Tübingen, made upon me ', Grossmann admitted, ' were so strong that I allowed the idea of trying ether myself, in a few cases, to drop. The impression was still fresh when, in March of this year [1893] I visited Dr. L. Landau's Clinic, in Berlin, and had the pleasure of learning how to administer ether by another method.

' What worlds apart the two methods are. Here was no trace of the state of affairs described above—the cyanosis, the froth on the lips, the stertorous breathing, the tracheal rattle (or if there was the least suspicion of them it was an indication that technique was faulty). . . .

' During June and July, through the kindness of Dr. Landau, to whom I offer my sincere thanks, I, acting as a house surgeon, had the pleasure of personally administering ether in about 60 cases and was present at about 80 cases.

' The advantages of this method of ether anaesthesia are so great that I most confidently advise every medical man to change over from chloroform to ether.'

After describing the inhaler used by Landau (see Fig. 114) —it consisted of a semi-spherical facepiece with an inflatable

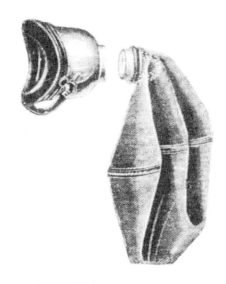

FIG. 114.—MODIFICATION OF WANSCHER'S
ETHER INHALER (cf. Fig. 113)

In use at Landau's Clinic in Berlin, c. 1894. The metal hoops which kept the walls of the rubber bag from falling together are indicated by dotted lines.

rubber rim and having an opening of ' two or three fingers' diameter ' in the floor of the dome, guarded on the outside by two metal hoops to keep the mouth of the rubber bag open, and the bag itself, which was about ' a span and a half in length '— Grossmann proceeded to describe an administration :

' From 50 to 100 g. of ether are poured through the facepiece into the bag and the inhaler is slowly approximated to the patient's face, which is turned to one side. As soon as the patient tolerates the vapour well and no further reflex spasm is manifest, which point is made immediately apparent by the onset of regular respiration, the facepiece can be more or less firmly applied. Even when the inhaler is firmly applied there is still sufficient space at certain points for atmospheric air to filter in between the rim of the facepiece and the face. But one is particularly careful to see that the lower border of the facepiece fits well, so that the ether vapour, which is heavier than air, cannot flow out there. At first the bag hangs down. In the bottom is the liquid ether in a pool, from the surface of which vapour rises and passes to the facepiece where it mixes with air and so will be inspired by the patient. As anaesthesia progresses one supplies the patient with an increasingly concentrated ether vapour by shaking the bag. Care must be taken, however, that breath holding does not occur ; should it do so it is a sign that the patient is not yet tolerating the concentrated ether vapour and this is particularly the case if reflex spasm occurs. Once tolerance is established the bag is shaken so that the patient breathes concentrated ether vapour until the corneal reflex is totally abolished, which may be regarded as a sign that anaesthesia is fully established. When surgical anaesthesia is complete the inhaler can be removed from the face, but not for very long, because the effect of ether is far more transient than that of chloroform, and the patient very quickly begins to wake. During deep anaesthesia the facepiece, in the majority of cases, is lightly applied, but the shaking is discontinued. The small amount of vapour rising from the surface of the liquid ether is sufficient, even when the apparatus is not shaken, to maintain anaesthesia.

' The point which distinguishes this from Julliard's mask is the way in which the ether vaporizes. In the first place, in Wanscher's inhaler the surface of the ether from which evaporation takes place is relatively small, but in Julliard's mask the whole of the inside of the mask is covered by ether-soaked flannel, providing a huge surface for evaporation. Secondly, in Julliard's mask the vapour descends, but in [Wanscher's inhaler] the vapour must rise. This circumstance is extremely important when one considers that ether vapour is heavier than air. If one allows ether to vaporize from an open dish the vapour diffuses to the floor of the room and collects there. If one pours ether into the Wanscher inhaler and immediately applies the face to it and breathes the vapour present in the bag, one draws in a large, suffocating quantity of ether.[1] But if one waits a few moments until the walls of the bag (freely moistened by the pouring in of the ether and thus presenting a much greater evaporating surface) have dried, one can then breathe easily and without that almost unbearable feeling of suffocation, the trifling quantity of

---

[1] Landau's assistant, Vogel, stated that this was, in fact, one way of producing narcosis with the inhaler—a way closely resembling Julliard's in effect. (*Berl. klin. Wschr.*, 1894, **31**, 406.)

14

ether vapour rising from the small surface of the pool of ether in the bottom. If the bag is held quite still, so that the pool of ether is not agitated, so remarkably little ether is vaporized that one can scarcely detect it on inspiration. But directly the bag is well shaken an almost suffocating quantity of ether vapour streams up.

' So, with the Wanscher inhaler, we are able to administer a very little ether to the patient ; or, by shaking the bag and thus increasing vaporization, we can allow a more or less concentrated vapour to be inspired. In other words Wanscher's inhaler permits of the graduated administration of ether. With Julliard's mask this is scarcely possible.'

Grossmann found one disadvantage in Wanscher's method— the fact that induction took, on an average, from 15 to 20 minutes ; very occasionally surgical anaesthesia was established in from 8 to 10 minutes, but often from 30 to 40 minutes were necessary. With Julliard's mask induction was certainly much quicker, but Grossmann, quoting Garré, explained :

' " The ether must be inhaled in as large and as concentrated a dose as possible, in order to ensure its prompt action. Through the use of this concentrated vapour unconsciousness supervenes in from 2 to 3 minutes . . . but it is only partly attributable to the ether ; far more is it the result of oxygen-lack producing asphyxia." ' [1]

In a subsequent article in May 1894 Grossmann amplified his previous statement.

' There are,' he wrote, ' as Wanscher has said, two ways in which ether can be used—the *asphyxiating* and the *intoxicating* methods. But it must not be imagined that the two are sharply distinct, for that is not the case. One can asphyxiate with every inhaler and will always do so if the patient is allowed too little air for the adequate provision of the oxygen which is essential to him. Wanscher himself touched upon the very kernel of the whole matter when he said " . . . the secret of good ether anaesthesia lies in giving as little air as possible, but in giving enough." '

In order to make certain that the patient received sufficient air in the inhaled mixture Grossmann, in 1894, modified Wanscher's inhaler. He greatly increased the diameter of the airway between the facepiece and the bag, and for the small hoops which kept the mouth of the bag open (cf. Fig. 114) he substituted a wire framework projecting farther into the bag so that its walls were kept widely separated. The bulk of the bag still hung down, however, ensuring that the level of the liquid ether in it was much below the level of the facepiece.[1]

While Wanscher's followers accused Julliard's of asphyxiating their patients, Julliard's followers, in turn, condemned Wanscher's inhaler as dangerous on the ground that with it the concentration of ether vapour could, and often did, rise to as much as 34 per cent. of the inspired mixture. Of the two methods, however, Julliard's had the wider following in Germany.[2]

Meanwhile another question was endangering the success of the revived use of ether in Germany—the question of post-operative complications following etherization, in particular damage to the kidneys and chest complications.

The first of these two considerations, damage to the kidneys resulting from ether anaesthesia, began to attract serious attention in America during the eighteen-eighties.[3] R. von Santvoord in 1883 published a paper on ' The danger attending the use of ether as an anaesthetic in cases of Bright's disease '.[4] T. A. Emmet in 1887 expressed the opinion that a careful examination of the urine ought to be made before anaesthesia in all cases where kidney disease was suspected. The presence of albumen or casts, he thought, should be taken as a positive contraindication to the use of ether and an indication for the use of chloroform.[5]

At the time of the revival of the use of ether in Switzerland, in 1888 Roux in Lausanne observed albumen in the urine in four instances after ether anaesthesia. In the same year Fritz Fueter, in Berne, influenced by the trend of American opinion, undertook an investigation of the effects of ether upon the kidneys of dogs.

' The results of this investigation . . .' wrote Fueter, ' so far as the function of the kidneys and urine are concerned, have proved completely negative ; nor could any change in the tissues of the kidney be detected microscopically. It was, indeed,

[1] Dtsch. med. Wschr., 1894, 20, 470–1.
[2] Cf. Dumont, F. L. 1903. Handbuch der allgemeinen und lokalen Anaesthesie. Berlin and Vienna. 42.
[3] Nothnagel (according to D. N. Eisendrath, of Chicago, writing in the Deutsche Zeitschrift für Chirurgie, 1895, 40, 467), in four experiments on etherized animals, observed in 1866 that although the tissues of the liver and heart under the microscope showed traces of fatty change the kidneys were normal and the urine albumen free. (Nothnagel, C. W. H. ' On the influence of ether and chloroform on the kidneys.' Berl. klin. Wschr., 1866, Nr. 4.)
[4] Med. Rec., N.Y., 1883, 23, 201.   [5] Ibid. 1887, 31, 199.

already assumed *a priori* to be improbable that pathologico-
anatomic appearances would be found where the urine had in
every respect been normal.

'Both after a single, prolonged administration of ether, for
as long as 2½ hours, and after several such administrations, at
intervals of from 1 to 2 and more days, no trace of albumen was
ever detected, and the quantity of the dogs' urine showed no
perceptible fluctuation—at all events, no decrease.

'If, then, after repeated and protracted anaesthesia . . .
not the least affection of the kidneys (in healthy animals, of
course) was manifest . . . I believe I am right in concluding
that the danger of etherization to the patient with only a slight
degree of disease of the kidneys is not so serious as the Americans
assert.

'My experience with this anaesthesia in patients with albumen
in the urine completely supports this opinion ; for I have never
observed any alarming complications whatsoever during anaesthesia nor any increase of albumen nor other symptoms which
could be attributed to the aggravation of a kidney lesion.

'I can, therefore, find no positive contraindication to ether
anaesthesia in the presence of an abnormal urine content.' [1]

In 150 clinical cases tabulated by Fueter albumen was
observed to be present in the urine post-operatively in two only
—in one of which it was strongly marked for three days.

The majority of German surgeons were prepared to accept
Fueter's view that the danger of damage to the kidneys following
ether was not a serious one. A far more formidable deterrent to
its use was the possibility of subsequent severe chest complications. This aspect of ether anaesthesia attracted little general
attention in Germany during the first three years of the revived
use of ether there (1891–3). But in 1894 there was a widespread
increase in the number of medical men who, although unfamiliar
with the use of ether, decided to try it. The frequency with
which patients developed post-operative 'chests' after inhaling
ether now became apparent to everyone.

In September 1894 Poppert, of Giessen, precipitated a
discussion on the subject in the German medical journals by
writing an article, 'On a case of death from ether resulting
from lung oedema, together with remarks on anaesthetic
statistics', for the *Deutsche medizinische Wochenschrift*. He emphasized the fact that deaths due to oedema of the lungs following

[1] Fueter, F. 1888. *Klinische und experimentelle Beobachtungen über die Aethernarkose.*
Leipzig. 22–8, 29.

ether anaesthesia were not at all uncommon and that such deaths should be accounted anaesthetic deaths no less than those occurring on the operating table during chloroform anaesthesia. This point, he thought, had been largely obscured by Gurlt's statistics which, in assessing the comparative mortality from the two agents, ether and chloroform, did not take into consideration these delayed deaths directly attributable to the toxic effect of ether.[1]

Mikulicz [2] added the weight of his opinion to that of Poppert and soon a return to the use of chloroform was in full swing among those who had met with difficulty either in the administration of ether or in its post-operative consequences.

Mikulicz, a convert of Gurlt's, who had been using ether with Julliard's mask since the winter of 1893-4, wrote in November 1894 :

' I have several times seen cases which, both during and after ether anaesthesia, contradicted the much praised safety of this agent and led me, at Easter of this year, to return to the use of chloroform.'

These cases (none of which proved fatal) were : three cases of asphyxia in the course of anaesthesia ; two cases of collapse after anaesthesia ; four cases of acute bronchitis and two cases of lung oedema and pneumonia. Mikulicz repeated Poppert's assertion that the fact of the existence of inherent dangers in ether anaesthesia was obscured by Gurlt's statistics.

' The results of the inquiry made by the German Surgical Society ', wrote Mikulicz, ' have as yet furnished no positive information on the important question : chloroform or ether? But it has achieved one important end—it has brought clearly before our eyes the fact that every anaesthetic is dangerous, more dangerous, indeed, than many people have up till now believed.' [3]

In 1895 Grossmann (who now admitted that his initial enthusiasm for ether anaesthesia had been considerably moderated by experience), in an article on ' Bronchitis and pneumonia in ether anaesthesia ', put forward the theory that chest complications were due only indirectly to the irritant effect of ether on the respiratory tract. The primary cause, he maintained,

[1] Dtsch. med. Wschr., 1894, 20, 719-22.
[2] The Polish surgeon, Johann von Mikulicz-Radecki (1850-1905), who at this date (1894) was working in Breslau.
[3] Berl. klin. Wschr., 1894, 31, 1035-9.

was auto-intoxication through the inhalation, during the anaesthetic state, of an increased flow of bacteria-laden mucous secretion from the nose, mouth, and pharynx, a view previously advanced (in February 1895) [1] by Professor Nauwerck of the Institute of Pathological Anatomy at Königsberg.

To remedy this state of affairs Grossmann recommended placing the headpiece of the operating table in a horizontal position, removing the customary pillow or roll from under the patient's head and turning the head to one side so that saliva collecting in the oral cavity would drain out of the corner of the mouth. The pillow, particularly if a thick one, he pointed out, raised the back of the patient's head in such a way that the chin was thrust down towards the chest, obstructing the airway and making it difficult or impossible to turn the head so that the mouth drained properly. In such a position oral and nasal mucus slipped easily into the trachea.[2]

Bruns, of Tübingen, on the other hand, supported the theory that chest complications were due to the presence of impurities in the ether.[3]

So far as abdominal operations were concerned, however, Mikulicz observed, in a comparative series of patients operated upon between 1896 and 1900, that the incidence of post-operative chest complications was as high (or higher) after local anaesthesia as after inhalation anaesthesia.[4] Also in connection with abdominal operations and, indeed, ' all operations an effect of which is to cause pain on coughing . . . and to upset expect-oration and the free functioning of the abdominal pressure ', P. Campiche, of the University Surgical Clinic in Lausanne, referring specifically to chest complications following ether anaesthesia, wrote :

' It is not even necessary for the patients to be bronchitics or cardiacs to develop them ; we find that even healthy individuals contract bronchitis after a laparotomy or a radical cure of hernia, simply because they have not had the energy to breathe deeply and to cough vigorously in order to get rid of such bronchial secretions as the anaesthesia may have left them.' [5]

[1] Dtsch. med. Wschr., 1895, **21**, 121–4.
[2] Ibid. **21**, 462.
[3] Berl. klin. Wschr., 1894, **31**, 1147–9 ; Lancet, 1895, ii, 1641.
[4] Dumont, F. L. 1903. Handbuch der allgemeinen und lokalen Anaesthesie. Berlin and Vienna. 182–3.
[5] Campiche, P. 1902. Contribution à l'étude de la narcose à l'éther. Geneva. 104.

Although many surgeons continued to use ether anaesthesia, from 1895 onwards the German enthusiasm for it waned. Gurlt still compiled statistics by which he demonstrated that the annual death-rate from chloroform anaesthesia far exceeded that from ether, but he no longer made converts.[1] This decline of interest was, to a considerable extent, due to the recent introduction of C. L. Schleich's new method of local anaesthesia by the infiltration of weak solutions of cocaine (see pp. 42–3), which increasingly attracted the attention given at the beginning of the decade to questions of inhalation anaesthesia.[2]

France

In France the first unmistakable sign that a revival of the use of ether anaesthesia had begun was a paper on the subject by Chaput, Angelesco, and Lenoble. The paper was read by Chaput at a meeting of the Surgical Society of Paris in May 1895. From the list of references appended to the paper it is clear that Chaput and his colleagues had been following, with particular interest, the development of the revived use of ether in Germany. Chaput had, however, been in direct communication by letter with Wanscher in Copenhagen, and it was the latter's apparatus and technique which were used by Chaput, Angelesco, and Lenoble in their clinical experiments (numbering 135) which were begun at the Salpêtrière in 1894. The results of these 135 cases decided the investigators in favour of ether and in their opinion the only formidable disadvantage of its use lay in the possibility of subsequent chest complications. The risk of explosions, they thought, had been greatly exaggerated.[3]

More interesting than Chaput's paper was the discussion which followed the reading of it. The discussion was opened by Ollier, of Lyons, and for the first time for some forty-five years the words of a Lyonnais etherist were received with attention by the Parisian chloroformists (cf. pp. 204–7).

' For more than thirty years ', said Ollier, ' I have, on numerous occasions, shown my preference for ether as an anaesthetic [4] and my conviction in this connection has become increasingly

[1] Cf., e.g., Berl. klin Wschr., 1897, **34,** 459.
[2] Cf. Kolaczck : ' Zur Narkosenfrage,' Dtsch. med. Wschr., 1896, **22,** 179–80.
[3] Bull. Soc. Chirurgie Paris, 1895, **21,** 358–80.
[4] An aphorism of Ollier's ran as follows : ' Ether is to chloroform as wine is to spirits '.

firmer as my experience has grown longer. During thirty-five years I have administered, or rather have had administered on my responsibility, 40,000 anaesthetics (comprising all cases in my department carried out by my deputies, assistants, heads of clinics or house officers)—though this figure is an under-estimation—. . . . and I have not had a single death during anaesthesia or a post-operative death which could be directly laid at the door of the anaesthetic itself. . . . Of this number . . . six or seven hundred cases at the most, have been anaesthetized with chloroform. Although I have not actually had a death among these last-mentioned cases, yet I have had occasion to fear for the lives of several patients and the alarms have been more frequent and more acute than has been proportionately the case with ether. . . .'

Speaking of the technique of administration used for ether Ollier continued :

' If one seeks to put the patient to sleep rapidly with ether by completely preventing the admixture of fresh air with the vapour, one is liable to have accidents. . . . I have never used the specialized and more or less complicated types of inhaler. . . . I always use Jules Roux's " sac " [see Fig. 24], which is simply a pig's bladder in a cloth envelope with an opening in the lower back part, closed with a stopper, for pouring in the ether. This is the apparatus which has been used for more than 40 years in the hospitals of Lyons. . . . Where there is a fear of carrying infection, I use a pig's bladder tobacco pouch, such as one finds cheaply everywhere, which is used only once.'

Ollier differed from Chaput and his two associates in having no fear that ether would adversely affect the lungs. He considered that, other things being equal, ether was less dangerous than chloroform even in cases where a lesion of the thoracic organs existed and might be expected to influence the patient's condition. But he made an exception to this general rule in cases where the reaction of the trachea or bronchi to the irritant effects of ether was very pronounced.[1]

This discussion was continued during subsequent meetings of the Society, and in the course of it another Lyonnais, Poncet, stated that he also used a Roux's *sac*, but of a type in which bladder and envelope could be separated and sterilized. His personal experience of ether anaesthesia extended to 25,000 cases, but he did not use it exclusively, preferring chloroform for children and for bronchitics.

[1] *Bull. Soc. Chirurgie Paris*, 1895, **21**, 380–3.

The experience in the use of ether of the dozen or so other members of the Society who spoke was of about a year's duration. Most of them used Julliard's mask and the majority of opinion was definitely in favour of ether anaesthesia given by that means. Many disagreed, however, with Ollier's statement that chest complications were less to be feared after ether than after chloroform and with Chaput's statement, made in his paper, that ' true vomiting was extremely rare after ether '.

Lucas-Championnière suggested that since both ether and chloroform had intrinsic advantages and disadvantages the best solution of the anaesthetic problem, after all, might be to use an anaesthetic sequence, beginning with ether and continuing with chloroform.

Only one member, named Reynier, said that after making a trial of ether, both clinically and in comparative experiments with chloroform on dogs, he had returned to the exclusive use of chloroform.

Reynier had used ether clinically both from Roux's *sac* and from an inhaler designed by Cusco (the details of which he did not describe, but in which ether was mixed with air). ' I returned to chloroform ', he said, ' when I saw that, after all, ether affords *just as many dangers* as chloroform, in spite of what people say.'

Poncet, in closing the discussion, summed up as follows :

' In judging the comparative frequency of pulmonary complications following ether and chloroform one meets in practice, it is true, with very real difficulties in interpreting the facts. These complications, so frequent in the old, are indeed often observed after chloroform as well as after ether, but the degree of responsibility which must be laid at the door of the anaesthesia itself is not always easy to define. . . . I believe that ether is undeniably likely to effect the bronchi and on this score I consider that its use is dangerous in the two extremes of life. As for my convictions as to the value of etherization and as to the method of anaesthetizing in general, they are as definite as can be, and without entering further into the reasons which ought, in my opinion, to make ether the anaesthetic of choice, I will call to mind only that for all those who have had experience of this drug, its harmlessness is beyond dispute. Herein lies the true cause of the superiority of ether—it is less dangerous than chloroform. Round this unique and peremptory argument all other arguments must group themselves.' [1]

[1] *Bull. Soc. Chirurgie Paris*, 1895, **21**, 453.

14*

PART SIX

THE BEGINNING OF MODERN ANAESTHESIA

Chapter XV

HYDERABAD COMMISSION AND ITS CONSEQUENCES

The Glasgow Committee—The Hyderabad Commission—The Commission's
Effect upon Physiological Research in Anaesthesia—Goodman Levy's Work.

The Glasgow Committee

AT the forty-third Annual Meeting of the British Medical
Association, held in Edinburgh in 1875, the Section of Surgery
passed a resolution :

'. . . that it is desirable that a committee be appointed to
inquire into and report upon the use in surgery of various
anaesthetic agents, and mixtures of such agents ; that it be part
of the object of such committee to collect and summarise the
experience of British practitioners of surgery and medicine as to
the relative advantages of chloroform, ether, nitrous oxide gas,
and other agents, and to carry out suitable experimental investigations ; that Professor Lister of Edinburgh, Professor Pirrie of
Aberdeen, Mr. Annandale, Dr. Thomas Keith, Dr. J. Duncan,
Dr. M'Kendrick, and Dr. Crum-Brown, of Edinburgh ; Dr.
Burdon Sanderson, Mr. Spencer Wells, Mr. Ernest Hart, and
Mr. Clover, of London ; Dr. Macdonnell and Mr. J. Morgan, of
Dublin, be requested to act as a committee for this purpose, with
power to add to their number.'[1]

This Committee in fact did not meet until 1877, in the
course of the forty-fifth Annual Meeting of the British Medical
Association, held in Manchester. On that occasion it was
suggested by T. Spencer Wells that ' as the committee is a very
large one, and is made up of members from Aberdeen, from
Edinburgh, from Dublin, as well as London, it is almost impossible for them to do what is required in the words of the
resolution '. It would be, Spencer Wells thought, ' far better
to expend any sum devoted to the purpose by the Scientific

[1] *Brit. med. J.*, 1875, ii, 214.

Grants Committee—and this sum ought to be a sufficient one—so as to encourage one really competent investigator to do the work thoroughly well, bearing the full responsibility and taking the credit which is due to work well done '.

The outcome of this suggestion was the appointment of ' a Subcommittee of research, to consist of the following medical gentlemen, all of whom belong to Glasgow : Dr. Ramsay [whose place was afterwards taken by David Newman, Pathological Chemist to the Western Infirmary], Dr. [Joseph] Coates [Pathologist to the Western Infirmary], and Dr. McKendrick, Professor of Physiology at Glasgow University ; the latter gentleman to act as Chairman and Convener. It was also recommended that for the purposes of this Subcommittee of research the Scientific Grants Committee should make a fresh grant of £50 '.[1]

This Subcommittee, which from the fact that all its members were connected with Glasgow became known as the Glasgow Committee, published the results of its researches in 1880. The report, which was made quite independently of the main Committee, whose functions remained nominal throughout the investigation, chiefly reaffirmed the findings of the Royal Medical and Chirurgical Society's Chloroform Committee of 1864 (see pp. 253–8). The aims and the principal conclusions arrived at by the Glasgow Committee were summarized in a leading article in the *British Medical Journal* on the occasion of the publication of the Report :[2]

' In conducting these investigations, two lines were followed : first, to discover wherein the special dangers of chloroform consist ; and, second, to attempt to find some safer anaesthetic. Observations made on rabbits showed that chloroform had a most disastrous action on the heart as well as upon the respiratory centre ; that, while ether might be administered for an indefinite period without affecting the heart, no sooner was the inhalation of chloroform commenced, than the right ventricle began to distend, and, in the course of time, the cardiac contractions ceased. In every respect but one, ether was superior to chloroform. It had, however, one disadvantage—viz., the length of time which was required to obtain its action ; and, on this account, the Committee proceeded to search for some other anaesthetic.'[3]

[1] *Brit. med. J.*, 1877, ii, 176, 224.
[2] *Ibid.* 1880, ii, 957–72.   [3] *Ibid.* ii, 984.

Whereas the Chloroform Committee in 1864 had recommended the substitution of the use of anaesthetic mixtures for chloroform as the sole anaesthetic, the Glasgow Committee in 1880 recommended the use of ethidene dichloride ($CH_3CHCl_2 =$ 1,1-dichloroethane) (see also pp. 215-6) as standing ' in an intermediate position ' between ether and chloroform, ' causing more lowering of [blood] pressure than ether, but less than that produced by chloroform. The same relation between these three anaesthetics is observed in regard to respiration : complete arrest of the pulmonary circulation being obtained most rapidly by chloroform, and with the smallest dose ; least rapidly by ether, and with the largest dose ; ethidene standing intermediate, whether as regards the time required, or the dose needed to produce the arrest of pulmonary circulation.

'. . . In the face of the constantly recurring notices in medical journals, and even in the public prints, of deaths during the administration of chloroform, it cannot fail to be patent to everyone that there is danger in the administration of that drug. It will be observed that it does not affect our argument whether such deaths were unavoidable, or were the result of faulty administration, or of administration of an insufficient quantity, as we believe to be not infrequently the case. The fact remains that deaths do occur ; and, in such circumstances, is it not the duty of the medical profession to endeavour to find a more safe anaesthetic ? and, further, if, as this valuable report goes to show, ethidene-dichloride be a safer drug, is it not, then, incumbent on our profession to make use of it ? Ether, while safe, has the alleged disadvantage of needing to be given in large quantities, and for a considerable time. Ethidene has no such disadvantages, and it may be given with the same feeling of security as attends the administration of ether.' [1]

In spite of Clover's championship of ethidene dichloride (cf. p. 216 footnote) the profession, as a whole, did not follow the Committee's advice—just as in 1864 it did not, as a whole, adopt anaesthetic mixtures.

The Glasgow Committee's Report, indeed, did no more than reassure both those who used ether and those who used chloroform and confirm them in their separate ways. For the majority who, during the eighteen-seventies, had adopted ether on the grounds that it was safer than chloroform found ether still acknowledged to be ' in every respect but one, . . . superior

[1] *Brit. med. J.*, 1880, ii, 984.

to chloroform'—and that that one respect, 'the length of time required to obtain its action', was immaterial to the etherist. Those, on the other hand, who had persisted in the use of chloroform in spite of the very general readoption of ether found that no additional deterrent to its use had been discovered since 1864 ; the recognized deterrent, the paralyzing effect of chloroform upon the heart, was unimportant to the chloroformist because he believed the danger to be avoidable. Then suddenly, in 1889, the whole vexed question of chloroform anaesthesia was reopened.

The Hyderabad Commission

' On the 25th ult.', stated the Lancet on February 23, 1889, ' their Royal Highnesses the Duke and Duchess of Connaught distributed the prizes to the students of the Hyderabad Medical School. Surgeon-Major Lawrie, M.D., [sic] the Principal of the School, delivered a short address on the occasion, in the course of which he said the male and female students at that institution enjoyed, in many respects, practical advantages of which very few European schools could boast. They had made experiments with reference to the effects of chloroform, which had conclusively decided a question which has been in dispute ever since chloroform was first introduced. They had killed with chloroform 128 full-grown pariah dogs averaging over 20 lb. weight each. What they found was that, no matter in what way it was given, in no case did the heart become dangerously affected by chloroform until after the breathing had stopped. The speaker added that, in the 40,000 or 50,000 administrations which he had superintended, he had never seen the heart injuriously or dangerously affected by chloroform. He had no doubt deaths would go on occurring until the London schools, which of course influence the whole world, either entirely changed their principles and ignored the heart in chloroform administration, or else confined themselves exclusively to the use of an anaesthetic like ether, which, with all its disadvantages, they know how to manage.' [1]

The Lancet was not prepared to let these provocative remarks go unchallenged. The editor, on March 2, 1889, wrote :

' In a report of the recent prize distribution at the Hyderabad Medical School, which appeared in our issue of Feb. 23rd, some remarks of Surgeon-Major Lawrie, M.B., [sic] M.R.C.S., of the Bengal Army Medical Service, are mentioned, which deserve

[1] Lancet, 1889, i, 394.

some comment. We learn that a commission [1] had been appointed to investigate the action of chloroform, and that the result of the researches made upon pariah dogs was that these animals were killed from respiratory failure, and in no case did cardiac syncope occur directly.   Unfortunately Mr. Lawrie contents himself with bare statements of results, adding that these results tally with his own experience, which he believes to be uniquely large.   Mr. Lawrie, as a disciple of Simpson and Syme, arrives at conclusions consonant with the teaching of those great clinicians, but utterly at variance with the experience alike of experiment and practice as carried out in Europe.   We should require more than the scanty statements of experiments performed upon dogs—notoriously non-susceptible to chloroform syncope—before we could accept the conclusions of the Hyderabad Commission when they appear to go in the very teeth of those at which the Commission appointed by the Royal Medical and Chirurgical Society and by the British Medical Association [the Glasgow Committee] arrived, and, further, are opposed to the careful and painstaking experiments of such scientific observers as Snow, Claude Bernard, McKendrick, and others too numerous to mention.   All those who are familiar with chloroform are well aware that syncope, when primary, as a rule supervenes in the initial stages of inhalation, while secondary syncope due to respiratory embarrassment is the result of accumulation of chloroform in the blood leading to paralysis of the medullary centres, and occurs in a late stage of the administration.   The primary syncope it is rarely, if ever, possible to induce in dogs, although, unfortunately, it is this form of chloroform heart failure which does occur in human beings, and which it is almost impossible to remedy.   While welcoming the attention paid to the subject by the Hyderabad Commission, we cannot but feel that, should the Commission inculcate a disregard of the heart as a factor in chloroform dangers, it will do harm and provoke a slipshod carelessness in the use of that valuable anaesthetic, which must in the long-run do damage to the cause the Commission has espoused.' [2]

Lawrie accepted the *Lancet's* challenge.   In a letter to that journal, published on May 11, 1889, he wrote :

'. . . I hold . . . that there is no such thing as chloroform syncope.

' It is conceivable that syncope may occur in the initial stages of inhalation of chloroform, but in the course of a very large

---

[1] This Commission, which was appointed by the Nizam of Hyderabad's Government during 1888 at the request of Lawrie, came to be known as the ' First Hyderabad Commission '.

[2] *Lancet*, 1889, i, 438.

experience I have never met with a single instance of such an accident, and if it ever does occur it cannot be due to chloroform poisoning, though it might be caused by fright or shock. Owing to the numerous accidents that have happened with chloroform, to the discussions prevalent in the profession, and to the mistaken notion that the risk of heart failure is inseparable from its use, the public dread its administration much more than they dread surgical operations, and fainting from mere fright in the early stages of inhalation is no less intelligible than it is easy to prevent, in cases where it is likely to occur, by a preliminary dose of alcohol. On the other hand, it is equally intelligible that syncope may be induced if an operation be commenced in the initial stages of chloroform administration, before the patient is rendered insensible to shock by being brought fully under its influence. In poisoning by chloroform the heart fails when the respiration ceases, and never before. . . . The heart rapidly or gradually stops beating, as a direct result of the stoppage of respiration, and as an indirect effect of the poisoning with chloroform.

' The *Lancet* asserts that the statements made in my address are utterly at variance with the experience alike of experiment and practice as carried out in Europe. They are, nevertheless, based on the principles taught by Syme and Simpson, and I hope by their successors, in Edinburgh ; and long before the Hyderabad Commission was formed I had satisfied myself that they are entirely true. . . .

' Neither I nor the Hyderabad Commission have any desire to inculcate a disregard of the heart as a factor in chloroform dangers. . . . The *Lancet* would trust to the heart and circulation for signals of danger in chloroform administration. Our contention is that if the administration is ever pushed far enough to cause the heart to show signs of danger, the limits of safety have already been exceeded, and a fatal result must almost inevitably ensue. . . . But we say, further, that the respiration invariably gives warnings when a dangerous point is approached, and consequently that it is possible to avert all risk to the heart by devoting the entire attention to the respiration during chloroform administration.' [1]

This letter drew from the *Lancet* the following annotation :

' It is a matter of regret that, instead of complying with our request for fuller information, Mr. Lawrie has contented himself with mere dogmatic assertion and iteration of his former statements. Whatever may be the value of the work done by the Hyderabad Commission—and Mr. Lawrie seems inclined to accept the conclusions arrived at, rather than those of well-known

[1] *Lancet*, 1889, i, 952.

and tried scientists—it is quite impossible for those who have neither seen the experiments to which Mr. Lawrie refers, nor received an authoritative statement as to the methods employed and precautions taken, to accept as evidence the results to which he refers. No mere *ipse dixit* can shake the weight of the large accumulation of facts of which we are now possessed concerning the depressant action of chloroform upon the heart.' [1]

The somewhat acrimonious character of this discussion happily changed in August 1889, when in a further letter Lawrie ' stated that he was directed by his Highness the Nizam to offer the *Lancet*, as the leading medical journal, the sum of one thousand pounds to send out a representative to repeat the experiments of the Hyderabad Chloroform Commission. We could not ', said the *Lancet*, ' decline an offer showing such commendable interest in a matter of enormous human and scientific importance. We therefore proposed to Dr. Lauder Brunton that he should represent us in this matter.[2] He accepted the offer. . . .' [3]

The *Lancet* gave as its reasons for choosing T. Lauder Brunton, F.R.S., that he was a pharmacologist of international repute and that in his book, *Pharmacology and therapeutics*, he ' very decidedly stated that one of the dangers resulting from chloroform is death by stoppage of the heart '.[4] Despite this emphatic pronouncement, the first important telegram received from Lauder Brunton in Hyderabad read as follows :

' " Four hundred and ninety dogs, horses, monkeys, goats, cats, and rabbits used. One hundred and twenty with manometer. All records photographed. Numerous observations on every individual animal. Results most instructive. Danger from chloroform is asphyxia or overdose ; none whatever heart direct." '

' These results ', said the *Lancet*, ' apparently indicate such a complete reversal of the view held by Dr. Lauder Brunton at the time he left England . . . that the details of the experiments made by Dr. Brunton, and the reasons for the conclusions he has evidently arrived at, will be awaited with the greatest interest by the profession.' [5]

---

[1] *Lancet*, 1889, i, 949.

[2] This new Commission, under the presidency of Lawrie, of which Lauder Brunton was a member, came to be known as the ' Second Hyderabad Chloroform Commission '.

[3] *Lancet*, 1889, ii, 601, 1351–2.   [4] *Ibid.* ii, 606.   *Ibid.* ii, 1183.

The eagerly expected report of the Second Hyderabad Chloroform Commission was completed in December 1889 and published in sections in the *Lancet* between January and June 1890.[1] All Lawrie's original contentions appeared to be substantiated by this Report :

'Chloroform, when given continuously by any means which ensures its free dilution with air causes a *gradual* fall in the mean blood-pressure, provided the animal's respiration is not impeded in any way, and it continues to breathe quietly without struggling or involuntary holding of the breath—as almost always happens when the chloroform is sufficiently diluted. As this fall continues the animal first becomes insensible then the respiration gradually ceases, and lastly, the heart stops beating. If the chloroform is

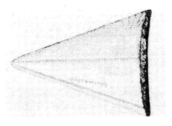

Fig. 115.—THE HYDERABAD CHLOROFORM CONE
Invariably used by Lawrie and his assistants.

less diluted the fall is more rapid, but is always gradual, so long as the other conditions are maintained ; and however concentrated the chloroform may be, it never causes sudden death from stoppage of the heart. The greater the degree of dilution the less rapid the fall, until a degree of dilution is reached, which no longer appreciably lowers the blood-pressure or produces anaesthesia.'

On the question of the influence of the vagal nerves upon the heart's action as a factor in chloroform anaesthesia the Commission stated :

'The experiments in which deliberate irritation of the vagi was carried on during anaesthesia show unmistakably that irritation of these nerves diminishes rather than enhances the danger of anaesthetics. . . .

'The theory which has hitherto been accepted is that the danger in chloroform administration consists in the slowing or stoppage of the heart by vagus inhibition [cf. pp. 396–8]. This

[1] *Lancet*, 1890, i, 149–59, 421–9, 486–510, 1140–2, 1369–88.

is now shown to be absolutely incorrect. There is no doubt whatever that the controlling influence of the vagus on the heart is a safeguard, and that it is the exhaustion of the nerve which is dangerous.

'It can be readily understood how a condition in which the pulse is rapid and bounding, with high blood-pressure, leads to more rapid absorption of chloroform from the lungs, and a more rapid propulsion of the chloroformed blood to the medulla oblongata, and consequently to a more rapid paralysis of the respiratory and vasomotor centres and precipitous fall in the blood-pressure.'

The first section of the Report ended with a list of fourteen ' practical conclusions which the Commission think may fairly be deduced from the experiments :

' 1. The recumbent position on the back and absolute freedom of respiration are essential.

' 2. If during an operation the recumbent position . . . cannot . . . be maintained during chloroform administration, the utmost attention to the respiration is necessary to prevent asphyxia or an over-dose. If there is any doubt whatever about the state of respiration, the patient should be restored to the recumbent position. . . .

' 3. To ensure absolute freedom of respiration, tight clothing of every kind . . . is to be strongly avoided ; and no assistants or bystanders should be allowed to exert pressure on any part of the patient's thorax or abdomen, even though the patient be struggling violently. . . .

' 4. An apparatus is not essential, and ought not to be used, as, being made to fit the face, it must tend to produce a certain amount of asphyxia. Moreover it is apt to take up part of the attention which is required elsewhere. . . . A convenient form of inhaler is an open cone or cap with a little absorbent cotton inside at the apex.

' 5. At the commencement of inhalation care should be taken, by not holding the cap too close over the mouth and nose, to avoid exciting, struggling, or holding the breath. If struggling or holding the breath do occur, great care is necessary to avoid an over-dose during the deep inspirations which follow. . . .

' 6. In children, crying ensures free admission of chloroform into the lungs ; but as struggling and holding the breath can hardly be avoided, and one or two whiffs of chloroform may be sufficient to produce complete insensibility, they should always be allowed to inhale a little fresh air during the first deep inspirations which follow. . . . Struggling is best avoided in adults by making them blow out hard after each inspiration during the inhalation.

' 7. The patient is, as a rule, anaesthetised and ready for the operation to be commenced when unconscious winking is no longer produced by touching the surface of the eye with the tip of the finger. . . . When once the cornea is insensitive, the patient should be kept gently under by occasional inhalations, and not be allowed to come out and renew the stage of struggling and resistance.

' 8. As a rule, no operation should be commenced until the patient is fully under the influence of the anaesthetic, so as to avoid all chance of death from surgical shock or fright.

' 9. The administrator should be guided as to the effect entirely by the respiration. His only object, while producing anaesthesia, is to see that the respiration is not interfered with.

' 10. If possible, the patient's chest and abdomen should be exposed during chloroform inhalation, so that the respiratory movements can be seen by the administrator. If anything interferes with the respiration in any way, however slightly, even if this occurs at the very commencement of the administration, if breath is held, or if there is stertor, the inhalation should be stopped until the breathing is natural again. . . .

' 11. If the breathing becomes embarrassed, the lower jaw should be pulled, or pushed from behind the angles, forward, so that the lower teeth protrude in front of the upper. . . .

' 12. If by any accident the respiration stops, artificial respiration should be commenced at once, while an assistant lowers the head and draws forward the tongue with catch-forceps, by Howard's method, assisted by compression and relaxation of the thoracic walls. . . . [Cf. Appendix C.]

' 13. A small dose of morphia may be injected subcutaneously before chloroform inhalation, as it helps to keep the patient in a state of anaesthesia in prolonged operations. There is nothing to show that atropine does any good in connexion with the administration of chloroform, and it may do a very great deal of harm.

' 14. Alcohol may be given with advantage before operations under chloroform, provided it does not cause excitement, and merely has the effect of giving the patient confidence and steadying the circulation.

' The Commission has no doubt whatever that, if the above rules be followed, chloroform may be given in any case requiring an operation with perfect ease and absolute safety so as to do good without the risk of evil.' [1]

In spite of the 588 carefully described experiments on the lower animals—animals either healthy or deliberately made diseased and submitted to a variety of the most rigorous tests

---

[1] *Lancet*, 1890, i, 149-59.

under strict experimental conditions ; in spite of the supporting evidence of kymographic records ' reproduced by photography ' ; in spite of Lawrie's personal assurance that in all his large experience he had never seen a death from heart failure due to the direct action of chloroform ; and in spite of Lauder Brunton's conversion to Lawrie's beliefs,[1] the *Lancet* remained to some extent sceptical.

' We thought that it would be well to supplement the work of that Commission as far as possible by a consideration of the results arrived at by clinical observations ', wrote the editor. ' Our investigation into the relative safety of anaesthetics as usually administered to human beings was therefore commenced as soon as the Second Hyderabad Commission's report was received.'

The inquiry was directed for the *Lancet* by Dudley Wilmot Buxton (cf. pp. 464, 469).

A carefully drawn-up series of questions was sent to individual members of the British medical profession and a more detailed questionnaire to every hospital (of over ten beds) in the United Kingdom. This latter form together with a circular letter, ' couched in the language of the country to which it was sent ', was despatched to the larger hospitals on the Continent, in the Colonies, the United States, and India. The form which members of the profession were asked to complete, ' desired information on the following points :

' What anaesthetic do you usually employ, and how ? (Apparatus ?). Average number of times a year ? Do you keep an accurate register ? What class of cases (operation, midwifery, etc.)? Can you give particulars of any deaths ? Agents used ? Apparatus ? Nature of operation ? Age, sex, and peculiarities of patient ? Posture ? How long under ? Did heart or respiration stop first ? If a post-mortem, particulars ? Can you give particulars of any dangerous cases and means used for resuscitation ? '

Similar information was required from the hospitals at home and abroad.

---

[1] Lauder Brunton's conversion, it seems, was not quite wholehearted, for Lawrie in 1901 wrote of him : ' Dr. Lauder Brunton proceeded [at the end of the Second Hyderabad Commission] to England to convert Europe and America, but he could not entirely divest himself of the opinion he had held and taught for so many years that " one of the dangers of chloroform is death by stoppage of the heart " and ' Lawrie admitted, ' the conversion of Europe and America devolved to a large extent upon me '. (Lawrie, E. 1901. *Chloroform*. London. 11.)

The gathering of material was completed by the close of 1891 ;[1] the analysis of it took until 1893. From this analysis many interesting generalizations were made.

It was found that by far the most prevalent method of administering chloroform was ' poured on a handkerchief ', and in descending order of frequency : on lint, on a towel, a napkin, into an extemporized cone, or on a sponge. This, the *Lancet* pointed out, offered a possible explanation of the fact that ' the recorded deaths resulting from chloroform being administered without an inhaler are rather more than double those occurring when an inhaler is used '.

When an inhaler was used deaths occurred in the following order of greatest to least frequency :

Inhaler, type unspecified ; Skinner's (or similar) inhaler (see Fig. 56) ; Snow's inhaler (see Fig. 41) ; Junker's inhaler (see Fig. 63) ; Clover's inhaler (see Figs. 53–5) ; Esmarch's inhaler (see Figs. 58–9) ; metal cone ; Guy's Hospital inhaler ; Morton's ether inhaler (see Fig. 12) ; Weiss's inhaler (see Fig. 52).

The *Lancet* commented :

' We have, however, no figures to show the number of times these inhalers are used, and, in the absence of these, there is no accurate basis for comparison in regard to their safety or danger. . . . Skinner's apparatus, from its simplicity and portability, is probably used very much more frequently than any other. Snow's and Clover's inhalers are seldom, if ever, employed at the present time. Skinner's, Junker's (in one of its modifications), or some form of cone, containing a sponge or piece of lint, probably represent the inhalers at present in vogue in order of their frequency of employment.'

Although it was possible to generalize from the information provided by the answers to the questionnaire, the *Lancet* found it necessary to add : ' It is a remarkable fact that, in more than half the cases of fatalities reported to us, no mention is made of the method which was followed in giving chloroform '.

The *Lancet* complained also of a looseness of terminology. The term ' open method ', for instance, was used by some people to designate ' chloroform " poured " on lint " after the manner

---

[1] ' In order to arrive at a continuous series of cases from 1847 . . . not only were the above sources of information used ', the *Lancet* stated, ' but the records of Snow. . . .' (See Appendix C.)

of Syme ", who taught that plenty of the drug should be used ',
while others used the same term to designate ' chloroform
" dropped " on lint after the manner advocated by the dosimetric school, who teach that by dropping chloroform literally
guttatim on lint the utmost safety is ensured '.

In considering the *Lancet's* finding ' that chloroform was
employed some six times more frequently than ether ', it must
be remembered that a proportion of the answers to the questionnaire came from the Continent where (in 1891) ether was virtu-
ally not used (cf. Chapter XIV), and from parts of Scotland
' where chloroform is used almost exclusively '. Furthermore
the *Lancet* found that ' an examination of the record of private
practice indicated . . . that chloroform is used more frequently
in that department of practice than is any other anaesthetic '.

As a general conclusion the *Lancet* stated :

' It would, therefore, appear that in England and Wales
chloroform is responsible for a larger number of deaths and of
dangerous cases than is ether. In India, and the Tropics generally, ether is not used, and chloroform is very largely employed,
with a very low death-rate ; on the Continent, the death-
rate is in favour of ether [1], but it is at present difficult to gauge
the relative frequency with which the two substances are employed. In the United States ether is widely used, but here again
we cannot estimate the number of times that anaesthetics in
general and chloroform in particular are used with sufficient
accuracy to draw conclusions. In Scotland . . . there is
no reliable evidence of how many deaths under chloroform
really occur, although it is believed that deaths are fairly
frequent.' [2]

As to the determining causes of death under chloroform, the
answers to the *Lancet's* questionnaire bore out the findings of the
Chloroform Committee of 1864 and the Glasgow Committee of
1880 :

' The larger proportion of deaths are reported as having
resulted from initial heart failure, in opposition to the view to
which the physiological researches of the Hyderabad Commission
have led.'

[1] This assertion was based on Julliard's figure for mortality under ether, viz. one
death in 14,987 administrations.
[2] ' As regards Scotland ', the *Lancet* stated, ' the present condition of the law as
to inquiries into the circumstances of deaths under anaesthetics greatly interferes with
accurate information being obtained upon this matter.'

A possible explanation of why the observations of the Hydera-bad Commission differed from those made during the *Lancet's* own survey was suggested :

' That these conflicting views are reconcilable seems to us to be possible, at least in many cases. The reports of numerous cases refer to *failure of the pulse* as occurring before that of respira-tion, and it is undoubtedly true that although the pulse does fail, yet the actual heart action continues for some time after pulse failure. This explanation, however, seems hardly to apply to those cases of *sudden death* which occur at the commencement of chloroform anaesthesia, nor can these deaths be explained . . . as being due to fright, and not to the anaesthetic.' [1]

The Commission's Effect upon Physiological Research in Anaesthesia

When the commotion caused in the field of practical anaes-thesia by the Report of the Second Hyderabad Chloroform Commission thus quietly subsided in 1893, it was noticeable that the beliefs as to the dangers of chloroform anaesthesia held by the opposing parties remained essentially unshaken. But for the investigator in the laboratory the problem of the physiological action of chloroform remained unsolved. In particular no satisfactory and conclusive answer had been supplied by the Commission to the question : ' What is the reason of the fall of blood pressure which always occurs when a large dose of chloroform is administered ? ' It was this question which W. H. Gaskell, Lecturer in Physiology in the University oɪ Cambridge, and his colleague, L. E. Shore, set themselves to answer.[2]

At the outset of their researches Gaskell and Shore admitted two possibilities : either that ' the fall of blood pressure may be due in the first instance to failure of the vasomotor centre, the heart not being affected until a very excessive dose has been given '—this was Lawrie's view ; or that ' the fall of blood pressure may be due from the very first to a weakening of the

[1] *Lancet*, 1893, i, 629, 693, 761, 899, 971, 1111, 1236, 1479.
[2] In the summer of 1890 Lawrie was in England, and because of the controversy which the Second Hyderabad Commission's Report had aroused here he asked Gaskell to undertake on behalf of the Nizam's Government a supplementary report on the blood-pressure curves recorded during the Hyderabad experiments. It was as a preliminary to this further report that Gaskell undertook the above-mentioned investigation. (*Brit. med. J.*, 1893, i, 105.)

heart's action, the vasomotor centre not being affected until a very excessive dose has been given '.[1]

The first series of experiments undertaken by Gaskell and Shore dealt with the effects of liquid chloroform injected into the vascular system and they compared the results with the effects of chloroform administered by inhalation.

' These experiments ', wrote Gaskell and Shore, ' point directly to the conclusion that chloroform causes a fall of blood pressure by the weakening of the heart's contractions and not by a paralysis of the vasomotor centre ; when, however, we attempt to explain the effects of chloroform inhalation by the experience thus gained we must always remember that liquid chloroform possesses a much more powerful irritant action upon the tissues than the vapour of chloroform. This is naturally only a question of degree, for the stimulating action of strong chloroform vapour is shown most markedly by the reflex effects produced upon the nasal and pharyngeal membranes. Although, then, we should expect . . . that injection of chloroform into the vascular system should produce stronger signs of irritant action than its inhalation, yet there can be no doubt that these experiments show that such injections of chloroform, whether brainwards or heartwards, do produce also anaesthesia and paralysis of respiration resembling in effect the symptoms seen upon inhalation of the drug. We are therefore, it seems to us, justified in concluding that although these experiments are not of themselves absolute proof of the action of chloroform when inhaled, yet they support rather than oppose the view that chloroform when inhaled differs in its action from chloroform when injected in degree rather than in kind. . .

' Experiments upon the effect of injection of chloroform into the brain arteries on the one hand, and into the jugular vein on the other, point strongly to the conclusion that the fall of blood pressure observed when chloroform is inhaled is due to a weakening of the heart's action, and not to a primary paralysis of the vasomotor centre ; still, however, as already mentioned, they cannot be regarded as a conclusive proof that such is the action of chloroform when inhaled. We require, therefore, as a supplement to these experiments, some method by which chloroform can be inhaled in the usual manner, and the blood containing chloroform thus inhaled can be sent either to the heart alone or the brain alone at will. . . . We have devised the method of cross circulation between two animals in order to test this point. . . .

' These cross-circulation experiments confirm absolutely the previous experiments in which chloroform was injected directly

[1] *Brit. med. J.*, 1893, i, 105–6.

into the circulation. In both cases the blood containing chloroform excites the vasomotor centre and raises the blood pressure when it reaches the medulla oblongata, while it depresses the heart's action and lowers the blood pressure when it reaches the heart.

'It is, then, clearly proved that the primary fall of blood pressure seen during chloroform administration is not due to paralysis of the vasomotor centre. We must, then, look beyond the central nervous system for an explanation of this fall—that is, to a direct paralysing action of the drug upon the vascular system—a direct action, therefore, upon the heart and blood vessels.' [1]

Lawrie, not unnaturally, was perturbed by the results of these experiments, which he himself had commissioned. Assuming with characteristic self-confidence, however, that since Gaskell's conclusions contradicted his own views there must, somewhere, be a fallacy underlying Gaskell's experiments, Lawrie repeated the cross-circulation experiments ' under almost insuperable difficulties, in Hyderabad '. The results he obtained were reassuring to himself, for they appeared to show yet again that chloroform had no direct influence on the heart. At a meeting of the British Medical Association at Montreal in September 1897 he had the further satisfaction of hearing Gaskell admit that true cross-circulation had probably not been obtained in the Cambridge experiments. Lawrie was never able to comprehend, however, Gaskell's subsequent refusal to agree that on this account all the observations made during the Cambridge experiments and the conclusions drawn from them were rendered completely valueless.[2]

Commenting on the work of Gaskell and Shore, Leonard Hill (Lecturer in Physiology at the London Hospital), in an address on ' The causation of chloroform syncope ' delivered before the Society of Anaesthetists in February 1897, said :

' The most brilliant part of Gaskell and Shore's work is the contrivance of their cross-circulation experiments. They take two dogs, " the fed and the feeder ". In the fed dog the carotid and the subclavian arteries are ligatured. One or more of these vessels are then connected by rubber tubes to one or more of the same arteries of the feeder. The jugular veins of the two animals are also put in connection. The blood of the feeder is rendered

---

[1] *Brit. med. J.*, 1893, i, 164-71.
[2] Lawrie, E. 1901. *Chloroform*. London. 12-20.

incoagulable by the injection of peptone or leech extract. By this means the circulation through the brain of the fed dog is maintained by the blood propelled from the heart of the feeder. The circulation through the rest of the body of the fed dog remains in its normal condition. If chloroform be now inhaled by the fed dog the drug circulates through the heart and the blood vessels of the lungs, abdomen, and the limbs of the dog. Its brain is supplied by the uncontaminated blood of the feeder. Under these conditions the heart of the fed dog passes into paralytic dilatation, while its respiratory movements are maintained unimpaired by the respiratory centre in the spinal bulb. If, on the other hand, the feeder be made to inhale chloroform, while the fed is given none whatever, the arterial pressure in the feeder will then fall, and the bulbar centres in the fed dog are first excited and then paralysed by the drug derived from the feeder which circulates through them. In this case the arterial pressure of the fed dog rises while its respiration is paralysed. . . .

' In reference to the cross section experiments, the objection has been raised that the blood supply to the spinal bulb is not entirely cut off by a ligation of the carotid and subclavian arteries. This objection carries no weight. It is perfectly true that by way of the anterior spinal artery a certain amount of blood does reach the spinal bulb. This does not to the slightest degree invalidate the main results of the research. On giving chloroform to the fed animal, the circulation is rapidly paralysed, while the respiratory centre is maintained in full activity by the blood of the feeder. This is the one fact of importance, proved without any possibility of controversion, that while the respiration remains in full force the circulatory mechanism poisoned by chloroform fails in a very short space of time to maintain its efficiency. If some of the blood of the fed animal did reach the spinal bulb, so much the worse for the respiratory centre, but we see that in spite of such contamination the respiration continued to act in an efficient manner. If the Hyderabad Commission failed to obtain these results on repetition of this experiment . . . the failure is only a further proof of the incompetence of the experimenters employed by the Commission.' [1]

Gaskell and Shore's finding that chloroform acted primarily on the heart, causing dilatation and paralysis, bore out the work of J. A. MacWilliam, Professor of the Institutes of Medicine at Aberdeen. In 1890 MacWilliam made a report to the Scientific Grants Committee of the British Medical Association on an experimental investigation, begun in 1888, ' of the action of chloroform and ether '. In the report he stated that experiments,

[1] Brit. med. J., 1897, i, 958-9.

chiefly on cats, showed that ' dilatation of the heart occurs to an appreciable extent, even when chloroform is administered gently, mixed with abundance of air (under 4 per cent. of chloroform vapour in the air) ', and ' may occur even before the conjunctival reflex is abolished ' and before there is any fall of blood pressure. ' Moreover ', MacWilliam found, ' when the dilatation has followed a fall of pressure it is not removed by artificially raising the pressure, for example, by compression of the abdominal aorta. There is no distinct change in the rate of the heart's action when dilatation occurs. A sudden and complete cessation of the cardiac rhythm is never caused by the inhalation of chloroform. Cardiac failure occurs by a more or less sudden enfeeblement and dilatation of the organ. . . . The tone of the heart muscle is depressed, the cardiac walls become relaxed, and . . . it fails to be an effective force in keeping up the circulation, while its rhythmic movement still continues—though so feebly as to be inefficient. . . .

' The depressing influence of chloroform on the heart—leading to dilatation of its cavities—is not exerted through the vagus nerves,' MacWilliam stated, ' but is a direct effect of the drug upon the cardiac mechanism. Section of both vagi does not obviate the weakening and dilating influence of chloroform upon the heart.'

Although MacWilliam stressed the point that the dilatation of the heart by chloroform was quite independent of the vagus nerves, he stated that ' a temporary slowing of the heart's action sometimes occurs—from asphyxial conditions or from sensory stimulation during imperfect anaesthesia—which is indirectly brought about through the vagus nerves '. He added that ' it does not appear to be dangerous in the healthy animal '.[1]

The Hyderabad Commission's contention that chloroform never affected the heart primarily had been based solely upon the evidence of kymographic tracings. MacWilliam pointed out that ' blood-pressure tracings by themselves, or taken along with respiratory traces, are entirely untrustworthy guides to the state of the heart under anaesthetics. The oscillations in blood-pressure tracings caused by the heart-beats do not give accurate indications as to the state of even the left ventricle—much less of the other parts of the organ. And even the general level of the blood-pressure does not prove a reliable guide to the cardiac

[1] *Brit. med. J.*, 1890, ii, 949–50.

condition. For it is obvious that the pressure may be profoundly affected by changes in the heart's action, by changes in the peripheral resistance (systemic or pulmonary), or by both these causes combined ; and the kymograph, while demonstrating the occurrence of alterations in the height of the pressure does not afford the data necessary for analysing the causation of such alterations '.[1]

MacWilliam, referring to ventricular fibrillation (a phenomenon first observed by him about 1889[2]), stated that ' the occurrence of fibrillar contraction (delirium cordis) does not appear to be a primary mode of cardiac failure from the inhalation of chloroform in the healthy animal, though it may sometimes supervene when the heart has become distended and incapacitated through chloroform '.[3]

MacWilliam differed from Gaskell and Shore in maintaining that apart from the dilatation of the heart caused by the direct action of chloroform upon it the drug could also cause depression of the vasomotor centre.

' The relative occurrence of cardiac dilatation and vasomotor depression varies. Sometimes the heart begins to dilate early— before there is any fall of pressure ; at other times a large fall of pressure may occur before cardiac dilatation becomes marked. The lowering of the blood pressure is in a certain sense protective ; it retards the access of more chloroform to the vital organs. But, on the other hand, the fall of pressure may become excessive and produce dangerous effects.'

He agreed (as indeed did other observers, both clinicians and physiologists) with the Hyderabad Commissioners in thinking that ' changes in the respiration exerted a most powerful influence upon the effects of chloroform administration. An amount of chloroform which can be given with safety during easy breathing ', he wrote, ' may speedily become dangerous during deep, rapid respiration. . . . Changes in respiration may be excited by sensory stimulation (operative interference, too strong chloroform vapour, etc.) during imperfect anaesthesia. Rapid, gasping respiration occurring in such circumstances is usually accompanied by a rise in the blood pressure, and, as there may be already a considerable amount of chloroform in the circulation, there occurs a combination of circumstances specially

[1] J. Physiol., 1892, **13**, 860.
[2] Brit. med. J., 1889, i, 6.   [3] Ibid. 1890, ii, 950.

favourable for the speedy and sudden development of dangerous collapse '.[1]

Leonard Hill agreed with MacWilliam in thinking that chloroform exercised a depressing action upon the vasomotor centres. In 1897 he reported experiments carried out on a morphinized dog, fixed to a board which could be swung round a horizontal axis, and with cannulae inserted into the jugular and carotid arteries and connected with manometers. ' This research ', Hill explained, ' forms one of a series of researches which for the past few years I have been carrying out on the influence of gravity on the circulation.'

From the results of his experiments he concluded that ' chloroform, more than any other known agent, rapidly abolishes the vascular mechanisms which compensate for the hydrostatic effect of gravity. Chloroform abolishes these mechanisms by paralysing the splanchnic vasomotor tone, and by weakening the action of the respiratory pump. When the mechanisms are totally abolished the circulation is impossible if the subject be in the feet-down position '.

Hill also stated that ' in the condition of shock or emotional fear the compensatory mechanism for the effect of gravity is almost abolished, and chloroform may easily be the last straw to completely paralyse the circulation '.[2]

At the Annual Meeting of the British Medical Association in 1897, held in Montreal, the Section of Anatomy and Physiology was under the presidency of Augustus D. Waller, Lecturer on Physiology at St. Mary's Hospital Medical School, London. The subject which he chose for his presidential address was ' the action of anaesthetics upon nerve '.

In the first part of his address Waller dealt with the action of various anaesthetic agents upon isolated nerve. In the second part of his address he turned to ' considerations bearing upon practice.

'. . . In accordance solely with the data acquired upon isolated nerve,' said Waller, ' and putting on one side for the moment all the mass of clinical knowledge slowly and expensively acquired during the last fifty years, the two agents one would select as most certain and effective in their action are precisely the two clinically selected agents, ether and chloroform. . . .

---

[1] *Brit. med. J.*, 1890, ii, 950.   [2] *Ibid.* 1897, i, 959–62.

' With regard to the two principal reagents the most important results have been these :

' (a) Using ether and chloroform at an indefinite but high degree of concentration (about 40 per cent. and 10 per cent. respectively) the nerve has nearly always been anaesthetised (=temporarily immobilised) by ether, killed (=finally immobilised) by chloroform.

' (b) Using ether and chloroform at various definite degrees of concentration (5 to 40 per cent. of the former, 1 to 5 per cent. of the latter) *the action of chloroform has been seven times that of ether. . . .*'

Alluding to the reputed danger of carbon dioxide in chloroform anaesthesia against which Lauder Brunton had recently given the warning : ' Chloroform vapour pure and simple is not nearly so dangerous as chloroform vapour with carbonic acid ',[1] Waller stated that ' in so far as concerns the electromobility of nerve, my observations distinctly traverse this statement. Carbon dioxide, while it may somewhat accelerate the immobilising action of chloroform, very distinctly accelerates and favours the recovery of mobility subsequent to such immobilisation. . . . I am persuaded . . . of the great danger of impeded respiration during chloroform anaesthesia. . . . But it is not the accumulation of noxious CO_2 by impeded respiration that is the source of danger . . . it is the accumulation of chloroform itself '.[2]

Early in the following year, 1898, at a meeting of the Society of Anaesthetists Waller returned to the question of chloroform anaesthesia. Referring to his Montreal address he said :

' Whereas on that occasion I very deliberately laid principal stress upon the great power of chloroform and upon the absolute certainty of a considerable percentage of avoidable and therefore unjustifiable deaths if chloroform is administered without adequate recognition of this fact . . . on the present occasion . . . I am about to urge the importance of a complementary principle in the practice of anaesthesia by chloroform—namely, upon the paramount necessity for dosage in its administration. Many practical anaesthetists, I know, admit this principle ; others, I believe, do not, or at least hold it to be . . . practically impossible. . . .

[1] Brunton, T. L. 1897. *Lectures on the action of medicines.* London. 219.
[2] *Brit. med. J.*, 1897, ii, 1474-5.

' In my view, the desideratum to aim at is a continuous production of chloroform vapour in pulmonary air of 1 per 100. This percentage will be got if with each 100 c.cm. of inspired air the patient inspires 1 c.cm. of chloroform vapour. Taking the inspiratory volume per minute at 6000 c.cm. more or less, the requisite volume of chloroform vapour per minute is 60 c.cm. more or less.' [1]

In February 1901 Waller strongly criticized the recently published findings of an ' Anaesthetics Committee ' appointed by the British Medical Association (see pp. 458–64) as being ' meagre and unsatisfactory, and even . . . incorrect in certain essential particulars.

' What has the ordinary administrator of anaesthetics learned from this clinical inquiry ? ' asked Waller. He himself gave the reply :

' That chloroform is more dangerous than ether, but that as regards methods of administration, rate of use, methods of restoration, clinical evidence has not warranted any conclusion. . . . And . . . that by far the most important factor in the safe administration of anaesthetics is the experience of the administrator, and that in many cases the anaesthetisation is of such importance and gravity that it is absolutely essential that an anaesthetist of large experience should conduct the administration.

' This last, and evidently most desirable, condition is not always easy to fulfil, and we must above all look to increased diffusion of precise knowledge for diminution of the death-rate by chloroform. For knowledge to be diffused it must first be acquired. To this end certain definite steps should be taken :

' 1. An experimental examination of the statement that by proper application of a volumetric method anaesthesia can be certainly effected of any required degree.

' 2. An experimental comparison of the relative power of various anaesthetics.

' 3. The determination of the best method of quantitative estimation of anaesthetics in various fluids and tissues of the body.[2]

' 4. A careful redetermination of the statement made by

[1] *Brit. med. J.*, 1898, i, 1057, 1061.

[2] At Waller's suggestion the British Medical Association, during 1898 and 1899, granted a sum of money for research on the quantitative estimation of chloroform in animal tissues. The work was begun by Dodgson, working under Waller in the physiological laboratory of St. Mary's Hospital Medical School. (*Brit. med. J.*, 1901, ii, 1859.)

Snow [cf. pp. 188-90], Gréhant [1], Paul Bert, and Dubois [cf. pp. 370, 374] with reference to the percentage of chloroform required for various degrees of anaesthesia, and the percentage of chloroform in the fluids and tissues of animals variously anaesthetized.' [2]

In July of the same year, 1901, a new Chloroform Committee, under the chairmanship of Waller, was appointed by the British Medical Association. The Committee was originally composed of Doctors Barr, Dudley Buxton, Sherrington, Waller himself, and Sir Victor Horsley. Its aim was ' to investigate methods of quantitatively determining the presence of chloroform in the air, and in the living body '. The Committee co-opted A. G. Vernon Harcourt, the physical chemist of Christ Church, Oxford, ' who has devised an accurate and comparatively expeditious method of combustion by means of a platinum wire raised to incandescence by an electric current. The method was originally applicable to mixtures of chloroform and air enclosed in a flask.[3] In connexion with the present inquiry Harcourt has devised a modification by which the combustion and acidimetry can be effected on a mixture in transit '.[4]

The chief practical outcome of the Committee's work was the production of Vernon Harcourt's regulating apparatus for delivering low percentages of chloroform. It was claimed that the maximum strength of chloroform vapour in the chloroform-air mixture was thereby automatically limited to about 2 per cent.[5]

In 1902 E. H. Embley, Honorary Anaesthetist to the Melbourne Hospital, published a detailed account of his researches on ' the causation of death during the administration of chloroform '. He believed that he had succeeded in demonstrating what Dastre, for example, had previously maintained (cf. p. 397), namely, that ' vagus inhibition is, in dogs, the great factor in the causation of sudden death under chloroform '.

[1] Waller apparently referred to a short series of experiments made by Gréhant in 1874. The latter anaesthetized animals by making them breathe from a balloon a quantity of chloroform which he had found to be proportionate to their body weight ; e.g. for a dog weighing 10 kilograms Gréhant introduced into the bag 100 litres of air and 20 grams of chloroform. This quantity, he claimed, produced tranquil anaesthesia indefinitely, whereas a smaller quantity of chloroform failed to produce anaesthesia and a greater quantity was liable to produce death. (*C.R. Soc. Biol. Paris*, 1874, **1**, 269–70.)   [2] *Brit. med. J.*, 1901, i, 447–8.
[3] *J. chem. Soc.*, 1899, **75**, 1060–6.   [4] *Brit. med. J.*, 1902, ii, 116–17.
   Ibid. 1903, ii, Supplement, cxli-clxi ; *ibid.* 1904, ii, 169.

Embley concluded from his experiments (which were all made upon morphinized dogs) that :

'chloroform raises the excitability of the vagus mechanism particularly in the early part of the administration. . . . The increased excitability of the vagus mechanism is due to the action of chloroform on the centres. . . . Chloroform vapour, not stronger than 1·5 per cent., in the air administered to morphinized dogs, after a period of mild excitation, slowly depresses vagus excitability. Above 2 per cent. in the air inhaled may occasion dangerous or persistent inhibitions in dogs.

'The failure of many experimenters to recognize the importance of vagus inhibition of the heart appears to depend upon the fact that the inhibitory mechanism was paralysed or exhausted by the previous induction of chloroform anaesthesia before the records of the experiments were commenced. This especially applies to the Hyderabad Commission. . . . A dog becomes, in fact, quite another animal after the induction of chloroform anaesthesia without morphine ; from being an animal with a very sensitive vagus control of the heart, he becomes one almost wholly devoid of this function, that is, if he lives through the induction. Consequently vagus inhibition from chloroform alone, or from chloroform and asphyxia combined, or from reflexes arising from surgical procedures, are difficult to demonstrate in dogs so prepared. . . .

'The recovery of vagus function after the depression resulting from the induction of chloroform anaesthesia, is slow, and I wish to emphasize the fact that transient recovery followed by reinduction does not represent the conditions of a primary induction.

'Section of the vagi or atropinization of dogs absolutely abolishes sudden heart arrest from chloroform.'

In Embley's opinion ' the cause of the fall of blood pressure from the administration of chloroform is paralysis of the muscle cells of the heart and of the arterioles, the fall may be further augmented by slowing of the heart's rate. . . .

'Failure of respiration in inhalation experiments is mainly due to fall in blood pressure. With a good blood pressure, failure of respiration by inhalation of chloroform is practically impossible. . . .

'I do not wish to discuss the practical application of these results at present ', Embley stated, ' but one obvious moral is, use only weak vapour of chloroform (less than 1 per cent.) in the early stages, until the initial increased excitability of the

15

vagus mechanism has given place to diminished excitability ;
in other words take time in putting the patient under.' [1]

Commenting upon Embley's experiments and results A.
Goodman Levy remarked :

' It appears evident that the large doses of morphia employed
played an important part in the production of the inhibition
phenomena in the early stages of the chloroform administration,
and as it is upon these morphia experiments that Embley bases
his theory of cardiac syncope and death through vagal action,
this cannot be regarded as a satisfactory explanation of sudden
death.' [2]

So the present century advanced with the understanding of
the physiological action of chloroform still unclarified. ' For
many years past the attempt has been made to prevent death
under chloroform by the restriction of the percentage administered, on the theory that death is caused by overdose alone ',
wrote Levy. ' This teaching has failed to decrease the incidence
of death, which has indeed tended to increase rather than
otherwise.' [3]

In 1893 Robert Kirk, a physician on the staff of the Glasgow
Western Infirmary, had carried out a series of fifty experiments
on animals and made clinical observations on the occurrence of
syncope during the emergence of the anaesthetized subject from
the effects of chloroform vapour. Although those who followed
the Edinburgh method of chloroforming (cf. p. 204) had always
stressed the point that in administering chloroform light and
intermittent anaesthesia was particularly to be avoided, Kirk's
work on the intrinsic dangers of waning anaesthesia remained
isolated from the main body of research and its full significance
was not appreciated until 1911, after A. Goodman Levy had
made his classic demonstration of ventricular fibrillation in
lightly chloroformed cats (see pp. 452–4).

Referring to his fifty experiments Kirk wrote in the *Lancet* : [4]

' The result . . . is believed to prove that when chloroform
is inhaled there is an action exerted by the vapour on the respiratory tract, and that a reaction ensues when the inhalation is
discontinued ; whilst it is maintained that both experiment and
clinical observation combine to show that this reaction is the

[1] *Brit. med. J.*, 1902, i, 817, 885, 951–61.
[2] Levy, A. G.   1922.   *Chloroform anaesthesia*. London.   37.
[3] *Ibid.* 103.   [4] *Lancet*, 1893, ii, 429.

cause of primary syncope when allowed to take place at certain stages of the inhalation. . . .

'. . . In four experiments four cats [enclosed in jars] inhaled 4 per cent. of chloroform for one minute. In one instance the observation was a failure owing to the resistance of the animal, and in another the cardiac rate, which had been 140 before the inhalation, was extremely rapid when the cat was taken out of the jar ; but there was a sudden stoppage in half a minute which lasted for about five seconds, and this was followed by extreme irregularity for a minute and a half, when the cat recovered. There were pauses between individual beats in this case ; sometimes after every third beat, whilst the sounds were very weak during this irregular action. . . . In the other two experiments the results were similar, rapid but regular action of the heart ending in sudden stoppage and irregularities in about half a minute.'

Very similar results were obtained in further experiments in which cats breathed 3½ per cent. of chloroform vapour for from two to eight minutes. ' More or less irregular cardiac action occurred during recovery in all.'

' These results ', Kirk remarked, ' showed that very deep anaesthesia in the cat did not always modify reactionary effects on the heart, but the fact that these stoppages were longer in occurring after deep anaesthesia proved that the latter were not due to absorption of the chloroform and that they could only be accounted for by the vapour reaction. . . . The irregular action commences when the last drop of chloroform has left the blood, but as long as it continues the animal is as passive as if under the influence of a profound dose of the agent.'

Dogs submitted to the same experimental conditions

' showed that the dog was liable to similar stoppages of the heart as the cat, and that they were almost invariably associated with spasms of the respiratory and other muscles. They further showed that deep anaesthesia modified or altogether prevented these effects on the heart, and this is a vital part of the inquiry. It was found, moreover, that immediately after the struggling stage and when the animal was quiescent the anaesthesia was nevertheless not deep enough to prevent irregular cardiac action. . . .

' It is maintained that the stoppages and irregularities of the heart, as above described in experiments on cats and dogs, correspond with and explain the fall of blood pressure to zero which has been observed by some other experimenters after the administration of chloroform has been discontinued, and also the syncope or sudden failure of the pulse which has been so often noted clinically in the human subject. According to this view chloroform syncope is analogous to syncope from other causes. The sudden removal of pressure from a large blood vessel—*i.e.*, the cessation of a force previously acting—may cause syncope. . . . Further, it has been seen that chloroform syncope coincides with a sudden transition from a quick to a slow cardiac rate, and the same has been observed in some other forms of syncope. Some clinical observations that have been made at the Western Infirmary, Glasgow, with a binaural stethoscope, may be briefly noticed. In one case the heart's action rose from 100 to 152 in half a minute, and in another it rose from 84 to 132 during the first minute, and to 152 before the expiration of one minute and a half, and similar results were seen in other cases. In all instances the cardiac rate returned to normal just as the patient was pronounced " over " and only one case occurred which tended to prove that the quickened cardiac rate, instead of gradually slowing, may suddenly drop to a slow action, just as we have seen it do in dogs and cats. In this case the cardiac rate rose in two minutes to 132, and so continued for the next minute, but during the fourth minute there was an instantaneous fall to 96, although the action continued to be tolerably regular. I told the chloroformist that he had allowed a vapour reaction to occur by not renewing the dose of chloroform soon enough. What were the consequences ? The patient began to talk loudly and to struggle violently, and within a minute his breathing gave cause for anxiety. If it be objected that the reaction did not give rise to syncope in this case the answer is that it was less in degree than it might have been, and there can be no doubt that these milder instances occur frequently. The coincidence with experimental results to be remarked is the instantaneous transition from the quick to the slow cardiac action, and this has been found to be associated in other cases in the human subject with irregular action and actual syncope. Deep anaesthesia in dogs and in the human subject prevents this untoward result, but space forbids the discussion of the question why this should be so. The chloroformisation ought to go on to deep anaesthesia in spite of coughing, struggling or apnoeal pauses of even a whole minute's duration. . . .'[1]

Goodman Levy's Work

In 1911 A. Goodman Levy ' communicated a note to the Physiological Society [2] describing a hitherto unrecognized form of sudden cardiac failure which occurred in cats under chloroform, and stating that he had, acting upon a suggestion

---

[1] *Lancet*, 1893, ii, 429–30.   [2] *J. Physiol.*, 1911, **42**, iii.

made by Professor Cushny, looked for and found ventricular fibrillation in such cases. At the same time he showed that an exactly similar form of death could be reproduced by injecting small dozes of adrenalin into the vein of a cat lightly anaesthetized with chloroform. These observations became the starting-point of a series of experiments elucidating the conditions under which ventricular fibrillation occurs, and showing that it happens only in light chloroform anaesthesia, never in full or deep anaesthesia.' [1]

' The ventricles of the mammalian heart are in an irritable condition when affected by chloroform. This irritability is most marked when they are lightly affected by chloroform, and is progressively diminished under conditions of deepening anaesthesia.

' Although thus made irritable, extrasystoles of ventricular origin are not evoked by the chloroform *per se*, but an exciting cause must be superadded ; [2] such exciting causes are :

' (1) Conditions which stimulate the ventricles.

' (2) Conditions which remove or reduce depressing influences and are thus the equivalent of a stimulation.

'. . . In the most intense exhibition of extrasystoles the sequence is a rapid succession which in the cat [chosen as a good subject in which to demonstrate the condition] may attain the rate of 300 per minute (the normal heart-beat having a rate of about 120 per minute). In such a condition every beat is an extrasystole, there being no longer any normal beats to be found. . . . The serious interest which this latter condition possesses for the anaesthetist is that it is a condition of potential fibrillation, for it is liable to pass suddenly, by an acute transition, into the condition known as ventricular fibrillation, with a consequent and frequently permanent cessation of the circulation. The onset of ventricular fibrillation is marked by a precipitate fall of blood-pressure, for the preceding irregular tachycardia is a sequence of co-ordinate (although abnormal) heart-beats, which sustain the blood-pressure, but with the onset of fibrillation the ventricles do not beat at all, and become entirely inert in respect of their capacity of emptying their cavities.' [3]

' These observations . . . provide an explanation of sudden cardiac failure as it occurs at any stage of the administration of chloroform, and in fact the only wholly acceptable explanation. The acceptance of this view involves the corollary that all clinical deaths occur under light anaesthesia.' [4]

[1] Levy, A. G. 1922. *Chloroform anaesthesia.* London. 96.
[2] *Heart*, 1912–13, **4,** 319.
[3] Levy, A. G. 1922. *Chloroform anaesthesia.* London. 23, 24.
[4] *Ibid.* 96.

Describing the clinical manifestations of ventricular fibrillation Levy stated :

' This form of syncope is extremely sudden in onset, and the patient is plunged from life into death in an instant. There is one preceding sign of danger which must invariably be present, but which is rarely actually observed. The pulse is accelerated, and at the same time becomes irregular ; the irregularity may in some instances be difficult to follow, but it is frequently well pronounced, and the short pauses convey a flickering impression to the finger on the pulse. The heart-beat then ceases absolutely suddenly, the face is blanched white, the pupils dilate extremely, and drops of sweat may form on the face and body. . . .

' The respiratory centre is never strongly depressed by the chloroform at the moment of syncope, and therefore the respirations continue until the centre fails from want of blood. Generally there are a few respirations only, and these may take the form of deep gasps ; . . . but whether or no the respirations are exaggerated depends upon the precise degree of anaesthesia. There may, however, be a persistent tendency towards recovery of the respiration, . . . and should the heart recover, the breathing is immediately resumed. A second cardiac syncope, with its attendant gasping respiration may in some circumstances supervene on such a recovery, and thus there may occasionally arise considerable confusion in the clinical interpretation of the true order of events. . . .

' The conditions under which ventricular fibrillation occurs during the administration of chloroform in man are in accordance with the theoretical considerations . . . and may be summarized as follows :

' (1) During struggling or excitement.

' (2) On the cessation of the administration, temporary or permanent.

' (3) On the abrupt re-administration of chloroform, after partial recovery from anaesthesia.

' (4) By strong sensory stimulation (some operative procedure) under light anaesthesia.

' (5) Some combination of the foregoing conditions.

' (6) Following the injection of adrenalin for surgical purposes under light anaesthesia, or in order to combat shock after the total withdrawal of chloroform.

' (7) Following recovery from an asphyxial condition.' [1]

' The study of the cause and conditions of death by ventricular fibrillation under chloroform has revealed the essential principles of the safe administration of chloroform to be :—

' (1) *To maintain a full degree of anaesthesia.*

' (2) *To make the administration continuous.*' [2]

[1] Levy, A. G. 1922. *Chloroform anaesthesia.* London. 97, 99.   [2] *Ibid.* 103–4.

' There can be no question that excitement during induction is reduced to a minimum when the induction of anaesthesia is performed by the delicate and gradual increase of the vapour from a low concentration up to the maximum. . . .

' If, in spite of all precautions, much excitement or struggling takes place, it is most essential not to remove the chloroform if it can possibly be avoided ; this is directly contrary to the old teaching, but the removal of the chloroform at this stage is a distinct danger. In order to continue the administration it is undoubtedly necessary sometimes to restrain the patient forcibly. . . .' [1]

'. . . A 1 per cent. vapour is comfortably respirable, but the greatest freedom from excitement is attained by beginning lower in the scale. . . .' [2]

' It is impossible to lay down any guide to a maximum percentage for all individuals for the induction of anaesthesia, as the range of individual differences is too great. In my personal experience 2 per cent. suffices for a small minority, 2·5 per cent. to 3 per cent. suffices for a good number, but 3·5 per cent is required not infrequently, and a maximum of 4 per cent. is essential for exceptional individuals, and an inhaler should be capable of supplying this latter amount in order to meet all emergencies. . . .

' The highest percentage found necessary to induce anaesthesia in any one case is generally sufficient to maintain it, and when the former has been high, e.g. 4 per cent., more than sufficient. . . . The strength of the vapour must be regulated entirely according to clinical requirements, and whereas 2 per cent. is frequently sufficient for all purposes, 3 per cent. and rarely more, is requisite under exceptional circumstances. In the later stages of a prolonged operation 1·5 to 1 per cent. is sufficient. It is doubtful if it is safe to use less than 1 per cent. except in cases of prolonged and severe operations.' [3]

Referring to the belief which, from 1848 to 1911, had conditioned the approach of both anaesthetists and physiologists to the problem of chloroform anaesthesia, namely that death under chloroform was due to overdosage, Levy wrote :

' J. Snow carefully observed the sequence of events in overdosed animals. He came to the conclusion that death never happens in man from overdosing with ordinary percentages of chloroform for it occurs in another fashion, the heart stopping suddenly before the breathing is affected. He claimed, however, that the heart could be suddenly overdosed by from 10 per cent. to 12 per cent. of vapour, and performed some experiments which he considered

[1] Levy, A. G. 1922. *Chloroform anaesthesia.* London. 139.
[2] *Ibid.* 140.   [3] *Ibid.* 77, 78, 79.

demonstrated this fact. It is certain that in this latter point he was in error.' [1]

' Overdosage never occurs suddenly. It has been held that rapidly charging the lungs with a high percentage of vapour may produce sudden syncope from overdosage, but this theory has no experimental support. Sudden overdosage cannot be produced in this way experimentally. It is true experiments of this nature have been described . . . but they are subject to fallacy ; the sudden administration of a high percentage to a *lightly anaesthetized* or *partially recovered* subject will sometimes lead to sudden cardiac syncope, as also indeed will a moderate percentage, but the mechanism involved is fibrillation of the ventricles and not over-dosage.[2]

' Ever since the introduction of chloroform as an anaesthetic it has been patent that if it be given in sufficient quantity for a sufficient time the breathing is first depressed and finally suppressed, and shortly afterwards the heart likewise stops.

' The process of overdosage is a gradual one, and the onset of respiratory and circulatory depression is progressive. The complexion assumes a cyanotic tinge owing to the reduced pulmonary ventilation combined with deficient circulation, but an ashy grey tint follows when the circulation ceases. The pupils dilate progressively until they become widely dilated from an excess of the poison. The corneal reflex generally disappears at a comparatively early stage.' [3]

' Overdose is a common enough occurrence in the practice of inexperienced practitioners ; it is a distressing condition, but it need not occasion acute alarm, for the appropriate remedial measures [placing the patient in the head-down position, pulling forward the tongue and keeping the airway clear, and applying artificial respiration promptly by Silvester's method] are simple and efficacious.' [4]

---

[1] Levy, A. G. 1922. *Chloroform anaesthesia.* London. 94.
[2] *Ibid.* 90, 91.   [3] *Ibid.* 90.   [4] *Ibid.* 91.

CHAPTER XVI

ANAESTHETIC TRENDS IN ENGLAND 1890–1900

General Survey—Influence of the New Leaders, Buxton and Hewitt

General Survey

ANAESTHETIC progress in England had reached a high level during the eighteen-seventies. Chloroform as the sole anaesthetic was then almost generally laid aside in major surgery in favour of ether or a nitrous oxide-ether sequence, and in minor surgery and dentistry nitrous oxide was used (cf. pp. 330–9). But in 1882 J. T. Clover died and after the removal of his firm yet gentle guidance a decline in effort is perceptible in English anaesthetic practice as a whole, which was not effectively checked until about 1890, when the influence of the new leaders of the profession, Dudley Wilmot Buxton and Frederic William Hewitt (who during this interregnum had been quietly preparing themselves for their task), began to make itself felt.

Clover had exerted his influence upon the trend of anaesthetic development principally through his researches carried out for various committees investigating anaesthetic questions (cf., *e.g.*, pp. 253, 285) and through the active part which he took in the meetings of learned societies, particularly the annual meetings of the British Medical Association (cf., *e.g.*, p. 296).

By delivering papers and by promoting discussion at these meetings Clover kept whatever was of importance in anaesthesia constantly before his medical and surgical colleagues. The removal of this influence happened at a critical time, when the non-specialist anaesthetist was faced with a mass of new material —the results of recent advances in anaesthesia—the significance of which he could not assimilate unaided ; its removal was the more abrupt because Clover had never collected together and published his opinions in book form.[1] In fact no first-class

[1] In an undated MS jotting of Clover's (now in the Nuffield Department of Anaesthetics, Oxford), in a paragraph describing the advantages of the peculiar mechanism of his ' portable ' ether inhaler, I came upon the following sentence, which had been deleted : ' In writing the history of Anaesthesia it would be a very difficult thing

monograph on anaesthesia had appeared since the publication of Snow's book, *On chloroform and other anaesthetics*, in 1858, so that by 1882 the want of a straightforward *vade mecum* of modern anaesthetic practice was acutely felt. To this lack both of a mentor and of written authority may be attributed, at least in some measure, the sudden falling off in the general level of anaesthetic practice in England during the eighteen-eighties. A characteristic feature of this deterioration was the return of the inexpert and the occasional (and, it must be admitted, the lazy) anaesthetist to the routine use of chloroform (cf. pp. 437–8).

By 1890 a sharp line of demarcation had become apparent between the methods of the specialist anaesthetists who, during the eighteen-eighties, had persisted in the discriminating use of various anaesthetic agents, each administered from an appropriate apparatus, and the methods of the rank and file of anaesthetists. These two classes of anaesthetists—specialist and non-specialist—had existed side by side in England since the adoption of surgical anaesthesia had become general, but until about the time of Clover's death the difference between them had appeared rather in the degree than in the kind of skill which each possessed. This suddenly remarkable divergence gave rise to the professional outcry, during the eighteen-nineties, for improved facilities for training the non-specialist anaesthetist (see p. 524 *et seq.*).

In 1891 the British Medical Association met at Bournemouth. During the meeting members of the Section of Therapeutics heard T. Lauder Brunton read a paper entitled ' Remarks on death during chloroform anaesthesia ', which stated the case, in modified form, from the Hyderabad Commissioners' point of view. The members also heard L. E. Shore, Demonstrator of Physiology at Cambridge and colleague of Gaskell, read a paper entitled ' Remarks on the effect of chloroform on the respiratory centre, the vasomotor centre and the heart ', which stated the contrary point of view. Following these two papers, on July 30, 1891, members of the Section of Therapeutics took part in a lively discussion on anaesthetics.[1]

for me to do justice to fellow workers in the same field '. The fact that Clover both wrote and deleted this seems to offer a revealing glimpse of his character. Some such thought may indeed have influenced him, who was remarkable for ' his gentle modesty ' (cf. Obituary Notice, *Lancet*, 1882, ii, 597), against attempting anything in the nature of a textbook.

[1] *Brit. med. J.*, 1891, ii, 1088–95.

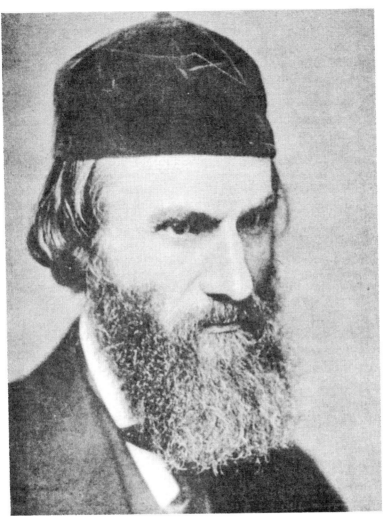

FIG. 116.—JOSEPH THOMAS CLOVER (1825–82)

After qualifying as a surgeon Clover decided to specialize in anaesthetics, a profession which he combined with private practice as a physician. From about 1862 onwards he came to be acknowledged as the leader in anaesthetic practice and research in England.

The discussion was opened by D. W. Buxton and he is reported as having said in the course of his remarks :

' The work of the Hyderabad Commission, as far as it went, was excellent, and it was only to be regretted that its so-called conclusions were permitted to be framed in such a way as to mislead those not sufficiently familiar with the matter to assume that it had settled, once and for all, the question whether chloroform caused primary heart failure. The Commission failed to observe it in their experiments, and this only was the Commission entitled to state. It however went beyond this, and stated emphatically that primary heart failure never occurred either in the lower animals or in man, and practically told the profession that deaths from chloroform need never occur save through carelessness or when the Commission's directions were not carried out. In so saying the Commission assumed a grave responsibility which had lulled many persons into a feeling of dangerous security when employing chloroform, and had led to a reckless use of the agent in a way open to the most severe criticism. He (the speaker) thought it the duty of the Section to state most distinctly that the clinical evidence before them contradicted the findings of the Hyderabad Commission, and showed its conclusions to be at variance with common experience.' [1]

Towards the close of this discussion Dr. Christopher Childs, of Weymouth, ' moved " that a committee be formed to investigate the clinical evidence with regard to anaesthetics, especially the relative safety of the various anaesthetics, and the best methods of administering them ". In addition to Dr. [W. V.] Snow (the President of the Section), they should be very glad to have the names of Dr. Lauder Brunton, Mr. Pridgin Teale [of Leeds, a great advocate of Clover's ' small machine ' for ether], Dr. Dudley Buxton, and Mr. [George] Eastes [assistant anaesthetist at the Great Northern Hospital] as members of the committee '.[2] Brunton declined membership and the Committee, as finally constituted, included Jonathan Hutchinson, Chairman ; Teale, Chairman of the Executive Committee ; and Childs, Secretary.

' To obtain evidence the Committee requested all anaesthetists throughout the kingdom to record their cases during 1892.' [3] In order that the observations might be as uniform as possible record books were drawn up containing columns for noting the consecutive number, date, hour, sex, age, general

[1] *Brit. med. J.*, 1891, ii, 1090–1.   [2] *Ibid.* ii, 1093.
[3] *Trans. Soc. Anaesth.*, 1901, **4,** 48.

state of the patient, nature of the operation, anaesthetic employed, method, duration, quantity used, source where anaesthetic obtained, and after effects in each case.

In January 1893, 156 books were returned with details of 25,920 cases in hospital and private practice. Each book and case was carefully investigated by the Analysis Subcommittee, consisting of Buxton, Hewitt, George Rowell, and George Eastes. The final Report of the Committee was not ready for publication by the British Medical Association until late in 1900.

On February 15, 1901, at a meeting of the Society of Anaesthetists,[1] George Eastes explained ' the chief points of the report, and more particularly the conclusions at which the Analysis Subcommittee had arrived.

' The report ', said Eastes, ' bristles with figures, but I will endeavour to introduce them only when they seem necessary. . . .

' The 25,920 cases in the record books were first separated in two great divisions—the uncomplicated (A) and complicated (B) cases. Those anaesthetics that were most frequently used appear in the following table, with the number of cases of the administration of each anaesthetic which were recorded.

No.	Anaesthetic	Total Records	No. of Cases in Division A	Ratio of Division A to Total	No. of Cases in Division B	Ratio of Division B to Total
1	Chloroform . . .	13,393	12,955	96·730	438	3·270
2	Ether	4,595	4,455	96·953	140	3·047
3	' Gas and ether ' . .	2,071	2,026	97·827	45	2·173
4	A.C.E. mixture . .	678	660	97·345	18	2·655
5	Mixtures of chloroform and ether . . .	418	406	97·129	12	2·871
7	Chloroform followed by ether	208	196	94·230	12	5·770
8	Ether followed by chloroform . .	225	216	96·000	9	4·000
9	A.C.E. followed by ether	155	148	95·484	7	4·516
14	Chloroform followed by A.C.E. or some similar mixture . .	275	270	98·182	5	1·818
28	Nitrous oxide . .	2,911	2,888	99·210	23	0·790
29	Nitrous oxide mixed with oxygen . .	597	596	99·832	1	0·168

[1] The Society of Anaesthetists was founded in 1893 by J. F. W. Silk : ' For some years preceding that date,' Silk stated, ' the subject of anaesthetics had occupied a very prominent position in the professional controversies of the period, and its importance as a branch of medical education and special practice was becoming more

'The details of every case, both in the complicated and uncomplicated divisions, were submitted to elaborate tabulation.

'Records of the administration of 43 distinct anaesthetics, mixtures, or successions of anaesthetics administered in different ways were contained in the books.   But, although the number was thus large, the administrations in over 21,000 cases were confined to chloroform, ether, gas and ether, A.C.E. mixture, and mixtures of chloroform and ether in various proportions ; whilst nitrous oxide and the same gas with oxygen accounted for over 3500 cases, leaving only about 1200 cases [1] to be distributed amongst the remaining 38 anaesthetics.

.   .   .   .

'It was only when the departure from the normal in any case was held to be due partly or entirely to the anaesthetic, that the case was placed in the " complicated " division. . . .

'In the next table are found the *cases of danger (including deaths)* *considered to be due entirely to the anaesthetic.* . . .

No. of Anaesthetic [2]	Total Cases A and B together	Cases of Danger		Total Cases of Danger	Ratio of Danger to Total Administrations
		Recovered	Died		
1	13,393	75	3	78	0·582
2	4,595	3	0	3	0·065
3	2,071	2	0	2	0·096
4	678	1	0	1	0·147
5	418	2	0	2	0·478
7	208	1	0	1	0·480
8	225	4	1	5	2·2
9	155	0	0	0	0·000
14	275	1	0	1	0·36

generally recognized. It seemed to me, therefore, that the time had arrived when an attempt should be made to form a special Society of Anaesthetists ; I accordingly placed myself in communication with the leaders of the profession in this branch, by whom the suggestion was received with much favour, both in London and the Provinces. . . . The Society started with a membership roll of forty, and the first list of Officers was as follows : President, F. Woodhouse Braine ; Treasurer, Dr. Dudley W. Buxton ; Secretary, Dr. Silk ; Council, Dr. Stallard and Mr. G. E. Norton. . . . The first [annual volume of *Transactions*] . . . was published in 1898. . . .'
In June 1908 the Society amalgamated with the new Royal Society of Medicine as the Section of Anaesthetics. (*Trans. Soc. Anaesth.*, 1908, **9**, 1–5.)

[1] Many of these cases were accounted for (by twos and threes) by the use of various ingeniously complex, but sometimes pointless and often dangerous sequences of the anaesthetics and anaesthetic mixtures listed from 1 to 14 in the table on p. 461. A few cases were accounted for by similar sequences supplemented by subcutaneous injections of morphine or atropine and morphine.

[2] These numbers correspond to the anaesthetics similarly numbered in the table on p. 461.

· ' This is probably the chief lesson taught by the report, namely, that chloroform, alone or in combination, caused in the reported cases a danger-rate six-fold higher than the danger-rate produced by ether. Or, contrasting chloroform alone with ether alone, chloroform had, in the opinion of the Subcommittee, a danger-rate . . . more than eight times higher than the danger-rate of ether.'

With regard to methods of administration the Subcommittee found :

' As to chloroform, the towel [1] was the most frequently used method, and it also showed the highest complication and danger-rates ; at the same time, of 65 danger cases occurring under this method only 5 died. There was a striking diminution in both the complication and danger-rates in the cases in which lint was employed ; but of the 23 cases of danger occurring when lint was used no fewer than 7 ended fatally. With Junker's apparatus there was a low complication-rate, and an absence of " danger " from the 422 cases recorded under this heading. But in the " combined methods " there were 3 danger cases recorded, and all 3 happened whilst Junker's apparatus was in use ; further, one of the 3 was a death.
' The recorded cases of ether administration were 4455 [2] and in over 4000 of these, including 13 " danger " cases, Clover's inhaler was used. There were 6 deaths among these 13 danger cases ; but in two of them death followed (from apoplexy and uraemia respectively) some days after the operation.
' Gas and ether was usually given with Clover's or Ormsby's [3] apparatus ; and . . . the complication and danger-rates were not very different under the two methods.
' With A.C.E. mixture the more " open " methods of towel, lint, and Skinner's mask gave far lower complication and danger-rates than the " mask and sponge " [4] or Clover's ether apparatus.'

¹ The B.M.A. Report noted that ' " Towel " includes cases in which a single layer of towel was apparently used as well as cases in which the towel was in more than one layer '.
² According to the Subcommittee's table (see p. 461) this figure (4455) represented only the number of uncomplicated cases ; the total number of cases was 4595. Further, of the six deaths referred to in this paragraph none was *entirely* due to ether (cf. table on p. 462). This latter remark applies also to the fatalities mentioned in the paragraph before, dealing with chloroform.
³ *i.e.* Anaesthesia was induced with the ordinary nitrous oxide apparatus and ether anaesthesia was then maintained with Ormsby's inhaler.
⁴ The B.M.A. Report stated that ' mask with sponge ' signifies Rendle's inhaler (see Fig. 67).

On the ' clinical evidence regarding anaesthetics generally ' the Subcommittee concluded :

' Anaesthetics are more commonly associated with complications and danger in males than in females.

' Excluding infancy . . . the complications and dangers of anaesthesia increase *pari passu* with advancing age.

' Anaesthetics are notably more dangerous in proportion as the gravity of the patient's state increases. . . .

' Danger to life is especially likely to be incurred in early periods of the administration of anaesthetics, while the tendency to less grave complications increases directly with the duration of anaesthesia.

' The tendency for complications, dangerous and otherwise, to occur, increases *pari passu* with the gravity of the operation. . . .

' From the evidence before the Subcommittee they are convinced that by far the most important factor in the safe administration of anaesthetics is the experience which has been acquired by the administrator.

' In many cases the anaesthetisation completely transcends the operation in gravity and importance, and to ensure success, particularly in these cases, it is absolutely essential that an anaesthetist of large experience should conduct the administration.

' As to this final recommendation, it may be possible to act upon it in hospitals and big towns, but practitioners everywhere must, in emergencies, be prepared to administer anaesthetics. No one, therefore, should be allowed to qualify until he or she has shown proficiency in this very important branch of medical work.' [1]

The picture of anaesthetic practice which this Report gives is representative only of the year 1892, to which year the cases analysed belong ; by the time that the Report was published, in 1901, various innovations had made their appearance in anaesthesia and many of them were due to the efforts of two men —Dudley Buxton and Hewitt.

Influence of the New Leaders, Buxton and Hewitt

In 1888 Buxton published (in H. K. Lewis's ' Practical Series '), his textbook, *Anaesthetics : their uses and administration.* This was a serious attempt to raise the general standard of

[1] *Trans. Soc. Anaesth.*, 1901, **4,** 48 *et seq.* ; see also, British Medical Association *Report of the anaesthetics committee (appointed in 1891).* London 1900.

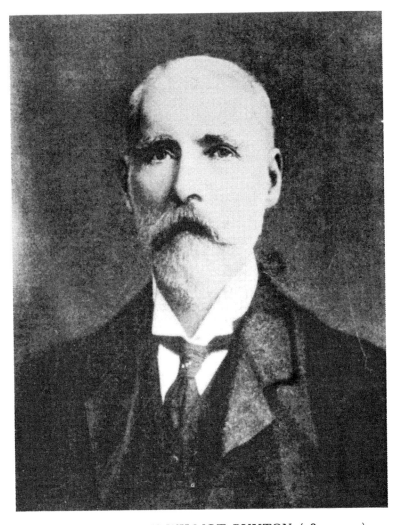

Fig. 117.—DUDLEY WILMOT BUXTON (1855–1931)
He decided to specialize in anaesthesia in 1885 and was subsequently
appointed anaesthetist to University College Hospital, London. He
greatly improved both the standard and the method of teaching
anaesthesia to the medical student.

anaesthetic practice to its former level. The book was well-received by the critics.[1]

'Personally I do not believe', wrote Buxton in his preface, 'that the perusal of any book will enable a medical man to do more than learn the rudiments of anaesthetising ; but a book may be of undoubted service to the thoughtful student or practitioner, in enabling him to appreciate the dangers incident to, the caution necessary in anaesthetising, and to grasp the rationale of the various methods of procedure.

'Unfortunately the subject of anaesthetics has for some years escaped the notice of the scientific side of the profession, and as a natural result has been relegated to the domain of routine.

'In this book, which has been written purely from the standpoint of everyday practice, I have attempted to indicate that the matter dealt with has a scientific as well as a work-a-day aspect, and that he who desires to be more than a mechanical (and hence dangerous) administrator of anaesthetics, must be scientifically as well as practically educated in his art.'

In a dozen chapters Buxton briefly dealt with the history of anaesthesia ; the preparation of the patient and choice of anaesthetic ; nitrous oxide ; ether ; chloroform ; amylene and other inhalation anaesthetics of secondary importance ; anaesthetic mixtures, mixed anaesthesia—the combination of alkaloids and chloral with inhalation anaesthetics—and some anaesthetic sequences ; anaesthesia in obstetrics and in 'special surgery', e.g. brain, ophthalmic, abdominal, rectal, and dental surgery, and operations in the facial region and on the respiratory tract ; anaesthetic accidents ; local anaesthesia, i.e. by cocaine (cf. pp. 39–40) and the ether spray ; and the 'medico-legal aspects of the administration of anaesthetics'.

The book contained little new material. Its value lay in the fact that it supplied, simply and concisely, a much-needed recapitulation of the essentials of sound anaesthetic practice. In particular Buxton drew attention to the various possibilities of choice in regard to anaesthetic agents and methods of administration and described the advantages and disadvantages generally recognized as attaching to each.

Buxton wrote :

'*The choice of an Anaesthetic* must depend on
   '1. The condition of the patient.
   '2. The necessities of the operation.'

[1] See, e.g., Brit. med. J., 1889, i, 138.

Thus he avoided the tendency to standardize the use of chloroform and of ether in certain clearly defined types of patient and classes of case (cf. pp. 340–2). A typical example of Buxton's attitude towards the selection of the anaesthetic is this :

' Emphysematous individuals with large (bullock's) hearts are always anxious cases requiring great nicety of treatment. On the one hand lies the possible danger of ether producing a water-logged condition of the rigid chest, and on the other a more than probable danger of syncope through the depressant action of chloroform on the enfeebled, dilated heart. In this dilemma I have found the A.C.E. mixture to answer well, though it needs careful watching as many and grave symptoms may occur during its use.' [1]

Buxton recommended the use of ether wherever possible, or of a gas-ether sequence. For the former he considered Clover's portable inhaler (see Fig. 88) and for the latter Clover's gas-ether apparatus (see Fig. 83) as being superior to other types of apparatus. He gave only brief descriptions of the A.C.E. and other mixtures which had become popular during the eighteen-eighties ; but he considered the A.C.E. mixture a useful substitute for chloroform in certain cases, notably in the radical cure of hernia in young children, because of the tranquillity of respiration obtainable with it.

A comparatively large section of the book was devoted to chloroform anaesthesia in its physiological as well as its clinical aspects. Buxton described two main types of administration : the ' Scotch method ', as recommended by Lister (see p. 536), and administration from an inhaler. Three of the inhalers of which he gave details, Snow's (see Fig 41), Clover's (see Figs. 53–4), and Sansom's (see Fig 51) must have been at least obsolescent in 1888, but the fourth, Junker's inhaler, Buxton himself had recently modified by substituting a foot-actuated bellows for the hand-bellows (see Fig. 118). ' Junker's inhaler . . .', he wrote, ' is of value, though it must not be supposed that by its use the patient is placed outside the range of danger.' [2]

With reference to the use of alkaloids with chloroform Buxton found ' the addition of gr. 1/120 of atropine to gr. 1/4 of

[1] Buxton, D. W. 1888. *Anaesthetics : their uses and administration.* London. 14.
[2] *Ibid.* 74–8.

morphine to be an advantage, when that last alkaloid is employed synergetically with chloroform '.

With reference to the use of morphine with ether, however, Buxton stated that ' the method possesses disadvantages in its liability to induce prolongation of the stage of excitement. It

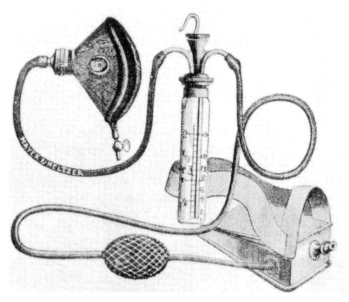

FIG. 118.—BUXTON'S MODIFICATION OF JUNKER'S
CHLOROFORM INHALER

In use *c.* 1888, showing the foot-bellows which he added to free one of the administrator's hands from the purely mechanical task of pumping a stream of air through the apparatus. The other hand was still needed to hold the facepiece in position.

may induce very violent struggling and increase the after-headache, prostration, and vomiting. Kappeler,' Buxton added, ' who has experimented with this mixed method, states that he has completely failed in several cases in which he attempted to narcotize patients with ether subsequently to hypodermic injections of morphine.

' It is not, however, clear whether Kappeler's results should be considered quite so absolute as his statements would lead one to suppose [cf. p. 399, footnote]. Certainly in cases at University

College Hospital in which the method was employed, no great struggling or inconvenience was observed.'[1]

The second edition of Buxton's *Anaesthetics*, considerably amplified both in text and illustrations, appeared in 1892, and the third edition, still further amplified, in 1900. Thereafter edition followed edition at intervals until by 1920 six had appeared.

From the first three editions of Buxton's book one may gain a clear picture of how, during the last ten years of the nineteenth century, anaesthetic development gradually gathered fresh momentum. Buxton's choice and treatment of his subject matter, too, is indicative of a new spirit in anaesthetic practice— a spirit which called upon the anaesthetist to be prepared to employ whatever agent or method of administration promised to give the best results in any particular case, irrespective of precedent. By contrast Clover's attitude typified the old fashioned ; for he maintained (with justification) that he could achieve satisfactory anaesthesia in almost any case simply by using nitrous oxide and ether, delivered to the patient from his favourite gas-ether apparatus.

When the first edition of Buxton's *Anaesthetics* appeared in 1888 anaesthetic practice in this country, so far as it was moving at all, was on the down grade. The turning-point in this decline appears to have come with the publication of the Report of the Second Hyderabad Commission (see Chapter XV), which startled anaesthetists out of their lethargy and set them arguing, and, for the first time for almost a decade, observing and testing their observations. Dudley Buxton undoubtedly exercised a powerful influence in guiding this revival in interest and endeavour. This he did through his work on various committees on anaesthetics, appointed either directly or indirectly as a result of the Hyderabad Report, and, more important still, through the steadily increasing amount of teaching to students which Buxton gave. Buxton himself was neither clinically nor in the laboratory an originator, but he possessed a remarkably keen sense of what was important in the trend of anaesthetic practice and his inestimable value to his contemporaries lay in his powers of expounding and demonstrating and in his cleverness in improving apparatus.

[1] Buxton, D. W. 1888. *Anaesthetics : their uses and administration.* London. 105.

In this last-mentioned sphere of activity Buxton had to his credit by 1900 :

1. An improved apparatus for giving nitrous oxide alone. It was essentially composed of a tripod, a fifty-gallon steel cylinder of compressed gas, a length of wide-bore ' mohair ' tubing, a Cattlin's bag fitted with a hook to suspend it from the lapel, and a Clover's facepiece with an ' expiratory valve of peculiar [but unspecified] construction '. Speaking of the apparatus as a whole Buxton stated :

'. . . Its main peculiarities are that (1) it is provided with an efficient " silencer " [fixed to the outlet tube of the cylinder] which ensures absolute quietude, (2) it is adapted for gas only, and so offers no temptation to the administrator to give " only a whiff of ether ", (3) it possesses a special contrivance to filter the air, and, if necessary, to impregnate the gas with aromatic or other vapours.'

This ' contrivance ', which was situated between the bag and the facepiece, consisted of ' a chamber made in metal and opened or closed by a valve, permitting either air or nitrous oxide gas to enter. In this chamber are placed pieces of fine honey-combed sponge or teased-out medicated cotton-wool. These substances can be moistened with lavender water, eau de Cologne, or with sal volatile, or liq. ammoniae dil.—if a stimulating action is needed '.

2. A Clover's gas-ether inhaler ' the feature of which is that it can be taken entirely to pieces and completely cleansed after use '.

3. A Junker's chloroform inhaler which, Buxton stated, ' I have now employed for some years and which I have found to answer better than any of the older patterns. It consists of a somewhat larger Junker's bottle than usually supplied. The Skinner's mask [a substitute suggested by Krohne and Sesemann for the original half-spherical vulcanite type of facepiece] is re-placed by a glass face-piece (after Vajna of Buda-Pesth) to which is fixed a metal rim carrying the air supply tube, and this delivers into a perforated tube running from back to front of the metal frame. There is a hinged rim, which can be raised to allow a piece of lint or domette being placed over the opening on the upper aspect of the mask. When this rim is shut down it locks itself and keeps the lint in position. This apparatus can be rendered sterile by boiling '.[1]

[1] Buxton, D. W. 1900. *Anaesthetics : their uses and administration*. London. 58–9, 118, 176.

Buxton had also added a trigger-action ratchet to Mason's type of gag, and had devised a mouth spoon 'which is safer than its archetype, the invention of Mr. T. S. Carter, in that

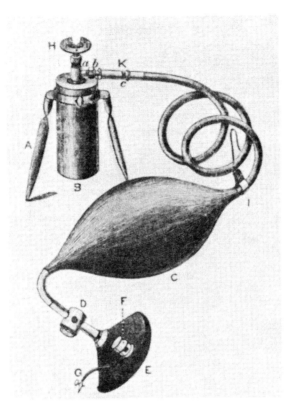

FIG. 119.—BUXTON'S APPARATUS FOR NITROUS OXIDE
In use during the eighteen-nineties.

A. Tripod. B. Steel bottle containing liquefied nitrous oxide. C. India-rubber bag. D. Chamber containing sponge or cotton-wool. E. Facepiece fitted with (F) cap expiration valve. G. Tube for inflating the air cushion. I. Hook attaching tube to administrator's buttonhole. K. Silencer.

the shank of the spoon in the latter instrument is liable to separate from the bowl, and then a risk is run of the detached bowl getting impacted in the gullet or windpipe. By carrying the shank to the distal end of the bowl as in my pattern [see Fig. 122], this danger is obviated. The use of the oral spoon is to catch any teeth or roots which may fall out of the forceps. . . .

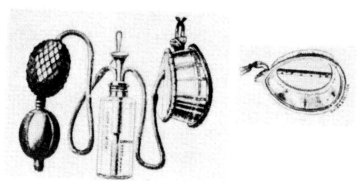

FIG. 120.—BUXTON'S 'IMPROVED' JUNKER'S
INHALER (*c.* 1900)

The efferent tube can be seen ensheathing the upper part of the afferent tube within the bottle, 'just so far as not to enter the chloroform, thus preventing the patient aspirating the chloroform through it when a nasal tube is used. It also prevents chloroform entering the tubes even if the bottle is inverted or laid upon its side'.

The facepiece is a modification of Vajna's mask (see Fig. 121). The stream of air charged with chloroform entered the mask, from the supply tube, through 'a perforated tube running from back to front' of a supporting metal rim added to the original mask.

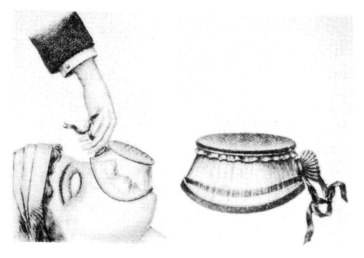

FIG. 121.—VAJNA'S CHLOROFORM MASK (Buda-Pesth)

The side walls were of glass, with a rubber rim. The chloroform was dropped on to the surgical gauze cover. This mask was designed for easy sterilization.

The spoon is held below the seat of operation [by the anaesthetist, acting as the dentist's assistant], care being taken not to allow it to get in the way of the operator '.[1]

F. W. Hewitt

In 1893 another manual of anaesthetics appeared. This was Frederic W. Hewitt's *Anaesthetics and their administration* ; its influence was as great or greater than that of Buxton's book, and it, too, passed through many editions.

Comparing the second edition (1892) of Buxton's book with Hewitt's (1893) one finds that the scheme chosen and general

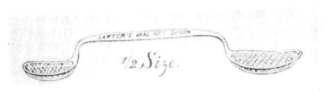

FIG. 122.—CARTER'S ' ORAL NET SPOON ' (*c.* 1900)
Used by the anaesthetist, in assisting the dental surgeon, to catch tooth fragments and prevent them being aspirated by the patient.

approach to the subject matter in both is very similar. Hewitt, however, did not concern himself either with the history or the legal aspects of anaesthesia,[2] but his treatment of his material was otherwise more comprehensive than Buxton's and his text abounded with diagrams, paradigms, illustrative case histories, and round black spots graphically indicating the state of dilatation or contraction of the pupil of the eye in given anaesthetic circumstances (cf. Fig. 123). Hewitt very frequently quoted the opinions of others and in so doing he rarely failed to give an adequate reference to the literature.

When his book was first published in 1893 Hewitt held, among other similar appointments, those of anaesthetist and instructor in anaesthetics at the London Hospital, and anaesthetist and lecturer on anaesthetics at the Charing Cross Hospital.

[1] Buxton, D. W. 1900. *Anaesthetics : their uses and administration.* London. 78, 84.
[2] It was mainly through Hewitt's efforts, however, that a Bill which sought to make it an offence for an unqualified person to administer an anaesthetic was actually drafted. That the Bill was never introduced was said to be due to the advent of the war of 1914–18. (Cf. *Brit. J. Anaesth.*, 1926–7, **4**, 118.)

In his preface he stated that he 'commenced collecting materials for this work just ten years ago. During this period I have taken as accurate notes as possible of every case which has presented points of interest, and have made comparative trials of all the best known methods of producing anaesthesia. . . . No attempt has been made, either to discuss the action of anaesthetics from a purely experimental point of view, or to harmonize clinical and physiological facts. All these aspects of the subject, although of great interest *per se*, are beyond the aim of the present volume '.

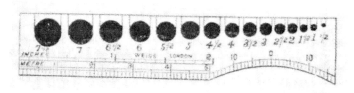

FIG. 123.—PUPILLOMETER (*c.* 1900)
Gauge used by anaesthetists for judging the degree of dilatation or contraction of the patient's pupil, as a guide to his condition and to the depth of anaesthesia.

Hewitt acknowledged that in addition to his own notes, ' about a year before going to press I received . . . the collection of Note-books left by . . . the late Dr. C. E. Sheppard, one of the anaesthetists at the Middlesex Hospital and at Guy's Hospital Dental School. These Note-books contain most carefully recorded notes of 2350 administrations. I felt that I could pay no better tribute to the memory of one whose friendship it was my privilege to enjoy, and whose loss so many must regret, than by going most thoroughly through these notes, and extracting what I considered to be most important. By the kind assistance and guidance of Dr. W. J. Sheppard, I have been able to bring together all the valuable observations made by his brother upon the pupil under chloroform, and upon many other points connected with the effects of anaesthetics ; and I have incorporated these observations with my own '.[1]

[1] During a discussion on the history of ether anaesthesia at a meeting of the Section of Anaesthetics of the Royal Society of Medicine on November 7, 1941, a member stated that Hewitt was accused by certain of his colleagues of plagiarism from Sheppard's work, an accusation which had grieved and embittered him.

CHAPTER XVII

SOME NEW DEVELOPMENTS

Nitrous Oxide—Ethyl Chloride—Minor Developments

TWO important practical developments in inhalation anaesthesia during the last years of the nineteenth century were the
adoption of various improvements in the technique of nitrous
oxide anaesthesia and the introduction of the use of ethyl chloride
as a general anaesthetic.

Nitrous Oxide

After its introduction into British practice in 1868 nitrous
oxide remained the anaesthetic of choice for short dental operations (although in difficult cases it was customary to use ether—
either alone or in conjunction with nitrous oxide—chloroform,
or the A.C.E. mixture).

For some fifteen years after 1868 the occasional as well as
the specialist anaesthetist continued to administer nitrous oxide
free from any admixture of air, using the same type of apparatus
which Clover and his colleagues had devised (see Fig. 74).
About 1885, however, fundamental changes in technique began
to become apparent.

Hewitt, for instance, made a special study of the various
methods then in use for administering nitrous oxide. He reached
the following conclusions :

' (1) That accurately fitting valves were essential at the commencement of the inhalation, in order to make sure of the rapid
exit of atmospheric air from the lungs ;
' (2) that, so far as the available resulting anaesthesia was
concerned, there was a decided advantage in allowing a certain amount of re-breathing of nitrous oxide towards the *end* of
inhalation ;
' (3) that although there were certain hygienic objections
[' it is next to impossible ', Hewitt stated in this connection, ' to
thoroughly cleanse nitrous oxide bags after every administration ']
to this re-breathing, it was nevertheless convenient to be able to

resort to it as a measure for securing a longer anaesthesia, or for successfully terminating an administration when the supply of nitrous oxide had unexpectedly fallen short. There was no apparatus which would allow of two valves being in action for the earlier or middle stages of the administration and would subsequently permit re-breathing. I therefore devised and used a face-piece with thin rubber valves which could,' he wrote, ' at the will of the administrator, be thrown out of action, and allow of the gas-bag being used very much as Clover's " supplemental bag " [see Fig. 71] was used, i.e. for to-and-fro breathing. Subsequently I placed these rubber valves in a little box between the stopcock and the face-piece, so that plain valveless face-pieces could be attached. The valves were thrown into and out of action at will by turning a small handle surmounting the valve-box. A short trial of this apparatus led to my placing the valves and the two-way stopcock *in one chamber*.' [1]

In the first edition of his book, *Anaesthetics and their administration* (London. 1893), Hewitt described and illustrated the final form which this apparatus took :

[Fig. 124] ' From the single union (su) the tube (t) passes to join the bag (B). A little stopcock (s) is useful in case it should be wished to disconnect a full bag from the rest of the apparatus. The bag (B) has a capacity of from 2 to 2½ gallons. There is certainly an advantage in having the bag as near as possible to the face-piece ; for not only can its movements be readily watched, but the patient can take the most forcible inspirations without any of that impediment which is likely to be experienced when a tube exists between the bag and the face-piece. The valved stopcock (VS), which is the most important part of the apparatus, connects the gas-bag (B) to the face-piece (F). This stopcock [see Fig. 125] . . . contains two thin valves of sheet india-rubber, which may be thrown into or out of action by turning the tap T. The handle H determines whether air or gas is admitted to the face-piece. When T and H are arranged as in . . . [the diagram on the left, Fig. 125] air enters the stopcock and is breathed out through valves in the direction shown by the arrows. [Fig. 125, diagram on right] . . . shows in diagrammatic section the mechanism of the valved stopcock. It has two slots cut out of its circumference, an upper slot (US) and a lower slot (LS). There are two inner cylinders which revolve immediately inside the outer casing of the stopcock. The upper inner cylinder (UIC) is worked by T, the lower (LIC) by H. The upper cylinder carries the

[1] Hewitt, F. W. 1893. *Anaesthetics and their administration*. London. 94–5 ; see also *Lancet*, 1885, i, 840–1 ; *J. Brit. dent. Ass.*, 1886, **7**, 86–91 ; *Brit. med. J.*, 1887, ii, 452–4.

inspiratory and expiratory valves (IV and EV). The lower has
a slot in its walls (shown in dotted lines) which can be made to
correspond with LS by turning H. When T is turned as in the
diagram the upper slot is open, both valves act, and expirations

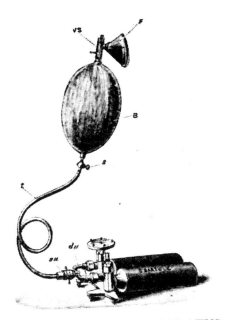

FIG. 124.—HEWITT'S APPARATUS

for administering nitrous oxide gas, in use in 1893.

    du. double union linking two cylinders of nitrous oxide to
    su. single union, from which
      t. tubing led the gas through
      s. small stopcock into
     B. bag, capacity 2 to 2½ gallons.

Between the bag, B, and the facepiece, F, was
Hewitt's Valved Stopcock, VS (shown in diagrammatic section in Fig. 125).

escape as shown by the arrow. When T is turned completely
round the upper inner cylinder rotates, the valves are thrown
out of action, the upper slot is closed (as shown by dotted line),
and to-and-fro breathing results. Whether air or nitrous oxide
is admitted to the face-piece is determined by the position of H.
When H is placed as in the diagram [right] the inner cylinder
which it controls allows of a free passage of gas from the bag to
the face-piece (as shown by the long arrow). Should H be

moved round, the inner cylinder would cut off the way to the
bag, and would open the air slot (LS), so that air and not gas
would be respired [Fig. 125, diagram on left]. . . .

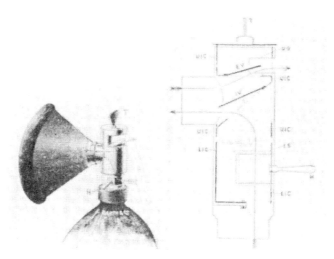

FIG. 125.—HEWITT'S VALVED STOPCOCK
(VS in Fig. 124)

    (*Left.*)   External view—the arrows show the direction
of the current when the patient was allowed to inhale
and exhale air only.
    (*Right.*)   The stopcock in section.   The lower arrow
shows the direction of gas passing from the bag to the
facepiece ; the upper arrow shows the path of the exhaled
mixture when the valvular system was in use.

' The valved stopcock therefore permits :

' (1) Air to be breathed $\left\{\begin{matrix}(a)\\(b)\end{matrix}\right.$ through valves, or
                                   backwards and forwards.

' (2) Nitrous oxide to be breathed $\left\{\begin{matrix}(a)\\(b)\end{matrix}\right.$ through valves, or
                                                 backwards and for-
                                                 wards.

' In actual practice ', explained Hewitt, ' we arrange the
stopcock so that the patient may first of all breathe air through
valves, and then nitrous oxide through valves ; and we only call
into play the to-and-fro breathing of nitrous oxide under special
circumstances . . . *towards the end of the administration, i.e.* when
most of the air has been washed out of the air-passages of the

patient. . . . Let us suppose that we have six gallons of nitrous oxide ready for administration. We allow the patient to breathe four gallons of this through valves . . . and all expirations escape into the surrounding atmosphere. The valve-action is now stopped, and the patient is made to breathe the remaining two gallons of nitrous oxide backwards and forwards into the bag. Anaesthesia will take a little longer to become established than

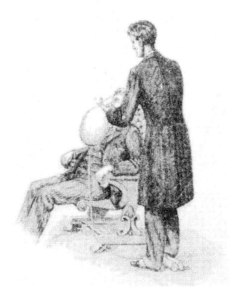

FIG. 126.—ADMINISTRATION OF NITROUS
OXIDE WITH HEWITT'S APPARATUS

(See also Figs. 124–5.)

usual, because of a small percentage of oxygen (probably from the residual air of the lungs) being still in the to-and-fro current. Had no to-and-fro breathing been permitted, the phenomena of nitrous oxide anaesthesia would have come on earlier, because of the quicker expulsion of all oxygen. Now, the longer inhalation leads to a longer anaesthesia, so that from some points of view this plan of administering nitrous oxide has distinct advantages. That the re-breathing *towards the end of the administration* has no bad effect upon the patient I have proved by a very large number of administrations. I have found, it is true, that the recovery is not quite so rapid as when nitrous oxide is continuously inhaled in the usual manner ; but this slight difference is connected with

480 BEGINNING OF MODERN ANAESTHESIA

the longer period of inhalation. . . . Some have objected that this method of re-breathing towards the end is more " asphyxiating " than the ordinary method. But the reverse is probably more correct if by asphyxiating is meant the occurrence of symptoms dependent upon the deprivation of oxygen. Were it not, therefore, for the hygienic objections . . . the plan of administering nitrous oxide just described would certainly have advantages over others.' [1]

George Rowell, meanwhile, was experimenting with ' the increase in the length of anaesthesia, which is in most cases obtainable when small quantities of air are administered with nitrous oxide. . . . The method ', he stated in a chapter specially written for A. S. Underwood and C. Carter Braine's *Notes on anaesthetics in dental surgery* (London. 1893), ' is useful whenever an extra ten to fifteen seconds' anaesthesia is desirable, always provided that the patient is a suitable subject '. Patients regarded as unsuitable were :

' (1) Quite robust and strong adult males ; (2) Marked alcoholics ; and (3) Those patients, occasionally though rarely met with, who invariably struggle or become very rigid under nitrous oxide alone. . . . The most favourable patients, and those in whom we see best the benefits derived from the air, are anaemic girls, weakly persons generally, and children.

' The main essential in the giving of air with nitrous oxide appears to be that the patient shall first have several breaths of gas free from air. If some air is admitted from the beginning, the risk of . . . excitement occurring is much greater. . . . Any apparatus with an inspiratory valve, which shuts off the gas-bag from the patient's expirations may be used.'

Various devices were adopted about the year 1890 for admitting air to the patient during nitrous oxide anaesthesia.

' Mr. Woodhouse Braine admits it ', wrote Rowell, ' by the simple contrivance of pulling aside the india-rubber expiratory valve of the facepiece, which is accomplished by means of a piece of silk attached to the valve. This allows a certain quantity of air to enter with each inspiration that is taken while the silk is pulled upon. Mr. Carter Braine has a number of small holes, covered with an airtight cap, adjusted to the side of the facepiece. By rotating the cap he is able to uncover any number of the holes, and thus not only to permit of the entrance of air through them when the patient takes a breath, but to vary the quantity admitted.

[1] Hewitt, F. W. 1893. *Anaesthetics and their administration.* London. 95–101.

' The plan which I have adopted ', Rowell stated, ' is to occasionally interpose a complete breath of air between the breaths of gas, by turning the stop-cock of a Hewitt's gas apparatus off and on again before and after an inspiration. . . .
' When air has thus been carefully given, the resulting anaesthesia, is practically as deep and good as when nitrous oxide alone is employed, and it is, I believe, always lengthened.' [1]

Since 1878 attention had been attracted also by Paul Bert's detailed researches relating to nitrous oxide anaesthesia, first upon the effects of the gas when administered under increased pressure, then in 1883 when mixed with oxygen at normal pressure (cf. pp. 356–63). These latter researches in particular were soon followed up, not by Bert himself or his French colleagues but by a few Austrian and German workers, notably H. T. Hillischer, a Viennese dentist. When Hewitt became interested in the subject of nitrous oxide-oxygen mixtures in 1886, it was Hillischer's practical application of Bert's suggestion which directly influenced him in carrying out his preliminary researches.

Hillischer gave the name *Schlafgas* (' because of the sleeplike condition it produces ') to his mixture, which contained from 10 to 15 per cent. oxygen. His apparatus was described by Hewitt as follows :

' Dr. Hillischer's apparatus consists of a kind of cabinet which contains iron cylinders of nitrous oxide and of oxygen. Two large bags of Chinese silk are kept supplied from the cylinders by an assistant. Two short exit tubes pass from the bags to join a specially made inhaling tube. This latter tube is in reality a double tube, nitrous oxide passing along one half, and oxygen along the other. In cross section the double tube shows two semicircular tubes, one for each gas. The exit tubes from the bags join the double inhaling tube at the wall of the cabinet ; so that the double inhaling tube (looking like one tube) passes from the cabinet to the patient. At the free end of the inhaling tube there is a stop-cock containing valves, through which the mixed gases are breathed. The proportion of oxygen and of nitrous oxide respired is regulated by a revolving semi-circular plate guarding the orifices of the tubes, that is, it is interposed between the orifices and the stop-cock. The revolving plate is furnished with an indicator and dial to show the extent to which each semi-circular orifice is opened. When the nitrous oxide orifice is fully opened

[1] Underwood, A. S., and Braine, C. Carter. 1893. *Notes on anaesthetics in dental surgery*. London. 74.
16

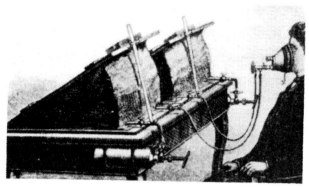

FIG. 127.—APPARATUS FOR ADMINISTERING A
MIXTURE OF NITROUS OXIDE AND OXYGEN
(*c.* 1890)

Of the type designed by Hillischer. The reservoir bags
were kept filled from the cylinders at the sides of the table.
One bag contained eleven gallons of nitrous oxide, the
other seven gallons of oxygen.

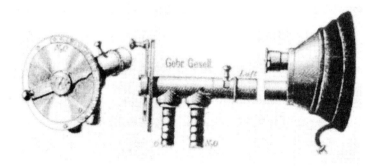

FIG. 128.—NITROUS OXIDE AND OXYGEN
APPARATUS

Mixing chamber into which the tubes from the reservoir
bags led, percentage indicator, handle controlling the
opening and closing of the air port (this part of the
apparatus shown, on the *left*, front view, *centre*, side view),
and *right*, the facepiece with expiratory valve and
inflatable rubber rim.

482

the oxygen one is quite closed—100 per cent. nitrous oxide. When the nitrous oxide orifice is half open the other is half open —50 per cent. of each gas. When the nitrous oxide tube is three-quarters open the oxygen tube is only a quarter open—25 per cent. of oxygen. A mouth-piece, to fit between the teeth, is used instead of the face-piece generally employed in this country.' [1]

' Hillischer's apparatus is portable enough ', said Hewitt, ' but it has one great drawback, viz. that the oxygen cannot be regulated with that nicety which is necessary in actual practice ; in other words, a very small movement of its oxygen indicator means a considerable increment or decrement in the gas. This difficulty I have overcome, . . . for the oxygen on its way from the bag to the face-piece, is made to pass through minute circular holes, any number of which may be opened at a time.

' Two india-rubber bags are employed : one for nitrous oxide, the other for oxygen. These, which are fed from cylinders worked by the foot, are attached to two metal tubes T' and T. Where the tubes join there is an arrangement by which oxygen may be added to the current of nitrous oxide to the desired extent. Above this regulating arrangement with its dial (D), indicating handle (H), and indicator (i), there is a two-way stop-cock, which allows, by the movement of its handle (H'), either of air or of the mixed gases being breathed. In order to permit the free escape of each inspiration, two flap-valves, one an expiratory (EV), and one an inspiratory (IV) are provided. The tubes (T and T') also possess flap-valves (v and v') to prevent the contents of one bag passing over to the other. The oxygen tube T is considerably expanded above, so that the nitrous oxide tube may pass up through its middle. Oxygen thus travels along the circular channel left between the tubes, whilst nitrous oxide passes along the inner tube. . . . The space left between the nitrous oxide tube and the expanded oxygen tube is closed by two circular plates, the upper of which (P) revolves by means of the handle (H) upon the lower, which is fixed. The upper plate has thirteen holes in it. The lower has a long slot (S) shown in dotted lines. When the handle (H) is turned, so that P revolves, one or more holes can be brought over the slot in the lower plate, and be thus rendered available for the passage of oxygen. . . . *By this plan a very small increment or decrement in oxygen is represented by a very considerable excursion of the indicator along the dial plate.* Notwithstanding that I have made a large number of experiments with the object of ascertaining what percentages of oxygen pass through these holes, I find it impossible to give any reliable

[1] Hewitt, F. W. 1893. *Anaesthetics and their administration.* London. 120.

averages, owing to the variations in pressure which must to some extent occur in the bags during the administration. All that I can say is that when both bags are kept partially distended, [Hewitt admitted that ' considerable practice is necessary to keep both bags equal in size throughout '] and one hole is

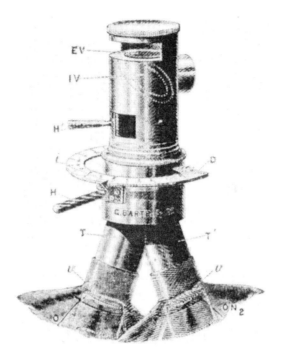

FIG. 129.—REGULATING STOPCOCK OF HEWITT'S NITROUS OXIDE AND OXYGEN APPARATUS (c. 1893)

O. oxygen bag. ON_2 nitrous oxide bag. v and v'. flap-valves in the tubes, T and T'. H. handle controlling the proportions of oxygen and nitrous oxide in the mixture. i. indicator on H, passing over D, dial. H'. handle of two-way stopcock allowing either air or the anaesthetic mixture to reach the facepiece. IV and EV. inspiratory and expiratory valves.

open, a very small percentage (something between $3\frac{1}{2}$ and $6\frac{1}{2}$ per cent.) of oxygen will come through, and that each additional hole turned on represents something like an additional 1 per cent. or $1\frac{1}{2}$ per cent. of oxygen. . . . The apparatus here described allows (1) air, (2) nitrous oxide, or (3) nitrous oxide mixed with a proportion of oxygen, to be freely respired through valves at the will of the administrator.' [1]

[1] Hewitt, F. W. 1893. *Anaesthetics and their administration.* London. 122-4.

'. . . It is important not to charge the bags till immediately before the inhalation. The face-piece should be one which is capable of being applied to the face with the utmost accuracy, as a want of co-aptation . . . would, in the case of the mixture, be likely to lead to partial or complete failure. . . . After passing a small quantity of the gases through the bags, in order to free them from all traces of air, the anaesthetist should turn off the two-way stop-cock, and place the oxygen indicator at " o." Both

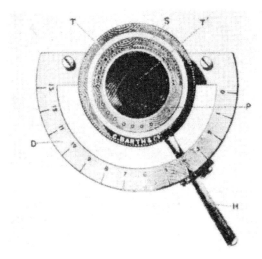

FIG. 130.—THE REGULATING MECHANISM OF HEWITT'S NITROUS OXIDE-OXYGEN APPARATUS

T'. nitrous oxide tube. T. expanded oxygen tube. P. circular plate revolved, by means of the handle, H, over the lower, fixed plate with slot, S, cut in it, indicated by dotted line. 'When the handle, H, is turned, so that P revolves, one or more holes can be brought over the slot in the lower plate, and be thus rendered available for the passage of oxygen.' In Fig. 130 the indicator points to ' 4 ' on the dial, i.e. four holes are opened for oxygen.

bags should now be filled to about one-half with their respective gases, and the face-piece applied. Air will now be breathed freely through the apparatus, and the sound of the acting valves will prove that the face-piece fits well. The patient should be instructed to breathe freely and moderately deeply, " in and out through the mouth." This is important, for as he commences to breathe, so he will probably continue when the mixture is admitted. When the administrator sees and hears that breathing is free . . . he should fix the oxygen indicator at " 2," and turn on the mixture at the two-way stop-cock. . . . It is best to commence with a comparatively small percentage of oxygen, as we have to allow for that originally present in the lungs and blood. . . . The objection to giving pure nitrous oxide itself at the beginning, is that it is sometimes difficult to quickly neutralise the effects thus

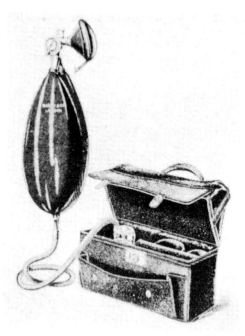

FIG. 131.—HEWITT'S IMPROVED APPARATUS FOR NITROUS OXIDE AND OXYGEN (1897)

It consisted of a carrying bag, 'two nitrous oxide cylinders, one oxygen cylinder, a combined stand and union, double india-rubber tubes (one running inside the other) for conducting the two gases from the cylinders to the . . . two india-rubber bags joined together by a septum common to both, a combined regulating stopcock and mixing chamber [see Fig. 132], and a face- piece '. The bags were filled before the patient entered the room and the readily-attachable foot-key was kept on one of the nitrous oxide cylinders during the administration. The foot-key can be seen in the carrying bag.

produced without going to the other extreme and administering too much oxygen. After two or three seconds the oxygen indicator may be turned to " 3," and in a few seconds more to " 4." In children, anaemic subjects, and debilitated persons, the indicator may be moved to " 3 " and " 4 " more quickly than in strongly-built or alcoholic individuals. During these manipulations

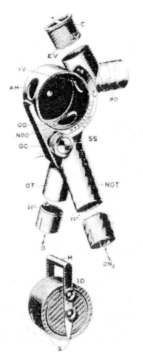

FIG. 132.—REGULATING STOPCOCK AND MIXING CHAMBER OF HEWITT'S APPARATUS FOR NITROUS OXIDE AND OXYGEN, 1897 (see also Fig. 131)

Arrows show the direction of oxygen and nitrous oxide flowing from the bags into OT, oxygen tube, and NOT, nitrous oxide tube, respectively. *iv* and *iv′*, valves acting during inspiration.

(*Upper figure.*)

NOO. Orifice for nitrous oxide.

OC. Chamber in which a small amount of oxygen was allowed to accumulate.

OO. Ten small orifices for oxygen (three showing) ' any number of which may be opened by moving the inner drum [ID, lower figure]. All the 10 oxygen orifices are of the same size except the first, and by means of the supplementary stopcock, SS, this can either be made of the same size as the other 9 (1st position of SS), or it can be made equal to the 10 orifices collectively (2nd position of SS), or to 20 such orifices (3rd position of SS).' In its third position SS gave the administrator the equivalent of thirty oxygen orifices.

IV Inspiratory, and EV, expiratory valve (with chimney, C).

PD. Partial diaphragm directing the patient's expirations towards EV.

(*Lower figure.*)

ID. Inner drum, revolving within the mixing chamber, with

H. Handle and pointer, which passed over the index on the side of the mixing chamber (see upper figure).

S. Slot in ID.

When H was at its lowest point (cf. Fig. 131), air entered the mixing chamber through AH, air hole, and slot, S, and was breathed in and out through IV and EV, NOO and OO being closed by ID. As ID was revolved by raising H, AH closed and first NOO and then an increasing number of oxygen inlets, OO, were made to coincide with slot, S, thus allowing nitrous oxide and oxygen to enter the mixing chamber. By means of SS the equivalent of any number of oxygen orifices between one and thirty could be opened.

the two bags must be kept as nearly as possible equal in size. It is rarely, if ever necessary to replenish the oxygen bag during the administration, but the foot must be constantly kept on the nitrous oxide key. . . . Should phonation, laughter, excited movement, or struggling assert itself, the administrator should withhold more oxygen for the present, or even . . . turn . . . back the indicator for a few breaths. In forty or fifty seconds from the commencement of the inhalation the indicator may usually be got as far as " 5," and in twenty seconds or so more may be allowed to point to " 6," or even " 8." Generally speaking, it is not advisable to give more oxygen than this. . . . It is impossible to formulate any definite rules. Considerable practice is necessary . . . to know when to give more, and when to give less oxygen. Whilst too much oxygen will be likely to induce laughter, excited movement, stamping, screaming, &c., . . . the anaesthetist must be careful not to proceed too far in the opposite direction. In regulating the increase or decrease of oxygen we must reckon what the *future* effects of any procedure will be. . . . On the one side we wish to avoid the clonic respiratory movements, &c., which prevent a free and lengthy intake of the anaesthetic ; and on the other any inconvenient signs of incomplete anaesthesia.' [1]

In 1897 Hewitt published what he described as a ' small treatise on *the administration of nitrous oxide and oxygen for dental operations*, dealing more particularly with the practical aspects of the subject '.

' Eleven years have elapsed since I commenced working at this subject ', wrote Hewitt. ' The first eight years were mainly devoted to conducting preliminary experimental administrations of various mixtures of nitrous oxide and oxygen and to devising and perfecting apparatus. The last three years have been occupied in ascertaining the precise influence exerted by this or that percentage of air or of oxygen upon the usual asphyxial phenomena of pure nitrous oxide.'

Although Hewitt claimed that the apparatus used by him in 1897 was a ' perfected ' version of that described in 1893, the two did not greatly differ in essentials ; nor had the three years' additional research seriously modified Hewitt's opinion on the correct percentages of oxygen to be administered.

' There is, unfortunately, no rule ', he wrote, ' which will apply to every case. . . . A little practice will enable him [the anaesthetist] to avoid the Scylla of asphyxia on the one hand,

[1] Hewitt, F. W. 1893. *Anaesthetics and their administration.* London. 124–6.

and the Charybdis of excitement on the other. He will find, after a time, that he is able to detect even slight deviations from the proper course, almost before such deviations have taken place.

' Generally speaking . . . the best results will be obtained by starting the inhalation . . . with from 2 to 4 per cent. of oxygen, and then progressively increasing this proportion to 8 or 9 per cent. It seems to me ', he added, ' that it is a mistake to adopt the plan which is customary in Germany [1], and to begin with as much as 10 per cent. of oxygen. . . . If a 10 per cent. mixture be used from the commencement, excitement is liable to ensue from the undue proportion of oxygen. Witzel, for example, who follows this course in his administrations, finds it necessary to employ arm-rings, foot-straps, and other appliances to restrain the patient's movements, and to have at hand, on all occasions, strong and trained assistants. Such precautions are unnecessary when the method here advocated is followed.' [2]

In 1898, in a paper read at a meeting of the Society of Anaesthetists, Alfred Coleman revived an idea which both he and J. T. Clover had put into practice thirty years earlier, namely, the administration of nitrous oxide through the nose (cf. p. 285, footnote) ' with the object of prolonging unconsciousness during operations on the mouth '. Without referring to the earlier experiments with nitrous oxide given nasally Coleman said :

' I had long found that by forcing air mixed with ether into the nostrils after the removal of the face-piece [he did not explain how he did this, but cf. p. 604] when gas had been administered, some prolongation of the anaesthesia was obtained, but the slight delay in changing the apparatus, combined also with interference with the operator, were drawbacks to its employment. To avoid these I have constructed the apparatus now before you [see Fig. 133]. It consists of a nose-piece made to loosely cover the nose and fit accurately to its base, and which is connected with a very flat tube also adapted to fit accurately over the forehead. To the latter is attached a piece of stout rubber tubing having at its further extremity a very lightly constructed two-way stopcock which is connected with the ordinary gas-bag, but between the two is placed a valve which opens towards the nose. The gas-bag is connected by a long tube to the gas-bottle. When using the apparatus it is well, as Dr. Hewitt, who has very kindly

---

[1] The plan was originally introduced in Germany by Adolph Witzel, of Essen, who was a disciple of Hillischer's.

[2] Hewitt, F. W. 1897. *The administration of nitrous oxide and oxygen for dental operations.* London. 48–50.

16*

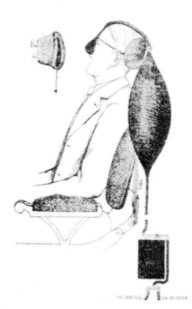

Fig. 133.—COLEMAN'S APPARATUS FOR MAIN-
TAINING NITROUS OXIDE ANAESTHESIA
THROUGH THE NOSE DURING DENTAL
OPERATIONS (1898)

Anaesthesia was induced with the extra-large facepiece
applied over the nose-piece and mouth.

The patient is shown leaning back, his head supported by the head-rest of the dental chair (seen behind
his ear). The nose-piece is held in place by a strap passing
round his head. From the nose-piece a flat tube passes
back over the crown of the head to the reservoir bag, a
small stopcock being interposed between the two. The
function of the square piece of apparatus seen below the
reservoir bag was not explained by Coleman, nor was the
direction ' to blower ' ; ' to bottle ' means ' to cylinder '.

assisted me in some experiments [1], suggests, to instruct the
patient to breathe in at the nose and out at the mouth for a few
times, and then to adapt the nose-piece, the same form of breathing
being continued. An air-padded face-piece, rather larger than is

[1] J. Blomfield has stated that ' although he described it in his book Hewitt never
practised . . . the nasal administration of nitrous oxide, . . . so keen was he on the
constant use of the oral respiration in all inhalation anaesthesia '. (Brit. J. Anaesth.,
1926–7, 4, 122.)

SOME NEW DEVELOPMENTS   491

ordinarily employed, and having only the outlet valve, is placed over the nose-piece and mouth and the gas turned on.   When the patient is fully narcotised the face-piece is removed and the opera-tion commenced, whilst sufficient gas is admitted into the bag to slightly distend it beyond its normal capacity.   My friend Mr. Paterson, one of the anaesthetists at St. Bartholomew's Hospital, has kindly employed my apparatus. . . . He says, " I have used your apparatus in fifteen dental cases. . . . In all the cases the administration could, I believe, have been continued for a longer period had it been required.   The longest case was exactly five minutes, and during this time 13 teeth were removed, several of them difficult extractions ".' [1]

Coleman's paper was followed, at the same meeting of the Society (March 17, 1898), by a paper on ' The continuous administration of nitrous oxide ', read by Stephen A. Coxon : [2]

' In 1888 ', said Coxon, ' I commenced to try if anaesthesia could not be lengthened by allowing a small stream of gas to pass into the mouth by means of a bent tube.   This proceeding certainly lengthened the anaesthesia.   Encouraged by this, I employed a larger tube . . . with the result that there were few dental operations that could not be completed with one inhalation of the gas, and in many there is no sign of returning consciousness as long as the injector is kept going.   The method of administering is to anaesthetise the patient in the ordinary way with nitrous oxide ; then on removing the face-piece to place the curved tube into the mouth until it is a short distance from the uvula (for preference the injector is passed to behind the prop) ; then, with the gas-bag well filled up, a steady stream of gas is maintained. The patient with every inspiration inhales a mixture of gas and air, and is of necessity kept under for a longer period than would otherwise be the case if he were only inspiring air.   There is one thing upon which stress must be laid, viz. that the gas-bag be kept well filled with gas, so that the gas comes out under pressure, or otherwise only partial success will be obtained.   It is of neces-sity rather wasteful, but the results you get will more than compensate you for this.

' One day ', continued Coxon, ' when giving gas in this fashion, I found the patient's mouth unusually cold.   This undoubtedly arose from the stream of nitrous oxide gas that was being sent into it.   On the patient leaving I tried by placing the bulb of a thermometer in the gas-bag.   The result was that, in a room regis-tering 64°, the thermometer in the bag was a shade under 50°.

[1] *Trans. Soc. Anaesth.*, 1898, **1**, 117–21.
[2] Coxon, according to William McCardie (who for a time used the apparatus recommended in Coxon's paper quoted above), was a dentist practising at Wisbech.

Since that time I have made a practice of letting the gas traverse a small copper coil as it passes to the bag, and of placing the coil in hot water. This method heats the gas and prevents it causing possible trouble to the lungs of a delicate patient. . . .

' During the time of using the injector there is very little jactitation, and the patient is nearly as quiet as he would be under chloroform. Now, after using the tube for a while you can make it of great service to the operator ; it will act as a tongue depressor [cf. Dubois's tube, p. 372] and obstruct the entrance of teeth into the throat that have slipped out of the forceps. . . . During no part of the time, after once getting the patient under, do you obstruct any of the air-passages.'

During the general discussion of these two papers Herbert Paterson offered several friendly criticisms of Coleman's nasal apparatus. Paterson suggested that if both nose- and facepiece were made of celluloid instead of ' rigid material ', ' pressure marks on the patient's face could be avoided '. He had also ' found the bag rather in the way, and would suggest that there should be only a small reservoir bag at the back of the patient's head, and that the main bag should be on the floor, out of the way of the operator. . . . Mr. Coleman [sic, but probably in error for ' Coxon ', cf. p. 491] had spoken of the importance of maintaining a pressure of gas, which he thought was a point requiring special attention. It was true that in maintaining pressure a considerable waste of gas ensued ; this, however, was inevitable if satisfactory anaesthesia was to be obtained '.[1]

A month later, at a meeting of the Society of Anaesthetists on April 21, 1898, Harvey Hilliard described a method of prolonging nitrous oxide anaesthesia by means of a nasal tube. He used an ordinary nitrous oxide apparatus (cf. Fig. 126), except that the exit tube from the gas cylinders was bifurcated and controlled by a stopcock. To one arm of this tube was attached the tubing leading to the reservoir bag, stopcock, and facepiece of the apparatus, to the other was attached a similar length of tubing, at each end of which was a small reservoir bag (like the bag of a hand-bellows), that farthest from the cylinders being surrounded by a net. This length of tubing terminated in a flexible nasal tube.

' The administration ', said Hilliard, ' is conducted in the usual way until the patient has lost consciousness ; then, taking the precaution that the ordinary gas bag is full, the stopcock

[1] *Trans. Soc. Anaesth.*, 1898, **1**, 123-9.

having been turned on to it, and choosing the end of an inspiration, the face-piece is removed, the nasal tube is rapidly passed
(this can be done during a single expiration), the face-piece is
reapplied, and the stopcock is turned so that the gas now flows
through the nasal tube ; at this stage the inhalation is continued
by both nasal tube and face-piece up to full anaesthesia ; the
face-piece is now finally removed, the operation is begun, and
narcosis is maintained by the nasal tube alone. To prevent the
return of consciousness the " netted bag " must be kept fully
distended, the gas being supplied at considerable pressure.' [1]

On May 5, 1899, Paterson, who had been developing
Coleman's method and apparatus for nasal nitrous oxide along
independent lines, demonstrated, at a meeting of the West
London Medico-Chirurgical Society, a new type of nasal cap
and his own technique for administering nitrous oxide nasally,
which is, essentially, that commonly used at the present time.

' The apparatus . . . [see Fig. 134] ', he said, ' consists of a
small metal cover made to fit the nose accurately, with the aid of
a rubber pad. The pad is detachable, so that the cover can be
readily sterilised by boiling. Two small metal tubes are let into
the nose-piece, and to these are attached two rubber tubes which
lead to an ordinary gas bag, a twoway stop-cock intervening. In
using the apparatus, the nose-piece is placed *in situ*, the bag being
filled with gas, and the stop-cock turned on. After the patient
has taken a few breaths of gas a celluloid cover is placed over the
mouth. At the top of the mouth cover is an expiratory valve.
The patient is now breathing gas through the nose only and
expiring through the mouth. I may say that the use of the mouth
cover is not absolutely necessary. Its function is twofold. It
diminishes the period of inhalation necessary for the production
of anaesthesia, and consequently economises gas. In about thirty
seconds the mouth cover is removed and the operation proceeded
with. The patient is now taking in gas through the nose, and a
limited amount of air through the mouth, and there is no difficulty
in maintaining anaesthesia, indeed, the stop-cock has often to be
turned off occasionally in order to allow the patient to obtain
more air than is admitted by the mouth. . . .

' So far as I know ', said Paterson, in conclusion, ' there is
only one disadvantage with this method, and that is, that owing
to the anaesthetist being engaged in giving gas all through the
operation, he is not so able to assist the operator as in giving gas
in the ordinary way. It is, however, quite possible, although
somewhat inconvenient to manipulate the gag when required.
. . . I venture to maintain ', added Paterson, ' that the ordinary

[1] *Trans. Soc. Anaesth.*, 1898, **I,** 170.

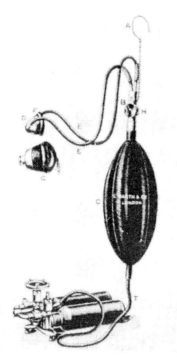

FIG. 134.—PATERSON'S APPARATUS FOR MAIN-
TAINING NITROUS OXIDE ANAESTHESIA
THROUGH THE NOSE (1899)

A. Hook for suspending the apparatus from the anaesthetist's person.
B. Stopcock. By turning off the flow of gas about once in every
   four or five breaths the patient was allowed to draw in air
   through the aperture, H.
C. Bag, into which gas flowed through the tubing, T, from the foot-
   actuated cylinders.
E, E'. Tubes leading nitrous oxide, and once in every four or five
   breaths, air, to the metal nose-piece, D, rimmed with an air-
   filled rubber pad, F.
G. Celluloid mouthpiece, with expiratory valve, used, if necessary,
   to shorten the induction period.

method of dosing the patient with gas to the utmost limit, so as
to maintain the anaesthesia as long as possible after the removal
of the face-piece, is unscientific and wrong in principle. In this
method the administration need not be pushed so far, the anaesthesia is carried only to the stage of unconsciousness, and the
patient maintained gently under the influence of the gas without
pushing it to an extreme degree.' [1]

[1] *West Lond. med. J.*, 1899, **4,** 211–13.

Another innovation made during 1899, but one which did not survive the test of time, was George Belben Flux's 'administration of nitrous oxide gas by an open inhaler'. 'The objects of the method', Flux explained to a meeting of the Society of

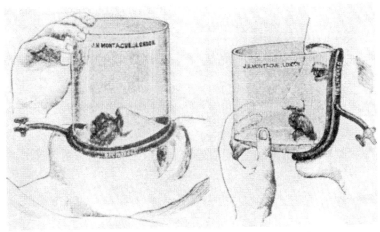

FIG. 135   FIG. 136

FLUX'S 'OPEN METHOD' OF ADMINISTERING
NITROUS OXIDE (1899)

Fig. 135. The open-ended, celluloid cylinder, with inflatable rubber rim, used when the patient was in the recumbent position.

Fig. 136. The celluloid 'cup' used when the patient was in the sitting position.

With both types of inhaler an ordinary nitrous oxide apparatus (cf. Fig. 126) was used; the facepiece was detached and the free end of the tubing connecting with the reservoir bag and gas cylinders was simply held over the side of the celluloid inhaler and a gentle stream of gas allowed to flow in during the patient's inspiration.

Anaesthetists on February 17, 1899, 'are, in addition to the induction of anaesthesia :

' 1. To save the patient from the discomforts of the accurately fitting air excluding face-piece.

' 2. To enable the patient to breathe the gas at the atmospheric pressure.

' 3. To maintain free access of air to the patient.

' 4. To admit the gas *to* the inspired air, only in such amount as circumstances may require.'

' In using the open inhaler, it is the gas which is admitted to the air ', said Flux, ' and not air which is admitted to the gas—the air is permanently present, the gas is merely a temporary addition.'

Flux's open inhaler was made of thin, pliant celluloid [1] and two different forms were available (see Figs. 135 and 136). One form was for use when the patient was lying down. It was cylindrical, with open ends, one end having an inflatable rubber rim to fit accurately over the face, from below the mouth to the bridge of the nose. The other form, for use when the patient was sitting, was shaped like an oval, flat-bottomed beaker, but with an aperture in the side, also rubber rimmed, to admit the patient's face. The rim ran round the cheeks and chin from temple to temple.

Neither form of the inhaler was directly connected with the supply of nitrous oxide—the end of the tubing of ' an ordinary gas apparatus, without the face-piece ' was merely held over the side of the celluloid inhaler. To induce anaesthesia ' a gentle but sufficient stream of gas ' was allowed to flow, during inspiration only, from the cylinder through the reservoir bag and tubing and so ' into the wide mouth of the inhaler '. ' When anaesthesia has been once induced ', said Flux, ' it can be kept up indefinitely by allowing the patient an occasional breath of GAS—the inhaler being moved or not in the intervals between the breaths as may be convenient.'

Flux explained the rationale of his method as follows :

' When a suitable open inhaler is accurately applied to the face, there cannot be any escape of gas unless due to overflow resulting from too free a supply. The weight of the gas prevents escape upwards, and unless leakage is permitted between the margins of the inhaler and the face, there can be no escape downwards. The gas as it falls into the inhaler ', he added, ' is warmed by the breath of the patient, and by the surrounding atmosphere. . . .

' To render an ordinary adult anaesthetic by this method, an average expenditure of from seven to eight gallons of gas is required ; a further amount of three or four gallons for each additional minute will suffice to maintain anaesthesia.'

[1] The use of celluloid for facepieces was first introduced by J. F. W. Silk about 1891. In the ' New Inventions ' column of the *Lancet* he wrote in 1894 : ' The value of celluloid . . . is gradually being recognised. For the last two or three years I have had in constant use a set of face-pieces and masks made of this substance." (*Lancet*, 1894, i, 198–9.) These included facepieces of the ordinary type for nitrous oxide administration (cf. Fig. 125, diagram on left) and a Rendle's mask (see Fig. 67). In 1897, however, Silk recommended metal facepieces for hospital use as being less fragile than celluloid. (*Lancet*, 1897, i, 892.)

Flux claimed that in addition to the pleasant freedom from constraint during the induction period, the patient suffered no distressing after-effects of anaesthesia ; from the anaesthetist's and the surgeon's point of view anaesthesia was equally satisfactory, because at no time was there ' excitement, stertor, lividity, or convulsive movement, or any sign of asphyxia '. Moreover the patient's face was always clearly in view and the inhaler was in the highest degree hygienic.

The discussion of Flux's paper was opened by H. Bellamy Gardner whose remarks were reported as follows :

' While fully appreciating the advantage of the forms of face-piece . . . and the simplicity of the whole method, he was convinced that there must be some fallacy in the fact stated by Dr. Flux, namely, that a large quantity of air and a very small quantity of gas was necessary for that form of anaesthesia. He helped Dr. Hewitt with a large series of experiments with a mixture of known percentages of air and nitrous oxide gas, and when they got up to certain percentages over 30 per cent.—the air being mixed most accurately and carefully in a gasometer—they found that true anaesthesia was almost unobtainable. In breathing into both forms of face-piece which had been exhibited he found that the air taken in was, after the first breath, extremely warm, and he had no doubt that for some reason—either due to the amount of aqueous vapour present in the expirations or some other physical reason—the expirations did not escape to the degree which at first sight one would expect. He thought, therefore, that it was very probable that both these face-pieces were open to any amount of atmospheric mixture, that expirations containing CO_2 were mixed with the gas, and though probably Dr. Flux and others who had tried it could very nicely adjust the gas and air mixtures, it seemed that less than twenty per cent. of air was mixed with the gas.'

Carter Braine, however, stated that he

' had had the pleasure of seeing Dr. Flux administer the anaesthetic by the method he explained, at the Dental Hospital of London, and he was very much surprised at the state of the patients. Although he watched very carefully, he was unable to tell when they were anaesthetised. They simply seemed to remain in a sort of normal sleep, and he would not have known when to stop the administration. . . . He obtained Dr. Flux's permission to be himself anaesthetised. . . . The face-piece was put into position, and the gas fell in from the top. He breathed perfectly naturally, and did not seem to be taking gas ; he thought the whole thing was a farce. . . . The next thing he was aware of was that he was simply in the chair, staring straight in front of him. . . . At the time he was convinced he had not been under the anaesthetic at all. But very shortly afterwards he found he had been under it, because his knees seemed very shaky . . . he was afterwards told that the anaesthesia had lasted two and a half minutes. He could, therefore, bear out the statement that it was a most pleasant way of taking nitrous oxide. As to the degree of anaesthesia obtained, of course he could not give an opinion.' [1]

Ethyl Chloride

The last important inhalation anaesthetic to be generally adopted during the nineteenth century was ethyl chloride. Although its powers as an inhalation anaesthetic had been demonstrated both by Flourens in the laboratory and by Heyfelder clinically during 1847 and 1848 (see p. 170), ethyl chloride was not finally accepted in practice until after 1896, and this acceptance took place in a curiously roundabout way.

In 1890, at the International Congress of Medicine held in Berlin, Redard, of Geneva, recommended (in the Section of Dentistry) the use of an ethyl chloride spray for producing anaesthesia by refrigeration in minor and, more particularly, dental surgery. He explained that it was necessary to use pure ethyl chloride and that he himself obtained the drug from the firm of Gaillard, P. Monnet, and Cartier, of Lyons.[2] It was supplied in small glass phials, each fitted with a special nozzle (cf. Fig. 146) easily opened and closed by a lever, and ' the warmth of the hand was sufficient to vaporise the liquid and project it on to the skin in a fine jet '.[3]

In the following spring Redard again recommended the ethyl chloride spray, this time at the Fifth Congress of French Surgeons in Paris. On that occasion he reported that Reverdin and Vulliet, of Geneva, had used it successfully in 300 cases.[4]

During 1891 the use of ethyl chloride for local anaesthesia in dentistry spread widely in Europe, and in England Underwood was reported to be using it in the dental department of King's College Hospital ' with a large amount of success '.[5]

---

[1] *Trans. Soc. Anaesth.*, 1899, **2**, 140–50.
[2] A year or two later this firm changed its name to the *Société chimique des Usines du Rhône* and the name of its pure ethyl chloride product to *Kelene*.
[3] *Trans. int. Congr. Med.*, 1891, **5** (xiv), 71.
[4] *Sem. méd. Paris*, 1891, **11**, 133.   [5] *J. Brit. dent. Assoc.*, 1891, **12**, 780.

In America the editor of the *Dental Cosmos*, in the late spring of 1892, submitted a sample of ethyl chloride to Professor H. C. Wood, asking him to investigate its physiological properties ' sufficiently to determine the question whether . . . [it] can be of service as . . . [a] practical anaesthetic '.

On June 22 Wood described the results of the investigation of ethyl chloride which he and his associate David Cerna had made before a meeting of the Philadelphia County Medical Society. He stated that owing to the smallness of the sample submitted for testing only a few experiments, on dogs, could be made. These showed ' that the chloride of ethyl is capable of acting as an anaesthetic [by inhalation] provided that its vapor be given in concentrated form '. The results obtained were not consistent, however, for in one instance, after producing two minutes' complete anaesthesia with ten grams of ethyl chloride, given from a cone ' almost impervious to the air and so flexible that it could be ligatured around the dog's nose ', a second application of the cone recharged with ten grams of ethyl chloride inexplicably failed to produce anaesthesia. In two other cases in which ten grams of the drug were administered through a tracheal tube, one administration lasting about three minutes, the other being made as rapidly as possible, no anaesthesia resulted.

Wood stated in conclusion :

' As the result of the various experiments which we have made with chloride of ethyl, we believe that the fugaciousness of the action of the drug must interfere with its use as a general anaesthetic, and that its depressing effect upon the circulation is too pronounced for it to be a safe anaesthetic. It is most probable that if it should come to be employed in practical medicine as an anaesthetic there would be a record of sudden deaths through cardiac failure proportionately even more numerous than those caused by chloroform.' [1]

During 1894, however, H. Carlson, a Gothenburg dentist, accidentally produced general instead of local anaesthesia with ethyl chloride in two cases. One of the patients had been anaesthetized on previous occasions, once with ethyl bromide (see p. 212) and once with chloroform. This man emphatically stated that of the three anaesthetics ethyl chloride was by far the most pleasant, producing no feeling of suffocation or

[1] Wood, H. C., and Cerna, D. ' Chloride of ethyl and pental ', reprinted from *Trans. Philadelphia County Medical Society*, 1892.

embarrassed breathing. He remained in Carlson's surgery for an hour after recovering from the ethyl chloride anaesthesia, without experiencing any after-effects.

In the following year (1895) another dentist, Thiesing, of Hildesheim, told members of a dental congress in Hanover that he too had accidentally produced general instead of local anaesthesia with ethyl chloride in five out of about fifty cases.

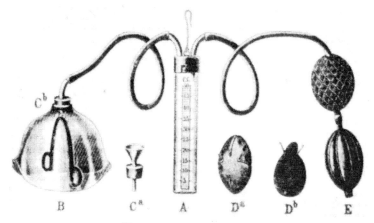

FIG. 137.—SCHÖNEMANN'S ' UNIVERSAL MASK '

Used for various volatile anaesthetics.

A. Junker's bottle (Kappeler's pattern).
B. Glass facepiece, detachable from A and then used alone, as an anaesthetic mask.
Cᵃ and Cᵇ. Rubber corks. Cᵇ for use with A ; Cᵃ pierced by a funnel through which the liquid anaesthetic was dropped or sprayed when B was used alone.
Dᵃ and Dᵇ. Small frames, covered with surgical gauze and inserted into B to receive the liquid anaesthetic.
E. Hand-bellows of Junker's apparatus.

This had led him to carry out a series of experiments with ethyl chloride used as a general anaesthetic, first on animals and finally upon himself and his assistant. The results were very satisfactory.

Meanwhile at a dental congress held in Strasbourg Billeter, of Munich, reported further satisfactory cases of general anaesthesia deliberately induced with ethyl chloride. In administering ethyl chloride Billeter made use of Schönemann's ' universal mask ', commonly used for ethyl bromide anaesthesia (see Fig. 137). He detached the glass facepiece (B in Fig. 137) from the rest of the apparatus, inserted the cork and funnel, Ca, into the aperture in its dome, and sprayed ethyl chloride through on to the surgical gauze-covered wire frame, Da, fixed inside the mask.[1]

Billeter's example was followed by Reugg and Respinger, of Basel, Brodtbeck, of Frauenfeld, Seitz, of Constance, and others,

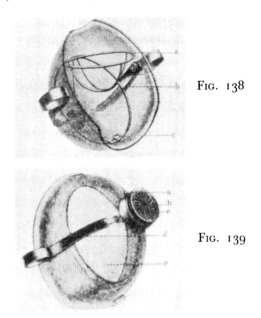

FIG. 138

FIG. 139

BRODTBECK'S MASK

(A modification of Schönemann's, see Fig. 137).
Used for ethyl chloride (1895).

(Fig. 138. *Interior view.*)
 a. hinged frame (over which surgical gauze was laid to receive the ethyl chloride) clipping on to the inner frame at *c.*
 b. metal bands screwed to the glass walls, one on either side of the mask, supporting the wire framework.

(Fig. 139. *Exterior view.*)
 a. handle opening or closing the aperture, *b*, in the iris diaphragm, *c.*
 d. metal bands, the ends bent to form ring handles, for holding the mask in position.
 e. gauze-covered frame, seen through the glass walls of the mask.

most of whom made their own modifications of the ' universal mask '. Brodtbeck's, for instance, had an iris diaphragm in the dome to control the admixture of air with the ethyl chloride vapour in the mask, and a hinged frame covered with surgical gauze to receive the liquid anaesthetic (see Figs. 138 and 139).[2]

---

[1] Dumont, F. L. 1903. *Handbuch der allgemeinen und lokalen Anaesthesie.* Berlin and Vienna. 98.   [2] *Ibid.* 90, 99.

At a medical congress held in Bordeaux in 1895 Soulier and Brian, of Lyons, described a series of laboratory and clinical experiments which they had recently carried out, using as a general anaesthetic ethylidene chloride, a drug similar to ethyl chloride (C_2H_5Cl) but having the formula ($C_2H_4Cl_2$). They stated that the drug was swifter in action than chloroform and could be given in smaller doses. Out of 100 clinical cases they reported ninety-nine successful anaesthesias and one death, in an alcoholic patient.

Soulier and Brian's researches aroused considerable interest ; but it appears that owing to the fact that the drug was referred to as ' Aethylchlorid ' in the brief German report which appeared in the *Münchener medizinische Wochenschrift* in 1896,[1] many German-speaking people very naturally assumed that ethyl chloride had been used. Through this error they themselves were, in many cases, led to make a trial of ethyl chloride anaesthesia. G. F. Henning, a member of a Berlin firm of pharmaceutical manufacturers, pointed out the mistake in 1896 :

' While studying the experiments of Soulier and Brian, I read the French account and found that Aethylidenchlorid to which they referred had become confused with Aethylchlorid. Aethylidenchlorid (CH_3—$CHCl_2$) has long been recognized as a narcotic, but the use of ethyl chloride (C_2H_5Cl), which is so useful as a local anaesthetic, in inhalation anaesthesia was new to me and interested me so much that I made chemically pure ethyl chloride. . . .' [2]

Georg Lotheissen, of Professor von Hacker's Clinic in Innsbruck, was one of those who read the German report and was impressed by Soulier and Brian's high percentage of successes but who mistakenly identified the drug used by them with ethyl chloride.[3] In August 1896, without preliminary trial, Lotheissen administered ethyl chloride (' Kelene ') at the Clinic, cautiously spraying it on to an Esmarch's mask (see Figs. 58–9).

The first patient was a young girl with a whitlow. ' We were astonished ', wrote Lotheissen, ' when after one minute, without any trace of preceding excitement, complete anaesthesia was established and the operation could be begun immediately. Scarcely was the mask removed than the patient opened her eyes and after a few seconds was completely herself and would not believe that the operation could be over so soon. This

[1] *Münch. med Wschr.*, 1896, **43**, 646.   [2] *Ibid.* **43**, 859.   [3] *Ibid.* 1900, **47**, 601.

favourable result led Professor von Hacker to make further trials with ethyl chloride at his Clinic.'[1]

Sixty-six further cases at the Clinic were reported by Alfred Ludwig in 1897,[2] and by 1898 the number had increased to 170. 'This figure', said Lotheissen, 'may, perhaps, seem relatively small, but this is easily explained because wherever possible we prefer to avoid general anaesthesia and use Schleich's infiltration anaesthesia.'[3]

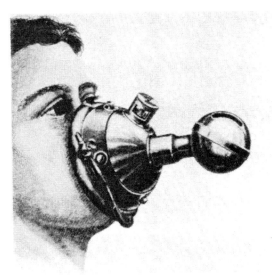

Fig. 140.—BREUER'S INHALER

Designed for administering pental (see p. 222), but used for ethyl chloride by Lotheissen, of Innsbruck (c. 1898).

Describing the evolution of the method of administering ethyl chloride at Innsbruck Lotheissen stated :

' It became apparent that an inhaler which makes an airtight junction with the face [4] was necessary in order to produce reliable anaesthesia in all cases. For a time we used Julliard's ether mask [see Fig. 107]. But the fact that the patient must rebreathe the expired mixture is not a matter of indifference and we discontinued the use of this mask and changed to the Breuer

[1] *Arch. klin. Chir.*, 1898, **57**, 865–6.
[2] *Beitr. klin. Chir.*, 1897, **19**, 639–64.   [3] *Arch. klin. Chir.*, 1898, **57**, 866.
[4] William McCardie (see p. 508 *et seq.*) translated this article and in the margin of the copy which he used for this purpose (now in the Nuffield Department of Anaesthetics, Oxford) he wrote at this point : ' Try Ormsby inhaler '.

inhaler [see Fig. 140] (using it in 125 cases, so far [1898]). This is a modification of Clover's inhaler [*Clover'schen Maske* [1]]. It consists of a metal dome, furnished with a rubber rim, which makes it possible to fit the dome tightly to the face, covering nose and mouth. It has an inspiratory and an expiratory valve. Over the former is attached a hollow ball, made in two pieces

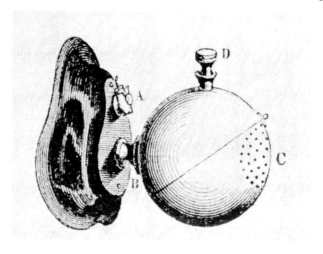

FIG. 141.—CHLOROFORM INHALER

designed by Elser, of Strasbourg, *c.* 1848, which appears to have influenced the design of Breuer's inhaler (Fig. 140).

A. Expiratory valve.
B. Inspiratory valve at the screw-junction between the facepiece and the body of the inhaler.
C. Hollow sphere, in two pieces screwing one into the other ; the lower piece pierced with holes to allow air to enter the inhaler.
D. Stoppered filling aperture, for chloroform.

Within the sphere, just behind the rosette of holes, was placed a strip of sponge, previously wrung out of hot water. On to this the chloroform was dropped through D.

which fit accurately one into the other. This can be opened and a piece of lint inserted to receive the drug. A slot in the ball enables the drug to be sprayed in without lifting the inhaler. Breuer originally devised this inhaler for pental anaesthesia in Professor von Hacker's Surgical Department at the Sophien Hospital in Vienna.

[1] Clover's portable regulating ether inhaler (see Fig. 92) was so referred to in German-speaking countries, and in France as *masque de Clover* (cf. p. 543). It is difficult to imagine why Lotheissen should have stated that Breuer's inhaler was a modification of Clover's.

' The preparation of the patient is the same as for chloroform anaesthesia. Whenever possible the patient should be fasting, but we have anaesthetised a few out-patients, when the operation was urgent, although they had had a meal. Heart and lungs were always carefully examined and the urine tested. Pulse and breathing were kept under observation throughout anaesthesia.'

Lotheissen stressed the advisability of having everything in readiness for the operation before beginning induction because ' the onset of anaesthesia is rapid and it passes with equal rapidity '. He stressed the need for quiet during the induction period because any disturbance delayed the onset of anaesthesia and so entailed a greater expenditure of ethyl chloride.

Describing administration Lotheissen wrote :

' From 3 to 5 grams of ethyl chloride are sprayed on to the gauze, the patient is asked to breathe normally and the facepiece is applied to the face and pressed lightly home, so that it fits airtight. This quantity of ethyl chloride is sufficient for 3 to 4 minutes ; for longer anaesthesia more anaesthetic must be sprayed in just before the end of this period.

' The rapid onset of anaesthesia is characteristic ; about 1 to 1½ minutes after the application of the facepiece (and in children ½ to 1 minute after) the operation can be begun. The excitement stage is usually absent or trifling—in only 13 per cent. of our Kelene anaesthesias was the excitement worth recording. Complete analgesia is established with the induction of anaesthesia, although corneal and pupillar reflexes are usually completely retained, so that the patient moves his eyeballs and so to speak " looks around ". As we never needed deep anaesthesia, in the few cases where these reflexes were abolished we immediately raised the facepiece until pupil and cornea again reacted briskly.

' The quality of the pulse does not alter during anaesthesia, although the rate changes slightly, as a rule somewhat decreasing. The number of respirations is generally increased, but without being otherwise disturbed. Cyanosis is almost always absent ; we observed it in only 3 cases.

' Recovery from ethyl chloride anaesthesia, by comparison with that from other anaesthetics, is very swift, but the return to consciousness is not quite so rapid as the onset of anaesthesia. . . . We noticed [vomiting] in a few (18) cases, but it was quickly over. Many patients, indeed, feel so well after anaesthesia that they can eat with appetite. In any case Kelene anaesthesia leaves no unpleasant after effects, such as the nausea following chloroform anaesthesia ; in fact, some patients (and not only adults but children also) are quite anxious to take Kelene again should operative procedure be necessary.

' Like the corneal and pupillar reflex, muscle tonus persists and complete relaxation is generally absent. This on the one hand, and on the other the rapid return to consciousness immediately the supply of the drug is discontinued, makes ethyl chloride anaesthesia unsuitable for long operations or for operative procedure where muscular relaxation is essential. We use it chiefly in dealing with suppurations, particularly in extensive cellulitis where it would be difficult to use local anaesthesia ; in scraping away carious bone ; in cases of suppurating lymph glands, and in the reduction of fractures and dislocations (particularly those of long standing). . . . In these latter instances muscular relaxation is quite sufficient for reduction, as it is, also, for the manipulation of contractures and pes varus. Ethyl chloride is also very suitable for dilating the female urethra in order to sound the ureters. To these operations must be added such operations as, for example, the extirpation of small tumours, when, although infiltration anaesthesia could easily be used, the patients themselves request general anaesthesia. . . .

' As a rule anaesthesia is maintained for from 5 to 10 minutes ; in oniy 18 cases did it last 15 minutes, and in only 2 cases 20 and 25 minutes. The usual quantity of Kelene used varied between 8 and 10 grams but differed in individual cases. The smallest quantity used was 3 grams in a child one and a half years old. This was our youngest subject for Kelene anaesthesia ; the oldest was a man of seventy-two. The time of life, however, did not affect the character of the anaesthesia.

' We never observed any undesirable symptoms—signs of the heart weakening, of respiratory disturbance, still less of actual asphyxia. . . . Nor did we observe any ill effects upon the kidneys and although, in almost all cases, the urine was tested after anaesthesia, albumen was never found.' [1]

Professor von Hacker was sufficiently pleased with the results of ethyl chloride anaesthesia at his Clinic to encourage its use there. Between 1898 and 1900 it was administered in more complicated types of operation, e.g. in gastrostomies, colostomies, radical operations for hernia, mastectomies, amputations of limbs and rib resections. Lotheissen stated, however, that since longer operations under ethyl chloride had been undertaken, vomiting was noticed to be more frequent, although it was never so violent in character nor so persistent as after chloroform or ether and once it was over the patient felt very well.

[1] *Arch. klin. Chir.*, 1898, **57,** 868–71.

' Lately ', wrote Lotheissen in 1900, ' we have liked to combine a subcutaneous injection of heroin sulphate with Kelene anaesthesia, when the patient is an alcoholic and if complete muscular relaxation is necessary throughout anaesthesia.' [1]

Lotheissen emphatically recommended that, as a safety measure, ethyl chloride should be sprayed into the inhaler in only small quantities at a time and that the dose should never be repeated until the anaesthetist had satisfied himself (by sniffing at the expiratory valve) that the previous dose was exhausted. In order to control the size of the dose more easily, Lotheissen advised that ethyl chloride bottles with wide-bored outlets should be rejected. He also warned against making use of masks intended for ether (which at that time had an impermeable covering, cf. Figs. 107–8) and the valveless, helmet-shaped type of mask used for ethyl bromide (cf. Fig. 44).

Lotheissen had good reason to give these warnings because the first death from ethyl chloride anaesthesia at von Hacker's Clinic had occurred in October 1899. The patient was a forty-one year old labourer, very thickset and a heavy drinker. The proposed operation was a skin graft to an extensive ulceration of the leg. After two minutes' anaesthesia the man became very excited and during the third minute more Kelene was sprayed into the inhaler to quieten him. While this was being done he became cyanosed and the inhaler was removed from his face. The eye reflexes were now absent. As cyanosis appeared the patient struggled and there was tonic spasm of the jaw muscles, respiration was jerky but the pulse was still palpable although, owing to the muscular rigidity, it could not be counted. Suddenly, however, it ceased. Artificial respiration by Silvester's method was immediately begun and kept up for an hour. Supplementary methods of resuscitation, such as the subcutaneous injection of camphorated oil, cardiac massage, and galvanization of the phrenic nerves were also tried. All these measures were completely unavailing (cf. Appendix C).

In this case about ten grams of ethyl chloride had been sprayed from a bottle with a wide outlet tube, but the tip of the tube was thickly frosted up and Lotheissen estimated that probably not more than five grams could have been inhaled.

[1] *Münch. med. Wschr.*, 1900, **47**, 603.

The post-mortem examination revealed extensive disease of the heart. ' I believe ', said Lotheissen, ' that in this case the principal cause of death was not dilatation of the heart but the arterio-sclerosis of the coronary arteries.'

At this time, 1900, Lotheissen mentioned that ethyl chloride was useful for inducing anaesthesia, which was then maintained with ether, or more frequently, chloroform.[1]

The Continental reports of the use of ethyl chloride as a general anaesthetic in dentistry, and in particular Lotheissen's reports of its use in minor surgery, were read by William J. McCardie, anaesthetist to the Birmingham General and Dental Hospitals. ' Being much interested ', wrote McCardie, ' I translated and published Lotheissen's papers [in the *Birmingham Medical Review*, in January and December 1900], but waited till some 2500 cases (with one fatality [Lotheissen's case]) had been reported abroad before I began to administer ethyl chloride myself. I published my first cases in 1901.'

In this report on his first ten cases anaesthetized with ethyl chloride at Birmingham during the early months of 1901 McCardie stated :

' Before I tried ethyl chloride on others I asked Mr. Charles St. Johnston, M.R.C.S., to administer it to me experimentally in a dental chair, and I can say that the subjective effects were like those of nitrous oxide in every respect and not at all unpleasant. . . .

' I used Breuer's mask for all these patients and found it very convenient to manipulate. At no time had I anxiety, nor did I see any change for the worse either in respiration or circulation. I have several times used ethyl chloride instead of nitrous oxide as a preliminary to etherisation and with the same successful effect. The few cases which I have briefly and imperfectly recorded have been so successful that I shall lose no suitable opportunity of testing the drug in carefully selected patients for longer and more difficult operations.' [2]

McCardie's first seven cases were for dental extractions ; in the third case ethyl chloride anaesthesia was a failure and the operation was completed under nitrous oxide. In cases eight and nine the patients were children and the operation the removal of tonsils and adenoids. Case ten was that of an adult with granulations of both ears, for scraping.

[1] *Münch. med. Wschr.*, 1900, **47**, 601-3.   [2] *Lancet*, 1901, i, 698.

In the early part of 1901 the value of ethyl chloride as a general anaesthetic was only just beginning to be appreciated in England. Hewitt,[1] in the newly published second edition of his *Anaesthetics and their administration* (London, 1901, p. 385), concluded a brief description of the use of ethyl chloride by Continental surgeons and by McCardie with the remark that ' further experience with this agent is necessary before any definite statements can be made as to the precise place it should occupy in the list of general anaesthetics.'

H. Bellamy Gardner also, in an article on anaesthesia in the *Medical Annual* for 1901 (pp. 113–16), gave a brief account of the Continental use of ethyl chloride as a general anaesthetic and he repeated Lotheissen's description of Breuer's inhaler as ' resembling Clover's ether inhaler '.

Whether or not Bellamy Gardner's statement influenced anaesthetists is uncertain, but during 1902 and 1903 several people in Great Britain began to administer ethyl chloride from Clover's portable ether inhaler (as modified for giving nitrous oxide and ether, see Fig. 94). For this purpose they dispensed with the ether chamber but kept the facepiece, Hewitt's two-way stopcock and bag, and sprayed ethyl chloride directly into the bag through the stopcock.

By 1904 there were on the market a number of inhalers of this type specially adapted for ethyl chloride ; of these G. W. Bampfylde Daniell's was a prototype.[2]

By the summer of 1901 McCardie himself was recommending the use of a modified version of Breuer's inhaler, about which he stated merely that it was obtainable ' from Messrs. Allen and Hanburys or from Messrs. Greeff '. He added, however : ' Probably an Ormsby's ether inhaler of the pattern made with an air-inlet would serve very well for short inhalations at any rate ' (cf. footnote, p. 503).[3]

Harvey Hilliard was one of those who, in fact, adopted Ormsby's inhaler for ethyl chloride administration ; he used Carter Braine's modification (see Fig. 142).[4]

The acceptance of ethyl chloride as a general anaesthetic in Great Britain was largely due, in the first instance, to McCardie's enthusiastic recommendation of it. His enthusiasm was con-

[1] Hewitt's introduction of the use of an ethyl chloride-nitrous oxide sequence dated from 1903. (See *Brit. dent. J.*, 1903, **24**, 615.)

[2] *Lancet*, 1903, ii, 1087–8.   [3] *Ibid.* 1901, ii, 123–7.

[4] *Practitioner*, 1905, **74**, 205.

siderably modified, however, between 1903 and 1906 by the number of recorded deaths following ethyl chloride anaesthesia.[1]

In 1901 Georges Rolland, Director of the Dental School at Bordeaux, and his associate Field Robinson, introduced into practice an anaesthetic mixture, ' Somnoform ', which was composed of '60 parts chloride of ethyl, 35 parts of chloride of methyl, and 5 parts of bromide of ethyl '. In the following year Rolland and Robinson read a joint paper on Somnoform at the May

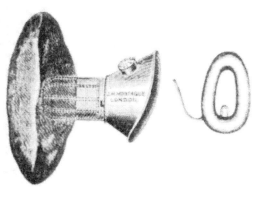

FIG. 142.—CARTER BRAINE'S MODIFICATION OF ORMSBY'S ETHER INHALER

Showing the bag, wire cage, and facepiece with adjustable air inlet and detachable rubber air-pad.

This inhaler was appropriated to the administration of ethyl chloride by Harvey Hilliard, (c. 1905).

meeting of the British Dental Association held in Shrewsbury. They described their method of administration as follows :

' The extremely simple and complete apparatus we use is first of all a small glass bottle, six inches in length, containing sufficient somnoform for 8 to 10 cases, and which is suspended by a piece of string or ribbon from the button-hole ; secondly, an ordinary linen handkerchief, in the folds of which is placed a piece of paper which must *not* be blotting paper, the object of which is to prevent the evaporation of the somnoform—in fact, a protective ; the handkerchief is then refolded in such a manner as to form a cornet hermetically closed, conical in shape, the whole being finally fixed either with an ordinary tie-clip or a trouser-clip as used for cycling. At the extreme bottom of the

[1] See McCardie, W. J. 1906. ' Remarks on the position of and mortality from ethyl chloride as a general anaesthetic.' (*Brit. med. J.*, 1906, i, 616–18.)

cornet, and completely filling the point, is placed a piece of cotton-wool. From the bottle, suspended as aforesaid, the nozzle of which should be placed well forward into the cornet, five cubic centimetres of somnoform is sprayed on to the cotton-wool and surrounding parts of the handkerchief . . . the nose and mouth are completely covered by the cornet, and as far as possible no air allowed to pass.' [1]

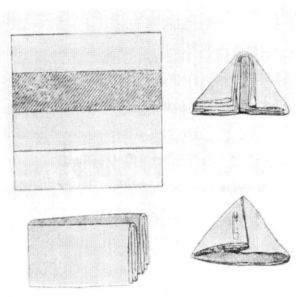

FIG. 143.—ROLLAND'S METHOD OF FOLDING A HANDKERCHIEF ROUND A STRIP OF PAPER (shaded diagonally, in the top figure on the left), to form a closed cone, for the administration of ' Somnoform '.

The vogue for Somnoform anaesthesia was comparatively short-lived, but ' cornets ' similar to Rolland's were for a time used for administering ethyl chloride alone, particularly in America.[2]

In 1902 Aristide Malherbe, a Parisian ear, nose, and throat surgeon specializing in children's cases, introduced what he called the ' compress method ' of giving ethyl chloride.

[1] J. Brit. dent. Ass., 1902, 23, 331.
[2] Cf., e.g., Erdmann, A. F. ' Ethyl chlorid anesthesia'. Med. News, N.Y., 1904, 84, 1024–30.

' All that is necessary, indeed ', wrote Malherbe, ' is a simple compress folded into four thicknesses, or even a handkerchief.

' The compress covers the inside of the right hand, which is held deeply hollowed. This is to avoid too great an evaporating surface.'

According to the age of the patient and the depth of anaesthesia required, from two to three c.c. of ethyl chloride were sprayed on, and the compress, still cupped in the hand, was immediately applied tightly over the patient's nose and mouth. If necessary the compress was removed from the face and the dose repeated just before the effects of the previous dose wore off; in this way anaesthesia could be maintained for from fifteen to twenty minutes.

Malherbe recommended the practice of inducing anaesthesia with ethyl chloride, and then maintaining it with chloroform dropped in small doses on to another compress similarly held in the cupped hand to prevent the free admixture of air.[1]

Nieriker, of Zurich, also used a compress for ethyl chloride, particularly when anaesthetizing children ; but his compress allowed a freer access of air and exit for the exhaled mixture.[2] It consisted of a square pad of woven material laid diamond-wise over nose and mouth and held in position by a band passing round the head. The corner of the pad next the bridge of the nose was caught on the inside by a safety-pin, to form a groove, and into this the nozzle of the ethyl chloride bottle was introduced (see Fig. 144).[3]

In America the use of ethyl chloride as a general anaesthetic seems to have been adopted by a few surgeons about 1900. In February 1900 J. P. Tuttle, Professor of Rectal Surgery at the New York Polyclinic, described to the New York Medical Society his use (in more than fifty cases) of ethyl chloride as a preliminary to ether and to chloroform anaesthesia.

' The time required ', Tuttle said, ' has been less than that required with nitrous oxide as a precedent to ether. There have been no accidents and no physical symptoms which would lead us to believe the drug, thus administered, anything but perfectly safe. The amount of ether has been greatly lessened ;

---

[1] *Bull. méd. Paris,* 1902, **16,** 551.

[2] The practice of spraying ethyl chloride on to an open mask began to be developed about 1911.

[3] Dumont, F. L. 1903. *Handbuch der allgemeinen und lokalen Anaesthesie.* Berlin and Vienna. 101–4.

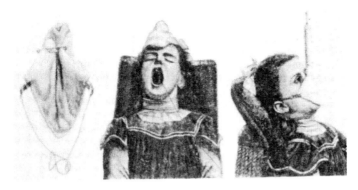

FIG. 144

(*Left.*)   The square pad of woven material, with clips and head-band ; a safety-pin holds the material so that a groove is formed.

(*Middle.*)   The pad pushed up on the forehead to show the gag in place in the patient's mouth.

(*Right.*)   The nozzle of the ethyl chloride bottle inserted into the groove in the pad.

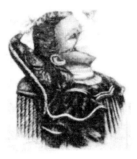

FIG. 145

As an alternative to the ethyl chloride spray, the liquid anaesthetic could be poured directly into a measuring funnel inserted into the groove.

FIGS. 144, 145.—NIERIKER'S METHOD OF ADMINISTERING ETHYL CHLORIDE TO CHILDREN

the recovery from anaesthesia much hastened ; nausea and vomiting are practically obliterated, and the elements of shock have been greatly reduced. Moreover, we have had no experts, but simply an operative surgeon—the author [Tuttle]—and the ordinary house surgeon to administer it. There is no complicated, cumbrous, and costly apparatus necessary for its administration, and it does not require a Saratoga trunk to carry it around. If such experiences with Kelene shall be verified, it seems to me its use will probably supersede that of nitrous oxide, and much of the dread shock and disagreeable experiences of general anaesthesia be done away with.' [1]

The man who appears to have done most to popularize the use of ethyl chloride as a general anaesthetic in the United States, during the early years of the twentieth century, was Martin W. Ware, surgeon to the Good Samaritan Dispensary, New York.

Ware's inhaler (see Fig. 146) consisted of a dome-shaped facepiece having a three- to five-inch, open-ended tube fitted into it. Over the end of the tube, where it entered the facepiece, a few layers of gauze were laid ; on to this gauze a stream of ethyl chloride was intermittently directed down the tube itself.

The main disadvantages of this inhaler were said to be that if the layers of gauze were not sufficiently thick ethyl chloride fell on to the patient's face, whereas if they were too thick hoar frost formed on them and occluded the opening of the tube.[2] Referring to this ' layer of " hoar frost " resulting from the combination of the vapor of the breath with the ethyl chlorid, which forms on the gauze ', Ware himself said:

' I have now learned to regard this rather as a favorable than a deterrent factor, provided the frost be not allowed to form in too thick a layer so as to intercept all access of air. This " hoar frost " constitutes a storage depot for much of the ethyl chlorid and thereby facilitates narcosis. . . . No untoward experience has resulted from the inspiration of air chilled in its passage over the frost, since the vapor of ethyl chlorid is dispelled, expanded and warmed in the pharynx before being taken up in the lungs.'

When muscular relaxation was necessary, and to overcome the resistance of chronic alcoholic patients to ethyl chloride

[1] Quoted in *Kelene*, a brochure published by R. W. Greeff & Co., London, n.d. [1901].
[2] *Med. News, N.Y.*, 1904, **84,** 1026.

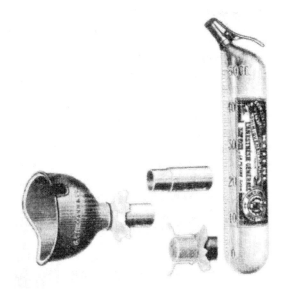

FIG. 146.—WARE'S INHALER FOR ETHYL
CHLORIDE
In use in New York (*c.* 1902).

(*Left.*) Inhaler assembled. Open-ended tube, fitting into
the facepiece. Part of the facepiece in section,
showing how the tube end covered with layers of
surgical gauze, was inserted into it.

(*Right.*) Graduated 'Kelene' bottle, showing the lever
releasing the stopper of the nozzle so that, when
the bottle was held downwards, ethyl chloride
issued in a fine spray.

When used with Ware's inhaler, the nozzle of
the bottle was inserted into the free end of the
tube, so that the ethyl chloride droplets fell
down the tube on to the surgical gauze placed
over its other end.

anaesthesia, Ware gave a preparatory dose of morphine
sulphate gr. ¼.

By the close of 1902 Ware had administered ethyl chloride
1000 times. He stated :

' Symptoms bordering on fatality I have in my series
encountered six times. In each instance they were those of
respiratory interference and they occurred as the outcome of
neglect of attention to the retro-placed tongue during the stage

of profound narcosis, of a disregard of sufficient admixture of air. The fact that all of these patients recovered under artificial respiration speaks very favorably for ethyl chlorid.' [1]

By 1904, in addition to Ware's inhaler, there were in use in the United States various types of Continental inhalers for ethyl chloride and modifications of them, the English type of bag inhaler, modifications of Allis's inhaler (see Figs. 98–101), cones (with gauze in the apex) made from rubber or from a towel folded round an impermeable layer, and simple pads of woven material on to which the drug was sprayed or poured.[2]

Minor Developments

During the late eighteen-nineties two minor developments in inhalation anaesthesia attracted attention ; these were the administration of oxygen with volatile anaesthetics and the anaesthetic mixture suggested by Schleich.

In 1887, possibly through the example set by Hillischer in using oxygen with nitrous oxide (see p. 481), Neudörfer, of Vienna, had proposed the routine administration of oxygen with chloroform vapour for general anaesthesia. His suggestion was soon afterwards adopted by Kreutzmann, in San Francisco, who attached a sixty-litre reservoir bag of oxygen to the afferent tube of a Junker's inhaler and pumped an oxygen-chloroform or oxygen-chloroform-ether mixture to the patient.[3]

The effects of such mixtures on the patient were found to be satisfactory, but the technical difficulties of devising a convenient apparatus for their administration were great, and both in Germany and in the United States, where experiments continued independently, it was some years before the problem was adequately solved.

In Germany it was not until 1901 that Wohlgemuth produced a potentially satisfactory apparatus for delivering a chloroform-oxygen mixture. This apparatus was directly based upon another, designed by L. Prochownick, of Hamburg, in 1895, for giving oxygen towards the end of chloroform or ether anaesthesia in order to improve the patient's general condition in the immediate post-operative period, or, in an anaesthetic emergency, for resuscitation.

[1] *J. Amer. med. Ass.*, 1902, **39**, 1160–2.
[2] Cf. Erdmann, A. F. 'Ethyl chlorid anesthesia.' *Med. News, N.Y.*, 1904, **84**, 1024–30.   [3] *Jber. Leist. ges. Med.*, 1887, i, 395.

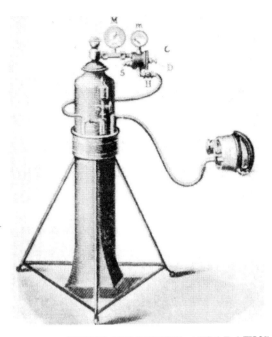

FIG. 147.—WOHLGEMUTH'S APPARATUS

for administering a mixture of oxygen and chloroform vapour, in use in Germany in 1901.

The apparatus consisted of a cylinder of oxygen, supported by a metal stand running on castors. The cylinder was opened by turning a finger nut and the pressure of the gas issuing was registered on the manometer, M. The pressure of gas passing through the reducing valve, beneath the small manometer, m, was regulated by turning the screw, D. When the stopcock, H was open oxygen flowed along the tubing, at a pressure of $\frac{1}{10}$ to $\frac{1}{5}$ of an atmosphere, to the chloroform vaporizing apparatus, which was protected by a tin fender.

The vaporizing apparatus consisted of a glass tube containing water to moisten the gas before it entered the glass U-tube into which chloroform was allowed to fall from a graduated drop bottle containing 50 c.c. of liquid chloroform. The chloroform vapour was taken up by the stream of oxygen and the mixture passed to the celluloid facepiece, which had an expiratory valve and an inflatable rubber rim.

Prochownick's apparatus consisted of a cylinder of oxygen mounted on a mobile stand, rubber tubing and a facepiece and, its most important features, a reducing valve and manometers for quickly and easily regulating the pressure of the gas reaching the patient. Prochownick stated that, as a rule, he gave the oxygen towards the end of anaesthesia at a pressure of one-quarter to one-third of an atmosphere, but in difficult and protracted operations the pressure might be increased from one-third to one-half an atmosphere.[1]

In adapting Prochownick's apparatus Wohlgemuth simply added a chloroform reservoir from which the liquid was dropped into a U-tube in the path of the gas. As he did not also add a reservoir bag, however, whenever the patient breathed deeply the supply of anaesthetic mixture available in the narrow tubing of the apparatus must have become temporarily exhausted (see Fig. 147).

This difficulty was overcome by Roth, of the Lübeck General Hospital, who, in 1902, substituted a chloroform bottle for Wohlgemuth's dropping device, and allowed the oxygen to bubble through the liquid. The resulting mixture passed into a small reservoir bag from which the patient was able to draw an adequate supply, even during deep respiration. This apparatus was manufactured by the Lübeck firm of Dräger.[2]

In America the administration of oxygen with ether began to attract widespread attention about 1898, the method having been under clinical observation in certain hospitals, notably in New York, Boston, and Philadelphia, for more than two years. Thomas S. K. Morton for example, President of the Philadelphia College of Physicians, told a meeting of his colleagues in 1898 'that he had been using oxygen and ether for inducing anaesthesia since December 1895, with increasing confidence and satisfaction. His cases now numbered in the hundreds, with but a single accident'.

The apparatus used by Morton consisted ' of a small wrought-iron tank containing 40 gallons of oxygen gas under pressure, a two-quart pressure-equalizing rubber bag, and a wash-bottle [containing ether] and rubber tubing, connecting with any suitable [valved] inhaling mask. . . . The amount of ether

[1] *Münch. med. Wschr.*, 1895, **42**, 721–3.
[2] Dumont, F. L. 1903. *Handbuch der allgemeinen und lokalen Anaesthesie.* Berlin and Vienna. 141–9.

carried over with the gas is regulated roughly by the depth of ether through which the gas is permitted to bubble up. . . . If it is desired at any time to give pure oxygen ', Morton explained, ' the tube is elevated above the surface of the ether or detached

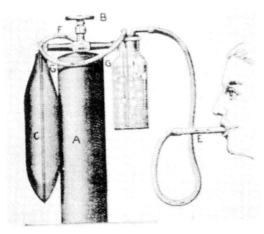

FIG. 148.—OXYGEN-INHALING APPARATUS
made by the American firm of S. S. White, in use during the eighteen-nineties.

A. Cylinder of compressed or liquid oxygen.
B. Handle opening the valve through which gas flowed into the tubing, F.
C. Rubber bag, holding three pints. Gas passed from C, along the tubing, G, into
D. Wash-bottle, half filled with water. The water served to wash and moisten the gas and also to indicate the rate of flow.
E. Mouth-tube.

T. S. K. Morton, of Philadelphia, about 1898, adapted this type of apparatus to the administration of a mixture of oxygen and ether vapour. This he did by replacing the water in the wash-bottle by liquid ether and substituting a valved facepiece for the mouth-tube.

entirely from the wash-bottle and directly connected with the mask. It has proved difficult ', Morton continued, ' to etherize children or nervous persons with the mixture, and the speaker usually prefers that all cases be etherized by the ordinary methods to the stage of primary anaesthesia before turning on the gas mixture. The latter is then generally sufficient to maintain thorough anaesthesia indefinitely. If otherwise, then a small bunch of gauze is introduced into the mask and additional ether poured upon it. At the termination of anaesthesia, or in a case of collapse or other accident, pure gas is always made use of '.

Morton stated that through the use of this mixture his patients were less cyanosed and secreted less mucus than when ether was used alone, and that respiration remained good throughout anaesthesia, and vomiting tended to be less frequent.'

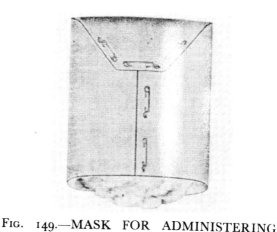

FIG. 149.—MASK FOR ADMINISTERING SCHLEICH'S MIXTURE OF CHLORO-FORM, SULPHURIC ETHER, AND BENZINE In use about 1896. The mask was made by folding a napkin round a sheet of paper and securing it with safety-pins. Into this case was put a handful of sterile cotton wool, on to which the anaesthetic mixture was poured. The mask was then held over the patient's nose and mouth, which had previously been smeared with a protective layer of vaseline.

The anaesthetic mixture proposed by C. L. Schleich in 1895 and 1896 was composed of chloroform, sulphuric ether, and petroleum ether (benzine). When the proportion of the three constituents was : chloroform 45 parts, sulphuric ether 180 parts and benzine 15 parts, Schleich claimed that the mixture boiled at 38° C., i.e. at body temperature. By decreasing the proportion of sulphuric ether to 150 parts, Schleich obtained a second mixture boiling at 40° C. and by further reducing the sulphuric

---

[1] Ann. Surg., 1898, **28**, 272–4.

ether to 80 parts and the chloroform to 30 parts, he obtained a third mixture boiling at 42° C. Schleich claimed that the first of these three mixtures would produce light anaesthesia, the second a medium depth, and the third deep anaesthesia. He argued that as the boiling-point of his mixtures (*i.e.* the point of most rapid evaporation) so nearly coincided with body temperature, elimination of the anaesthetic from the lungs would be sufficiently rapid to avoid overdosage by accumulation of the drug in the body tissues. It would not be so rapid, on the other hand, as to cause over-distension of the air-cells of the lungs with consequent post-anaesthetic chest complications.

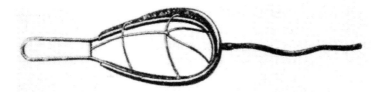

FIG. 150.—ROSTHORN'S OPEN MASK

Designed for chloroform, but used by Wertheim, of Vienna (*c.* 1897), for administering his own version of Schleich's mixture of chloroform, sulphuric ether, and benzine.

To the trough-shaped rim of Rosthorn's mask, intended to catch liquid chloroform, Wertheim added a length of tubing through which, if too large a dose of the anaesthetic mixture were poured on to the gauze cover of the mask, the surplus would flow away.

Schleich recommended administration from a closed cone, made from a towel folded and pinned over a paper lining. The cone was filled with sterile cotton wool on to which the mixture was poured (see Fig. 149). He advised smearing the patient's face with vaseline to protect the skin from the chilling and chafing effects of the anaesthetic-soaked mask.[1]

On the Continent the use of Schleich's mixtures persisted for some years in German-speaking countries, the most important modification of the method being that of the gynaecologist, Wertheim, of the Elisabeth Hospital in Vienna.

In the autumn of 1897 Wertheim proposed the use of a mixture composed of one part each of chloroform and petroleum ether to two parts of sulphuric ether. This most nearly resembled

[1] Schleich, C. L. 1899. *Schmerzlose Operationen.* Berlin. 66 *et seq.*

17*

Schleich's mixture number three.   Wertheim tried administering
the mixture from a Skinner's chloroform mask but found its area
too small.   He then adopted the use of Rosthorn's open chloroform mask (see Fig. 150), inserting into its trough-shaped rim,
at the side opposite to the handle, a length of tubing through
which surplus liquid would flow away should too large a quantity
of the anaesthetic mixture be poured on to the gauze cover of
the mask.[1]

In America Schleich's mixtures aroused much interest during
1898 and 1899.   During 1898 Willy Meyer and a New York
chemist named Weidig found that although in the three variations of the mixture all the chloroform was combined, ' a certain
amount of sulphuric ether is in a free state '.   They therefore
made what they termed a ' molecular solution ' in which, they
claimed, all the constituents were in combination.

M. L. Maduro, introducing a discussion on Schleich's
mixture at a meeting of the College of Physicians of Philadelphia
in April 1898, stated that he himself ' always used the No. 1
mixture to begin with, and rarely found much indication to use
Nos. 2 or 3.   In laparotomies lasting one and a half hours he
had kept his patient completely under with No. 1 '.

Maduro gave the mixture from an open-ended cylinder
made with a towel folded round paper and having a pad of
gauze in the end farther from the face.   The gauze was first
saturated and then kept moist by a steady dropping in of the
mixture through the open end of the cylinder.   The advantages
of the mixture noticed by Maduro were : freedom from the
choking sensation usual with ether, rapidity and comparative
tranquillity of the induction period, reduced mucous secretion
and, in most cases, at any rate short ones, absence of vomiting.[2]

Another American, H. Rodman, writing in the *Medical
Record* in 1898, severely criticized the mixture, however, basing
his criticism on the results of 700 cases.   He agreed that the
mixture was easier to inhale than ether, but so also, he pointed
out, was chloroform.   He found that induction, far from being
rapid, lasted from fifteen to twenty minutes and that the face
was frequently ' burnt ' by the mixture.   He also noticed some
degree of cyanosis in many patients and definite asphyxial

---

[1] Dumont, F. L.   1903. *Handbuch der allgemeinen und lokalen Anaesthesie.* Berlin and
Vienna.   123–4.
[2] *Ann. Surg.,* 1898, **28,** 266–9.

symptoms in six. In one case syncope occurred and in a few others bronchitis supervened upon the administration.[1]

Schleich himself came to the conclusion, during 1898, that the benzine in his mixture was uncertain in its action and caused undesirable symptoms in the patient. He accordingly substituted ethyl chloride and adjusted the three forms of the mixture still to boil at 38° C., 40° C., and 42° C.[2]

In England Dudley Buxton, after testing Schleich's original mixture in its three forms, expressed himself as being doubtful of its worth, but R. J. Probyn-Williams in 1901, and in the following year J. F. W. Silk, reported favourably on the use of Wertheim's mixture and method of administration.[3]

[1] *Med. Rec., N.Y.*, 1898, **54,** 478 ; *Lancet*, 1897, ii, 1671 ; *ibid.*, 1898 ii, 1784 ; *ibid.*, 1899, ii, 1832 ; Buxton, D. W. 1900. *Anaesthetics : their uses and administration.* London. 222–4.
[2] Schleich, C. L. 1899. *Schmerzlose Operationen.* Berlin. 67 *et seq.*
[3] *Trans. Soc. Anaesth.*, 1901, **4,** 98–123 ; *ibid.*, 1903, **5,** 138–45.

CHAPTER XVIII

THE JUBILEE OF ANAESTHESIA

Anaesthetic Education in England, the United States, Scotland, and on the European Continent—The Status of the Anaesthetist in England at the Close of the Nineteenth Century

Anaesthetic Education

IN 1896 the jubilee of ether anaesthesia was celebrated. All over the civilized world medical men met to consider the art and science of anaesthetics in retrospect and in prospect. At meetings of the learned societies in America, in Great Britain, on the Continent, and as far afield as Japan, fresh tribute was paid to W. T. G. Morton's initiative, and stories of anaesthesia in 1846 and of the almost indescribable horrors of surgical operations before that date were retold. In the following year the jubilee of chloroform anaesthesia was marked with similar though less widespread tributes to Simpson's contribution.

The majority of anaesthetists were well content with the half-century's achievement in controlling pain and making possible ' countless advances and developments in surgical science ' ; but the more progressively minded, because they considered the initial benefits bestowed by the universal introduction of inhalation anaesthesia in 1846 to have been so tremendous, found cause for disappointment in the relatively slight progress in anaesthesia made between 1847 and 1896.

' Although the present state of our knowledge leaves much to be desired ', wrote Hewitt in 1896, ' we may, I think, congratulate ourselves upon the advances which have been made during recent years.

' With all these additions to our storehouse of knowledge ', he continued, ' the question may well be asked " Why do not deaths from anaesthetics show signs of diminution ? " '

The answer which he himself gave to this question was one which had already been given not only by other anaesthetists in England but, indeed, by the Americans as well. ' The reply ', said Hewitt, ' is that the responsibilities involved in administering

524

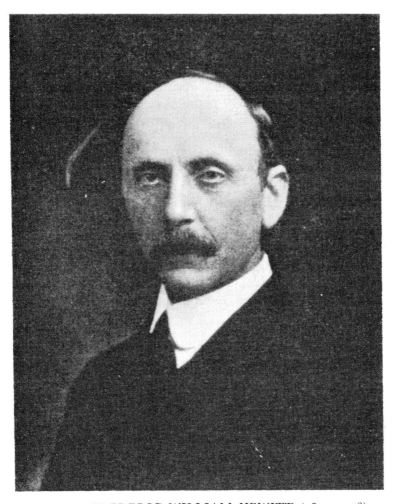

FIG. 151.—FREDERIC WILLIAM HEWITT (1857–1916)

Knighted in 1911. Graduated in medicine at Cambridge in 1883, decided to specialize in anaesthesia and was elected anaesthetist to the Charing Cross Hospital in 1884, to the Royal Dental Hospital in 1885, and to the London Hospital in 1886. Did much to raise the general level of efficiency in anaesthetic practice and to improve the teaching given to the student, and the status of the qualified anaesthetist.

anaesthetics are not yet fully realised ; that the administration is too often placed in the hands of comparatively unskilled men. . . . The first step should be an educational one. By sending out into practice men who have a proper appreciation of the responsibilities and requirements in anaesthetising, an improved position of the subject, and a notable saving of human life will inevitably result.' [1]

This point of view had first been strongly advanced by J. F. W. Silk in March 1892. Silk at that time was assistant anaesthetist to Guy's Hospital and anaesthetist to the Dental School and to the Royal Free Hospital. In a paper read before the Thames Valley Branch of the British Medical Association, entitled *Anaesthetics a necessary part of the curriculum : a plea for more systematic teaching*, he said :

' I propose . . . to discuss very briefly—(A) the nature and character of the instruction in anaesthetics at present offered to the student ; (B) some reasons for thinking this instruction should be improved upon ; (C) a brief indication of the direction in which it is both possible and desirable to make this improvement.'

With regard to (A) Silk stated :

' It may, I think, be assumed at the outset that at every medical school in the United Kingdom where lectures on surgery are delivered, some allusion is made in the course of those lectures to the subject of anaesthetics. I think, too, that it may be assumed that at every hospital attended by students the respective surgeons occasionally direct attention clinically to their administration. But this can hardly be called "systematic teaching ". With these general exceptions it does not appear, if one may judge from the prospectuses issued by the respective medical schools, that any special instruction in anaesthetics is afforded in Scotland, Ireland, or the provinces. In some instances, it is true, anaesthetists are attached to the several hospitals, but it would seem that their duties are, if I may use the term, functional rather than academic—limited, that is, to the mere administration, and not concerned with the teaching. In the metropolitan schools things are a little better ; in London there are, including the Women's School, twelve medical schools, and these twelve schools are responsible for the education of between 40 and 50 per cent. of all the students registered at the Medical Council. To eleven out of these twelve schools special anaesthetists are attached ; at the twelfth an " administrator of

[1] *Practitioner*, 1896, **57**, 347–56.

anaesthetics " is included among the appointments open to the student immediately after he has become qualified ; and at one school, in addition to the anaesthetist to the hospital there are two junior appointments open to students, the holders of which are qualified and resident in the hospital. In nine out of these eleven schools it is definitely stated in the prospectuses that instruction in anaesthetics is given ; but the actual amount of instruction afforded varies considerably, and, of course, it is almost as impossible as it would be invidious to estimate the exact value of the instruction given in the several instances. In some few schools, for example, lectures and demonstrations are given ; in some the teaching appears to be limited to instruction simply, and this, of course, may mean almost anything. At some schools, too, the teaching is not included in the general course of study, but an extra fee is charged, and at some a certificate of instruction is required before the student can hold any or certain of the resident appointments. However, assuming that the instruction given at these nine hospitals is the best and most systematic possible, and that all the students attached to the respective hospitals sought for and obtained it, that would, after all, represent but 76 per cent. of the London students alone. As a matter of fact, however, at six of the largest of these nine hospitals an average of about 51 per cent. attend the classes and lectures. Assuming, then, that a similar percentage of students attend at the remaining three schools, which I very much doubt, this means that of all the London students only 35 per cent. are instructed in any special manner. This percentage . . . applies merely to the London schools, and it would be reduced to under 18 per cent. if we took into account the students of Scotland, Ireland, and the provinces ; and a still greater reduction would be required if we were to attempt to estimate the quality as well as the quantity of the instruction given ; but the figures as they stand are quite sufficient for my present purpose. It results almost as a necessary corollary from this that many students must obtain almost their first experience in administering anaesthetics after they have qualified, and after they have gone beyond the reach of supervision and instruction.'

The main argument adduced by Silk under (B) was as follows :

' Generally speaking, the art of surgery may be said to have improved precisely in proportion to the certainty with which we can foretell results ; the possibility, however remote, of the death or subsequent illness of a patient as the direct result of the anaesthetic introduces an element of doubt which I think we ought to attempt to remove, and I think that if we taught anaesthetics more systematically, not only would the standard of average skill in administering them be raised, but we should soon get to know more about the subject.'

Silk outlined under (C) a plan of campaign for bringing about such an improvement in anaesthetic education :

' In the first place, candidates for the various degrees and diplomas should be required to produce evidence of proper instruction in the subject ; this might well take the form of a certificate of having attended a definite course of lectures and demonstrations, and of having personally administered in a certain number of cases. This is, I think, the least that can be done by the examining bodies. In the second place, I think that at the hospitals the system of teaching anaesthetics should be the same as that adopted in respect to medicine, surgery, and other branches—that is, that after attending the classes the student should be appointed " clerk to the anaesthetist ", when, under the direct supervision and guidance of his teacher, he should administer to the necessary number of cases, and should keep whatever notes and records it may be thought advisable. Finally, in the large hospitals especially, it would be of advantage to appoint resident anaesthetists to take charge of the administrations in the absence of the honorary officer. Some such plan as this would, I think, do much to place the teaching of anaesthetics upon a proper basis, and that, too, without dislocating existing arrangements, and, if generally adopted, I feel sure that good results would follow.' [1]

An equally strong plea ' for better instruction in the administration of anaesthetics ' was made in the jubilee year, 1896, by Marmaduke Shield, then assistant surgeon at St. George's Hospital.

' Much of what I may term, without offence, the neglect of the teaching of anaesthetics in our schools ', wrote Shield, ' is due to the manner in which the subject is sometimes looked at from the operator's point of view. The extraordinary opinion " that a good deal too much is made of anaesthetics " is still expressed by some surgeons who ought to know better ; and even in these modern days the aid of a nurse or the surgery porter is sometimes thought ample and sufficient ! It is this spirit and education of this kind that produce the haphazard methods of practice which are so often experienced, or which, on the contrary, produce such dislike of the responsibility of giving anaesthetics, that medical men refuse to administer them at all.

[1] *Lancet*, 1892, i, 1178–80.

'It will not be out of place to mention here one's actual experience of the administration of anaesthetics as too often conducted in private practice in remote districts. The patient, in a state of much nervous terror, has had a full meal, probably also some alcohol ! The administration of chloroform is commenced, without undoing the corset in a woman, and without examining the mouth for foreign bodies or " false teeth ". A transient application of the stethoscope suffices to assure the patient that the " heart is all right ". The operator notices with quiet dismay that the administrator has no gag at hand in case of spasmodic closure of the jaws, no forceps to pull forward the tongue, while that universal accompaniment of all anaesthetic apparatus, a tracheotomy-tube, is conspicuous by its absence. We all know that by a mixture of good fortune and careful supervision on the part of the operator such cases commonly do well. On the other hand, disaster is simply courted, and the patient may be rescued from the jaws of death by prolonged artificial respiration. A piece of vomited meat may be hooked out of the larynx "just in time", and other exciting adventures may occur, which are most embarrassing and condemnable, especially to an operator whose hands are already full. We hear of the deaths from anaesthetics ; we do not hear of the " narrow escapes " ! These are probably sufficiently numerous and, I need hardly say, should be avoided altogether. . . .

'It is perhaps singular that the public take a more accurate view of the matter than many medical men. In my own experience it is not so much an operation that the patients fear, as the anaesthetic. As a profession, it is our bounden duty to lessen this apprehension ; and I have said enough to prove that there is a strong and pressing case for the education of all medical men in the theory and practice of the administration of anaesthetics.'

Shield's description of the facilities then existing in London whereby the medical student could gain at least some knowledge of anaesthesia was very similar to Silk's. Shield also stressed the fact that the majority of students did not take advantage even of these few facilities.

'Indeed,' wrote Shield, ' we are forced to the old inevitable conclusion : that unless the subject of instruction in the administration of anaesthetics is made compulsory, and the examination spectre haunts the rest of student and teacher, regular education in this most important practical duty will be relegated to the limbo of obscurity. It is a somewhat humiliating statement to make, but I know it is a true one, that students work for examinations and examinations alone. . . . Considering that the vast bulk of the candidates pass into general practice, they will not commonly be called upon to remove stones from the cystic duct, or to pronounce a definite opinion upon a complicated scrotal tumour ! It is manifest, however, that such ordinary routine duties as the administration of anaesthetics will . . . certainly fall to their lot ; and it seems to me, speaking with all diffidence, that the tendency to examine in difficult and obscure subjects to the neglect of common and ordinary ones, is a serious defect in modern medical education. . . .

' It would be too much to expect that every medical man could be rendered a highly-skilled anaesthetist. He should, however, be able and competent to select an appropriate anaesthetic for any given case of operation, and he should be competent to administer the common agents with confidence and celerity. Especially should he be prepared with a good knowledge of such preliminary measures as are essential to the safety of the patient—emptying the stomach of food, removal of thoracic constrictions by tight clothing, inspection of the mouth for artificial dentures, and the like. The remedial measures to be employed in cases of sudden symptoms of danger should be clearly understood, and the administrator should be prepared with the requisite apparatus. . . .

' There can be no doubt that this subject should at once receive the earnest attention of the General Medical Council. . . . In concluding this article, I am expressing the feelings of many by a sincere wish that Mr. Teale [1] or some other enlightened and influential member of the General Medical Council will seriously consider the advisability of the adoption of compulsory education in the subject of anaesthetics. This must not be an addition to the curriculum. It should rather be looked upon as the proper carrying-out of an important part of it. Besides attendance upon a certain number of lectures and demonstrations, it should be compulsory for every medical man before qualification to produce evidence that he has administered anaesthetics to a given number of cases under the supervision of a skilled person.' [2]

Shield's plea for the compulsory training and examination of students in anaesthesia was echoed by the *Lancet* in a leader on October 17, 1896 ; [3] but nobody seemed prepared directly to approach the General Medical Council and try to force a decision.

---

[1] Pridgin Teale had recently criticized the existing system of medical education as a whole.

[2] *Practitioner*, 1896, **57**, 387–93.

[3] *Lancet*, 1896, ii, 1093.

Exactly three years later, in October 1899, H. Bellamy Gardner, anaesthetist to Charing Cross Hospital, reopened the subject in an annotation in the *Medical Times and Hospital Gazette*.[1] After quoting some of Shield's most pertinent statements made in the *Practitioner* for October 1896 Gardner wrote :

' Since Mr. Shield's article, no action has been taken by the examining bodies, and the same condition of incompetence exists among newly-qualified men ; yet the very first duty— when such an one becomes assistant to a doctor in a private practice—is to give the anaesthetic ; to take the patient's life in his hands while the senior performs, perhaps, some minor operation attended with no danger to health or existence. The worst of this is not yet disclosed, for he probably picks up a bottle of chloroform and a towel—being prepared with neither tongue-forceps nor mouth-gag for use in emergency—and administers the most powerful and most lethal of all the narcotic vapours, because he has neglected to learn and practise the use of nitrous oxide gas or ether, and is utterly at sea when the necessary apparatus are placed in his hands.

' Surely the possibility of letting such practitioners experiment in anaesthetics is now thirty or forty years behind the requirements of the year of grace 1899.

' The lecturers and anaesthetists on the staffs of the London Hospitals are doing their utmost at the present time to convince their colleagues of the vital necessity of making tuition in anaesthetics a compulsory part of the students' curriculum. Under existing rules, however, the most that has been done is to render the absence of such instruction a bar to the holding of resident house appointments ; but it is to be hoped that this move will gradually open the eyes of the Councils of the Colleges and Universities to the need for early action in the matter.' [2]

From 1847 onwards the English alone had persisted in asserting that anaesthesia was a task for the expert and that his knowledge and his skill were far more important factors in successful anaesthesia than the drug and the method of administration which he chose to employ. For this reason the medical student in England had been given little opportunity to try his hand at administration. Although it was only in England

[1] *Med. Times*, Lond., 1899, 663.
[2] It was not until 1911, however, that the General Medical Council was able to state that every such body in Great Britain included evidence of instruction in anaesthetics among its requirements from candidates for the qualifying examination. (*Brit. J. Anaesth.*, 1926–7, **4**, 117.)

that the profession of anaesthetist was generally recognized, specialization in anaesthesia almost invariably took place some years after qualification.[1] More often than not an anaesthetic practice was combined with general practice, as in Clover's case, or with dental surgery, as in Alfred Coleman's case. Even in the hospitals it was usual for the post of anaesthetist to be held by a man who was also in general practice privately.

It was not the potential specialist anaesthetist who occasioned the outcry for better education but the potential general practitioner who would not specialize and yet who, from the very nature of his profession, could scarcely avoid giving an occasional anaesthetic. It was at last recognized, during the eighteen-nineties, that the only way to make such a man into a reasonably efficient anaesthetist was to inculcate upon his mind during his student days the essentials of anaesthetic theory and practice.

Because anaesthetic development in England had always been largely in the hands of specialists, who for half a century had been constantly experimenting clinically and in the laboratory, inhalation anaesthesia in this country at the close of the nineteenth century was both intricate and highly organized. Different drugs and methods of procedure, often entailing the use of complicated apparatus, were considered appropriate according to the nature of the operation and the condition of the patient. The need for the specialist anaesthetist was indeed greater than ever before ; but although the demand outstripped the supply an acute shortage was not anticipated. There was, however, evident cause for anxiety in the low average degree of skill shown by the non-specialist practitioner when forced to act as an anaesthetist. It was considered desirable that he should reach at least a reasonable standard of proficiency in the simpler routine anaesthetic procedures, be able to satisfy a surgeon or dentist performing a minor operation, and himself be prepared adequately to deal with an anaesthetic emergency. Moreover, and this was particularly stressed, he ought to possess sufficient knowledge to recognize his own limitations in the field of anaesthesia.

---

[1] In the case of Clover, who suffered from general ill-health, and Hewitt, whose eyesight was very poor, the career of anaesthetist was adopted because it promised to be less arduous than the originally-chosen careers of surgeon and physician respectively.

In America also the prevailing standard of anaesthetic administration began to cause concern about 1894. In England the aim was to give a basic education in anaesthesia to every medical student before qualification because his profession made him potentially an occasional anaesthetist, whether he was interested in the subject or not. He was left free to specialize in anaesthesia after qualification if he chose. In the United States, although a certain proportion of the surgical profession had always been interested in the science of anaesthesia, the actual administration of an anaesthetic had hitherto never been considered sufficiently important to need an expert. It had indeed been entrusted to students or to junior house officers who, in preparation for this task, received only the barest of empirical instruction. Now, however, the aim was to create a class of professional specialist anaesthetists.

The New York *Medical Record* took an active interest in promoting this idea. A leading article appeared in this journal in 1894 entitled ' A plea for public anaesthetizers ' :

' To an observant spectator of operations in our hospitals it is a matter for surprise and wonder that fatal accidents so rarely result during the administration of anaesthetics. No stronger argument could be furnished to the advocate of the use of ether in preference to chloroform than the fact that the former is recklessly administered in hundreds of instances by inexperienced anaesthetizers, yet without any immediate ill consequences. We use the word " immediate " advisedly because we are convinced that not a few of the fatal cases of acute pulmonary and renal troubles which have followed ether-anaesthesia, might have been avoided, not by substituting chloroform but by administering ether in a proper manner, instead of saturating the patient with it. Strange as it would appear to the intelligent layman, hospital surgeons continue to delegate this important duty to junior assistants, dressers, and medical students, even in the most serious operations, in which the constant and skilful surveillance of the patient is a matter of vital consequence. . . .

' We are not exaggerating when we affirm that the average junior interne does not take the trouble to make a scientific study of the variation in the pulse and respiration ratio, the changes in the pupils and muscular reflexes, &c., in a perfectly healthy subject, while the danger signals in the case of weak patients are often unheeded, or are not recognized until the close of a long operation, when the patient is in actual collapse. . . .

' The entire responsibility of watching the patient devolves upon a young fellow, fresh from the medical school, whose knowledge is almost entirely theoretical, however great may be his aptitude and powers of observation. The rest of the house-staff are expected to devote their attention entirely to the operation, and it must be admitted that the junior's mind is too often absorbed in its details. . . .

' We are far from asserting that the young gentlemen . . . do not in many instances become expert anaesthetizers, but this requires time, so that as a rule, they have only become really proficient when they are replaced by green men. If this criticism applies to the giving of ether, how much more forcibly does it apply to the administration of chloroform ! Doubtless this valuable anaesthetic would be employed much more frequently than it is at present [1] if surgeons had sufficient confidence in the skill and experience of the anaesthetizer. . . .

' Now this state of things ought not to be allowed to continue. We believe that the time will come when every large hospital will have a regular salaried anaesthetizer who will always be available and who will enjoy the same confidence in his department as the pathologist does in his own. Operations will certainly proceed more smoothly and safely ; we shall hear of fewer deaths from " heart failure " ; and cases of " ether pneumonia " and of " acute uraemia from ether " will be almost unknown. The advantage to the operator will be immense. Instead of having his mind distracted by the struggles of a half-anaesthetized patient . . . he will be able to give his entire attention to the operation, relying on the anaesthetizer to note the danger signals, to administer stimulants when they are needed, and to keep him informed as to when he must hasten or when he can proceed deliberately. . . .' [2]

In the closing paragraph of the same article the *Medical Record* severely censured also the practice common in some American hospitals of allowing a nurse to induce anaesthesia.

Three years elapsed before the *Medical Record* (in 1897) followed up this first article with a second entitled ' The professional anaesthetizer '.

' So far as we are informed in the matter, there exists in this city [New York] no physician who makes a specialty of administering anaesthetics. There would seem, however, to exist a demand in this direction. Surgeons are constantly at a loss to find at short notice men of experience in ether and chloroform administration, no less than in other forms of general and local

---

[1] Some American surgeons held that ether was contra-indicated in patients with pulmonary or renal disturbance and instead used chloroform. (Cf. *Med. Rec., N.Y.,* 1895, **47**, 720 ; see also p. 419.)

[2] *Med. Rec., N.Y.,* 1894, **46**, 239.

anaesthesia, upon whom they can call for assistance in their important operations. . . . Large surgical hospitals might at times with advantage avail themselves of the services of such a professional anaesthetizer. . . .

' The probable explanation for the fact that this important field remains uncultivated . . . is to be sought in the unwillingness of young men to enter upon a career which would seem at first glance to offer so little for the future, whatever the emoluments of the present might be. This objection is, however, more imaginary than real. . . . Who will be the first to engage in this new specialty ? ' [1]

The first American so to engage himself seems to have been Dr. W. Oakley Hermance who, in 1897, was ' appointed instructor in the administration of anaesthetics in the Philadelphia Polyclinic and anaesthetizer in the Polyclinic Hospital '. Commenting on this appointment the *Medical Record* remarked : ' The faculty and trustees recognize the growing sentiment among the profession that the administration of an anaesthetic should be trusted to skilled hands only, and in providing for the proper instruction of the incoming residents of the hospital, they at the same time afford an opportunity to the pupils of the College to gain similar knowledge and experience '.[2]

Soon after the launching of this new career of ' anaesthetizer ', America entered with a will into the field of anaesthetic development. The large contribution which she has made to anaesthesia during the present century is entirely distinct in character from that which she made during the preceding fifty years.

Throughout the earlier period her role was a curious one. She acted both as an occasional innovator of vital importance and as a constant champion of primitive (although not ineffectual) anaesthetic methods. In 1846 the use of ether anaesthesia was established in America and from her shores it spread over the whole world. In 1862 and 1863 the American, Colton, revived the use of nitrous oxide and Colton and his fellow-countryman, Evans, were directly responsible for establishing it abroad (see Chapter X). In 1872 another American, B. J. Jeffries, brought about the revival of the use of ether in England (see Chapter XI), and yet another, H. C. Wood, was instrumental in furthering a similar revival in Germany during the eighteen-nineties (see p. 412).

[1] *Med. Rec.*, *N.Y.*, 1897, **51**, 522.   [2] *Ibid.*, **51**, 574.

Early in 1847 it was decided at Boston that an eminently practical way of giving ether was from a conical sponge ; soon afterwards the sponge was enclosed in a cone made from a folded towel, and for the next fifty years the majority of Americans saw no need for improving upon this method (cf. p. 125, footnote, p. 313). When nitrous oxide was reintroduced into practice by Colton the apparatus adopted for administering it was little more than an improved version of an apparatus used once by Bigelow in 1848 (see pp. 274–6).

Akin to the American attitude towards the administration of anaesthetics was the Scottish or, more precisely, the Edinburgh attitude.

The technique used at Edinburgh and, under Lister, at Glasgow was both simple and stereotyped and, except in comparatively minor details, remained constant during the half century 1847 to 1897. It consisted in pouring an estimated, but not measured, quantity of chloroform either on to a pad or on to a single layer of some woven material (the kind of material and the proportions of the evaporating surface were variable) and quickly applying it over the patient's nose and mouth, but not so as to exclude atmospheric air, until anaesthesia was established. Thereafter the material was replenished with chloroform and reapplied as the occasion demanded. Because the technique was both simple and stereotyped it was considered that, in hospital practice, administration could safely be entrusted to a medical student or junior house officer.

Joseph Lister (see also pp. 28–30, 191–2) contributed the article on anaesthesia to each of the first three editions of Holmes's *System of surgery* (London. 1861, 1870, and 1882). As a general survey of contemporary British anaesthetic practice these articles were somewhat limited in scope ; what they did furnish, however, was a clear picture of Scottish anaesthetic practice and they showed how slight were the changes in method made during the twenty years under review.

In 1861 Lister gave ' a short account of what ordinarily occurs in the mode of administration with which I am most familiar ' (see p. 247). By this method chloroform, sufficient to moisten a surface ' as large as the palm of the hand ', was poured upon a towel folded in six to form a square, which was then held over the patient's face, more chloroform being added when necessary.

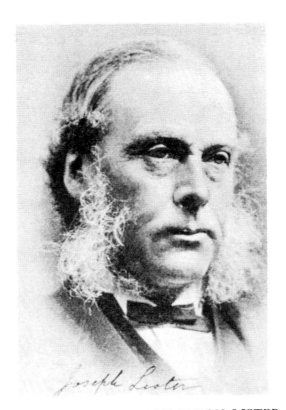

FIG. 152.—JOSEPH, FIRST BARON LISTER,
OF LYME REGIS (1827-1912)

Surgeon and founder of the antiseptic method in surgery.
Went to Edinburgh from University College, London, to
study under James Syme, in 1853. Became Professor of
Surgery at Glasgow in 1860 ; Professor of Clinical Surgery
at Edinburgh, 1869–77 ; Professor of Surgery at King's
College, London, 1877–92. In anaesthesia Lister was guided
by Syme's teaching that the effect of chloroform upon the
respiration was a more important factor than its effect upon
the heart. He himself taught that the services of a professional anaesthetist were unnecessary if a simple routine
was followed during administration.

Referring to anaesthetic administration in general Lister wrote in this article :

'The very prevalent opinion that the pulse is the most important symptom in the administration of chloroform is certainly a most serious mistake. As a general rule, the safety of the patient will be most promoted by disregarding it altogether, so that the attention may be devoted exclusively to the breathing. The chance of the existence of heart disease may seem to make this practice dangerous, but having followed it myself . . . for the last eight years, and knowing that it has been pursued all along by Mr. Syme, . . . I feel no hesitation in recommending it. . . .

'From these considerations it appears that preliminary examination of the chest, often considered indispensable, is quite unnecessary, and more likely to induce the dreaded syncope, by alarming the patients, than to avert it.'

Since 1853 the importance of drawing forward the tongue should the least sign of impending danger to the patient appear (see Appendix C, p. 570) had always been stressed at Edinburgh. In this connection Lister wrote :

'I am anxious to direct particular attention to the drawing out of the tongue because I am satisfied that several lives have been sacrificed for want of it. In order that it may be effectual, firm traction is essential. . . . Whether pulling the tongue operates by inducing or relaxing muscular contraction in the larynx may be a matter for discussion, but the main conclusion, that it does not act merely *mechanically*, but through the nervous system, appears satisfactorily established.' [1]

In his next article for the *System of surgery* (2nd ed., 1870) Lister stated :

'The nine years which have passed since the above article was written have tended to confirm its main doctrines. . . . I believe I am correct in stating that no case of death from chloroform has occurred during these nine years in the operating theatre of either the Edinburgh or the Glasgow Infirmary, two of the largest surgical hospitals in Great Britain. Yet in both these institutions a folded towel on which the anaesthetic liquid is poured, unmeasured and unstinted, is still the only apparatus employed in the administration ; preliminary examination of the heart is never thought of, and during the inhalation the pulse is entirely disregarded ; but vigilant attention is kept upon the

[1] Lister, Joseph, Baron. 1909. *The collected papers of Joseph, Baron Lister.* Oxford, I, 135–49.

respiration, and, in case of its obstruction, firm traction upon the tongue is promptly resorted to. And it is worthy of special notice,' Lister continued, ' that success is due to soundness of the principles acted on, rather than any particular skill, that the giving of chloroform, instead of being restricted to a medical man appointed for the function, as is elsewhere often thought essential, is entrusted to the junior officers of the hospital. In Edinburgh each of the five surgeons has two " clerks ", intermediate in position between the house surgeon and the dressers. They, besides other duties, take it in turn to administer the anaesthetic ; and if I had to be placed under its influence I would rather trust myself to one of these young gentlemen than to the great majority of " qualified practitioners ".

' The appointment of a special chloroform-giver to a hospital is not only entirely unnecessary, but has the great disadvantage of investing the administration of chloroform with an air of needless mystery, and withholding from the students the opportunity of being trained in an important duty, which any one of them may be called upon to discharge on commencing practice, and which, though certainly simple, is better performed after some practical initiation.' [1]

When Lister made his third contribution to Holmes's *System of surgery*, in 1882 the report of the British Medical Association's Glasgow Committee on anaesthetics, published in 1880 (see p. 426 *et seq.*), was fresh in his mind.

' These researches,' he wrote, ' by placing before the profession in an exaggerated form the effects of chloroform as a cardiac sedative, have tended to foster the idea that if chloroform kills, it always does so from the heart, and that the pulse is the main thing to be attended to in its administration.

' Against this pernicious error I have endeavoured in the earlier parts of this article [*i.e.* in 1861 and 1870] to raise an emphatic protest. I have pointed out how liable the breathing is to become obstructed under chloroform. . . . I have contended that if the breathing is carefully observed, and the obstructions referred to [the falling back of the relaxed tongue, and closure of ' the valve of mucous membrane which guards the orifice of the larynx '] are removed as soon as they occur, due care being taken to avoid pushing the agent beyond what is needful to produce its anaesthetic and relaxing effects, the chloroform being given well mixed with air by means of a folded towel held loosely over the face, all fear of primary failure of the heart may be dismissed from the mind.

[1] Lister, Joseph, Baron. 1909. *The collected papers of Joseph, Baron Lister.* Oxford. I, 149–50.

'The experience of the last twelve years', he continued, 'has confirmed me in the success of this doctrine. . . . In my hospital cases I have still entrusted the administration of the chloroform . . . to a succession of senior students, changing from month to month, whose only qualification for the duty is that they must previously have served the office of dresser, and that they strictly carry out certain simple instructions, among which is that of never touching the pulse, in order that their attention may not be distracted from the respiration.'

Lister also discussed chloroform administration with Junker's inhaler (see pp. 265–6), which he thought acted ' admirably in experienced hands ', but was apt to get out of order, and by the open-drop method with Skinner's mask (see pp. 247–8). The latter, Lister thought, was too large, and ' the closely fitting bag ' seemed to him ' liable to the danger of giving the chloroform too strong, especially when the breathing is shallow '. On this account Lister

' made trials with a piece of flannel stretched over . . . [a] small frame, but having an interval of about half an inch between its border and the skin of the face ; and I found that a piece with an area of nine square inches . . . kept constantly moist with chloroform . . . answered the purpose well if a piece of rag was thrown lightly round the interval between the flannel and the skin, so as to check, but not altogether prevent, the flowing away of the heavy vapour of the chloroform. . . . As there was no special virtue in flannel, as compared with a single layer of linen of coarse texture, I substituted for the frame and flannel the corner of a towel, pursed up systematically into a concave mask to cover the mouth and nose by pinching it together [1] at such a distance from the corner that, when the pinched-up part is held over the root of the nose, the corner extends freely to the point of the chin.

' The cap formed in this manner being so arranged upon the face, chloroform is gradually dropped upon it till the greater part of it is soaked, the edges being left dry to avoid irritation of the skin by the liquid ; and the moist condition is maintained by frequent dropping until the requisite physiological effects are produced. . . . When the cap is made as above directed, . . . the part which is moistened during the production of anaesthesia has an area of about nine square inches (that of a circle three and a half inches in diameter) in the case of the adult male. But the apparatus is self-adjusting in so far that the cap varies

---

[1] Soon after this Lister hit upon the more expedient method of drawing the corner of the towel through a large, closed safety-pin.

in dimensions with the face, which again, is more or less proportionate to the size of the body. . . . It is further self-regulating in this respect, that when the breathing is shallow . . . the percentage of chloroform is not correspondingly increased, because a smaller amount evaporates . . . than when the air is moved freely over the cloth in deep inspiration ; and further, when the vapour is not drawn into the chest, its density causes it to flow away under the loose margins of the cap, instead of accumulating as it would do under a closely fitting bag. . . .

' This method is a little more troublesome than our old plan ; . . . but the constant attention which it necessitates is an additional element of safety. During the last five months I have proceeded on these principles, and have been much pleased with the results. . . .

' If chloroform carefully given in the simple manner above recommended ', Lister concluded, ' is really as safe a means of producing prolonged anaesthesia as we possess, a conviction that such is the case will be a great relief to the majority of our practitioners throughout the country ; all special apparatus being avoided, and selection of cases needless. . . .' [1]

In Scotland the majority of practitioners were convinced of the rightness of Lister's contention and ten years later a modified version of Syme's teaching was still the method exclusively employed at Edinburgh.

A brief account of the current procedure at Edinburgh was given in 1892 by Laurence Turnbull, a visitor to Great Britain from Philadelphia :

' Prior to all operations in the Royal Infirmary, the heart, lungs, and kidneys are examined. In the morning before the operation, nothing is given to the patient but a cup of beef-tea. If there has been constipation, a purge is given the evening before. The chloroform is administered on a towel by a senior student, who has been under instruction for six weeks.'

Turnbull then tabulated the directions which the students were expected to memorize :

' *Action of Chloroform*

' Is (1) stimulant ; (2) sedative.

(a) Abolishes sensation.
(b) Abolishes power of motion and reflex action.
(c) Stops heart's action.
(d) Kills patient.

[1] Lister, Joseph, Baron. 1909. *The collected papers of Joseph, Baron Lister.* Oxford. **1**, 155–75.

' *Methods of Administration*

' Towel *versus* engine.   Brains *versus* valves.

(1) Give all your attention.
(2) Have your artery forceps ready [for pulling forward the tongue].
(3) Watch the breathing.
(4) Watch the patient's appearance.

' *How do you know when the Patient has had enough ?*

(*a*) Insensibility of conjunctiva.
(*b*) Muscular relaxation.
(*c*) Local insensibility of part to be operated upon.

' *How do you know when the Patient has had too much ?*

(*a*) Tongue falling back.
(*b*) Glottis closing.
(*c*) Fainting.
(*d*) Vomiting.
(*e*) Respiration and heart's action stopped.' [1]

Although Scottish and American anaesthetic practice had in common the custom of entrusting administration to students, there was a marked difference in the working of this system in the two countries.   This was largely due to the fact that in Scotland chloroform was invariably used in surgery while in America ether was used.

The Scots maintained that so long as certain clearly defined rules were observed chloroform anaesthesia was absolutely safe. Accordingly they strictly drilled each student in the application of those rules before he was allowed to undertake administration. Within these narrow limits the result was an efficient anaesthetist and for this reason the Scots remained satisfied with their system.

The Americans, on the other hand, maintained that ether anaesthesia was reasonably safe in any hands, so that it was unnecessary to rehearse the student once he had been shown his part ;   more often than not the result was an inexpert anaesthetist.

On the Continent of Europe the routine of administering an anaesthetic resembled American or Scottish, never English, methods ;   that is to say administration was entrusted to a medical student or to a house surgeon to whom adequate pre-

[1] *Brit. med. J.*, 1892, ii, 936.

liminary instruction might or might not have been given. The professional anaesthetist did not exist anywhere on the Continent, although some Continental surgeons deeply interested themselves in anaesthesia.

In France conditions most nearly approached the Scottish. A surgical assistant of subordinate rank was thoroughly drilled in an inflexible routine, and once he had mastered his duties he continued to act as administrator until it became necessary, for any reason, to replace him by another similarly trained assistant (cf. pp. 16–17, 207).

J. A. F. Dastre, Professor of Physiology at the Sorbonne, writing in 1890 stated :

' Abroad, surgeons, particularly those who use ether, willingly employ special inhalers : Clover's [portable] inhaler (*masque de Clover*), Junker's and Ormsby's apparatuses. In France the various methods all consist in pouring chloroform on to a compress which is placed in front of the patient's mouth and nostrils, in such a way as to make him breathe air mixed with the anaesthetic vapour. The compress is covered over on one side by a waxed cloth which prevents the surgeon from inhaling as much chloroform as the patient ; the size of the compress varies ; its approximation to the respiratory orifices also varies ; so does the quantity of chloroform poured on, according to the needs of the operation, the patient's condition and the customary procedure of whoever is administering the anaesthetic agent.[1]

' For some years past, surgeons have tended to relieve themselves of the anxious business of personally superintending the administration of chloroform : they leave this task to an assistant, always the same one, who through constant practice, finally acquires a considerable degree of reliability. Thus, and not unprofitably, a new function has been created, that of chloroformist (*médecin chloroformiseur*), lieutenant *ad latus* to the surgeons in the large towns.'[2]

As this system was proving reasonably efficient there was no great outcry for reform in anaesthetic education in France at the close of the nineteenth century.

[1] Dastre stated : ' Among these methods there are two which merit mention : 1. Procedure by *massive doses*, or the procedure by *sideration* ; 2. the dosimetric, or *drop* method '. He further distinguished between the strong initial dose, *dose anesthésique*, for establishing anaesthesia and the weaker dose, *dose d'entretien*, for maintaining anaesthesia. (Dastre, A. 1890. *Les anesthésiques, physiologie et applications chirurgicales*. Paris. 103.)

[2] Dastre, A. 1890. *Les anesthésiques, physiologie et applications chirurgicales*. Paris. 10:.

Theodor Billroth, Professor of Surgery at Vienna, in describing anaesthetic procedure in his own practice in 1872 showed an attitude of mind which was typical of many Continental surgeons. Once he had instituted what he considered to be reasonable precautions to protect the patient from the most obvious dangers of anaesthesia the subject ceased to have any further interest for him ; the routine which he followed, however, was, within its limitations, a sound one and not unlike the Scottish.

' Unfortunately ', wrote Billroth, ' in 1870, I was upset by having another chloroform death, the second in my practice. The deep impression which these two cases made upon me, moved me thereafter to try mixtures of chloroform, ether and alcohol, although I was very little convinced of their complete safety and in spite of the fact that I had formerly spoken against the use of such mixtures. I now allow anaesthesia to be produced with a mixture of 3 parts of chloroform, 1 part of ether and 1 part of absolute alcohol. The only advantage which I see in this method is that it is not possible for too much chloroform to be inhaled at one time ; the other ingredients serve, as I see it, merely as diluents of the chloroform. It is unavoidable that in a hospital such as this in Vienna, among 8 dressers (Assistenten) and 2 house surgeons (Assistenzärzten) a turn must be taken in the quite uninteresting business of chloroforming. Whoever gives the chloroform often sees little or nothing of the operation ; I cannot very well condemn one of my dressers to this post for a whole semester. If, however, a rota of duty is established, so that each dresser anaesthetises for a month in turn, then by changing thus often I can rely with absolute certainty upon whoever anaesthetises. It is, on this account, expedient for chloroform to be administered in such a diluted state that it cannot easily become dangerous even if, on any occasion, it should be shaken on in too great a quantity at once.' [1]

In Germany until the eighteen-nineties, although as elsewhere certain surgeons devoted time and thought to anaesthetic problems, the general attitude towards anaesthesia was one of apathy, so that administration was entrusted to students and junior house officers, many of whom came to the task without having been prepared by even the most rudimentary instruction. Furthermore, so far as practice in the hospitals was concerned, no responsibility was attached to the surgeons either for the conduct of administration or for the results of anaesthesia (cf. p. 546).

[1] Billroth, T. 1872. *Chirurgische Klinik, Wien, 1869-70.* Berlin. 35.

During the eighteen-nineties, however, an increasing number of German surgeons, realizing that the administration of an anaesthetic, even in minor surgery, called for a greater skill and judgment than a student or house surgeon without special training could be expected to show, began to agitate for a reform in medical education.

One of the first in Germany to stress the need for a recognized course of training in anaesthesia was Jean Borntraeger who, in a thesis on the legal responsibility of the medical man in using chloroform and other inhalation anaesthetics, looked forward to a time when adequate opportunities for study would be available and when, in the surgical part of the state medical examination, the candidate would be expected to carry out an administration in all its details.[1]

Soon afterwards C. L. Schleich (see also pp. 42–3, 520–1) emphatically expressed his belief in the need for educating the medical student in anaesthesia.

' Each year hundreds of medical men qualify and can practise anywhere in Germany, but how small a proportion of them has ever received a single word of instruction in chloroforming, at the university, and how very small a proportion has ever handled an anaesthetic apparatus before qualifying. Thus all of them, for want of having received individual instruction, must complete their studies after graduation upon suffering humanity. At whose expense ? ! So it comes about that the danger of anaesthesia, through lack of systematic teaching, is considerably increased. For even in the big hospitals members of the staff who are scarcely more than learners, administer anaesthesia— novices, whom nobody directs, nobody systematically controls, nobody instructs ; novices so young that they must meekly accept the possibly impatient, irritable, fault finding of the surgeons. And so it comes about that these latter, the surgeons themselves, mostly consider chloroform as being dangerous only because " so few people know how to give chloroform ", " scarcely one in a hundred ". These are the complaints, made with a shrug of the shoulders, that are so often heard. But do not these gentlemen, who make this as it were an excuse for the danger of anaesthesia, realise that they themselves thereby increase the difficulty ? It is undeniable that there are very few people who thoroughly understand the art of administering chloroform but this is because only a very small proportion of students is ever in a position to anaesthetise hundreds of times. If he has been

---

[1] Borntraeger, J. 1892. *Ueber die strafrechtliche Verantwortlichkeit des Arztes bei Anwendung des Chloroforms und anderer Inhalations-Anästhetika.* Berlin. 5.

18

endowed by nature with judgment and powers of observation, then in the course of these anaesthesias the student can gradually work out his own technique for himself along empirical lines. Nobody else will furnish him with understanding. And yet proper teaching could be effected in a much smaller number of cases, if only the whole problem of chloroform were not treated so irresponsibly. If only the senior surgeons, the clinical teachers and the house officers would resolve to hold proper courses in anaesthesia, then the state administrative authorities would soon be convinced of the necessity of creating anaesthetic specialists, but on condition that they themselves must give instruction in their specialty. This would quickly bring about the freeing of anaesthesia from the fetters of empiricism and of apathetic tradition. One should hold courses in chloroforming ; one should ask for testimonials of efficiently carried out anaesthesias ; one should make it an examination subject ; then one would have done more for the chloroform question than by publishing, as a sop to one's conscience, two or three lots of statistics covering a 50-year period.'[1]

Contrasting private practice with hospital practice in Germany Schleich pointed out that the private practitioner was wholly responsible for the safety of the patient undergoing prescribed treatment, whereas the surgeon on the staff of an institution, although he actually performed the operation, accepted no responsibility for the anaesthetic, which he considered to be quite outside his province. ' This is certainly not what patients expect ', Schleich commented, ' they tacitly assume that the surgeon whose authority they have consulted will protect them with both his experience and his reputation, from all dangers during the operation. What would happen if all patients knew that the anaesthetic is often infinitely more dangerous than the biggest operation !

' And this most dangerous undertaking is, for the most part, entrusted to the hands of—well, let us say the youngest house officers ! . . . Indeed ', Schleich continued, ' one can be a great surgeon and in the front rank of diagnosticians and specialists in operative treatment without understanding any more of the technique of chloroforming than a dresser or a junior house surgeon.'[2]

Schleich's comments on the existing system of administering anaesthetics in Germany made a considerable impression upon the more receptive among his surgical colleagues.

[1] Schleich, C. L. 1899. *Schmerzlose Operationen*. Berlin. 137.   [2] *Ibid.* 7, 9.

F. L. Dumont, of Berne, in his *Handbuch der allgemeinen und lokalen Anaesthesie*, wrote :

' Nothing is more ridiculous than the diffidence with which he [the administrator of an anaesthetic] accepts a subordinate role in the operation. He is just as important a personage as the operating surgeon, for the patient's life depends upon him just as much as it does upon the latter. In our opinion the great short-coming of most medical teaching on the European Continent is that (unlike English and American teaching [1]), it makes no provision for instruction in anaesthetics. This latter subject is surely at least as important as, for example, bandaging, which is almost everywhere compulsory. It ought not to be forgotten that the achievement of smooth, perfect, and safe anaesthesia is a skilled art, which must be properly learned. How often have we failed to find this art in young colleagues, who come as house surgeons, fresh from the classroom, with top marks in surgery, yet who are not a little embarrassed if they have to undertake the administration of an anaesthetic.' [2]

The Status of the Anaesthetist in England at the Close of the Nineteenth Century

Although in England the anaesthetist had a recognized status in the medical profession which, during the eighteen-nineties, had come to be the envy of medical men of other nations, his position so far as the law was concerned was ill-defined. Since about 1885 anaesthetists had been perplexed by questions of etiquette in anaesthetic practice, particularly in cases where some legal difficulty was, or might be, involved.

The middle years of the eighteen-eighties form a sort of silly season in the history of anaesthesia in England (cf. p. 457 *et seq.*) ; creative effort was temporarily almost at a standstill and the journals, particularly the *British Medical Journal*, were full of questions and answers bearing upon correct procedure in various hypothetical cases having a legal or quasi-legal interest. For example, to the inquiry : is it legal for an anaesthetist to charge a fee of one guinea in a case of amputation of a pauper's leg ? the *British Medical Journal* replied :

' We advise that our correspondent should apply for the same [to the Local Government Board]. . . . It should be remembered

---

[1] This passage was published in 1903 after reform in anaesthetic education had begun in the United States.

[2] Dumont, F. L. 1903. *Handbuch der allegemeinen und lokalen Anaesthesie*. Berlin and Vienna 17.

that, when the scale of extra fees was drawn up, the value of anaesthetics in diminishing human suffering had not been discovered.'[1]

' A Member ', in 1887, asked

' what a medical man ought to do when summoned by a dentist to administer gas, &c., and he finds on arrival that the patient is a stranger to him ?   May he simply administer the gas without asking any questions, or ought he to ascertain the patient's usual medical attendant, and hand the case over to him ?   If the latter course is correct, what bearing on the point would the alleged unfitness of the ordinary medical attendant for giving gas, ether, &c., or the distance of his residence from the dentist's have ? '

' In the absence of any ethical rule ', replied the *British Medical Journal*, ' that directly bears on the exceptional case described by " A Member ", we are not in a position to do more than express the opinion, based on the general principle laid down in the *Code of medical ethics*, that, under the circumstances, it would be the duty of the practitioner to ascertain whether the patient was resident in the neighbourhood, and whether it was possible to procure the attendance of the family medical adviser without reference to his possible " unfitness for giving gas, ether, &c." In the event of the patient being a non-resident, and the case one of more or less urgency, " A Member " would in our opinion, be justified in administering the gas or other anaesthetic without previous communication with the ordinary attendant, but not otherwise.'[2]

' Tory ', also in 1887, asked :

' When called two miles into the country to see a man with crushed fingers, and I find it necessary to remove one digit, am I legally justified in chloroforming the man and operating without another surgeon being present : If the man should die under the anaesthetic, what would the law require—an inquest or simply my certificate ? '

The *British Medical Journal* replied :

' The law fixes no rules as to the administration of chloroform, but a medical practitioner may be held liable for the consequences of negligence in performing any operation. As there is a certain amount of risk attending the use of most anaesthetics, it is usual for a medical practitioner to get another qualified man, if possible, to be present, so as to avoid any imputations being made. But a qualified practitioner may, if he chooses, administer chloroform to a patient without the presence of a third person. If the patient

[1] *Brit. med. J.*, 1885, i, 206.   [2] *Ibid.* 1887, i, 650.

should die, it would be a question for the coroner whether an inquest should be held. This would to a great extent depend on what the certificate disclosed.' [1]

In 1893 'Practitioner' raised the point : should dentists administer anaesthetics ? To this the *Journal* answered :

'Anaesthetics should be administered only by duly qualified medical men. There is no law upon the subject, but only those who are able to perform tracheotomy in the event of asphyxia ought ever to administer nitrous oxide gas. Ether and chloroform should only be administered by medical men experienced in the use of anaesthetics. If a death were to occur in a dentist's chair the magistrate might consider it culpable negligence on the part of the dentist if he had no medical assistant present at the operation. The only safe rule is always to have a second person present, and, when possible, that person should be a doctor, or, better still, a skilled anaesthetist.' [2]

This correspondence on the subject of dentists acting as anaesthetists was reopened from time to time during the remaining years of the nineteenth century. It was complicated in 1895 by the further question : should unregistered dentists administer anaesthetics ? On this point the *British Medical Journal* refused to give an opinion and suggested referring the matter to the President of the General Medical Council.[3]

The General Medical Council took no part in this particular discussion, but in February 1899, as an outcome of a previous discussion upon the administration of anaesthetics by qualified medical men for unregistered dentists, the Council stated :

'Any registered medical practitioner who knowingly and wilfully assists a person who is not registered as a dentist, . . . either by administering anaesthetics or otherwise, will be liable . . . to be dealt with by the General Medical Council as having been guilty of infamous conduct in a professional respect.' [4]

At the time of the jubilee of anaesthesia celebrations in the autumn of 1896, when the past, present, and future of anaesthesia were under review, a legal opinion on ' The present state of the law as to the administration of anaesthetics ' was given in the *Practitioner* by R. W. Turner, a barrister-at-law.

' The present state of the law ', he bluntly affirmed, ' is one of lawlessness. Any man, woman, or child may administer

[1] *Brit. med. J.*, 1887, ii, 1406. [2] *Ibid.* 1893, i, 447.
[3] Cf. *Ibid.* 1895, i, 347. [4] *Ibid.* 1899, i, 624.

anaesthetics. But as the administration of anaesthetics is part of the duty of a qualified [1] man, it is clear that the unqualified administrator is liable to the penalties imposed by the Medical, Dentists and Apothecaries Acts on unqualified persons provided the case falls within the four corners of any of their Acts. These Acts do not directly forbid the general administration of anaesthetics. . . . Reform is necessary, not only to prevent quacks practising as doctors, but to prevent unqualified persons administering anaesthetics and other dangerous drugs. It is anomalous and absurd that this should not be a specific offence when the sale of poisons is prohibited to a certain extent.' [2]

Although from the legal point of view the liabilities of the administrator of an anaesthetic were not clearly defined,[3] from the medical point of view they were very definite and were categorically stated in a leader in the *Lancet*.

' The person who undertakes the control of the anaesthetic is responsible for the safety of the patient. It has been held by persons of great weight in the profession that the real person who bears the burden of the responsibility is the surgeon who operates. . . . But the responsibility of the actual conduct of the administration of the anaesthetic must in every case rest with the person whose allotted task it is to devote himself to it. The surgeon may be highly reprehensible if he permits a novice to undertake the administration of ether or chloroform, but the person giving the drug cannot be screened from his act by the surgeon. . . . The person who gives an anaesthetic, unless he be a student who does it under the eye of his teacher, who then assumes the responsibility, must always be a duly qualified medical practitioner. It may be urged that many ward orderlies or nurses are far more experienced than newly qualified men, but even were this so it is no valid reason for permitting unqualified persons to undertake the functions of medical practitioners.

.   .   .   .

' More than one action for damage has been brought against medical men who have lost patients under chloroform, and in such cases the only possible defence can be that everything was done for the unhappy patient which experience and skill could effect. Thus the fact must not be blinked that both from the point of view of medical ethics . . . and from the purely legal

[1] Turner stated that the term ' qualified ' included registered dentists, physicians, and surgeons.

[2] *Practitioner*, 1896, **57,** 398–400.

[3] These liabilities are still not clearly defined, cf. Macintosh, R. R., and Bannister, F. B. 1943. *Essentials of general anaesthesia*. Oxford. 322–3.

standpoint the responsibility of giving an anaesthetic should be borne wholly and solely by a registered medical man who is competent to select his anaesthetic and to administer it in the best possible way. Certain it is that anyone who wittingly violates these rules puts himself outside the pale of professional and legal right.' [1]

[1] *Lancet*, 1896, i, 634.

APPENDIX A

MORTON'S INHALERS

Patent Specifications

LETTER Patent No. 4848 in respect of a method and apparatus for etherizing (such as Morton used during the operation performed at the Massachusetts General Hospital on the morning of October 16, 1846) was issued by the United States Patent Office to Morton jointly with Jackson (who, however, assigned his rights to Morton) on November 12, 1846 (cf. p. 116). The specification for this patent (which is of importance in deciding what the ' original ' inhaler, used on October 16, 1846, was really like) was as follows :

' UNITED STATES PATENT OFFICE
' C. T. Jackson and Wm. T. G. Morton, of Boston, Massachusetts ; said C. T. Jackson Assignor to Wm. T. G. Morton.
' IMPROVEMENT IN SURGICAL OPERATIONS Specification forming part of Letter Patent No. 4848, dated November 12, 1846.

' *To All Whom It May Concern :*

' Be it known that we, CHARLES T. JACKSON and WILLIAM T. G. MORTON, of Boston, in the County of Suffolk and State of Massachusetts have invented or discovered a new and useful Improvement in Surgical Operations on Animals, whereby we are enabled to accomplish many, if not all operations, such as are usually attended with more or less pain and suffering, without any or with very little pain to or muscular action of persons who undergo the same ; and we do hereby declare that the following is a full and exact description of our said invention or discovery.

' It is well known to chemists that when alcohol is submitted to distillation with certain acids peculiar compounds, termed " ethers," are formed, each of which is usually distinguished by the name of the acid employed in its preparation. It has also been known that the vapors of some, if not all, of these chemical distillations, particularly those of sulphuric ether, when breathed or introduced into the lungs of an animal have produced a peculiar effect on its nervous system, one which has been supposed

552

to be analogous to what is usually termed " intoxication." It has never to our knowledge·been known until our discovery that the inhalation of such vapors (particularly of sulphuric ether) would produce insensibility to pain, or such a state of quiet of nervous action as to render a person or animal incapable to a great extent, if not entirely, of experiencing pain while under the action of the knife or other instrument of operation of a surgeon calculated to produce pain. This is our discovery, and the combining it with or applying it to any operation of surgery for the purpose of alleviating animal suffering, as well as of enabling a surgeon to conduct his operation with little or no struggling or muscular action of the patient and with more certainty of success, constitutes our invention. The nervous quiet and insensibility to pain produced on a person is generally of short duration. The degree or extent of it or time which it lasts depends on the amount of ethereal vapor received into the system and the constitutional character of the person to whom it is administered. Practice will soon acquaint an experienced surgeon with the amount of ethereal vapor to be administered to persons for the accomplishment of the surgical operation or operations required in their respective cases. For the extraction of a tooth the individual may be thrown into the insensible state, generally speaking, only a few minutes. For the removal of a tumor or the performance of the amputation of a limb it is necessary to regulate the amount of vapor inhaled to the time required to complete the operation.

' Various modes may be adopted for conveying the ethereal vapor into the lungs. A very simple one is to saturate a piece of cloth or sponge with sulphuric ether, and place it to the nostrils or mouth, so that the person may inhale the vapors. A more effective one is to take a glass or other proper vessel, like a common bottle or flask and place in it a sponge saturated with sulphuric ether. Let there be a hole made through the side of the vessel for the admission of atmospheric air, which hole may or may not be provided with a valve opening downward, or so as to allow air to pass into the vessel, a valve on the outside of the neck opening upward, and another valve in the neck and between that last mentioned and the body of the vessel or flask, which latter valve in the neck should open toward the mouth of the neck or bottle. The extremity of the neck is to be placed in the mouth of the patient, and his nostrils stopped or closed in such manner as to cause him to inhale air through the bottle, and to exhale it through the neck and out of the valve on the outside of the neck. The air thus breathed, by passing in contact with the sponge, will be charged with the ethereal vapors, which will be conveyed by it into the lungs of the patient. This will soon produce the state of insensibility or nervous quiet required.

*18

' In order to render the ether agreeable to various persons, we often combine it with one or more essential oils having pleasant perfumes. This may be effected by mixing the ether and essential oil and washing the mixture in water. The impurities will subside, and the ether, impregnated with the perfume, will rise to the top of the water. We sometimes combine a narcotic preparation—such as opium or morphine—with the ether. This may be done by any way known to chemists by which a combination of ethereal and narcotic vapors may be produced.

' After a person has been put into the state of insensibility, as above described, a surgical operation may be performed upon him without, so far as repeated experiments have proved, giving to him any apparent or real pain, or so little in comparison to that produced by the usual process of conducting surgical operations as to be scarcely noticeable. There is very nearly, if not entire, absence of all pain. Immediately or soon after the operation is completed a restoration of the patient to his usual feelings takes place without, generally speaking, his having been sensible of the performance of the operation.

' From the experiments we have made we are led to prefer the vapors of sulphuric ether to those of muriatic or other kind of ether ; but any such may be employed which will properly produce the state of insensibility without any injurious consequences to the patient.

' We are fully aware that narcotics have been administered to patients undergoing surgical operations, and, as we believe, always by introducing them into the stomach. This we consider in no respect to embody our invention, as we operate through the lungs and air-passages, and the effects produced upon the patient are entirely or so far different as to render the one of very little while the other is of immense utility. The consequences of the change are very considerable, as an immense amount of human or animal suffering can be prevented by the application of our discovery.

' What we claim as our invention is—

' The herein before described means by which we are enabled to effect the above highly important improvement in surgical operations—viz., by combining therewith the application of ether or the vapor thereof—substantially as above specified.

' In testimony whereof we have hereto set our signatures this 27th day of October, A.D. 1846.

' CHARLES T. JACKSON.
' WM. T. G. MORTON.

' Witness :

' R. H. Eddy.
' W. H. Leighton.' [1]

[1] Transcribed from Roth, G. B. 1932. *Ann. med. Hist.*, N.S. **4,** 393–5.

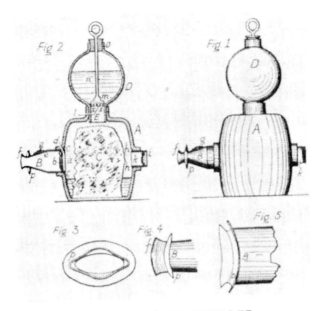

FIG. 153.—ETHER INHALER

Patented by Morton and Gould, in November 1847.
These drawings accompanied the patent specification
(No. 5365).

Exactly a year later, on November 13, 1847, Morton, this
time jointly with Augustus A. Gould, who had assisted him in
the designing of the inhaler used on October 16, 1846 (cf.
p. 107), took out a patent for a new inhaler. For this the
specification was as follows :

' (Patent No. 5365)
   ' Be it known that we, AUGUSTUS A. GOULD and WILLIAM
T. G. MORTON, of Boston, in the County of Suffolk and State
of Massachusetts, have invented an inhalation apparatus to be
used for the purpose of administering to persons or introducing
into their lungs the vapors of ether or various other chemical
matters ; and we do hereby declare that the same is fully described
and represented in the following specification and accompanying
drawings [shown in Fig. 153], letters, figures and references
thereof.
   ' Of the said drawings Figure 1 denotes an external side elevation of our said apparatus. Fig. 2 is a central and vertical section
of it.

' A, Figs. 1 and 2, exhibits a receiver or vessel, made of glass or other suitable material, and shaped as seen in the drawings, or in any other convenient and proper manner. It has a mouth or opening *a* formed in one side of it, into which mouth or opening a tube B is inserted and closely fitted, as seen in Fig. 2. The said tube B is formed at its opposite end, and in any proper manner to enable a person to place and hold it in or to his mouth. A valve *b* is adapted to and arranged within the tube B, and at or near its inner end. This valve should be made to open toward the mouth piece or that end of the tube B which is to be inserted in the mouth as aforesaid. The said valve is hinged to a partition *c*, *c*, which is inserted in and fixed across the tube and has a hole *d* made through it, over which the valve closes, and rests on the partition as a seat. Another hole or passage *e* is bored or made through the top or other proper part of the tube B, and between the valve *b* and end *f* of the tube. The said hole *e* is provided with a valve or flap *g* which is hinged to the outer surface of the tube, and closes over the hole *e*. The valve *b* may be termed the induction valve and the valve *g* the eduction valve of the mouth tube B. Through the opposite side or any other proper part of the vessel A we made another passage or opening *h*, *h*, which is intended to admit atmospheric air into the interior of the vessel A. This last opening may be provided with a valve opening inward or toward the interior of the vessel.

' In the drawing *i* denotes the valve as applied to a tube *k* which is fitted into the opening *h*, *h*. The object of the valve *i* is to prevent the vapor within the vessel A from escaping through opening *h*, *h*. Into the vessel A we insert a sponge C which on being wet with any volatile fluid, such as ether for instance exposes a large evaporating surface to the action of the current of air, made to pass through the vessel A while the person is in the act of using the apparatus. As a convenient addition to the vessel A we provide it with a supplying reservoir D which consists of a fountain or vessel of glass or other suitable material placed on the top of the vessel A, and secured or affixed to it in any proper manner.

' For the sake of convenience we terminate the lower end of the vessel D in a short tube or neck E which we insert in the top of the vessel A (which top is suitably formed to receive it) in the same manner as a cork is fitted into the neck of a bottle. A horizontal partition *l* is made to extend across the tube E and to have a series of small holes, *x*, *x*, *x*, bored or made downward through it. A small piston or valve *m* sustained on the lower end of a wire *n* is arranged over the holes of the said partition *l* and should be of such size as when forced down closely upon the partition to cover all the holes through it and prevent any liquid which may be in the vessel D from escaping into the vessel A.

The rod *n* and valve *m* are supported by a cork or plug *o* inserted in an opening suitably formed through the top of the vessel D. If the supplying reservoir D contains any liquid by raising the valve *m* above its seat the said liquid will trickle or pass through the opening of the partition *l* and fall on the sponge C or into the vessel A. The quantity of liquid required to keep up the necessary supply in the vessel A during inhalation may be regulated by raising the valve *m* to such height above the seat *l* as circumstances may require. The tube B may be made wholly or in part of a flexible material and of such length as circumstances may require, and for the purpose of more readily evaporating ether or any chemical material in the vessel A, heat may be applied to the said vessel in any convenient manner. It (the vessel) may be surrounded partially or wholly by a vessel of hot water, if desirable, but as a general rule it will not be necessary when sulfuric ether is to be evaporated in the vessel A.

'The manner of using the apparatus is as follows : Sulfuric ether or other material to be vaporized is poured into the vessel and the apparatus is carried toward the patient and the outer end *f* of the tube B placed in his mouth. By closing his nostrils and causing him to make an inhalation through his mouth, air charged with vapor will pass from the vessel A through the opening *d* of the induction valve *b* and thence into the mouth and lungs of the patient. When he expels air or the mixture of air and etheric or other vapor from the lungs it will pass into the tube B out of the opening *e* of the valve *g* the valve *b* closing upon its seat and preventing the vapor and expelled air from passing back into the vessel A. At each inhalation of the patient the valve *i* will open and admit air to rush into the bottle or vessel A.

'Fig. 3 represents on an enlarged scale a front view of the mouth piece or end of the tube B which is introduced into the mouth. Fig. 4 is a side elevation, and Fig. 5 is a top view of the same. By inspection of these figures it will be seen that the said end is provided with a curved flanch *p* which is made to extend partially or entirely around the tube and to project from it as seen in the figures. Such a curved form or shape should be given to the flanch as will not only cause it to fit closely to the lips and prevent the apparatus from being forced too far into the mouth, but prevent as far as practicable the passage of external air between it and the lips during respiration.

'We do not intend to limit ourselves to the peculiar shape or configuration of any or all the parts of our improved inhalation apparatus, as we have exhibited in the drawings, nor do we intend always to employ the supplying reservoir D, or the tube *k* and its valve, but we intend to make one of such shapes and forms, and such portions of our improvement as occasion may require, while we do not change the inventional character of the mechanism which may be considered as of our discovery and as peculiarly applicable to the inhalation and exhalation of etheric or other vapors in the manner as above set forth.

' Having thus described our improved inhalation apparatus, that which we claim therein is—

' 1. The system of induction and eduction valves (b and g) and openings (d and e) of the mouth tube B, (or any mechanical equivalent for such valves and openings) in combination with said tube and the vessel A, and made to operate therewith in the manner, and for the purpose substantially as specified.

' 2. We also claim the supplying reservoir D, or apparatus in combination with the evaporating vessel A, the same being arranged and made to operate together substantially as specified.

' 3. We also claim the supporting or lip flanch p as combined with or applied to the mouth piece of the tube B, and operating therewith in the manner and for the purpose, as above set forth.

' 4. And, for the purpose of inhaling a due portion of atmospheric air, while breathing the etheric vapors, and preventing the escape of the vapors when the apparatus is not in use, we claim, in combination with the reservoir A and air inlet or tube k, and its valve i, the whole being combined and operating together substantially as specified.

' 5. And we also claim, in combination with the vessel A and its air inlet and exhaustion pipes or contrivances, a sponge C, or other equivalent operating by capillary attraction or otherwise, to expose an extensive surface of liquid to the evaporative action of the air passing through the vessel A.

' Augustus A. Gould.
' W. T. G. Morton.

' Witnesses :

' R. H. Eddy.
' D. P. Wilson.' [1]

The ' Original ' Inhaler

Two variants of Morton's first ether inhaler are in existence, each of which has been claimed as representing that originally used by Morton at the Massachusetts General Hospital on October 16, 1846. These are the ' Wiksell Exhibit ' (with its stand), shown in Fig. 154, now in the Smithsonian Institution in Washington, and two inhalers, identical with each other, one in the Museum of the University of Harvard Medical School, the other in the Museum of the Massachusetts General Hospital in Boston (see Fig. 12).

---

[1] Transcribed from Roth, G. B. 1932. *Ann. med. Hist.*, N.S. **4**, 391–3.

The question which of these two variants more probably represents the prototype was carefully considered by G. B. Roth

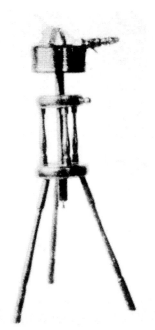

FIG. 154.—ETHER INHALER KNOWN AS THE 'WIKSELL EXHIBIT'

A two-necked glass flask with a wooden mouth-tube inserted into one neck ; the inhaler rests in a wooden stand, said to have been constructed for it.

This inhaler was presented to the Smithsonian Institution in Washington in 1911 and is claimed as representing the original type of inhaler used by Morton. Its construction agrees less well with Morton's own description of his first inhaler than does that of the inhaler (also claimed as the original type) one example of which (see Fig. 12, p. 108) is now in the possession of the Harvard Medical School, the other in the Museum of the Massachusetts General Hospital.

in 1932, in an article in the *Annals of Medical History*.[1] After weighing the evidence Roth came to the conclusion that the inhalers in the Harvard and Massachusetts General Hospital museums appear, in all essentials, to conform to the description

[1] *Ann. med. Hist.*, 1932, N.S. **4**, 390–7.

of the ether inhaler given by Morton himself in the patent specification, No. 4848, whereas the 'Wiksell Exhibit' does not.

Referring to the 'Wiksell Exhibit', Roth stated that it 'was placed in the Smithsonian Institution in 1911 by William J. Morton, the son of the discoverer of the anesthetic properties of ether, as a gift from Dr. Gustave P. Wiksell'. Roth's transcription of the label of this exhibit reads as follows :

'This is the only complete Morton Ether Inhaler known to exist. It was supplied to Dr. Wm. L. Johnson, of Boston, Dentist, in the fall of 1848 after the successful demonstration by Dr. W. T. G. Morton in the Massachusetts General Hospital on Friday, October 16, 1846.'

'Presented to the U.S. National Museum by Dr. Gustave P. Wiksell.'

The feature about the 'Wiksell Exhibit' which does not conform to contemporary descriptions of the inhaler originally used by Morton is its wooden mouthpiece, furnished with a spigot.

Morton, in his specification for the patent drawn up on October 27, 1846 (only eleven days after the initial use of his inhaler), stated :

'. . . take a glass or other proper vessel, like a common bottle or flask and place in it a sponge saturated with sulphuric ether. Let there be a hole made through the side of the vessel for the admission of atmospheric air, which hole may or may not be provided with a valve opening downward, or so as to allow air to pass into the vessel, a valve on the outside of the neck opening upward, and another valve in the neck and between that last mentioned and the body of the vessel or flask, which latter valve in the neck should open toward the mouth of the neck or bottle. The extremity of the neck is to be placed in the mouth of the patient, and his nostrils stopped or closed in such manner as to cause him to inhale air through the bottle, and to exhale it through the neck and out of the valve on the outside of the neck. . . .'   (See p. 553.)

Even the description of the 'temporary' apparatus hastily improvised for Morton by Wightman on the eve of the demonstration at the Massachusetts General Hospital (see pp. 106–7) gives no hint of any such mouthpiece as that attached to the 'Wiksell Exhibit'.

The evidence of Morton's description in the specification for Letter Patent No. 4848 is supported by the further evidence of

H. J. Bigelow's description of the inhaler originally used by Morton :

' A small two-necked glass globe contains the prepared vapour with sponges to enlarge the evaporating surface. One aperture admits the air to the interior of the globe, whence, charged with vapour it is drawn through the second into the lungs. The inspired air passes through the bottle, but the expiration is diverted by a valve in the mouthpiece, and escaping into the apartment is thus prevented from vitiating the medicated vapour.' (See p. 107.)

This description must be taken as authoritative. Bigelow was a member of the staff of the Massachusetts General Hospital at the time of the demonstration ; he was acquainted at first hand with Morton's methods of etherization and he was the first man to read a paper on the subject—at a meeting of the Boston Society of Medical Improvement (see pp. 118–20).

APPENDIX B

THE TERM 'ANAESTHESIA'—ITS INTRODUCTION AND DEFINITION

ON November 21, 1846, Oliver Wendell Holmes wrote to W. T. G. Morton :

'My Dear Sir,—Everybody wants to have a hand in a great discovery. All I will do is to give you a hint or two, as to names, or the name, to be applied to the state produced and the agent.

'The state should, I think, be called "Anaesthesia." This signifies insensibility, more particularly (as used by Linnæus and Cullen) to objects of touch. (See Good—*Nosology*, p. 259.) The adjective will be "Anaesthetic." Thus we might say, the state of anaesthesia, or the anaesthetic state. The means employed would be properly called the anti-aesthetic agent. Perhaps it might be allowable to say anaesthetic agent, but this admits of question.

'The words, antineuric, aneuric, neuro-leptic, neuro-lepsia, neuro-etasis, etc., seem too anatomical ; whereas the change is a physiological one. I throw them out for consideration.

'I would have a name pretty soon, and consult some accomplished scholar, such as President Everett or Dr. Bigelow, senior, before fixing upon the terms, which will be repeated by the tongues of every civilized race of mankind. You could mention these words which I suggest for their consideration ; but there may be others more appropriate and agreeable.

'Yours, respectfully,
'O. W. Holmes.' [1]

The word *anaesthesia*, implying loss of sensation as a result of disease or injury, but not loss of consciousness, was quite frequently used during the eighteenth and early nineteenth centuries. For example, Murray's *New English dictionary* (Oxford. 1888–1928) quotes : '1721 Bailey, Anaesthesia, a Defect of Sensation as in Paralytic and Blasted Persons '. In the *Edinburgh Medical and Surgical Journal* for April 1829 Alexander Reid reported a ' Case of Anaesthesia, or loss of Sensation ', and in the *London Medical Gazette* for 1832–3 Watson wrote on ' Anaesthesia and Facial

[1] Quoted by Rice, N. P. 1859. *Trials of a public benefactor.* New York.

Palsy . . .'. The adjective *anaesthetic*, however, appears to have been coined by Holmes himself.

The word *narcosis* was commonly used before 1846 to signify a state of stupor, either pathological or induced by drugs. Murray cites : ' 1693 Blancard's *Phys. Dict.* (ed. 2), *Narcosis*, a privation of Sense as in a Palsie, or in taking of Opium, &c. ; . . . 1753, Chambers *Cycl. Supp.*, *Narcosis*, a stupefaction or insensible state, whether brought on by medicines, or happening from natural causes '. Nicholas Culpepper, in *The English physitian* (London. 1656), stated : ' A sleeping Disease is got by the too frequent use of medicines called Narcoticks, that do produce sleep '.

Murray traces back the term *analgesia* to 1706 : ' Phillips, *Analgesia*, Indolency, a being free from Pain or Grief'. Its use to describe a conscious or semi-conscious state in which pain is obtunded by the administration of anaesthetic drugs does not seem to have occurred before 1870. John Snow, for instance, although he described the condition, did not employ the term analgesia (cf. pp. 193–4). The word *analgésie* to describe that state was, however, used by Guibert, of St. Brieuc, writing in 1872 in the *Comptes Rendus* of the Académie des Sciences (see p. 380).

As Holmes predicted, terms for the new state produced by the inhalation of ether were soon being repeated by the tongues of every civilized race. But *anaesthesia*, the word which he himself had suggested, although it was immediately accepted, was at first less commonly used than the word *etherization*.

After ether was superseded by chloroform in Europe the word *anaesthesia* came into general use, no doubt because of the clumsiness of the alternative *chloroformization* (although this word was sometimes used). In France the anomaly of referring to the administration of chloroform as *éthérisation* persisted for some years.[1]

John Snow, in his book *On chloroform and other anaesthetics*, wrote :

' Chloroform belongs to the large class of medicines known as narcotico-irritants. This and some other agents which have been inhaled for the prevention of pain are often called anaesthetics ; a name to which there is no objection, so long as it

[1] Cf., *e.g.*, Lallemand, L., Perrin, M., and Duroy, J. L. P. 1860. *Du rôle de l'alcool et des anesthésiques dans l'organisme.* Paris. 291, 292 ; cf. also p. 170.

does not lead to the idea that they have a different action from other narcotics, or more precisely speaking, narcotico-irritants ; there being no such medicines as pure narcotics. The term anaesthesia has been frequently employed to designate the insensibility and suspension of consciousness caused by chloroform and ether ; but, in describing the effects of these agents, I shall confine this term to its original meaning, privation of feeling, and I shall employ the term narcotism to designate the entire effects of these agents on the nervous system. This is the sense in which the term narcotism has always been employed. It has been the custom, however, to restrict the use of the word very much to cases in which stupor existed, but I shall apply it to designate the slighter, as well as the more profound effects of a narcotic, as I am entitled to do by strict etymology.'[1]

H. K. Beecher, in his book *The physiology of anesthesia*, wrote :

' Anesthesia and narcosis are conditions in which the normal response to stimuli of the whole or part of the body are temporarily depressed. While, strictly speaking, we have no right to assume that these conditions are identical, it is probable that they are manifestations of the same general process.

' The distinction between narcosis and anesthesia is not clear-cut. Claude Bernard (1875) applied the term narcosis, in a rather general sense, to the conditions in which the vital activity of lower forms of life is depressed by toxic agents (narcotics) provided the affected cells return to their original state when the narcotic is eliminated. " *Narcosis* ", then, designates a reversible reaction and should be limited to single cell organisms or groups of like cells from higher organisms. . . .

' " *Anesthesia* " may be reserved for the complicated reversible depression of the senses or automatic activity of higher forms of life, usually by drugs, but also, on occasion, by physical means. In man the primary characteristic of general anesthesia is loss of consciousness. The reversible nature of the process is one of its outstanding characteristics. It has points in common with the unconscious state produced by other means, as rhythmically recurring sleep, shock, or death.

' There is much evidence to indicate that anesthesia is more nearly akin to sleep than to shock or death. . . .'[2]

From October 1846 until the introduction of chloroform into practice in November 1847 the state induced in the patient by the inhalation of ether vapour was, perhaps more often

---

[1] Snow, J. 1858. *On chloroform and other anaesthetics.* London. 34.
[2] Beecher, H. K. 1938. *The physiology of anesthesia.* New York. 3.

than not, what would be recognized to-day as analgesia, or as an alternation between light anaesthesia and analgesia, rather than true anaesthesia. But after the introduction of the more powerful and therefore more easily administered agent chloroform, when Flourens in France and Snow in England had defined successive stages in anaesthesia and when Snow had, moreover, clearly described signs by which different phases of anaesthesia could be recognized clinically, then the term *anaesthesia* assumed its modern meaning.

APPENDIX C

RESUSCITATION

SINCE the last quarter of the eighteenth century some form of artificial respiration has been the sheet anchor of resuscitative measures. Early methods included mouth to mouth insufflation ; pumping a stream of air or oxygen into the lungs either through the mouth, with or without intubation, or through a tracheotomy wound ; and manual compression of the chest and abdomen. Of the supplementary measures the most common have been attempts to revive the patient by irritating the body in various simple ways, as for instance, by friction of the limbs and trunk ; by passing electric currents through the body and by the application of extremes of temperature ; by percussion ; by stimulants given by mouth ; and by bringing pungent vapours under the nostrils or introducing them into the rectum by fumigation. These measures, intended primarily for the resuscitation of the drowned, the suffocated, and the newborn,[1] were adopted by surgeons during 1847 and 1848 for use in cases of respiratory and circulatory arrest supervening on anaesthesia.[2]

An account of the first fifty recorded deaths from chloroform anaesthesia, collected from many parts of the world, was given by John Snow in his book *On chloroform and other anaesthetics*.[3] In almost all these cases an attempt was made at resuscitation by well-known methods.

The first of these cases was that of fifteen-year-old Hannah Greener (cf. pp. 195–7). Very little was done for her. Snow quoted the account of events given by the administrator of the anaesthetic, Meggison :

' I was proceeding to apply more [chloroform] to the hand-kerchief, when her lips, which had been previously of a good

[1] It may be mentioned here that John Snow's first published paper dealt with ' a double air-pump for supporting artificial respiration ' in still-born children. (*Lond. med. Gaz.*, 1841–2, i, 222–7 ; Snow, J. 1858. *On chloroform and other anaesthetics*. London. x.)

[2] Cf., *e.g.*, the suggestion made by Plouviez in a note on the insufflation of air into the lungs as a means of dealing with the asphyxia which sometimes results from the inhalation of ether or of chloroform. (*C.R. Acad. Sci.*, Paris, 1848, **26**, 106 (extract).)

[3] Snow, J. 1858. *On chloroform and other anaesthetics*. London. 123–99.

colour, became suddenly blanched, and she spluttered at the mouth, as if in epilepsy. I threw down the handkerchief, dashed cold water in her face, and gave her some internally, followed by brandy, without, however, the least effect, not the slightest attempt at a rally being made. We laid her on the floor, opened a vein in her arm, and the jugular vein, but no blood flowed. The whole process of inhalation, operation, venesection, and death, could not, I should say, have occupied more than two minutes.'

Case 2 happened in Cincinnati in February 1848, and the victim was a healthy, thirty-five-year-old woman. Chloroform was administered to her by two unqualified dentists from a Morton's ether globe (see Fig. 12) :

' The dentists gave nearly the same account, saying that the breathing was at first slow, and that the patient inhaled twelve or fifteen times, occupying from a minute to seventy-five seconds. They committed the great error of not placing the patient at once in the horizontal position, when the alarming symptoms came on, but kept her sitting in the chair, from five to ten minutes, whilst they sent out for restoratives. They thought the patient was living during this time, but her female friends [who were present] thought not. The patient was placed on a sofa, and sometime afterwards artificial respiration and galvanism were applied without effect.'

Case 4 happened at Boulogne in May 1848 ; the operation was the opening of a sinus in the thigh and the patient was a woman of thirty. She was given chloroform on a handkerchief ' placed over the nostrils ' by the surgeon performing the operation :

' M. Gorré . . . expressed the opinion afterwards that death had already taken place when he made the incision. Amongst the means used, with a view to resuscitate the patient, was inflation of the lungs, which was performed with such force as to produce permanent dilatation of the air-cells [1].'

In *case 9*, at the Hôtel-Dieu, at Lyons, in January 1849, the patient was a seventeen-year-old boy who was to have a finger amputated. Chloroform was administered on ' a piece of fine gauze '.

---

[1] Leroy warned against this type of accident in 1827, and suggested intermittent pressure on the chest and abdomen instead of the use of bellows. (*Journal de Physiologie expérimentale*, 1828, **8**, 97-135.)

'At the end of four or five minutes, the patient still felt and spoke. . . . The pulse was regular, and of normal strength. All at once the patient raised his body, and struggled . . . the assistants . . . however . . . seized . . . and replaced the patient in his position. Within a quarter of a minute, one of the assistants stated that the pulse at the wrist had ceased to beat . . . and the sounds over the region of the heart could no longer be heard. Respiration still continued but . . . ceased completely in the space of about half a minute.

'The extreme danger of the patient was manifest, and immediate and energetic means were employed to rouse him. Ammonia was held to the nostrils, and rubbed in large quantity over the surface of the chest and abdomen. It was also applied to the most delicate parts of the skin, *e.g.* the lips and the extremity of the penis, with a view to excite irritation. Mustard was used ; the head was inclined over the bed ; and, finally, an attempt was made to restore respiration by means of alternate pressure on the abdomen and chest. After two or three minutes, respiration reappeared, and even acquired a certain fulness, but the pulse nowhere returned. Frictions were continued. Respiration became again slower, and at length ceased. Artificial inflation was practised, at first through the mouth, and afterwards through the larynx, by passing a tube through the glottis [1], as it was perceived that air had passed from the mouth into the stomach. The precordial, epigastric, and laryngeal regions were energetically cauterised with a hot iron. The pulse did not return. For the space of half an hour every effort was made to resuscitate the patient ; but in vain.'

Case 12, according to Snow, was ' the first which occurred in any of the hospitals in this metropolis ' (London). The patient was a burly and alcoholic porter, forty-eight years old and suffering from an ingrowing toe-nail. Chloroform anaesthesia was uneventful until after the removal of the nail at about 2 p.m. Then :

' He continued insensible ; and, his face becoming dark, the pulse small, quick, but regular, respiration laborious, his neckerchief was removed, and the chest exposed to fresh air from a window near to the bed ; cold water was dashed in his face, the chest rubbed, and ammonia applied to the nose. After struggling for about a minute, he became still, the skin cold, pulse scarcely perceptible, and soon ceased to be felt at the wrist ; respiration became slow and at intervals, but continued a few seconds after the cessation of the pulse. Immediately on the

¹ Lozes recommended this method in 1818. It was a modification of the earlier intubation method of Chaussier (1806) for the new-born.

appearance of these symptoms, artificial respiration was commenced by depressing the ribs with the hands and then allowing them to rise again until the proper apparatus was brought, when respiration was kept up by means of the trachea tube and bellows, and oxygen [1] gas introduced into the lungs by the same means. Galvanism was also applied through the heart and diaphragm, but all signs of life ceased about six or seven minutes after the commencement of inhalation. These means were persisted in until a quarter past three, but to no purpose.'

In *case 17*, which occurred at the Seraphim Hospital, Stockholm, the patient was a man of thirty, suffering from hydrocele. About a drachm and a half of chloroform was administered to him on cotton in a cone made from a folded towel by Professor Santesson, who had previously seen James Young Simpson at work in Edinburgh.

' The patient died before the operation was begun, and within five minutes from the commencement of inhalation. During the application of various means of resuscitation, including the dropping of cold water *guttatim* on the epigastrium, the breathing returned . . . for the space of three or four minutes ; but the pulse and sound of the heart did not return.'

In *case 25*, at St. Bartholomew's Hospital, London, in March 1852, the patient, a young man, was suffering from ' aneurism by anastomosis, occupying the right ear and its neighbourhood '. Induction was somewhat turbulent and lasted five or ten minutes.

' The operation was then commenced ; but no sooner had Mr. Lloyd cut the skin, than it was stated that the pulse had suddenly ceased. The chloroform was at once removed ; but in a few seconds, the patient had ceased to breathe, and no pulsation could be felt at any of the arteries or the heart.

' Artificial respiration, as well as percussion and compression of the different parts of the body, were immediately employed with energy ; . . . with the use also of galvanism, the circulation and respiration were again restored. Quickly, however, the patient fell into the same state as at first, but was again restored by the same means.

' In a few minutes the state of inanimation again returned, when the external jugular vein . . . was opened, and tracheotomy was performed, and the lungs inflated. The patient was also placed in a warm bath, at the temperature of 104°, artificial respiration being kept up all the time. All, however, was of no avail.'

1 Inflation with oxygen for resuscitation had been suggested by John Hunter. *Philos. Trans.*, 1776, **66**, 481, *footnote.*

Tracheotomy and artificial respiration through a flexible tube, and an electric current 'sent by needles through the region of the heart' were also tried without avail in *case 31*, that of a soldier, twenty-five years old, in the Hôtel-Dieu at Orléans in 1853.

Case 32 occurred at the Edinburgh Royal Infirmary in September 1853. The patient, a man of forty-three, was about to be operated on for stricture of the urethra when the pulse became weak. Dr. Dunsmore, the operating surgeon, gave the following account of the accident :

'. . . A second or two after . . . [two assistants] exclaimed that the pulse was gone. I rushed from my seat to the patient's head, and found that his breathing had ceased. Those present who had an opportunity of observing the respiration . . . positively assert that the breathing did not cease before the pulse. The face was much congested, the jaws were firmly closed, and the pupils were dilated. I immediately forced open the lower jaw by means of the handle of a staff, and with catch forceps pulled out the tongue [¹]. Artificial respiration was had recourse to, and in a few minutes he made a long inspiration. This was soon followed by [four more] . . . when all attempts at natural breathing ceased. No pulsation could be felt in the radial arteries. The chest was noticed to be much contracted, to have apparently lost its elasticity, and not to expand when the ribs were forcibly compressed during the artificial respiration. . . . By the time the tracheotomy tube was inserted, the galvanic apparatus was in working condition, and it was applied on each side of the diaphragm. It acted remarkably well ; at each application of the sponges, the muscle descended as if the patient was in life ; air passed through the tube in the trachea, and for some time I was in great hopes that the man was to be saved ; but the muscle gradually lost its contractility, and although the galvanism was kept up for an hour, it was evident . . . that life was extinct.'

¹ This is the first mention among the fifty fatal cases listed by Snow of the tongue being drawn forward. In subsequent cases in this series the tongue is several times mentioned as having been drawn forward and the operator's finger passed round the root to make sure that the airway was clear.

The method of catching the tongue by its tip and rhythmically drawing upon and relaxing the whole member was suggested by J. V. Laborde in 1892 as a means of resuscitating the apparently drowned. He told a meeting of the Académie de Médecine in Paris how, during such an emergency, he called to mind that in the laboratory animals were revived in this way, particularly after anaesthetic collapse.

The method attracted considerable notice, but although its use in chloroform syncope was suggested accounts of early cases all related to other emergencies. (*Bull. Acad. Méd. Paris*, 1892, **28**, 9, 519 ; *ibid.*, 1894, **31**, 108.)

In *case 48* in February 1856 a boy of nine, a private patient of Paget (of St. Bartholomew's Hospital), collapsed immediately before the operation, the removal of a tumour of the scapula, was begun. Among resuscitative measures resorted to Marshall Hall's recently introduced 'postural' or 'ready' method of artificial respiration [1] was mentioned.[2]

This method was described by Snow as being 'the most ready and effectual mode of performing artificial respiration. It consists', he added, 'in placing the patient on the face and making pressure on the back; removing the pressure, and turning the patient on his side and a little beyond; then turning him back on the face and making pressure on the back again; these measures being repeated in about the time of natural respiration'.[3]

Marshall Hall's method was mentioned also in the fiftieth case of death from chloroform recorded by Snow; this death occurred at King's College Hospital in August 1857.

In addition to these fifty fatalities from chloroform anaesthesia Snow noted several cases in which the vital functions were successfully restarted.[4] In this connection Snow stated:

'It is probable that artificial respiration, very promptly applied, will restore all those patients who are capable of being restored from an overdose of chloroform. All the patients who are related to have been restored after this agent has occasioned a complete state of suspended animation, have been resuscitated by this means. It is only by artificial respiration that I have been able to recover animals from an overdose of chloroform, when I felt satisfied that they would not recover spontaneously. And under these circumstances I have not been able to restore them even by this means, except when a tube had been introduced into the trachea, by an incision in the neck, before giving them what would have been the fatal dose. . . .

'Where patients have recovered under the use of other measures, without artificial respiration, it is probable that animation was not completely suspended, and that the recovery was spontaneous. . . .

[1] E. A. Schäfer, himself the originator (c. 1903) of the 'prone pressure method' of artificial respiration, wrote of Marshall Hall's method: 'It has the advantage . . . that the tongue does not require to be drawn out of the mouth by a special operator'. (*J. Amer. med. Ass.*, 1908, **51**, 801.) Marshall Hall intended his method primarily for the resuscitation of drowned persons.

[2] See *Lancet*, 1856, i, 144, 229, 393; *ibid.*, ii, 654.

[3] Snow, J. 1858. *On chloroform and other anaesthetics.* London. 260-1.

[4] *Ibid.* 251 *et seq.*

' Such measures as dashing cold water on the patient, and applying ammonia to the nostrils, can hardly be expected to have any effect on a patient who is suffering from an overdose of chloroform ; for they would have no effect whatever on one who has inhaled in the usual manner, and is merely ready for a surgical operation, but in no danger. I have applied the strongest ammonia to the nostrils of animals that were narcotized by chloroform to the third or fourth degree [see p. 163] and it did not affect the breathing in the least. It is difficult to suppose a case in which the breathing should be arrested by the effects of chloroform whilst the skin remained sensible, yet it is only in such a case that the dashing of cold water on the patient could be of use. There is, however, no harm in the application of this and such like means, provided they do not usurp the time which ought to be occupied in artificial respiration ; for this measure should be resorted to the moment the natural breathing has entirely ceased. . . .

' Whether the artificial breathing is successful or not must depend chiefly on the extent to which the heart has been paralyzed by the chloroform. . . . The fact of the breathing continuing after the action of the heart has ceased, in some of the fatal cases, shows that the heart may be so paralyzed as not to be readily restored by the breathing. It is probable that in all cases in which artificial respiration can restore the patient, its action would be very prompt ; still it is desirable to persevere with the measure for a good while.'

Snow drew attention to the fact that ' when the breathing has ceased, the tongue is indeed liable to fall backwards, if the person in a state of suspended animation is lying on the back, and this circumstance requires to be attended to in performing artificial respiration '.[1] He did not think it likely, however, that ' the falling back of the tongue into the throat, under the deep influence of chloroform, might be the cause of death by suffocation . . . for the muscles of the larynx and neighbouring parts preserve their action as long as the diaphragm, and contract consentaneously with it '.

With reference to the fairly common practice of opening one of the jugular veins Snow [2] expressed the opinion that :

' there is every reason to conclude that the right cavities of the heart are distended with blood, in all cases of suspended animation by chloroform, and therefore it would be desirable to open one of the jugular veins if the artificial respiration does not

[1] Snow, J. 1858. *On chloroform and other anaesthetics.* London. 245.
[2] *Ibid.* 261.

immediately restore the patient. In opening animals, just after death from this agent, I have observed the contractions of the heart to return, to a certain extent, when the distension of its right cavities was diminished by the division of the vessels about the root of the neck.'

He added, however, that :

' Opening of the jugular vein has been resorted to in a few of the cases of accident from chloroform, but hitherto without success.'

Snow was sceptical also about the efficacy of electricity as a means of resuscitation :

' I have not succeeded ', he stated, ' in restoring an animal from an overdose of chloroform, by means of electricity, in any case where I felt satisfied that it would not recover spontaneously ; and I have not heard of a patient being restored by its means. . . . If electricity be used, it should be directed towards restoring the action of the heart. It is probable that the electric current would not reach the heart without the help of the acupuncture needle ; but it would be justifiable to use this in a desperate case, when other measures had failed. The needles should be coated with wax, or some other non-conductor of electricity, except near the points.' [1]

In France Jobert had reported in 1853 a series of experiments made to test the resuscitative effects of electricity on chloroformed animals. He, too, found that once the contractions of the heart had been abolished they could not be restored by electricity, but when the circulation was not yet completely suspended and the animal could still be said to live electricity applied to the mucous membrane of the mouth and rectum was, in his opinion, sufficient to revive the vital functions of the body. In extreme cases, he stated, a resort had to be made to electropuncture, for this alone was sufficiently powerful to overcome the sluggishness of the organs.[2]

About two years later Duchenne, using a faradic current on the phrenic nerves, succeeded, both in chloroformed human beings and in animals, in producing powerful diaphragmatic contractions even a considerable time after death.[3]

[1] Snow, J. 1858. *On chloroform and other anaesthetics.* London. 261-2.

[2] *C.R. Acad. Sci., Paris,* 1853, **37**, 344-6.

[3] Cf. Lallemand, L., Perrin, M., and Duroy, J. L. P. 1860. *Du rôle de l'alcool et des anesthésiques dans l'organisme.* Paris. 343-5.

In 1856 von Ziemssen reported a successful clinical case of resuscitation from chloroform syncope by applying a faradic current to the diaphragm.[1] Later authorities, however, considered the external application of faradic or galvanic currents to the region of the heart to be a useless procedure and electro-puncture to be a dangerous one.[2]

In 1889 J. A. MacWilliam, Professor of the Institutes of Medicine at Aberdeen, made a series of experiments on animals which, he thought, tended to show that when the heart was suddenly inhibited through the vagus, rhythmic contraction might be excited by ' a periodic series of single induction shocks sent through the heart at approximately the normal rate of cardiac action. A single induction shock ', MacWilliam stated, ' readily causes a beat in an inhibited heart, and a regular series of induction shocks (for example, sixty or seventy per minute) gives a regular series of heart beats at the same rate '. He added to this statement the important qualification : ' Never on any occasion have I seen fibrillar contraction [3] excited by such a mode of stimulation '. He found, on the contrary, that ' the application of strong galvanic and faradic currents to the ventricles is attended with disastrous results ; an immediate abolition of the normal beat, and the occurrence of a wildly inco-ordinated, arhythmic [sic] contraction of the ventricular muscle (fibrillar contraction or heart delirium) ' ; but ' galvanic and faradic currents, too weak to induce fibrillar contraction in a heart of depressed excitability, have a comparatively trivial influence in exciting or accelerating its beat '.[4]

In 1858 a new method of artificial respiration was introduced by Henry R. Silvester, of Clapham, London, which came to be almost universally used during the remainder of the nineteenth century.[5] The method was intended for resuscitation in any circumstances, but Silvester suggested a preliminary manœuvre particularly applicable in cases of chloroform syncope. This was ' immediately and suddenly to compress the front and

[1] Ziemssen, H. von. *Greifswalder med. Beitr.*, Danzig, 1863, i, 288–92 ; reference taken from : *Surgeon-general's library index-catalogue*, Washington 1891, **12**, 68.

[2] Cf., *e.g.*, *Trans. Soc. Anaesth.*, 1898, **1**, 52.

[3] MacWilliam first drew attention to the occurrence of ventricular fibrillation in 1889. (See *Brit. med. J.*, 1889, i, 6–8.) He reported on the occurrence of ventricular fibrillation during chloroform anaesthesia in 1890. (See *Brit. med. J.*, 1890, ii, 831, 890, 948 ; see also p. 444.)

[4] *Brit. med. J.*, 1889, i, 348–9.

[5] *Lancet*, 1858, i, 353, 616.

sides of the chest by the patient's own arms, the compression to be continued for about two seconds. By this means the poisoning vapour is expelled ; and upon the pressure being suddenly relaxed, the elastic parietes of the chest recoil, and give the primary impetus to inspiration '.[1] When this had been done an attempt was made ' to imitate natural respiration by raising the ribs and thus increasing the capacity of the thorax. This is effected by forcibly drawing the arms upward toward the head ; the muscles passing from the arms to the chest wall, which are attached to the ribs, are thus made to drag the ribs upward. Expiration is effected by lowering the arms and pressing them against the sides of the thorax '. The only formidable drawback to Silvester's method was considered to be the need for two assistants in addition to the operator, one to hold forward the tongue and another to steady the trunk and legs.[2]

In 1868 the third and last of the important nineteenth century manipulative methods of artificial respiration was introduced by Benjamin Howard, of New York. Like the other methods— Marshall Hall's and Silvester's—it was not especially intended for anaesthetic emergencies. It was most widely used in the United States.

' The method consists in laying the patient on his back, kneeling over the lower part of the body, and alternately pressing on the lower part of the chest and relaxing the pressure, repeating the operation eight or ten times a minute.'

According to E. A. Schäfer :

' The advantage of the method is that it is simple and that the patient on the operating table is usually in the supine position. The disadvantages are : that the tongue is apt to fall backward and block the pharynx ; . . . that the ribs in senile subjects are brittle and may be fractured ; and that the liver in asphyxia is congested and greatly enlarged and is liable to be ruptured.' [3]

Many modifications of these three methods, Marshall Hall's, Silvester's and Howard's, were made during the nineteenth century and were in a number of cases named after their adaptors.

[1] *Med. Times, Lond.,* 1863, i, 389.
[2] Schäfer, E. A. 1908. *J. Amer. med. Ass.,* **51,** 801.
[3] *Ibid.* 1908, **51,** 801.

For about twenty-five years after the adoption of these manipulative methods of artificial respiration the use of peroral intubation in adult patients, or the insertion of a tracheotomy cannula, and subsequent pumping of air or oxygen into the lungs as a means of resuscitation were discontinued.

In 1861 Auguste Nélaton successfully resuscitated a young woman, whose pulse and respiration had suddenly ceased during an operation for vesico-vaginal fistula under chloroform, by total inversion, assistants supporting her body by its legs and thorax so that it rested on the shoulders at right angles to the operating table. This drastic procedure was supplemented by artificial respiration and the tongue was held forward.

Nélaton, believing that chloroform syncope was due to cerebral anaemia, thought that this could be most speedily remedied by sending blood back to the head by the force of gravity.[1] H. C. Wood in 1890 pointed out that this theory was 'probably incorrect. The respiration in anaesthesia fails', he said, 'not through want of blood in the respiratory centres, but because the blood contains a poison which paralyzes these centres'.[2] Leonard Hill, after carrying out experiments during the early eighteen-nineties, found that when the heart itself was paralysed and in a state of dilatation from the action of chloroform the 'feet-up' position merely aggravated the condition and was, in fact, worse than useless.[3]

Although several successful cases of resuscitation were said to have resulted from the use of Nélaton's method the difficulties of inverting an adult were too formidable for the method to become popular. By 1901 it was usual to compromise (unless the patient happened to be a child), and after securing the patient by the feet to raise the foot of the operating table or bed with the patient on it.[4]

The combination of J. O'Dwyer's laryngeal tube with G. E. Fell's foot-bellows and tubing for producing forced artificial respiration (see Appendix E, pp. 609–10) was followed, during the early eighteen-nineties, by a revival of interest in methods of insufflation.

In 1894 T. Lauder Brunton, at the International Congress of Medicine held in Rome, 'demonstrated an instrument for

[1] Rottenstein, J. B. 1880. *Traité d'anesthésie chirurgicale*. Paris. 194–7.
[2] *Trans. int. Congr. Med.*, 1891, **1**, 149.
[3] *Brit. med. J.*, 1897, i, 957.
[4] Hewitt, F. W. 1901. *Anaesthetics and their administration*. London. 479.

keeping up artificial respiration with oxygen'. The gas flowed from a cylinder along tubing to a reservoir bag and thence to two accurately-fitting nasal tubes. The rate of flow was controlled by a stopcock behind the bifurcation of the tube. ' But ', wrote Brunton some years later, ' the account which appeared in the reports was not illustrated and attracted very little attention either at the time or afterwards.' [1]

During the last twenty-five years or so of the nineteenth century there was a growing tendency among anaesthetists, particularly in America, to supplement artificial respiration by injecting, intravenously or subcutaneously, certain drugs thought to have a stimulant action on the heart or upon respiration. Among these drugs were ether,[2] alcohol, ammonia, amyl nitrite, atropine, caffeine, digitalis, and strychnine.

Careful experiments on the effects of these drugs on anaesthetized animals were carried out by Professor H. C. Wood and his colleague, David Cerna, at the University of Pennsylvania about 1890. The majority of these drugs they dismissed as being useless or nearly so. Speaking of the injection of ether, for instance, Wood (in a paper read at the International Congress of Medicine in Berlin in 1890) said :

' Although, at least in America, hypodermic injections of ether have been frequently employed even in ether accidents, such use is so absolutely absurd that it does not seem to me to require any experimental evidence of its futility. Ether in the blood acts as ether, whether it finds entrance through the lungs, through the rectum, or through the cellular tissue ; and the man who would inject ether hypodermically to a patient who is dying from ether, should, to be logical, also saturate the sponge with ether and crowd it upon his unfortunate victim.'

Speaking on the same occasion of the action of digitalis on the circulation Wood stated that :

' The influence of injections of digitalis has been, in a number of experiments, very pronounced in producing a persistent gradual rise of the arterial pressure with an increase in the size of the individual pulse-wave. In several instances, death was apparently averted by its injection. . . .'

---

[1] Brit. med. J., 1912, i, 354.
[2] A. Fabre in 1856 claimed to have demonstrated by experiments on animals that ether could be used to act as an antidote to chloroform. (C.R. Acad. Sci., Paris, 1856. 43, 193–6.)

He suggested ' that in all cases of weak heart in man, a full dose of digitalis before the administration of chloroform, would greatly lessen the danger of cardiac collapse '.

In connection with the effects of strychnine on the circulation Wood stated :

' Of all my experimental results, those which have been reached with strychnine have been the most surprising. The injection of strychnine into the jugular vein sometimes produced a gradual rise of the arterial pressure, but always caused an extraordinary and rapid increase in the rate and extent of the respiration. Thus I have seen the respiration, which had ceased for ten seconds, suddenly, under the influence of an injection of two-tenths of a grain of strychnine, become at once very large and full, and reach a rate of 130 a minute.' [1]

Wood and Cerna, about 1892, made a separate study of the effects of strychnine and also of atropine and of cocaine upon respiration and reported as follows :

' The experiments which we have made prove that the three alkaloids, atropine, strychnine, and cocaine, are all respiratory stimulants, increasing the amount of air taken in and out of the lungs ; exerting action, apparently, by a direct influence upon the nerve-centres which preside over the respiratory movements. The question which of these alkaloids is the most powerful and reliable in practical medicine, can scarcely be answered positively by means of experimentation upon the lower animals. . . . [But] although the conclusions which we have reached have been based solely upon the results of experiments made upon dogs, we think they . . . apply to the man as well as to the dog. The difficulty with the use of massive doses of cocaine and strychnine in practical medicine is the danger that attends their action on other portions of the nervous centres than the respiratory tract, and atropine, though probably not the most certain and powerful, seems the safest drug of the three, when it has been determined to get to the fullest possible influence of the agent used. . . . We believe that the best results can be obtained in practical medicine, by the simultaneous use of two or more of the respiratory stimulants. Cocaine and strychnine have so much similarity of action upon the nerve-centres that the use of one will probably increase any danger that may have been incurred by the administration of the other. The relations of atropine to cocaine and strychnine, however, are different, and it would seem that by the consentaneous use of atropine and strychnine or of atropine and cocaine, may be obtained the advantages of

[1] *Trans. int. Congr. Med.*, 1891, **1**, 144, 147.

what has been denominated by Dr. H. C. Wood . . . as " crossed action " ; the two drugs touching and reinforcing one another in their influence upon the respiratory functions, and spreading wide apart from each other in their unwished for and deleterious actions.' [1]

Strychnine seems to have been the drug most in favour among anaesthetists in England during the eighteen-nineties, and indeed it was used by some as a routine prophylactic measure. Silk, for instance, stated in 1898 that ' for some time past [he] . . . had been in the habit of giving strychnine in all cases in which he contemplated a severe operation,—injecting a small quantity (gr. 1/20) immediately after the introduction of the anaesthesia . . . and repeating the dose once or twice if necessary '. Silk also stated that ' the general idea seemed to be, now-a-days, that the dose of strychnine given to counteract the ill effects of chloroform should be much larger than it had been the custom to give. . . . Recently as much as half a grain of strychnia had been given in a case of chloroform poisoning . . . '.[2]

In the course of a discussion held by the Society of Anaesthetists in January 1898 on resuscitation in emergencies under anaesthetics, E. A. Schäfer suggested the use of two drugs ' which might be effectual '—nicotine and extract of suprarenal gland.[3] Both drugs, but particularly suprarenal extract, used intravenously ' produced an enormous contraction in the arterioles ' and suprarenal extract ' also had an extraordinary effect upon the heart, causing an enormously increased rate and force of beat '. Schäfer suggested that, in the case of suprarenal extract, ' it might be perfectly possible to inject it with complete safety in extreme cases directly into the heart by means of a hypodermic syringe '.[4]

In 1893 Hewitt, in his book *Anaesthetics and their administration* (p. 324), directed the attention of anaesthetists to the intravenous injection of saline solutions. This method of raising the blood pressure was already well-known to the physician and surgeon in connection with the treatment of the exhausted or the shocked patient. It was, however, little used by the anaesthetist until

[1] *J. Physiol.*, 1892, **13**, 892–6.
[2] *Trans. Soc. Anaesth.*, 1898, **1**, 57–8.
[3] The physiological effects of extracts of the suprarenal capsules were investigated by E. A. Schäfer and G. Oliver in 1895. (*J. Physiol.*, 1895, **18**, 230–79).
[4] *Trans. Soc. Anaesth.*, 1898, **1**, 54–5.

after 1899 when G. W. Crile had drawn attention to the close inter-relation between anaesthesia and shock.[1]

During the last ten years of the nineteenth century interest was growing among anaesthetists in the possibility of reviving the chloroform-poisoned heart by massage. The method most commonly used was that of König modified by Maas, of Göttingen.

The operator, using Maas's method, stood at the patient's left side and resting the ball of the thumb of the open left hand on the clavicle, pressed quickly and strongly with the finger tips about 120 times a minute into the region of the heart. The operator's right hand gripped the right side of the patient's thorax to steady the body. König's procedure was identical with this, except that the fingers pressed only from thirty to forty times a minute into the heart region.

Maas first successfully demonstrated his method on children —a boy of nine and a half years and another of thirteen—in whom, presumably, the chest walls were more flexible than in an adult.[2]

The other, less commonly used, method was that of resecting the ribs and massaging the heart directly. The effectiveness of this drastic measure was demonstrated on dogs by Schiff working in Florence in 1874. Schiff found that when the heart, rendered inert by chloroform, was distended with blood it was impossible, with the thorax closed, to make the heart beat either by artificial respiration or by galvanic excitation. But if the thorax was opened and at the same time air was slowly insufflated into the lungs it was sometimes possible, by rhythmic manual compression of the heart (if the abdominal aorta was compressed so as to send a greater volume of blood towards the head and care was taken not to impede the coronary circulation), to restart the heart-beat even as long as eleven and a half minutes after its arrest. Schiff noted, however, that in his experiments the revival was only temporary and incomplete. The animals were convulsed and incapable of voluntary movement and generally died within a few hours.[3]

In experimenting on animals Schiff's method of direct massage of the heart suddenly arrested from any cause was

[1] Crile, G. W. 1899. *An experimental research into surgical shock.* Philadelphia.
[2] *Berl. klin. Wschr.*, 1892, **29**, 265–8.
[3] Quoted by Arabian, H. 1903. *Contribution à l'étude du massage du cœur dans la mort par le chloroforme.* Geneva. 7, 8.

quite frequently used ; but as a clinical procedure it was rarely attempted and then only as a desperate resort after other measures had failed. It is not known ever to have been successful. In 1898 Tuffier reported to the Société de Chirurgie in Paris a case of embolism in a young man in which he temporarily revivified the heart by direct massage, reaching it by resecting the ribs. In the discussion which followed Tuffier's report two other members of the Société de Chirurgie each mentioned an instance in which they had similarly and unsuccessfully massaged the heart of a patient who, in their cases, had died from the effects of chloroform.[1]

It was not until 1902 that W. Arbuthnot Lane and E. A. Starling completely restored a patient to life by massaging the heart directly ; they reached the heart not by rib resection but by making an abdominal incision and grasping it through the diaphragm, thus avoiding pneumothorax.[2]

In April 1893 Alexander Duke, of Cheltenham, directed attention to ' the value of stretching the sphincter ani in chloroform collapse '. At the time of writing Duke had used the method in a single case only, that of a child.

' Of course, one case cannot prove much,' he wrote, ' but I am so impressed by the value of the proceeding, I think it well to call the attention of the profession to such a simple and harmless plan as one, I am quite sure, not generally known.' [3]

[1] *Bull. Soc. Chirurgie Paris*, 1898, **24**, 937, 976.
[2] *Lancet*, 1902, ii, 1476.
[3] *Med. Times, Lond.*, 1893, **21**, 201.

APPENDIX D

WARM ETHER—OPEN ETHER

Warm Ether

THAT ether in volatilizing draws heat from its immediate surroundings and that where the supply of heat is inadequate vaporization is checked or arrested are self-evident facts which were clearly recognized by members of the ' Pneumatic School ' of medicine who advocated the therapeutic inhalation of ether, among other vapours, during the last decade of the eighteenth century. For instance Thornton recommended warming the ether container—he used a teapot—by holding it near a candle flame (see p. 64). The container used by Pearson, on the other hand, was a cup or wineglass with about a dessertspoonful of ether in it, which was held under the patient's nose and mouth. Although the warmth of the hand holding the vessel would have produced some heat for vaporization Pearson suggested that in cold weather the cup should be placed in a basin of warm water and a large funnel inverted over all (its rim being slightly raised to admit air). The patient then drew the vapour into his lungs through the tube of the funnel (see pp. 63–4).

After the general introduction of surgical anaesthesia into practice during 1846 and 1847 many people found it expedient to warm the inhalers which they used for ether, either by holding them near a flame or by means of warm water (see Figs. 20–2 ; pp. 140–3). John Snow, however, expressed the opinion that many of the early failures to produce satisfactory ether anaesthesia were due to the fact that the inhalers used had not been warmed, so that ' the patient breathed air much colder than the freezing point of water and containing very little of the vapour of ether ' (see p. 139).

Snow himself was the first man to put the warming of ether for inhalation purposes upon a scientific basis. Working on ' the formula for the elastic form of the vapour of ether ' given by Ure in a paper in the *Philosophical Transactions* in 1818, Snow ascertained by experiment ' the quantity of vapour of ether that

582

100 cubic inches of air will take up, when saturated with it, at various temperatures, the barometric pressure being 30 inches of mercury ' ; these results he tabulated and then ascertained by further experiments that the maximum percentage of ether vapour in air which ' the patient can be got freely to breathe ' was, as a rule, ' nearly 47 per cent. ' (see pp. 156–7).

Snow proceeded to devise an apparatus (see Figs. 29, 30) which delivered to the patient an ether-air mixture containing between 34 and 46 per cent. of ether vapour. The mixture could be diluted by allowing the ingress of atmospheric air through the expiratory valve of the facepiece.

To control vaporization Snow ' made use of the conducting power of the metals, and the great capacity of water for caloric ' ; he constructed his ether-vaporizing chamber from plated copper and placed it in a water-bath. The water-bath contained 100 cubic inches of water at between 50° and 60° F., *i.e.* water from the domestic cold-water supply was used and only occasionally was it necessary to warm or cool it (see p. 156).

For completing an average administration Snow usually found that about two fluid ounces of ether, poured into the vaporizing chamber before induction, were sufficient. He stated that 100 cubic inches of water ' will . . . supply the caloric necessary to the conversion of one or two ounces of ether into vapour without being much reduced in temperature ; and as the heat of the water employed differs little from that of the air of the patient's room, it is not much altered during an operation by radiation or other causes ' (see p. 156).

Before Snow's ' regulating ether inhaler ' had been extensively used, however, the use of ether as the sole anaesthetic was almost completely abandoned and remained so in England until the ether revival of 1872 (see Chapter XI).

In the northern states of America the use of ether as a general anaesthetic persisted. Between about 1850 and 1900 by far the most common method of administration was to pour the ether directly on to a conical sponge enclosed in a cone improvised from some material impervious to air, or nearly so. Usually the sponge was wrung out·of warm water immediately before the ether was poured on. Then the cone was held firmly over the patient's nose and mouth, the exhaled mixture being reinhaled, until he became insensible.

On the Continent of Europe, after about 1850, the only important stronghold of ether anaesthesia for some twenty-five years was Lyons. Throughout this period the surgeons there continued to use Roux's *sac* (see Fig. 24). This was a bag lined with a pig's bladder. A small quantity of ether was poured into the bottom and the mouth of the bag was held over the patient's nose and mouth and he breathed to and fro, with occasional intermissions, during anaesthesia (see pp. 146, 207, 424).

When the use of ether anaesthesia was revived in England in 1872 the American 'cone' method of administration at first prevailed ; but during 1873 the use of inhaling apparatuses gradually returned. J. T. Clover in 1873 introduced an inhaler in which the ether was warmed by leading back the patient's exhalations down a bent tube running through the interior of the vaporizing chamber (see pp. 323–5 ; Fig. 82).

In his apparatus designed between 1874 and 1876 for giving a nitrous oxide-ether sequence Clover surrounded his ether reservoir with a jacket containing cold water (see pp. 325–8), but immediately before use the ether vessel was 'dipped into a basin of warm water, and rotated until the thermometer [mounted in its wall] stands at about 68 deg. '—or, 'if the patient have thin cheeks and large whiskers, the temperature may be 73 deg.' (see p. 326).

The ether container of Clover's 'portable regulating ether inhaler' (1877) was also partly surrounded by a water-jacket (see pp. 342–4 ; Figs. 89 and 90). Clover stated of this container 'it does not need to be warmed before it is used '. Nevertheless Hewitt, who subsequently modified the inhaler, recommended that in very cold weather or in order to anaesthetize an alcoholic man the ether chamber should be briefly immersed in hot water immediately before induction was begun (see p. 346).

When using Ormsby's inhaler (1877), which consisted of a bag, a facepiece, and a sponge held in a wire case, the anaesthetist usually squeezed the sponge out of warm water before pouring the ether upon it (see pp. 349–50 ; Fig. 95). Hewitt, however, had a small water vessel made which was inserted into the sponge itself to prevent it becoming too cold during administration (see p. 352 ; Fig. 97).

In 1895 R. W. Carter, 'with the assistance of Mr. Krohne (of Krohne and Sesemann, the surgical instrument makers) ' devised an ingenious apparatus (Fig. 155), called the 'Thermo-Ether Inhaler', which worked upon the same principle as Junker's chloroform inhaler (cf. Fig. 120). The lower part of the ether bottle, through which a stream of air was driven to the

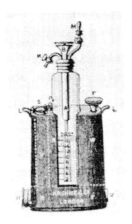

A. Bottle for ether holding two ounces. N. Connexion for facepiece or mouth-tube. M. That to bellows. RW. Water-jacket provided with funnel, F, for filling, and vent hole fitted with plug, P. H. Cylinder in which Japanese tinder is inserted into RT, the tinder chamber. V. Vent hole to chamber. S. Shutter which regulates the admission of air and so of combustion.

FIG. 155.—THE 'THERMO-ETHER INHALER'

Designed by R. W. Carter, about 1896. The design was based upon that of Junker's inhaler, *i.e.* a stream of air was driven, by hand-bellows, through the ether vessel to a facepiece. The ether in the vessel was warmed by a water-jacket, the temperature of the water being kept constant by a charge of 'Japanese tinder' (agaric) which was kept smouldering by a draught of air passing through its container. The ether bottle and its container hung from the administrator's neck by a strap passing through the rings, L, L.

facepiece by a hand-bellows, was surrounded by a water-jacket, the water being poured in at a temperature of 100° F. When the inhaler was to be used for a succession of administrations the water could be kept hot by means of a small charge of smouldering 'Japanese tinder' (agaric). 'One of these charges', Carter stated, 'lasts from one to two hours.' The rate of combustion

19*

was controlled by a shutter which regulated the draught of air passing over the ' tinder '.[1]

On the Continent the revival of the use of ether for general anaesthesia took place gradually during the last quarter of the nineteenth century. Two basic methods of administration were recognized. By the first—Julliard's or the Geneva method—use was made of a large, wire face-mask lined with surgical gauze and having a flannel pad on to which the ether was poured. The mask was covered over outside by waxed cloth so that the admixture of air was restricted. By the second method, Wanscher's, the patient breathed to and fro into a rubber bag resembling Ormsby's, but without the sponge, the liquid ether being poured directly into the bag (see pp. 405–6, 410 ; Figs. 109–12, 114).

The first of the Continental inhalers, during this period, deliberately designed to provide a source of heat to facilitate vaporization was the Wagner-Longard inhaler (Fig. 156). It consisted of a hollow metal cylinder, one end being rubber rimmed and adapted to fit over the face ; the other was furnished with a shallow ' funnel-shaped ' lid. At the lowest point of the lid were a few holes and beneath them, but within the cylinder, was a spring-loaded inspiratory valve. A spring-loaded expiratory valve was set in the wall of the cylinder behind the rubber rim of the facepiece. The upper half of the cylinder was partitioned off transversely by two layers of metal gauze (the top one removable) and between these surgical gauze was laid. Liquid ether was poured into the funnel-shaped lid and ran through into the inspiratory valve. When the valve was drawn down by the patient's inspiration the ether fell through the upper layer of metal gauze on to the surgical gauze where it evaporated and mixed with the stream of air.[2] This mixing of fresh air with the ether vapour at every inspiration, and the avoidance of rebreathing, were innovations in Continental practice which were very favourably received by many surgeons in Germany.

It was found, however, that in wet weather the moisture in the air drawn into the inhaler condensed (owing to the rapid cooling due to the evaporation of the ether), forming tiny ice crystals which encrusted the metal gauze partitions, the surgical gauze between them, and the inspiratory valve itself, impairing

---

[1] *Med. Times, Lond.*, August 24, 1895, reprint.   [2] *Zbl. Chir.*, 1898, **25**, 1193–5.

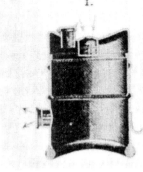 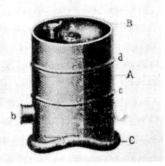

Fig. 156.—WAGNER-LONGARD ETHER INHALER

In use at Aachen, about 1900. Immediately before administration was begun a patent device for absorbing and retaining heat, called a 'Thermophor' (not shown), previously immersed in boiling water, was inserted into the uppermost compartment of the inhaler to prevent the excessive chilling of the inhaler due to the evaporation of ether.

I. The inhaler in section. Arrows indicate the direction of air entering the inspiratory valve and of the exhaled mixture leaving the inhaler through the expiratory valve.

II. Exterior view of the inhaler.

    A. Metal case of the inhaler.
    B. Funnel-shaped lid.
    C. Inflated rubber rim fitting the patient's face.
    a. Holes arranged in a rosette at the lowest part of the lid; beneath them was a spring-loaded inspiratory valve (seen in section in I.).
    b. Expiratory valve (seen in section in I.).
    c, d. Indicate the location of two layers of wire gauze partitioning the inhaler transversely (as shown in I.).

Between *c* and *d* surgical gauze was laid. Liquid ether was poured into the funnel-shaped lid and dropped through the rosette of holes into the inspiratory valve. When the valve was drawn down by the patient's inspiration, the liquid ether fell through on to the surgical gauze and its vapour mixed with the current of air drawn through the inhaler.

587

its action. To remedy this Longard[1] had made, by a Berlin firm specializing in such things, an ' annular *thermophor* ' (the precise nature of which was not disclosed). The *thermophor*, when immersed in boiling water for from one to two minutes, absorbed and subsequently retained heat; it was placed, immediately before induction was begun, between the upper layer of metal gauze and the lid of the inhaler, where it fitted accurately. By warming the incoming stream of air it effectively prevented the formation of ice crystals.[2]

All these methods of deliberately warming ether described above had one aim—to make the administration of ether vapour more readily controllable by the administrator. In 1876 Robert Lawson Tait, surgeon to the Birmingham Hospital for Women, suggested a very different motive for warming ether—the prevention or lessening of the danger to the patient of pulmonary and bronchial complications following the inhalation of ether vapour.

' For the last two years,' wrote Tait in 1876, ' I have had ether given in all my ovariotomies, and, indeed, in all operations where it was at hand. . . .

' About the time that my friend Mr. Jessop noticed in the *Lancet* [1875, ii, 326] that patients might suffer from the after effects of ether in the shape of pulmonary inflammation, I had a case of severe bronchitis in an aged person after the administration of ether. A few weeks after, I had another experience of a similar kind, and then became convinced that ether was not free from risk, and that the source of danger was the loss of heat on the pulmonary surface by the administration of air and ether vapour at a very low temperature. . . .

' Having twice experienced the danger from bronchitis, I tried various plans for removing what I believed to be its cause, and that which I found to be the best, is to give the vapour of boiling anhydrous ether [ether boils at 34·6° C., just below body temperature], pure and free from any admixture of air.'

Lawson Tait's apparatus (Fig. 157) and method of use were as follows : liquid ether was poured into a reservoir (capacity about ten ounces). The reservoir was fitted with a spring pump which at every stroke injected about one drachm of ether into a glass vaporizing chamber partly immersed in a water tank kept

[1] The inhaler itself was designed by Wagner alone. He appears to have based hi design on that of an American inhaler for ether devised by Joseph W. Hearn, os Philadelphia, about 1883. (Cf. Turnbull, L. 1880 (2nd ed.). *The advantages and accidents of artificial anaesthesia.* London. 233.)
[2] *Zbl. Chir.*, 1900, **27**, 857–8.

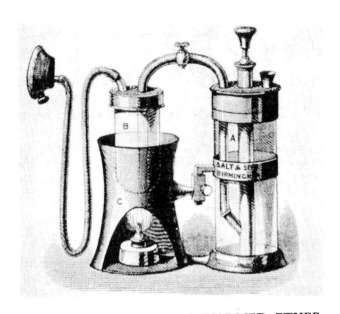

FIG. 157.—LAWSON TAIT'S WARMED ETHER
INHALER (1876)

For administering 'the vapour of boiling anhydrous
ether, pure and free from any admixture of air', in
order to reduce the risk of post-operative chest complications, believed by Lawson Tait to be due to the
cooling of the pulmonary surface by the mixture when
inhaled at a low temperature.

    A. Ether reservoir, with piston which injected, at each
        stroke, one drachm of liquid ether into
    B. Vaporizing chamber, partly immersed in
    C. Water tank, kept hot by the spirit lamp beneath.

The resulting vapour then passed through four or
five feet of rubber tubing to the facepiece, which was
fitted with an expiratory valve; it reached the patient
at a temperature of from 31°–33° C. The length of the
tubing was considered, by Lawson Tait, to be sufficient
to avoid the danger of ether vapour escaping from
the facepiece being exploded by the flame of the spirit
lamp.

589

hot by a spirit lamp beneath (Lawson Tait gave a warning that any leakage of ether might cause an explosion). The ether vapour was led off through four or five feet of rubber tubing (as a safeguard against explosion) to a facepiece ; it was claimed that the vapour reached the facepiece at a temperature of 31° C. to 33° C. For an ordinary induction about three drachms of liquid ether were pumped into the vaporizing chamber.

' The advance which we have made in our knowledge of anaesthetics since 1849,' wrote Tait, ' is in no way commensurate with the enormous amount of labour which has been devoted to the subject. We have, it seems to me, made no advance on ether for surgical work. . . .

' I think the method I have detailed will be found to be a substantial advance. . . . Dr. Lauder Brunton made to me the ingenious suggestion of having a steam-jacket round the boiler, but that I have not found to be practicable without greatly complicating the apparatus. The use of a hot iron bolt to boil the water, instead of the lamp, would probably be safer, but it would not be so handy, and would involve great wear and tear.' [1]

Although the incidence of bronchial and pulmonary complications following ether anaesthesia continued to disturb anaesthetists, no notice whatever was taken of Lawson Tait's recommendation. It was not until 1891 (so far as can be traced) that the administration of ether at 31° C. was again mentioned. The following brief account appeared as an annotation in the *British Medical Journal* :

' *Warm Ether as Anaesthetic*

' We learn from the *Independencia Medica*, of Barcelona, that on October 31st Dr. Giné y Partagás performed an operation for osteoma of the fibula on a woman . . . the anaesthetic used being ether warmed to 31° C., which was administered by Dr. A. Diaz de Liaño, with an apparatus of his own invention. Anaesthesia was rapidly induced and was kept up for fifty-five minutes. . . . The apparatus, which is called by its inventor an " Electro-thermo-etheriser," has since been used in several other cases with equally satisfactory results.' [2]

Still no great interest was aroused in warmed ether ; nor indeed was it aroused until after the publication of Gwathmey's researches on warmed and unwarmed anaesthetics in 1912.[3]

[1] *Practitioner*, 1876, **16**, 206–9.   [2] *Brit. Med. J.*, 1891, ii, 1322.
[3] See Gwathmey, J. T. 1912. ' The value of warmed anesthetics.' *New York Medical Journal*, **95**, 1130–3.

Open Ether

From 1873 onwards Lawson Tait, in his gynaecological practice, had been in the habit of giving methylene ether—a new anaesthetic introduced into practice by B. W. Richardson in 1872 (see p. 319)—in a manner precisely similar to J. Y. Simpson's later method of giving chloroform (see pp. 192-3) by dropping the liquid on to a single fold of towel held over the patient's face.[1]

Describing in 1882 his open-drop method of giving ' anhydrous methylated ether ' Lawson Tait wrote :

' It is always given for me after the simple fashion which Sir James Simpson introduced for the administration of chloroform, that is by dropping it on the outside of a single fold of a towel, laid upon the patient's face. Bearing in mind that ether is extremely volatile, and that its vapor is very heavy, the following directions must be attended to. The towel used must not be too thin, because it must retain a sufficient body of ether for the continuance of the current of vapor ; and yet it must not be so thick as to prevent the passage of air freely through it. The ether must be dropped on to the towel, not splashed on, but administered in a continuous stream, which must be allowed to drop from a small orifice on to the towel, above the level of the patient's nose, because the vapor of the ether will fall like a cataract over the patient's face. If the ether is dropped on the towel on a level with the patient's mouth, she will inhale, not the vapor, but a mixture of air and ether, which will act as a stimulant and not as an anaesthetic, and the ether must not be splashed on, for exactly the same reason. The towel should not be tightened over the face, but puffed out around it at a distance of an inch, or an inch and a half, from the skin, in order that it may enclose a body of vapor. The whole of the piece of towel covering the face must be kept continually moist with ether, and in this way a continuous volume of pure ether vapor will be inhaled by the patient. After a few minutes the part of the towel in use must be changed for another part, because anhydrous ether absorbs with intense avidity the moisture of the breath, and the towel will be found coated with ice, and thus, by its interference with rapid evaporation, prolongs the process : this is the chief argument against all ether inhalers. Only one other caution need be given, and that is to avoid bringing any light or red-hot cautery near the patient's face while the ether is being given, for it is explosive. . . .

[1] *Brit. med. J.*, 1873, i, 253, 254.

' The quantity of ether given during an operation, especially during ovariotomy, is necessarily very large, but no one need ever be alarmed on account of the quantity of ether administered. It is absolutely necessary to keep all the patient's abdominal muscles, except the diaphragm, perfectly quiet; and long before there is the least danger the patient's deep snoring will indicate that the stage of profound sleep has been reached. When the patient snores the administration should for a short time be discontinued. The quiet regularity of breathing which always characterizes the unconscious state induced by breathing the vapor of ether is quite enough to indicate to any one of any experience in its use that the patient is in a condition of profound insensibility, and this will also serve as the best indication of safety. There is, therefore, very little need for the pulse being watched, or for the conjunctiva to be experimented upon to determine unconsciousness. Should sickness come on during the operation, the ether should be pushed a little more and this will stop it, because sickness really is an indication of returning consciousness.' [1]

As in the case of his use of warmed ether Lawson Tait's use of the open-drop method of giving the drug was not followed by others.

During the eighteen-seventies also, O. H. Allis's ether inhaler (see pp. 352–5; Figs. 98–101) was introduced into American practice and attempts were made to popularize its use in England. But although this inhaler was designed to allow a freer access of air to the evaporating surface on to which the ether was dropped than was possible when the towel cone was used, the ' dead space ' of this inhaler prevents it from being classed as an open-drop inhaler in the generally accepted sense of the term.

It was not until the late eighteen-nineties that attention in America, and soon afterwards in Germany, began seriously to turn to the practicability of open-drop methods of giving ether.

The movement began with L. H. Prince, of Chicago. He stated in 1897 that for the past two years he had been using an ordinary Esmarch's chloroform mask on to which he dropped ether. The only disadvantage was the small evaporating surface, but he was already having a larger mask made. [2] It was several years, however, before the method gained much of a following in America.

[1] Tait, L. 1883. *The pathology and treatment of diseases of the ovaries.* Birmingham. 263–4, 266.   [2] *Chicago med. Rec.*, 1897, **12**, 232–40.

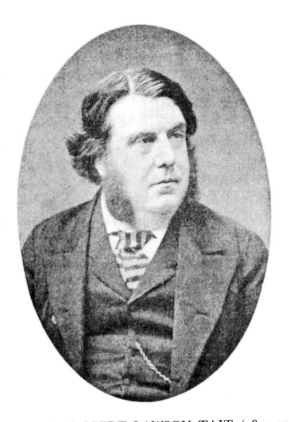

FIG. 158.—ROBERT LAWSON TAIT (1845-99)
Gynaecologist and surgeon, received his medical
education in his native city, Edinburgh, and was
a pupil of and later assistant to James Young
Simpson. In 1870 Tait removed to Birmingham,
and during the eighteen-seventies was at the height
of his career. An individualist in all that he did,
Tait adopted the open method of giving ether when
his contemporaries were developing closed methods.
It was he who first suggested warming ether not
merely to facilitate vaporization but as a possible
means of obviating post-operative chest complications, then considered the chief danger of ether
anaesthesia.

Among the first hospitals to adopt open ether was St. Mary's Hospital, Rochester, Min. (the Mayo Clinic), where S. G. Davis was the chief exponent of the method. The *Lancet*, quoting from the *Maryland Medical Journal* for May, 1907, described Davis's technique :

'. . . The inhaler consists of a wire frame like that of Esmarch's chloroform inhaler but larger. . . . It may be covered with one or two layers of stockinette or with several layers of gauze. The best covering is about six layers of ordinary gauze. . . . The inhaler is applied over the patient's face [a piece of 'rubber protective' having been placed over the eyes, and the rest of the face protected by a moist towel or gauze laid round it] and the ether is administered drop by drop, very slowly at first, then gradually more rapidly as the patient takes stronger vapour. Finally, at about the time when he will not respond to questions, a moist towel or some gauze is wrapped snugly round the mask, leaving a small area in the centre for the free passage of air through the gauze.' [1]

A report of similar methods in use at the Mount Sinai Hospital, Cleveland, had appeared in the *Journal of the American Medical Association* in 1906.[2]

An example of the typical European conception, during the eighteen-nineties, of how a mask should be used for chloroform anaesthesia and how it should be used for more volatile anaesthetics such as ether is furnished in an article, written in English, by Professor Dreser, of the University of Bonn, for publication in the *Johns Hopkins Hospital Bulletin* :

'Surgeons now try to substitute less dangerous agents, such as bromide of ethyl, ether or pental for chloroform, which is suspected of being a heart poison. The vapour of these fluids, which are more volatile than chloroform, must accumulate in the air, to be inhaled in a far greater quantity than in the case of chloroform. Therefore the simple Esmarch's mask used for chloroform is not efficient. The permeable cover of the Esmarch mask would bring about quite the contrary effect. The air exhaled by the patient being of a higher temperature than the surrounding atmosphere, a great quantity of ether would escape into the room ; whereas the cooler atmosphere of the room, passing through the cover of the mask at the next inhalation, will carry too little ether into the patient's lungs.

'For this reason the great basket mask of Julliard has an impermeable cover of waxed taffeta. . . .' [3]

[1] *Lancet*, 1907, i, 1585.   [2] *J. Amer. med. Ass.*, 1906, **47**, 1653.
[3] *Johns. Hopk. Hosp. Bull.*, 1895, **6**, 7.

Nevertheless from about 1901 onwards the open-drop method of ether anaesthesia began to be developed in Germany independently, it seems, of American influence.

In 1902 C. Hofmann, of Cologne, stated that he had completed a series of experiments in which he administered ether to animals by dropping it from a drop-bottle on to gauze stretched over a Schimmelbusch mask (see Fig. 61). He concluded from these experiments that in order to produce adequate surgical anaesthesia in the adult human being by the open-drop method it would be necessary to supplement the ether by an injection of morphine, given about an hour before the inhalation was begun. If this were done most satisfactory anaesthesia would result. Hofmann thought, however, that in certain cases a very small amount of chloroform might prove helpful in hastening induction.[1]

Also in 1902 Oscar Witzel, of Bonn, reported a series of clinical cases in which he had dropped ether on to an oval mask overlaid with four thicknesses of sterilized, loosely woven gauze held in place by a stout metal hoop. During administration a junior house surgeon held the mask in position and steadied the patient's head. The senior house surgeon, under Witzel's direction, allowed ether to fall drop after drop continuously from a bottle held with one hand one third of a metre above the mask ; with the other hand he followed the patient's pulse beat.[2]

In 1906 the Annual Meeting of the British Medical Association was held in Toronto. A number of members (perhaps at the invitation of W. J. Mayo who, as President of the American Medical Association, attended the Toronto meeting) took the opportunity of visiting the Mayo Clinic at Rochester, Minnesota. There they saw S. G. Davis anaesthetizing with ether by the open-drop method.

Some interest was aroused by this demonstration, particularly among a few anaesthetists who were in the habit of using Allis's inhaler or other methods which they considered equivalent to an open-drop technique.[3] But the man who exerted the most powerful influence in establishing open ether in England was H. Bellamy Gardner, and he was not led to make a trial of the method by any particular American example.

[1] Dtsch. Z. Chir., 1902, 65, 403–16.
[2] Münch. med. Wschr., 1902, 49 (ii), 1993–4.
[3] See, e.g., Brit. med. J., 1907, ii, 1823–4.

He reported three months' personal experience of open ether in the *British Medical Journal* for November 23, 1907, and made a further communication on the subject to the same journal in 1908.[1] In 1910 he read an important paper on ' The open system of ether administration ' at the Annual Meeting of the British Medical Association [2] in which he stressed the importance of a hypodermic injection of atropine before the administration of ether by the open method, in order to check the secretion of saliva and mucus.

[1] *Brit. med. J.*, 1907, ii, 1516 ; *ibid.* 1908, i, 145.
[2] *Ibid.* 1910, ii, 766–7.

APPENDIX E

INTUBATION AND THE GROWTH OF
ENDOTRACHEAL ANAESTHESIA

RALPH M. WATERS has assigned to the development of endotracheal anaesthesia what appeared to him to be three main causes : ' (1) the treatment of respiratory obstruction and resuscitation by artificial respiration ; (2) protection of the tracheo-bronchial tree from contamination by debris in surgery of the mouth and nose ; and (3) control of intra-pulmonary pressure in thoracic surgery '.[1]

So far as group (1) is concerned, intubation, both by passing a tube through the mouth into the larynx and by inserting a cannula into the trachea through an incision to allow air or oxygen to be blown into the lungs, was adopted during 1847 as a ready-to-hand means of resuscitation in anaesthetic emergencies (cf. p. 566 *et seq.*). The idea of introducing an anaesthetic vapour into the patient's lungs by such means as a routine procedure in certain types of surgical work was not, however, suggested until some twenty years later.

Nevertheless John Snow in 1852, ' in order to see more precisely the action of the vapour of chloroform on the heart, when not sufficiently diluted ', administered the drug to a young rabbit in a jar and then opened the trachea and tied in a tube through which the animal breathed air from a bladder until a return to consciousness was imminent when a second bladder, containing air and 10 per cent. chloroform vapour, was substituted for the first. Meanwhile the lungs and heart had been exposed and were under observation.[2]

Snow also recorded one clinical case of anaesthesia produced through a laryngotomy wound.

' I also administered it [chloroform], on four occasions, to a patient of Mr. Partridge, a boy four years old, who was believed to have a button in some part of the air-passages. The larynx had been opened a few days previously to the first occasion in

[1] *Anesth. & Analges.*, 1933, **12**, 196.
[2] Snow, J. 1858. *On chloroform and other anaesthetics.* London. 117.

which I gave chloroform, and I administered it on a sponge, held near to the tube in the larynx. It was necessary to give the vapour gently at first, just as if it was entering in the usual way. When it was given at all strong, whilst the patient was still conscious, he showed exactly the distress that a patient experiences when he says that the vapour produces a choking feeling ; which confirms my opinion that the feeling referred to the throat, from the action of pungent vapours and gases, is caused by their presence in the lungs. The chloroform was given to keep the child quiet whilst Mr. Partridge searched for the supposed button in the larynx and bronchi. When the child recovered from the chloroform, before the operation was concluded, the explorations in its air-passages embarrassed the breathing much more, and caused more apparent threatening of suffocation, than they did when he was under the influence of the vapour.' [1]

Packing off the throat (and hence the necessity for intubation) to prevent the entrance of blood and operative debris into the air-passages was never suggested by Snow. Referring to the removal of tumours of the upper jaw, for instance, Snow wrote :

' Mr. Syme, Mr. Lizars, and some other surgeons, expressed an opinion at one time that chloroform could not be safely used in this operation, as the blood would be liable to flow into the lungs. This is not the case, however, as the glottis retains its sensibility apparently unimpaired, if the influence of the chloroform is not too deep or long continued. It is only necessary to hold the head forward now and then, when the throat is very full of blood, in order to allow the patient the same opportunity of breathing that he would require if he were awake. A good deal of blood passes into the stomach in great operations about the mouth under the influence of chloroform ; and if a few drops pass into the wind-pipe they are coughed up again, as they would be in the waking state. . . . The glottis appears to retain some sensibility as long as a creature is capable of breathing. . . .
' I have always made the patient insensible in the usual way, with the inhaler, before the operation of removing tumours of the jaw, and have kept up the insensibility during the operation by means of a mixture of chloroform and spirit on a hollow sponge [2]. . . . Owing to the hands of the surgeon and

[1] Snow, J. 1858. *On chloroform and other anaesthetics.* London. 312.
[2] Whenever Snow was obliged for any reason to lay aside his regulating chloroform inhaler (see Fig. 41) he was in the habit of administering chloroform from a hollow sponge, and to prevent the possibility of giving an overdose he diluted the drug with alcohol (cf. p. 194).

assistants being very much in the way, I have not always been able to keep the patient quite insensible throughout the operation. He has sometimes struggled or cried out, but there has been hardly any case in which the patient afterwards remembered any considerable part of the operation.'[1]

The rather unsatisfactory state of affairs described by Snow in the latter part of this account provides an explanation of his contention that blood would not enter the lungs. For if the anaesthetist[2] was using a dilute mixture of chloroform with alcohol and air, and at the same time had constantly to be moving out of the way of the surgeon and his assistants, it would not be possible for him to maintain more than very light, intermittent anaesthesia ; consequently the patient's cough reflex would never be abolished during the operation.

A deliberate attempt to make use of the cough reflex in operations on the mouth under ' mixed anaesthesia' (morphine followed by chloroform) was made by Karl Thiersch about 1877. By maintaining only an analgesic state Thiersch was able to gain the patient's co-operation in coughing up and spitting out blood and debris when requested to do so.[3]

Friedrich Trendelenburg, however, while an assistant at Langenbeck's Clinic in Berlin, had already, in 1869, come to the conclusion that in all operations on the larynx and the buccal and pharyngeal cavities the trachea ought to be packed off to prevent the inspiration of blood and debris.

The method which he evolved was to anaesthetize the patient and, as the first step in operative procedure, to perform tracheotomy. Through the wound he then introduced a cannula with a tampon round it—' a delicate double-walled indiarubber tube of about 3·4 centimetres in length' which, ' when inflated within the trachea, thoroughly plugs the space between the cannula and the windpipe'. The tampon was inflated in situ, through ' a small tube opening into the external wall', by means of ' a small indiarubber balloon, with an ivory nozzle'.

---

[1] Snow, J. 1858. On chloroform and other anaesthetics. London. 280–1.
[2] Not every anaesthetist was so expert (or, perhaps, so fortunate) as Snow in anaesthetizing for this type of case. F. E. Junker in 1872 stated in the Medical Times (i, 510) :
    ' It has happened in the practice of some of the most eminent Surgeons that they had been obliged to perform tracheotomy and suck out the blood from the air-passages, often with but negative results, in order to save the life of the patient.'
[3] Lancet, 1877, ii, 861–2.

After inflating the tampon by gently pressing the balloon the latter was detached and the small tube was closed with a clip. The tampon was prevented from slipping by a raised shoulder of about one millimetre in thickness above and below it on the cannula itself.

Anaesthesia was kept up through the cannula during the operation. The anaesthetic apparatus (see Fig. 159) consisted of a japanned-tin funnel, with thin flannel stretched on a slightly raised wire frame over the mouth ; on to this the anaesthetic (Trendelenburg used chloroform) was dropped. Fresh air entered the funnel through a number of holes arranged in a ring

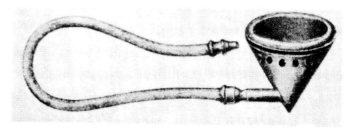

FIG. 159.—TRENDELENBURG'S CONE

For the administration of an anaesthetic vapour (chloroform) through a tube inserted into the trachea by tracheotomy. The method was introduced into German practice in 1869.

The chloroform was dropped on to the flannel cover of the cone. Air was drawn in through the ring of holes and the chloroform-air mixture passed along the tubing, the nozzle of which was inserted into the tracheotomy cannula.

just below its rim. To the outlet of the funnel was attached one end of from two to three feet of rubber tubing (this length enabled the anaesthetist to place himself out of the surgeon's way), stiffened with a spirally coiled wire to prevent kinking. The other end of the tubing was provided with a cone-shaped nozzle which fitted into the external aperture of the tracheotomy cannula. ' Before the removal of the plug, after the operation, the larynx—viz., the portion of the trachea above the tampon— has to be carefully irrigated with warm water by introducing into the trachea a delicate curved nozzle of the irrigation-tube through the superior angle of the tracheal incision.' [1]

The German physician F. E. Junker, who was for many years resident in England, was the first to give anaesthetists in this

[1] *Med. Times, Lond.*, 1872, i, 510–11.

country a detailed eye-witness account of Trendelenburg's tampon-cannula in use. He stated in 1872 that the apparatus could be obtained from Krohne and Sesemann, the London firm of surgical instrument makers. In place of the funnel and tubing, Junker said, Esmarch's or Skinner's masks (see Figs. 56, 58-9), moistened with chloroform, could be held against the external aperture of the cannula, or the afferent tube of his own chloroform inhaler (see Fig. 63) could be inserted and a chloroform-air mixture pumped in.

In England the use of Trendelenburg's tampon-cannula and method of anaesthesia was never more than occasional, but as late as 1900 D. W. Buxton mentioned its use ' in extensive removals of growths about the jaws ',[1] adding that ' it is quite possible to obtain a most satisfactory anaesthesia with ether.' [2] A year later, in 1901, Hewitt also described the method in connection with excision of the larynx and of laryngeal growths (see pp. 608-9).

In 1878 William Macewen, surgeon and lecturer at the Glasgow Royal Infirmary, decided to try the ' introduction of tracheal tubes by the mouth instead of performing tracheotomy or laryngotomy '. He intended the procedure to be used as a means of relieving such conditions as acute oedema of the glottis and also to allow the packing off of the throat and the administration of chloroform in operations where blood and operative debris were liable to be aspirated into the air-passages.

' *Post-mortem* experience showed ', wrote Macewen, ' that instruments of the tube kind could, after a little practice, be passed with facility through the mouth into the trachea. This was accomplished by introducing the finger into the mouth, depressing the epiglottis on the tongue, and so guiding the tube over the back of the finger into the larynx. In experimenting with various instruments, it was found more easy to introduce those of a large calibre [3], such as Nos. 18 to 20, than instruments

[1] Buxton himself had developed a method of rectal etherization for use in such cases. (Buxton, D. W. 1900. *Anaesthetics : their uses and administration*. London. 136-9.)
[2] Buxton, D. W. 1900. *Anaesthetics : their uses and administration*. London. 40.
[3] In a letter addressed to the Nuffield Department of Anaesthetics, dated 28/3/40, Dr. W. B. Primrose, of Glasgow, stated that he had discussed this method of endotracheal intubation with Sir William Macewen's son, who has in his possession two of the original tubes. ' One is a piece of flexible brass about 9 inches long and about ¾ inches diameter ending in a bevelled tip. The other is a wire coil about 4 inches long ending in a pointed nozzle with 4 lateral apertures : this looked like ½ in. or 1/16 in. diameter and presumably required some kind of introducer.' Dr. Primrose added that ' this seemed an extraordinarily large instrument to pass through the glottis '.

of the size of 8 to 10 catheters—the latter being more liable
to catch on the various irregularities on the internal laryngeal
surface.

'While it was easy to introduce instruments by the mouth
into the trachea, it was difficult to pass them through the nose
into the air-passages. . . . A catheter, having a strong properly
curved stilette, after considerable labour and many efforts, might
find its way into the larynx ; but even this could not be depended
on. . . .'

The first occasion on which Macewen passed a tube through
the mouth into the larynx clinically was in order to pack off the
throat and anaesthetize the patient. He described the case in
detail :

'*Case 1*.—Removal of Epithelioma from Pharynx and Base
of Tongue : Introduction of Tube into Trachea through Mouth
to occlude Haemorrhage from Larynx and for administration of
Anaesthetic.—

. . . .

'As it was an operation which would cause considerable
bleeding, precautions had to be taken to secure the air-passages
from occlusion. Hitherto this had been effected by opening the
windpipe, by laryngotomy, and the introduction of Trendelenburg's tampon-cannula. Instead of this, I had determined,
should an opportunity present, to introduce into the trachea, by
way of the mouth a tube, which would extend beyond the vocal
cords, and through which the patient would respire. The upper
laryngeal opening could then be plugged outside this tube, so
as to prevent the entrance of blood into the larynx. The plug
could then be effected in various ways, by causing the tracheal
tube to perforate a close sponge of suitable size, which, after the
tracheal tube had been introduced, could then be fixed in the
laryngeal orifice ; by fixing to the tube, at a convenient part, a
piece of fine muslin or other material, which would act as the
canule à chemise used after lithotomy ; by inflation of a closely
fitting bag, etc.

'Preparatory to the operation, a tube was several times
inserted through the mouth into the trachea, beyond the vocal
cords ; and it was found that, with the exception of the cough
which ensued immediately on its insertion, he [the patient]
bore the tube sufficiently well to warrant the success of the
procedure. . . .

'The operation was performed on July 5, 1878. The usual
cough followed the introduction of the tube ; but it ceased as
soon as he received a few whiffs of chloroform, and long before

he became constitutionally affected by the drug ; the chloroform seemed to exercise a local sedative effect. The upper opening of the larynx was stuffed with a sponge. . . . The tube projected several inches beyond the mouth, thus enabling the administration of the anaesthetic to be continued uninterruptedly during the whole operation, without in any way interfering with the manipulative procedure. The entrance and exit of air through the tube was both felt and heard distinctly, so that Dr. Symington (who administered the chloroform) had a ready guide to the state of the respiration. After the operation was finished, when the haemorrhage had ceased and the patient had regained consciousness, the tube was withdrawn, it having acted throughout without the slightest hitch. . . .

' The air, as it passes through the natural passages into the lungs, becomes warmed, moistened, and filtered. When a wound is made into the trachea through the neck and a short tube is inserted, the cold dry unfiltered air gets access to the lungs, and often produces fatal congestion. . . . The tubes introduced through the mouth do away with the necessity of supplying extraneous warmth and moisture.'

Among hints on the introduction of tubes Macewen noted that 'before introducing the tubes, an examination by the laryngoscope[1] ought to be made to ascertain the precise state of the parts '. Macewen advised also that ' if any hitch occurred at the level of the cords, it might be overcome by asking the patient to take in a deep inspiration, during which the instrument ought to be passed. The head ought to be thrown back during the insertion of the tubes '.[2]

Instances of peroral intubation to relieve oedema of the glottis and membraneous croup were reported by Macewen during 1880 and 1881 ; but apart from his first case of intubation and the fourth case in the same series, in which he intended to maintain chloroform anaesthesia through the laryngeal tube, but was prevented by the death of the patient during induction but before intubation was effected, no further mention of anaesthetic procedure in this connection appears to have been made by him.

In spite of Macewen's clear statement made in the *British Medical Journal* about his method of peroral intubation and its application in anaesthesia, his work in this field made no great impression upon his contemporaries ; it appears, indeed, to have been entirely overlooked by them.

---

[1] See note on the evolution of the laryngoscope, pp. 612–3.
[2] *Brit. med. J.*, 1880, ii, 122–4, 163–5 ; *ibid.* 1881, ii, 523.

British anaesthetists, until a year or two after the introduction into clinical practice of Meltzer and Auer's insufflation anaesthesia by Elsberg in 1910 (see p. 609), continued to prefer methods which evaded rather than countered the entry of blood and debris into the air-passages.

They were concerned, however, with the problem of how to prolong anaesthesia under the difficult conditions of operative procedure involving the region of the face and neck. J. T. Clover, for example, at the International Congress of Medicine held in London in 1881, showed new ' instruments for keeping up the anaesthesia in operations in the mouth—especially a bag with a nasal tube adjusted and firmly fixed into the nostril with a screw movement ; also funnel-shaped india rubber tubes for conveying the anaesthetic to the back of the mouth during operations on the jaw '.[1]

Another method for prolonging anaesthesia in operations in the mouth, which was used during the last twenty years of the nineteenth century in Great Britain and also in Germany, seems to have been proposed independently by Joseph Mills, anaesthetist at St. Bartholomew's Hospital, in 1878, and at about the same time by Edmund Rose, of Zurich and afterwards of Berlin (cf. p. 267.)

Both men detached the facepiece from a Junker's inhaler, passed the rubber afferent tube of the apparatus up through the patient's nostril and round into the pharynx,[2] and pumped in a chloroform-air mixture. Mills found, however, that in many cases a gum-elastic catheter had advantages over the soft connecting tube, ' first, on account of its more easy introduction ; second, because, as that part which remains out of the nostril is sometimes subjected . . . to pressure or bending, it is necessary to employ an instrument . . . which cannot easily be rendered impervious. When giving the vapour by the nostril ', he wrote, ' I use a gum-elastic catheter of the largest size that can be conveniently introduced, and do not pass it beyond the edge of the soft palate '. Neither Mills nor Rose attempted to pack off the throat.

---

[1] *Trans. int. Congr. Med.*, 1881, **2**, 392 ; see also pp. 321, 368, footnotes.

In the previous use of nasal intubation by, for example, Malgaigne (see p. 135), Faure (see p. 233), Richardson and Sansom (see p. 234) the tube was merely inserted into the nostril, not pushed round into the pharynx.

Crile in 1903 proposed ' double tubage of the nares into the pharynx, and packing of the oropharynx with gauze ' for operations in the mouth. (*N.Y. med. J.*, 1908, **88**, 112.)

In cases where nasal intubation was for any reason impracticable Mills advised anaesthetists to use a mouth-tube—' what is called a " flexible metallic catheter ", No. 12, with both ends cut off, and hold it in the mouth about on a level with the wisdom teeth '.[1]

Hewitt's account of anaesthetic procedure in ' operations within or about the mouth, nose, pharynx, and larynx (excluding the extraction of teeth . . .) ' which he gave in the second edition of his book *Anaesthetics and their administration* (London. 1901) may, perhaps, be taken as representing the opinion of the majority of British specialist anaesthetists at the end of the nineteenth century :

' Twenty years ago ', he wrote, ' delicate and prolonged operations within the oral cavity were not unfrequently abandoned owing to want of knowledge as to the principles upon which anaesthesia should be maintained. But with our present methods it is possible to safely and satisfactorily anaesthetise all patients requiring these operations, provided attention be paid to certain important details which may now be conveniently considered under the following heads :

' (1) The selection of the anaesthetic and the adjustment of the depth of anaesthesia.

' (2) The posture of the patient and the avoidance of asphyxial complications from the entry of blood into the larynx and trachea.'

Under (1) Hewitt expressed the opinion that where protracted unconsciousness was essential anaesthesia should be maintained first with ether and finally with chloroform, but should be induced with nitrous oxide or the A.C.E. mixture, ' in order to prevent the initial unpleasantness of the ether '. Anaesthesia having been established ' the patient can be safely " charged-up," so to speak, by considerable quantities of . . . [ether] vapour,' Hewitt explained, ' so that when the inhaler is withdrawn there is not that tendency to inconvenient recovery during the necessary initial manipulations of the surgeon which is so common when other anaesthetics have been used '.

Once the patient had been placed deeply under the influence of ether Hewitt advised suspending the administration and allowing ' a *slight* tendency towards recovery, *i.e.* the reappearance of slight conjunctival reflex, cough, or swallowing '. The

[1] *Lancet*, 1878, ii, 839 ; *Brit. med. J.*, 1883, i, 917, 969.

next step was to subdue this tendency by cautiously administering chloroform from Junker's inhaler, either through the nose or into the mouth, according to Mills's plan. Operative procedure was begun when the patient was deeply under the ether ; but the subsequent chloroform anaesthesia was kept only ' moderately deep '.

' Before changing to chloroform, the anaesthetist should ascertain whether respiration is taking place through the mouth or nose. It is obviously next to useless to insert the tube of Junker's apparatus into, or place lint sprinkled with chloroform over the mouth, when respiration is taking place through the nose. Generally speaking, it is best to pass a flexible silk catheter of fairly large bore through the anterior nares so that its free end may be felt just beyond the soft palate. It is easier to maintain anaesthesia by this means than by the use of a mouth tube. Should the anaesthetist prefer the latter . . . he must be careful to see that respiration is oral, and if necessary the anterior nares should be plugged with lint.[1] As regards the depth of anaesthesia during the chloroformisation, it may be said that, putting aside such delicate operations as those for cleft-palate, slight phonation, occasional cough, and frequent swallowing movements are to be encouraged, provided they be not accompanied by movement. . . .'

Under (2)—posture ; avoidance of blood entering the larynx and trachea—Hewitt enumerated eleven positions of the patient, in which operations on the mouth, nose, and throat ' may be and are performed '.

' Of all postures, however, the lateral is undoubtedly the best so far as the anaesthetist is concerned. The patient should be placed strictly upon his side, with his legs flexed and with one cheek resting on the pillow, the open mouth being turned so that it directly faces a window. Owing to the facility with which all blood flows out of the mouth, sponging is generally unnecessary ; and it is possible to keep up a deep and uninterrupted anaesthesia throughout by means of Junker's inhaler. . . . Semi-recumbent or " propped up " postures . . . are open to considerable objection from the anaesthetist's point of view, for when patients

---

[1] For inducing anaesthesia with chloroform in operations ' within or about the mouth, nose, or pharynx ', instead of the usual types of mouth-tube Hewitt preferred to use an apparatus of his own invention. This was first described by him in 1891 : ' bent metal tubes are brazed to the arms of an ordinary Mason's gag, and to one of these tubes the india-rubber piping of Junker's apparatus is attached. The chloroform vapour is thus transmitted to the back of the throat along the arms of the gag.' (See Figs. 160–1.). (Hewitt, F. W. 1901. *Anaesthetics and their administration.* 320.)

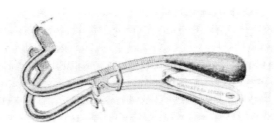

FIG. 160.—HEWITT'S MODIFICATION OF MASON'S GAG

For maintaining chloroform anaesthesia during operations within the mouth and nose. (This instrument was first described by Hewitt in 1891.)

Each arm of the gag had a bent metal tube soldered to it and to either tube the tubing of a Junker's inhaler could be attached and a stream of anaesthetic vapour blown towards the back of the mouth, in the direction of the arrows.

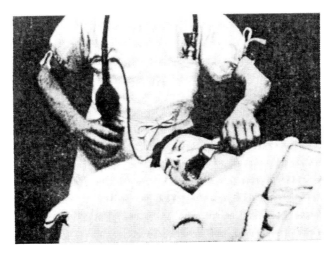

FIG. 161.—THE GAG SHOWN IN FIG. 160 IN POSITION

It may be noticed that in this illustration, which belongs to the year 1901, the anaesthetist no longer wears his street clothes when anaesthetizing, cf., *e.g.*, Fig. 65, p. 270 (1893).

607

are thus placed, all blood must, of necessity, drain backwards, and turning the head to one side does not permit the blood to escape as it would if the patient were flat.'

' The entry of blood into the larynx and trachea during these operations ', Hewitt stated, ' may be easily avoided by attention to the following simple rules :—(a) when practicable, the posture should be such that blood can easily flow out of the mouth ; (b) the head should be kept, as far as possible, in a line with the body, so that coughing and swallowing movements may effectually take place ; (c) the anaesthesia should not be too profound, otherwise the pharyngeal and laryngeal reflexes will be abolished ; and (d) the anaesthetist should have at hand several small, round, coarse sponges unattached to holders, so that, in the event of it being impracticable to adopt a posture favourable for the escape of blood, this fluid may be repeatedly removed by sponging.

' The cases in which asphyxial complications from blood are most to be feared are those in which the larynx has become, during the course of chronic throat or nose disease, comparatively insensitive. In such cases coughing and swallowing may not take place even during a comparatively light anaesthesia, and if the posture be faulty a moist expiratory râle will become audible, indicating that blood is present in the larynx. . . .

' In connection with . . . operations [upon the tongue] it may be well to say a few words as to the advisability of tracheotomy, for the anaesthetist may be consulted upon this point. Generally speaking, this measure is unnecessary if the lateral posture is adopted. But should the patient display any considerable embarrassment in breathing when the mouth is first opened to the requisite extent by the gag, it is, as a rule, advisable to open the trachea at this juncture, for such embarrassment to breathing will be liable to increase during the course of the case.'

Hewitt stated, however, that :

' For such operations as partial or complete *excision of the larynx, thyrotomy for the removal of laryngeal growths,* etc., the surgeon usually first performs tracheotomy, employing a Hahn's or Trendelenburg's tube with the object of preventing blood passing from the larynx to the trachea. In my experience Trendelenburg's plan of cutting off communication with the trachea by the distension of a small air-ball round the tracheotomy tube has given the best results. In one or two cases I have known the sponge surrounding the Hahn's tube to allow the passage of blood from above downwards. But whichever plan be chosen, it is certainly a mistake to adapt to the tracheotomy tube the long flexible tube and funnel generally supplied for maintaining anaesthesia ; for the additional tube greatly impedes breathing and tends to become choked by blood and mucus.   The simplest plan is to maintain anaesthesia by a Junker's apparatus, employing a small silk catheter, the end of which is passed a short distance down the tracheotomy tube.   Apnoeic pauses and almost imperceptible breathing are commonly met with immediately after the introduction of the tracheotomy tube.   It is advisable to keep up as deep an anaesthesia as possible in order to prevent reflex cough and movement.   Some surgeons employ an ordinary tracheotomy tube in these cases and insert a small sponge, directly the larynx has been opened, in such a way as to prevent blood passing towards the trachea.   There are practically only two postures available for these operations—the dorsal with the shoulders slightly raised and the head somewhat extended, and that of Trendelenburg. . . . The former, which is generally chosen, is not a good one from the anaesthetist's point of view. . . . The convenience of the anaesthetist must, however, give way to that of the surgeon.

' When Trendelenburg's posture is employed, precautions against blood entering the trachea need not be taken, and chloroform anaesthesia can be very efficiently kept up without in any way interfering with the manipulations of the surgeon, by holding a Skinner's mask, well charged with chloroform, horizontally and directly *above* the site of operation.   The neck being at about an angle of 45°, the operator will have no difficulty in working under the horizontally-placed mask, the side of which will touch the patient's sternum.' [1]

Hewitt stated in 1901 that ' intra-laryngeal operations are now generally performed under cocaine ', except in the case of children to whom ' no other agent than chloroform is applicable '.

The train of events which led up to the introduction into clinical practice of Meltzer and Auer's method of insufflation anaesthesia [2] by Elsberg in 1910 [3]—from which event modern methods of endotracheal anaesthesia date—was set in motion in New York in December 1885.   A woman suffering from chronic stenosis of the larynx consulted Joseph P. O'Dwyer because a colleague of his (who knew of his success in intubating diphtheritic children) had advised her that tracheotomy might be avoided if a tube could be passed through her mouth into the larynx.   ' So came to me the first case of chronic stenosis ever treated by intubation ', said O'Dwyer, and added : ' At this time there was no such thing as an adult intubation tube '

[1] Hewitt, F. W.   1901.   *Anaesthetics and their administration.*   London.   146–59.
[2] *J. exp. Med.,* 1909, **11**, 622–5.   [3] *Berl. klin. Wschr.,* 1910, **47**, 957–9.

(which, as an unqualified statement, was not true, for MacEwen had used one in 1878). ' I therefore had a set constructed.'

Soon O'Dwyer had successfully treated similar cases by intubation. He introduced his tube by gripping the end in the blades of a specially curved forceps.[1]

About eighteen months later, in July 1887, at the International Congress of Medicine held in Washington, George E. Fell, of Buffalo, N.Y., reported a series of cases of opium poisoning which he had successfully treated by forced respiration, using a foot-bellows joined by a length of tubing to a tracheotomy cannula. This apparatus was, in fact, precisely similar to contemporary apparatus used in the laboratory to produce forced respiration in animals for experimental purposes.[2]

Not long after 1887 O'Dwyer seems to have combined his method of intubation with Fell's apparatus to produce forced artificial respiration ; this Fell-O'Dwyer apparatus was extensively used by W. P. Northrup, of the Presbyterian Hospital, New York.

In a paper delivered at the Bournemouth meeting of the British Medical Association in 1894 Northrup quoted O'Dwyer as saying that ' in the performance of artificial respiration by any means it is important to remember that all we have to do is to get air into the lungs and give it sufficient time and room to escape, the power generated and stored up in overcoming the resistance to inspiration being amply sufficient to carry on expiration '.

Describing O'Dwyer's tube Northrup said :

' The laryngeal end of the metal intubation tube is curved on a right angle, tipped with a conical head, and is designed to be of the right size to wedge itself into the larynx and prevent air from returning between it and the laryngeal wall. The proximal end is practically bifurcated, one branch receiving the ingoing air from the bellows and tube, the other branch stopped with the operator's thumb (which is to act as a valve) serves for the exit of air.' [3]

None of Northrup's cases in which the Fell-O'Dwyer apparatus was used for producing artificial respiration was in any way connected with anaesthesia.

[1] *Brit. med. J.*, 1894, ii, 1478.
[2] *Trans. int. Congr. Med.*, 1887, **I**, 237—bare record that the paper was read.
[3] *Brit. med. J.*, 1894, ii, 697.

O'Dwyer's work on intubation suggested to Professor Maydl, of Prague, in 1893, that in order satisfactorily to prevent the entry of blood and debris into the patient's throat during operations in the oral and nasal cavities, it should be possible to pass a tube through the mouth into the larynx, to attach to this tube a Trendelenburg's cone for maintaining chloroform anaesthesia, and then to pack off the throat completely. This idea he successfully put into practice.

To a cannula adapted to fit the larynx he attached one end of a length of rubber drainage tubing ; the other end of the tubing was linked to a glass cone capped with woollen material on to which the chloroform was dropped throughout the operation.

The patient was first anaesthetized in the ordinary manner. Then the tongue was pulled forward and the cannula, grasped in a pair of forceps with specially adapted blades, was passed into the larynx with the help of an oral mirror, the anaesthetist's fingers acting as a spatula. When the tube was correctly placed, which fact was ascertained by the patient's breath passing to and fro through the tube and funnel, the throat was packed off with gauze.[1]

A fellow citizen of Maydl's, Victor Eisenmenger, was also working during 1893 on a similar idea. Eisenmenger used a curved, hard-rubber catheter which he, too, passed into the larynx with the aid of an oral mirror and then connected with a Trendelenburg's cone. Instead of packing off the throat with gauze, however, Eisenmenger adopted Trendelenburg's method of using a tampon to be inflated *in situ* by means of a small balloon of air (cf. p. 599). The tampon surrounded Eisenmenger's tube immediately behind its conical head, the slender inflating tube passing up the wall of the laryngeal tube and out of the mouth.[2]

A method of intubation and anaesthesia similar to Eisenmenger's was adopted a few years later by the Dutchman, van Stockum, who, about 1898, further packed off the throat above the inflated cuff by surrounding the laryngeal tube with a collar of sponge.[3]

In 1896 Tuffier and Hallion, working on problems of thoracic surgery in Paris, reported a number of experiments on dogs in

[1] *Wien. med. Wschr.*, 1893, **43**, 57, 102. [2] *Wien. med. Wschr.*, 1893, **43**, 199.
[3] Apparatus described by Kuhn : *Dtsch. Z. Chir.*, 1905, **76**, 155.

which they had passed an intralaryngeal cannula through the mouth and by means of it maintained at the same time continuous insufflation to prevent the lungs collapsing, and anaesthesia. So successful were these experiments that Tuffier and Hallion were confident that the method could safely be adapted to thoracic surgery in the human subject.[1]

After 1896 the needs of the thoracic surgeon increasingly influenced the development of intubation and forced respiration combined with anaesthesia. In this connexion pioneer work was done by E. L. Doyen in Paris and by Rudolph Matas, of New Orleans, and others. Matas in 1899 strongly recommended the use of the Fell-O'Dwyer apparatus.[2]

One of the dominant influences between 1902 and 1911 in developing peroral and nasal intubation in connexion with anaesthesia was that of Franz Kuhn, of Kassel. It was Kuhn who introduced the use of a flexible metal tracheal tube and curved introducer ; he also experimented with both positive and negative pressure insufflation in thoracic surgery.[3]

Note on the Evolution of the Laryngoscope

The use of a small piece of mirror set in wire at the end of a long shank, in partially successful attempts to see down the throat, can be traced back to 1829 when Benjamin Guy Babington showed such an instrument, which he called the ' glottiscope ', at a meeting of the Hunterian Society. When the ' glottiscope ' was to be used the patient was placed sitting with his back to the sun, and the observer concentrated the light on the back of the oral cavity by means of a hand-mirror. The tongue was depressed as the ' glottiscope ' was introduced.

In 1855 a distinguished London teacher of music, Manuel Garcia, published in the *Proceedings* of the Royal Society a paper on his experiments with auto-laryngoscopy, using mirrors. After reading Garcia's paper Türck, of Vienna, introduced the use of a laryngeal mirror into his hospital practice in 1857. In conjunction with the mirror Türck used a combined tongue forceps and depressor which the patient himself was made to hold. Türck claimed to be able to see ' the mucous surface of the

[1] *C.R. Soc. Biol.*, 1896, **3,** 951, 1047, 1086.
[2] *Ann. Surg.*, 1899, **29,** 426–34.
[3] *Dtsch. Ƶ. Chir.*, 1905, **76,** 148–207 ; *ibid.*, 1905, **78,** 467–520 ; Kuhn, F. 1911. *Die perorale Intubation.* Berlin.

posterior wall of the trachea as far down as the bifurcation of the trachea ' and even ' the six first circular cartilages of the bronchiae . . .'.[1]

By 1863 it was usual for the observer to wear a mirror on his forehead for concentrating the light, either of the sun or of a lamp, on to the pharynx.

Writing on the use of the laryngoscope in the *Medical Times* in 1863 George Johnson, Professor of Medicine at King's College Hospital, stated :

' I have never found it necessary to use the bromide of potassium, which has long been supposed to have the effect of lessening the reflex sensibility of the fauces, nor have I any experience of the bromide of ammonium. My friend Dr. Routh tells me that in one case, finding the throat very sensitive . . . he administered a small dose of chloroform by inhalation with the best results.' [2]

By 1878, at the time of Macewen's experiments with oral intubation, the use of the indirect vision laryngoscope had been further developed by George Johnson, Morrell Mackenzie, and others.

The first direct vision laryngoscope was not devised until 1895. Its inventor, Alfred Kirstein, of Berlin, called it the ' autoscope '.[3]

Kirstein's procedure was briefly described in the *Lancet* :

' The patient is placed on his back . . . with his head hanging down, and an oesophagoscope is introduced. A metal speculum in the form of a tube about 10 inches in length can then be passed behind the epiglottis and illuminated by a " Caspar's electro-scope " and through it the larynx viewed with the naked eye. . . . The tube itself acts as a tongue depressor, being a lever whose fulcrum is the edge of the upper incisors. Dr. Kirstein . . . asserts that it is by no means so severe a procedure as may be imagined, and that, especially if cocaine is employed, it caused the patient no distress either at the time or subsequently.' [4]

[1] *Med. Times, Lond.*, 1861, ii, 170. [2] *Ibid.* 1863, i, 585.
[3] *Berl. klin. Wschr.*, 1895, **32**, 476-8. [4] *Lancet*, 1895, i, 1132.

Summary of Events in Anaesthesia

1772–1911

1772 . . Nitrous oxide discovered by Priestley while working on nitric oxide.

1774 . . Oxygen discovered by Priestley while calcining red oxide of mercury with a burning glass.

1774–85 . Lavoisier, having been told by Priestley about the new gas (oxygen), used this knowledge to complete his theory of the nature of combustion. He proceeded to formulate his theory of respiration.

1785–c. 1800 Therapeutic inhalation in vogue ; oxygen, hydrogen, carbon dioxide, sulphuric ether, etc., inhaled for phthisis and other ailments.

1794–8 . . Beddoes founded the Pneumatic Institution at Clifton and appointed Davy Superintendent, to carry out research on the effects of therapeutic inhalation.

1800 . . Davy published his researches on nitrous oxide and suggested the possibility of using this gas to obtain analgesia for minor surgery.

1806 . . Sertürner isolated morphine from opium.

c. 1820 . . Magendie substituted morphine for opium in clinical practice. He prescribed it by mouth as a sedative and anodyne.

1824 . . Hickman formulated the principle of inhalation anaesthesia. He proposed surgical anaesthesia by the inhalation of carbon dioxide but failed to rouse interest either in England or in France.

1831 . . Atropine isolated.

1832 . . Hyoscyamine isolated (but hyoscine not isolated until 1871).

c. 1840 . . Esdaile, Elliotson, and others, claimed that they had operated painlessly on mesmerised patients.

1842–3 . . Long used ether successfully in several minor surgical cases, but lack of opportunity and apathy among his neighbours deterred him from publishing his results.

Note: Ether was discovered by Valerius Cordus in 1540. Faraday, in 1818, noted the similarity of the effects of ether and of nitrous oxide when inhaled.

1844   .   . Wells used nitrous oxide in dentistry after noticing its anaesthetic effects at a demonstration given by Colton.

1846   .   . Morton used ether. He gave it on a folded cloth for the extraction of Eben Frost's tooth (Sept. 30). At the Massachusetts General Hospital demonstration (Oct. 16) he used a valved glass flask filled with an ether-soaked sponge. The patient inhaled through a mouth-tube, his nostrils being pinched shut.
Jackson claimed that he suggested the use of ether to Morton.
Narcotic alkaloids increasingly used as hypnotics in acute mania and as analgesics in neuralgia, etc.

1846–7 .   . Ether established in surgical practice.

Dec. 1846 . Liston used Squire's inhaler at University College Hospital, London.

Jan. 1847 . Malgaigne, in Paris, having no proper inhaler, put some ether into a tube and inserted one end into the patient's nostril—the other nostril was plugged. The patient exhaled through his mouth.

Jan.–Feb. 1847   Snow's regulating ether inhaler. Snow (1813–58) was the first to control the amount of ether vapour which the patient received. He did this by surrounding the vaporising chamber with water at a temperature of 60–65° F. He substituted a valved facepiece for the mouth-tube.
Pirogoff, in Russia, administered ether rectally.

Nov. 1847   Chloroform introduced into practice by Simpson.
Note : Chloroform discovered in 1832, by Guthrie and Liebig independently.
Waldie suggested the use of chloroform to Simpson.

Dec. 1847   Snow's regulating chloroform inhaler delivered a maximum of 5 per cent. chloroform vapour.

1848   .   . Simpson overcame opposition to the use of anaesthesia in obstetrics.
Heyfelder used ethyl chloride in a few cases at the Erlangen Hospital, but abandoned it on account of the difficulty and expense of obtaining it (see also McCardie, 1901).

1848–c. 1854. The majority of practitioners in the northern States of America (but not in the southern States) and the surgeons of Lyons and Naples returned to the use of ether. Elsewhere the use of chloroform persisted.

1851–3 .   . Hypodermic syringes introduced by Pravaz and Wood independently.

1858 . . Richardson suggested the nasal administration of chloroform in dentistry.

1859 . . Niemann isolated cocaine from *Erythroxylon coca*.

1861 . . Ether anaesthesia revived at St. George's Hospital, London, but for specific cases only.
Pitha gave belladonna extract by enema during chloroform anaesthesia to obviate post-operative pain.

1862 . . Skinner introduced a wire frame covered with woollen fabric to fit over mouth and nose. On this chloroform was dropped from a bottle. Esmarch, and later Schimmelbusch, popularized this type of mask on the Continent.
Clover devised a chloroform apparatus to deliver a prepared mixture containing 4½ per cent. chloroform vapour in air.

1863 . . Colton (see also Wells, 1844) reintroduced nitrous oxide anaesthesia into American dental practice.

1864 . . Bernard in the laboratory and Nussbaum clinically found independently that morphine prolonged and intensified the action of chloroform.
Labbé and Guyon developed premedication with morphine (Bernard's 'mixed anaesthesia') 1864–72.
Royal Medical and Chirurgical Society's Chloroform Committee demonstrated that ether was safer than chloroform although its clinical use was inexpedient in existing circumstances. Mixtures, *e.g.* Harley's A.C.E. (1 pt. Alcohol, 2 pts. Chloroform, 3 pts. Ether) were recommended.

1867 . . Junker, then of the Samaritan Free Hospital, London, devised an inhaler for Richardson's recently introduced 'bichloride of methylene'. This inhaler was quickly appropriated to chloroform administration.

1868 . . Evans introduced nitrous oxide into British dental practice. Clover, Cattlin and others, developed apparatus. Clover and Coleman independently used a nasal cap for administration; this was soon abandoned but the method was revived by Coleman in 1898 and by Paterson in 1899.
Andrews, of Chicago, advocated the administration of oxygen with nitrous oxide and Bert independently suggested this combination in 1883, having previously (1879) advocated the administration of nitrous oxide and air under pressure. Hillischer adopted the use of oxygen with nitrous oxide *c.* 1885 and Hewitt, modifying Hillischer's technique, popularized this mixture *c.* 1892.

1869 . . Trendelenburg, in operations involving the mouth and neck, first performed tracheotomy and then introduced a tube with an inflatable cuff packing off the larynx. Through this tube he anaesthetized the patient with chloroform. This method was commonly used until about 1900.

1871 . . Mason invented his gag, but did not develop its use. Fergusson popularized the Mason-type gag during 1874–5.

Haward, of St. George's Hospital, London, suggested administering ether by the American method of an ether soaked sponge enclosed in a towel folded into a cone shape.

Clover stated, at a meeting of anaesthetists, that he was 'in the habit' of administering nitrous oxide followed by ether.

1872 . . Jeffries, of Boston, Mass., by a series of demonstrations given in London of the American towel cone method, re-established the use of ether in England.

1874 . . Oré, of Bordeaux, administered chloral hydrate intravenously.

Forné premedicated two patients with chloral hydrate given by mouth.

Clover improved his apparatus for administering nitrous oxide and ether. The apparatus received its final form in 1876.

1875 . . Allis's ether inhaler introduced into England. It had been introduced into American practice c. 1872. Although carbon dioxide accumulation in this inhaler must have been considerable, it appears to have initiated the trend in favour of open ether inhalers.

During the eighteen-nineties Prince and Herb in America and, about 1901, Hofmann and others in Germany, adopted the method of dropping ether on to an open mask. Little attention was paid to this method in England until about 1907, when Bellamy Gardner championed it.

1876 . . Lawson Tait administered 'the vapour of boiling anhydrous ether, pure and free from any admixture of air', in an attempt to mitigate postoperative chest complications. Hitherto ether had frequently been warmed, but only to facilitate vaporization.

20*

1877 . . Clover introduced his portable regulating ether inhaler into practice.

Ormsby's ether inhaler introduced into practice.

1878 . . Macewen, of Glasgow, disapproving of Trendelenburg's method (see 1869), passed a wide bore metal tube through the patient's mouth into the trachea, packed off the upper opening of the larynx with a sponge and anaesthetized with chloroform vapour. The method was not generally adopted, but peroral intubation for anaesthetic purposes was independently used in 1893 by Madyl and by Eisenmenger, both of Prague, and was developed, *c.* 1900, by Doyen (Paris), Matas (New Orleans), using the Fell-O'Dwyer apparatus, and Kuhn (Kassel). (See also Meltzer and Auer, 1909–10.)

Mills of St. Bartholomew's Hospital, London, used intrapharyngeal intubation, introducing the tube of a Junker's inhaler through the nose. Crile revived intrapharyngeal intubation in 1903 ; he packed off the throat.

1882–3 . . Cervello, of Palermo, gave paraldehyde by mouth as a hypnotic.

Paraldehyde was given intravenously by Noel and Souttar in 1912.

1883 . . Aubert, of Lyons, as an outcome of Dastre's researches (1878–83), used a pre-anaesthetic injection of atropine and morphine clinically (cf. Bernard, 1864).

1884 . . Koller used cocaine solution as an anaesthetic in ophthalmic practice.

Halsted operated on the brachial plexus, having first blocked its roots in the neck with cocaine. This is the first recorded case of regional anaesthesia. Regional anaesthesia was developed during the first decade of the twentieth century by Crile and Matas in America, and in Germany by Braun, in particular.

Mollière, of Lyons, revived rectal anaesthesia (see Pirogoff, 1847). He first used air and ether with an atomizer. Later he used ether vapour alone. Rectal anaesthesia was again revived by Cunningham (U.S.) in 1903 and Gwathmey developed his oil-ether colonic technique *c.* 1912.

1885 . . Corning laid the foundations of spinal anaesthesia in medicating the cord of a patient extradurally with cocaine. He recommended the type of anaesthesia obtained to the attention of surgeons.

1888–9 . . First and Second Hyderabad Chloroform Commissions. As a result of experiments made by the First Commission (1888), it was stated that chloroform could not affect the heart before affecting respiration. This statement was contested in England and a Second Commission (1889) repeated the experiments. The results appeared to support the original statement ; nevertheless English physiologists proceeded to disprove it.

1891 . . Schleich introduced infiltration anaesthesia. Reclus had been working on similar lines since 1886.

1893 . . Revival of the use of ether anaesthesia in Germany. Two methods were adopted : Wanscher's (introduced in Copenhagen, c. 1884), using an inhaler similar to Ormsby's (see 1877), and Julliard's (introduced in Geneva in 1877), using a large, impermeably covered, face-mask. A similar revival took place in France, c. 1896.

1895 . . Kirstein's autoscope, first direct vision laryngoscope.

1899 . . Bier established spinal anaesthesia in practice and Tuffier, c. 1900, did much to further its adoption.

1900 . . Schneiderlin introduced the use of morphine-scopolamine injection as the sole anaesthetic, but from 1903 onwards this was combined with inhalation anaesthesia.

1901 . . McCardie, in England, and at about the same time Ware, in America, popularized the use of ethyl chloride as a general anaesthetic. This form of anaesthesia had been established by Lotheissen of Innsbruck in 1896, ethyl chloride as a local anaesthetic in dentistry having been in use on the Continent since 1890. (See also Heyfelder, 1848.)

1902 . . Le Filliâtre suggested general spinal anaesthesia. A. W. Morton reported 60 successful cases of anaesthesia above the diaphragm, but fatalities soon caused the method to be abandoned until c. 1908, when Jonnesco of Bucharest revived it.

Vernon Harcourt's inhaler which, by limiting to 2 per cent. the maximum dose of chloroform vapour delivered to the patient, was believed to make chloroform anaesthesia innocuous.

1903 . . Fischer, of Munich, synthesized Veronal, the first of the barbiturates.

Hewitt combined the use of ethyl chloride with nitrous oxide anaesthesia.

1904 . . Fourneau synthesized Stovaine (an anglicized version of his own surname).

Babcock visited France to study spinal anaesthesia with Stovaine and proceeded to introduce it into American practice. Later he introduced the use of hypobaric solutions.

1905 . . Einhorn synthesized Novocaine.

1907 . . Barker introduced gravity control methods for spinal anaesthesia.

1909 . . Burkhardt popularized intravenous ether anaesthesia. Rood used his method in England.

Meltzer and Auer completed their experiments on intratracheal insufflation anaesthesia.

1910 . . Elsberg applied the Meltzer and Auer insufflation anaesthesia clinically.

Fedoroff, of St. Petersburg, used Hedonal for intravenous anaesthesia ; the drug had been much used in Russia since 1900, as a hypnotic given by mouth. Page used Fedoroff's method in England.

1911 . . Levy showed ventricular fibrillation to be the cause of death in lightly chloroformed subjects.

INDEX

Académie de Médecine (Paris), 5 ; and Hickman, 86, 88 ; and Wells, 88 ; discusses amylene, 222 ; and chloroform (1882), 367n.
— des Sciences (Paris), 5 ; and the discoverer of anaesthesia, 122-3, 125, 136.
A.C.E. mixture, 256-7, 461-3, 467, 605.
Acetone, anaesthetic use of, 166.
Adams, J. E., warmed ether apparatus, 332-3.
Adrenalin, 453, 579.
Alcohol, use in pre- and post-operative sedation, 375n., 376, 431, 435 ; in resuscitation, 567. *See also* Anaesthetic mixtures ; Chloric ether.
Allis's ether inhaler, 352-5, 412, 595 ; used for ethyl chloride, 516.
America (U.S.), contribution to anaesthesia (1846-1900), 535-6.
— Northern States, routine methods, for etherization, 11-13, 125, 181, 319-20, 352-5, 592, 594 ; use of nitrous oxide, 273-6, 307-9 ; ethyl chloride anaesthesia, 512, 514-16.
— Southern States, chloroform preferred in, 11-12.
Amyl nitrite, 577.
Amylene, Snow's researches on, 220-1 ; deaths from, 221 ; clinical use of, 221-2.
Anaesthesia, economic, social, and medical background, 1-9, 33-4, 36.
— legal aspects of, 232-3, 473n., 547-51.
— methods of prolonging, with chloroform, 234-6, 239, 368n., 541, 598-9, 604-5 ; with ether, 321n., 489 ; with nitrous oxide, 285n., 297, 489-94 ; Clover's methods (1881), 604 ; Hewitt's methods, 605-9. *See also* Endotracheal anaesthesia.
— physiological researches on, 15, 21-2, 157-64, 170, 188-91, 208-21, 253-5, 282, 284, 297, 307, 310, 356-7, 362-5, 379-80, 384-6, 389-98, 400, 419-20, 427-8, 429-32, 439-56, 497, 499, 502, 571-4, 576, 577-9, 597.
— professional etiquette in, 547-51.

Anaesthesia, relative dangers of, discussed, 461-4.
— religious controversy about, 177-8.
— routine practices, 10-11 ; in America (U.S.), 11-13, 125n., 181, 273-6, 307-9, 319-20, 352-5, 514-16, 592, 594 ; on the European Continent, 15-17, 33-4, 35-6, 181, 228-30, 404-11, 414, 542-7, 505 ; in Great Britain (Scotland), 13-14, 181, 536-42 ; (England), 17-22, 130-4, 139-57, 182-8, 192-3, 234-51, 285-93, 326-52, 457-8, 461-4, 475-81, 483-9, 508-9, 595-6.
— signs of, tabulated at Edinburgh, 542.
— stages of, Flourens on, 160 ; Snow on, 162-4.
— statistics relating to deaths under, 412, 413-14, 437-8, 461-4.
— terminology used in, 562-5.
'Anaesthesimeter', Duroy's, 225-7.
Anaesthetic agents, choice of, 330-41, 461-2 ; Buxton on, 466-7 ; Hewitt on, 605-6.
— — mode of action of, 'lipoid theory', 158 ; Flourens on, 160 ; Snow's theory, 161, 219-20 : Bernard's theory, 219n. ; Binz and the 'colloid theory', 219n.
— — proportion of in inhaled mixtures, Snow's researches, 188-91, 217 ; Bert's researches, 363-5.
— — warmed to obviate post-operative 'chest', 491-2, 588-90.
— car, Bert's, 360-2.
— mixtures (volatile), 14, 22, 179, 194, 255-65, 311, 331 *et seq.*, 413, 461-2, 467, 510-11, 520-3, 544, 598.
— room, at the Massachusetts General Hospital (Boston), 319 ; at St. Thomas's Hospital (London), 334.
— sequences, 22, 258-65, 285n., 331 *et seq.*, 425, 461-2, 508, 509n., 512, 605.
Anaesthetist, legal responsibility of, 232-3, 548-51 ; Bill to restrain the unqualified, 473n.

Hooke, Robert, on respiration, 52 ; on an active principle in nitre and air, 53*n*.
Hooper's ether inhaler, 131.
Hospitalism, 26 *et seq.*
Hospitals, survey of anaesthetic practice in London (1875), 330–9.
Howard's method of artificial respiration, 435, 575.
Hunter, John, and surgery, 9 ; and artificial respiration, 569*n*.
Hutchinson, Jonathan, 332, 460.
— S. J., swivel gag, 298, 300.
Hyderabad Commissions, 44 ; First (1888), 429 ; Second (1889), 432–5.
Hydrocarbons, as anaesthetic agents, 208–9, 212, 223.
Hydrogen, as a therapeutic inhalant, 68, 74.
Hyoscine. *See* Morphine and scopolamine.
Hypnotism, to produce anaesthesia, 38. *See also* Mesmerism.

Idiosyncrasy, a factor in death from chloroform, 196, 202.
Infiltration anaesthesia, 42–3 ; in England, 46–9 ; in Germany, 423 ; in America, 503.
Inhalation *versus* local anaesthesia, 43, 46–9.
Inhalers, English preference for, 17, 24–5, 181, 320 ; a contributory cause of death, 195, 437, 463 ; ' blow-over ' principle adopted in, 235, 267 ; in routine use in England (*c.* 1890), 463, 467.
— for anaesthetic mixtures, Ellis's, 258–64 ; Schleich's ' mask ' for, 520–1 : Wertheim's modified ' Rosthorn ', 521–2.
— bichloride of methylene, 264–72.
— chloroform (*c.* 1847–50), 182 *et seq.* ; Coxeter's, 182–3 ; Snow's facepiece adapted as, 182–3 ; Sibson's, 183, 184–5 ; Weiss's, based on one made by Coxeter, 184 ; Whitelock's, 184 ; of wickerwork, 185–6 ; Charrière's, 186, 225 ; Snow's, 186–8.
— — (*c.* 1850–70), Duroy's ' Anaesthesimeter ', 225–7 ; Coleman's nasal tubes, 234–5 ; Clover's nasal cap, 235–6 ; Coleman's nasal cap, 236 ; dosimetric, 236–44 ; ' modified Snow ', 236–7 ; Sansom's, 236–9 ; Weiss's dosimetric, 240–1 ; Clover's, 241–6 ; Junker's, 266–7 ; Kappeler's ' Junker ', 268–9 ; Millikin's, 333–4.

Inhalers, for chloroform, (*c.* 1885–1901), Hewitt's ' Junker ', 270–1 ; Dubois's ' anaesthetizing machine ', 370–3 ; Vernon Harcourt's, 448 ; Buxton's ' Junker ' with foot-bellows, 467–8 ; Buxton's ' improved Junker ', 470, 472 ; Elser's, 504.
— — ether (1846–7), defects of early types of, 9–10 ; 139–40 ; Morton's (1846), 11, 106–8, 552–4, 558–60 ; Morton's (1847), 126–7, 555–8 ; Hooper's, 131 ; Squire's, 132–4 ; Charrière's, 136–7 ; Dieffenbach's, 138 ; Smee's warmed, 140 ; Hoffman's warmed, 141 ; ' graduated-dose inhaler ', 141–2 ; Bell's ' simplified ', 143–4 ; Roux's *sac*, 145–6, 206–7, 424 ; Munaret's, 146 ; Tracy's, 147 ; Smee's ' portable ', 147–8 ; Heineken's, 148–9 ; Cloquet's, 150 ; Snow's, 154–7.
— — — (1872–7), Hawksley's (1872–3), 320–2 ; J. Morgan's, 322–3 ; Clover's ' double-current ', 323–5 ; Golding Bird's, 333–4 ; J. H. Morgan's, 337 ; Clover's ' portable regulating ', 342, 344–7 ; Hewitt's ' modified Clover ', 346–7 ; Ormsby's, 349–50 ; Hewitt's warmed ' Ormsby ', 351–2 ; Allis's, 352–5.
— — — (*c.* 1885–1900), Wanscher's, 410 ; Landau's ' modified Wanscher ', 416 ; Carter Braine's ' modified Ormsby ', 510 ; Carter's ' thermo-ether-inhaler ', 584–6 ; Wagner-Longard's, 586–8 ; Lawson Tait's warmed, 588–90 ; ' electro-thermo-etheriser ', 590.
— — ethyl bromide, 213.
— — chloride, Schönemann's ' Universal ', used for, 500–1 ; Brodtbeck's, 501 ; Breuer's, 503–4, 508, 509 ; Bampfylde Daniell's, 509 ; Ware's, 514–15.
— non-anaesthetic, Lavoisier's, 61 ; used for ether vapour, 63–4 ; at the Pneumatic Institution, used 66–9.
Inhaling bags, Watt's, for pneumatic medicine, 67 ; used by Davy, 70 ; Wells's, 98 ; Colton's, 76–80, 289 ; Andrews's, for nitrous oxide and oxygen, 307.
— — for measured chloroform-air mixtures, Snow's, 194–5, 221–2 ; Clover's, 241–4, 245.
Injector, Marston's, entraining air, 244*n*. *See also* Jetting methods.

action, 162, 219–20 ; on the anaesthetic properties of various agents, 212 *et seq.* ; on ethidene dichloride, 216 ; on chloroform and ether, 217–19 ; on the solubility of anaesthetics in blood, 217, 219 ; on the significance of volatility, 217 ; on amylene, 220–2.

Snow and resuscitation, air-pump for, 18*n.*, 566*n.* ; on methods used in first fifty chloroform deaths, 566–71 ; on artificial respiration, 571–2 ; on the use of irritants and of venesection, 572–3 ; on the tongue in anaesthetic emergencies, 572 ; on cardiac puncture, 573.

Society of Anaesthetists, history of, 461*n.*

Somnoform, 510–11.

Soubeiran, Eugène, and the discovery of chloroform, 171.

Soulier and Brian, of Lyons, researches on ethylidene chloride, 502.

Southey, Robert, inhales nitrous oxide, 75.

Spasm, laryngeal, disregarded during etherization, 320.

Spinal anaesthesia, 40–1 ; in England, 46.

Sponges, for administering ether, 11, 117, 125, 146, 148, 312, 319 ; for chloroform, 168–9, 194, 598 ; for swabbing the throat, 608.

Sprague's apparatus, for nitrous oxide, 274–6, 279, 289.

Spray, Lister's carbolic, 29–30, 32 ; Richardson's for local anaesthesia, 30, 39, 212, 265 ; ethyl chloride phial, 498, 515.

Squire's ether inhaler, 132–4.

Starling, E. A. *See* Lane, W. Arbuthnot.

Statistics relating to anaesthetic deaths. *See* Deaths.

Stelzner, of Dresden, and etherization, 410*n.*, 414.

Sterilization, and asepsis, 33, 35, 411.

Stopcock, Clover's, for nitrous oxide, 286–7, 292–3 ; for nitrous oxide and ether, 327, 329 ; Hewitt's valved, for nitrous oxide, 476–8 ; Hewitt's, for nitrous oxide and oxygen (1893), 483–5 ; Hewitt's (1897), 487.

Stockum, van, uses peroral intubation for anaesthesia, 611.

Strychnine, and restoration of blood-pressure, 578 ; as respiratory stimulant, 578–9 ; in pre-anaesthetic medication, 579.

'Supplemental bag', Clover's, for re-breathing nitrous oxide, 286–7, 292–3.

Surgery, anaesthesia adapted for, 36–7 ; conservative, 10 ; visceral, 33 ; thoracic, 37, 611–12 ; gynaecological, 332 ; ophthalmic, 332, 335, 410–11. *See also* Operations involving mouth and neck.

— without anaesthesia (1868), 16–17.

Switzerland, ether anaesthesia in, 35, 139, 146, 150 ; revived use of in, 405–7 ; research on renal effects of etherization, 419–20.

Syme, James, 31, 204–5, 247, 431, 538, 598.

Syringe, Pravaz's, 376*n.* ; Wood's, for injecting morphine, 378.

Tait, Robert Lawson, 593 ; and warmed ether, 588–90 ; and open administration, 591–2.

Tampon-cannula, Trendelenburg's, 599–600, 608, 611.

Taylor, S. J., on local *versus* general anaesthesia, 48–9.

Teale, Pridgin, 460, 530.

'Thermophor', used in the Wagner-Longard inhaler, 588.

Thiersch, Karl, and antisepsis, 31 ; uses analgesia, 599.

Thiesing, of Hildesheim, and ethyl chloride anaesthesia, 500.

Thomson, Thomas, and Dutch liquid, 171.

Thornton, R. J., and therapeutic inhalation of ether, 64.

Throat packs, MacEwen's use of, 602–3 ; Hewitt and, 608–9 ; Maydl's use of, 611. *See also* Tampon-cannula.

Thudichum, J. L. W., 293 ; arranges supply of nitrous oxide in Franco-Prussian War, 308.

Tomes, C. S., on anaesthesia at Boston Mass. (1873), 319.

Tongue, pulled forward in anaesthetic emergencies, 435, 538–9, 570, 572.

— forceps, Esmarch's, 250.

Towel cone. *See* Cones.

Tracheotomy and intubation, for anaesthesia, Snow's experimental use of, 597 ; Trendelenburg's method, 599–601 ; Hewitt's methods, 608–9.

— — for resuscitation, 570, 571.

Tracy, S. J., uses a sponge for anaesthetic administration, 146, 148, 169 ; his ether inhaler, 147.